Operative Standards
for Cancer Surgery

PRESENTED BY THE AMERICAN COLLEGE OF SURGEONS
AND THE ALLIANCE FOR CLINICAL TRIALS IN ONCOLOGY

Volume 3

Operative Standards *for* Cancer Surgery

PRESENTED BY THE AMERICAN COLLEGE OF SURGEONS AND THE ALLIANCE FOR CLINICAL TRIALS IN ONCOLOGY

Volume 3

EDITORIAL BOARD

KELLY K. HUNT, MD, FACS
American College of Surgeons Cancer Research
Program Director
The University of Texas MD Anderson Cancer Center
Houston, Texas

MATTHEW H. G. KATZ, MD, FACS
American College of Surgeons Cancer Research Program
Cancer Care Standards Development Committee Chair
The University of Texas MD Anderson Cancer Center
Houston, Texas

NIRMAL VEERAMACHANENI, MD, FACS
American College of Surgeons Cancer Research Program
Cancer Care Standards Development Committee Vice Chair
University of Kansas
Kansas City, Kansas

CHRISTINA L. ROLAND, MD, MS, FACS
Sarcoma Section Co-Chair
The University of Texas MD Anderson Cancer Center
Houston, Texas

AIMEE CRAGO, MD, PhD, FACS
Sarcoma Section Co-Chair
Memorial Sloan Kettering Cancer Center
New York, New York

BARBRA S. MILLER, MD, FACS
Adrenal Section Co-Chair
The Ohio State University
Columbus, Ohio

GERARD M. DOHERTY, MD, FACS
Adrenal Section Co-Chair
Brigham and Women's Hospital
Boston, Massachusetts

KAITLYN J. KELLY, MD, MAS, FACS
Neuroendocrine Section Co-Chair
University of California San Diego
San Diego, California

EDWARD JAMES KRUSE, DO, FACS
Neuroendocrine Section Co-Chair
Augusta University
Augusta, Georgia

PERRY SHEN, MD, FACS, FSSO
Peritoneal Section Co-Chair
Wake Forest School of Medicine
Winston-Salem, North Carolina

EDWARD A LEVINE, MD, FACS
Peritoneal Section Co-Chair
Wake Forest School of Medicine
Winston-Salem, North Carolina

KOSTANTINOS VOTANOPOULOS, MD, PhD, FACS
Peritoneal Section Co-Chair
Wake Forest School of Medicine
Winston-Salem, North Carolina

M. MINHAJ SIDDIQUI, MD, FACS
Urothelial Section Co-Chair
University of Maryland Marlene and Stewart Greenebaum
Cancer Center
Baltimore, Maryland

SHILAJIT KUNDU, MD
Urothelial Section Co-Chair
Northwestern University, Feinberg School of Medicine
Chicago, Illinois

FLAVIO ROCHA, MD, FACS
Hepatobiliary Section Co-Chair
Oregon Health and Science University
Portland, Oregon

CHING-WEI TZENG, MD, FACS
Hepatobiliary Section Co-Chair
The University of Texas MD Anderson Cancer Center
Houston, Texas

AMANDA B. FRANCESCATTI, MS
Senior Manager
American College of Surgeons Cancer Research Program
Chicago, Illinois

SUSAN DEMING
Project Manager
Associate Editor
American College of Surgeons Cancer Research Program
Chicago, Illinois

This manual was prepared and published through the support of the American College of Surgeons.

AMERICAN COLLEGE OF SURGEONS
Inspiring Quality:
Highest Standards, Better Outcomes

100+*years*

Wolters Kluwer

Philadelphia • Baltimore • New York • London
Buenos Aires • Hong Kong • Sydney • Tokyo

ALLIANCE
FOR CLINICAL TRIALS IN ONCOLOGY

Acquisitions Editor: Keith Donnellan
Development Editors: Lindsay Ries and Ashley Fischer
Marketing Manager: Kirsten Watrud
Senior Production Project Manager: Alicia Jackson
Manager, Graphic Arts & Design: Stephen Druding
Senior Manufacturing Coordinator: Beth Welsh
Prepress Vendor: Absolute Service, Inc.

9 8 7 6 5 4 3 2 1

Printed in Singapore

Library of Congress Cataloging-in-Publication Data

Operative standards for cancer surgery / presented by the American College of Surgeons and the Alliance for Clinical Trials in Oncology ; editorial board Heidi Nelson, Kelly K. Hunt, Nirmal Veeramachaneni, Sarah Blair, George Chang, Amy Halverson, Matthew Katz, Mitchell Posner.
  p. ; cm.
  Includes bibliographical references.
  ISBN 978-1-9751-5307-6
  I. Nelson, Heidi, editor. II. American College of Surgeons, issuing body.
III. Alliance for Clinical Trials in Oncology, issuing body.
  [DNLM: 1. Neoplasms--surgery. 2. Surgical Procedures, Operative--standards. QZ 268]
  RD651
  616.99'4059--dc23
                          2015011470

MKO522

SARCOMA

Waddah Al-Refaie, MD, FACS
John S. Dillon Professor and Regional Chief of
Surgical Oncology
Vice Chair of Research
Surgeon in Chief of Lombardi Comprehensive
Cancer Center
Georgetown University Medical Center
MedStar Georgetown University Hospital
Washington, DC

Dario Callegaro, MD
Surgical Oncologist
Department of Surgery, Sarcoma Service
Fondazione IRCCS Istituto Nazionale Tumori
Milan, Italy

Aimee Crago, MD, PhD, FACS
Sarcoma Section Co-Chair
Attending Surgeon, Associate Member
Department of Surgery
Memorial Sloan Kettering Cancer Center
New York, NY

Nicola Fabbri, MD
Attending Surgeon and Professor
Department of Surgery, Orthopaedic Surgery
Memorial Sloan Kettering Cancer Center
Professor, Weill College of Medicine,
Cornell University
New York, NY

Mark Fairweather, MD, FACS
Assistant Professor
Department of Surgery
Harvard Medical School
Associate Surgeon
Department of Surgery
Brigham and Women's Hospital/Dana Farber
Cancer Institute
Boston, MA

Rebecca Gladdy, MD, PhD, FACS
Associate Professor
Division of Surgical Oncology
Mount Sinai Hospital, Princess Margaret
Cancer Centre
Department of Surgery
University of Toronto
Toronto, Ontario, Canada

Matthew Houdek, MD
Associate Professor
Department of Orthopedic Surgery
Mayo Clinic
Rochester, MN

John M. Kane III, MD, FACS
Professor of Oncology
Chair, Department of Surgical Oncology
Chief, Sarcoma/Melanoma Service
Roswell Park Comprehensive Cancer Center
Buffalo, NY

Emily Z. Keung, MD, AM, FACS
Assistant Professor
Department of Surgical Oncology
The University of Texas MD Anderson
Cancer Center
Houston, TX

Kate J. Krause, MLIS
Senior Librarian and Research Specialist
Research Medical Library
The University of Texas MD Anderson
Cancer Center
Houston, TX

Alex Lazar, MD, PhD
Professor
Pathology and Genomic Medicine
The University of Texas MD Anderson
Cancer Center
Houston, TX

Valerae Lewis, MD
Professor and Chair
Orthopaedic Oncology
The University of Texas MD Anderson
Cancer Center
Houston, TX

Jessica E. Maxwell MD, MBA, FACS
Assistant Professor
Department of Surgical Oncology
The University of Texas MD Anderson
Cancer Center
Houston, TX

Benjamin Miller, MD
Associate Professor
Orthopedics and Rehabilitation
University of Iowa
Iowa City, IA

Carol Morris, MD, MS
Professor
Orthopaedic Surgery, Oncology and
General Surgery
Division Chief, Orthopaedic Oncology
Vice Chair, Orthopedic Surgery
Johns Hopkins University
Baltimore, MD

Chandrajit P. Raut, MD, MSc, FACS
Professor of Surgery
Harvard Medical School
Chief, Division of Surgical Oncology
Brigham and Women's Hospital
Surgery Director
Center for Sarcoma and Bone Oncology
Dana-Farber Cancer Institute
Boston, MA

Christina L. Roland, MD, MS, FACS
Sarcoma Section Chair
Associate Professor of Surgery
Vice Chair for Research
Department of Surgical Oncology
The University of Texas MD Anderson
Cancer Center
Houston, TX

Eric J. Silberfein, MD, FACS
Associate Professor
Department of Surgery, Division of
Surgical Oncology
Michael E. DeBakey Department of Surgery
Chief of Surgical Oncology and
General Surgery
Ben Taub Hospital
Baylor College of Medicine
Houston, TX

Sandra L. Wong, MD, MS, FACS
Professor and Chair
Department of Surgery
Geisel School of Medicine at Dartmouth
Professor and Chair
Department of Surgery
Dartmouth-Hitchcock
Lebanon, NH

ADRENAL

Herbert Chen, MD, FACS
Chair, Department of Surgery
University of Alabama at Birmingham (UAB)
Fay Fletcher Kerner Endowed Chair
Professor of Surgery and Biomedical Engineering
Surgeon-in-Chief, UAB Hospital and
Health System
Senior Advisor, O'Neal Comprehensive
Cancer Center at UAB
Birmingham, AL

Michael J. Demeure, MD, MBA, FACS, FACE
Director of Precision Medicine Program
Hoag Family Cancer Institute
Newport Beach, CA
Clinical Professor
Translational Genomics Research Institute
Phoenix, AZ

Gerard M. Doherty, MD, FACS
Adrenal Section Co-Chair
Moseley Professor of Surgery, Harvard
Medical School
Surgeon-in-Chief, Brigham Health and
Dana-Farber Cancer Institute
Crowley Family Distinguished Chair
Department of Surgery
Brigham and Women's Hospital
Boston, MA

Quan-Yang Duh, MD, FACS
Professor of Surgery
Chief, Section of Endocrine Surgery
Department of Surgery
University of California San Francisco
University of California San Francisco –
Mount Zion
San Francisco, CA

Douglas Evans, MD, FACS
Donald C. Ausman Family Foundation
Professor of Surgery
Chair, Department of Surgery
Medical College of Wisconsin
Milwaukee, WI

Douglas L. Fraker, MD, FACS
Jonathan E. Rhoads Professor of Surgery
Chief, Division of Endocrine and
Oncologic Surgery
Department of Surgery
University of Pennsylvania
Philadelphia, PA

Thomas J. Giordano, MD, PhD
Henry Clay Bryant Professor of Pathology
Department of Pathology
Director, Division of Molecular and
Genomic Pathology
University of Michigan
Ann Arbor, MI

Raymon H. Grogan, MD, MS, FACS
Associate Professor
Michael E. DeBakey Department of Surgery
Baylor College of Medicine
Houston, TX

Elizabeth G. Grubbs, MD, FACS
Program Director, CGSO Program
Department of Surgical Oncology
The University of Texas MD Anderson
Cancer Center
Houston, TX

Gary D. Hammer, MD, PhD
Professor
Internal Medicine
Director of Endocrine Oncology
Rogel Cancer Center
University of Michigan
Ann Arbor, MI

Marybeth S. Hughes, MD, FACS
Associate Professor
Chief, Division of Surgical Oncology
Department of Surgery
Eastern Virginia Medical School
Norfolk, VA

Electron Kebebew, MD, FACS
Professor of Surgery
Chief, Division of General Surgery
Harry A. Oberhelman, Jr. and Mark L. Welton
Endowed Professor
Stanford University
Stanford, CA

Jennifer H. Kuo, MD, MS, FACS
Associate Professor of Surgery
Columbia University
Attending Surgeon
New York-Presbyterian Hospital
New York, NY

Alexander Kutikov, MD, FACS
Professor, Surgical Oncology
Chief, Urologic Oncology
Fox Chase Cancer Center
Philadelphia, PA

Amanda M. Laird, MD, FACS
Associate Professor
Chief, Section of Endocrine Surgery
Department of Surgical Oncology
Rutgers Cancer Institute of New Jersey
Rutgers Robert Wood Johnson Medical School
New Brunswick, NJ

Jeffrey E. Lee, MD, FACS
Professor and Chair, Department of
Surgical Oncology
Vice President, Medical and Academic Affairs,
Cancer Network
The University of Texas MD Anderson
Cancer Center
Houston, TX

Travis McKenzie, MD, FACS
Associate Professor of Surgery
Division of Endocrine and Metabolic Surgery
Mayo Clinic
Rochester, MN

Barbra S. Miller, MD, FACS
Adrenal Section Chair
Professor of Surgery
Endocrine Surgery, Division of Surgical Oncology
Department of Surgery
The James Cancer Hospital and Solove
Research Institute
The Ohio State University Wexner
Medical Center
Columbus, OH

Matthew A. Nehs, MD, FACS
Assistant Professor, Harvard Medical School
Associate Surgeon, Department of Surgery
Brigham and Women's Hospital
Boston, MA

Sarah C. Oltmann, MD, FACS
Associate Professor of Surgery
Dedman Family Scholar in Clinical Care
Department of Surgery
University of Texas Southwestern
Medical Center
Associate Program Chief of Surgery—Quality
and Best Practice
Parkland Health and Hospital Systems
Dallas, TX

Jennifer E. Rosen, MD, FACS
Regional Chair of Endocrine Surgery, MedStar
Division of Endocrine Surgery, Department of
Surgery
MedStar Washington Hospital Center
Washington, DC

Allan Siperstein, MD
Professor and Chair
Department of Endocrine Surgery
Cleveland Clinic
Cleveland, OH

Carmen C. Solorzano, MD, FACS, FSSO
Professor of Surgery
Chair, Department of Surgery
Director, Endocrine Surgery
Vanderbilt University
Nashville, TN

Tracy S. Wang, MD, MPH, FACS
Professor of Surgery
Vice-Chair, Strategic and Professional
Development
Chief, Section of Endocrine Surgery
Department of Surgery
Medical College of Wisconsin
Milwaukee, WI

NEUROENDOCRINE

Volkan Adsay, MD
Professor
Chair, Department of Pathology
Head, Surgical Sciences Section
Koç University School of Medicine
Istanbul, Turkey

J. Philip Boudreaux, MD, FACS
Professor
Division of Surgical Oncology
Department of Surgery
LSU Health New Orleans
New Orleans, LA

Callisia N. Clarke, MD, MS, FACS, FSSO
Assistant Professor of Surgery
Division of Surgical Oncology
Medical College of Wisconsin
Milwaukee, WI

Armen Eskandari, MD
Fellow of Interventional Endoscopy
Division of Gastroenterology
Department of Medicine
University of California San Diego
San Diego, CA

Paul T. Fanta, MD
Professor
Co-Director, Gastrointestinal Medical Oncology
Department of Medicine
University of California San Diego
San Diego, CA

Syed M. Abbas Fehmi, MD
Professor
Division of Gastroenterology
Department of Medicine
University of California San Diego
San Diego, CA

Alexandra Gangi, MD, FACS
Assistant Professor
Director, Gastrointestinal Tumor Program
Division of Surgical Oncology
Department of Surgery
Cedars-Sinai Medical Center
Los Angeles, CA

Alan W. Hemming, MD, MSc, FACS
Professor
Surgical Director of Liver Transplantation
Transplantation and Hepatobiliary Surgery
Department of Surgery
University of Iowa
Iowa City, IA

James Howe, MD, FACS, FSSO
Professor of Surgery
Director, Division of Surgical Oncology and
Endocrine Surgery
University of Iowa Carver College of Medicine
Iowa City, IA

Kaitlyn J. Kelly, MD, MAS, FACS
Neuroendocrine Section Co-Chair
Associate Professor of Surgery
Division of Surgical Oncology
Department of Surgery
University of California San Diego
San Diego, CA

Edward James Kruse, DO, FACS
Neuroendocrine Section Co-Chair
Professor of Surgery
Medical College of Georgia at Augusta
University
Section Chief, Surgical Oncology
Augusta University
Augusta, GA

Robert C.G. Martin II, MD, PhD, FACS
Sam and Lolita Weakley Endowed Chair,
Surgical Oncology
Vice-Chair, Department of Surgery for Research
Director, Division of Surgical Oncology
Professor of Surgery
Director, Upper GI and HPB Multi-Disciplinary
Clinic
Academic Advisory Dean
University of Louisville School of Medicine
Louisville, KY

James M. McLoughlin, MD, FACS
Section Chief of GI Surgical Oncology
Professor of Surgery
The University of Tennessee Medical Center
Knoxville, TN

Sushanth Reddy, MD, FACS
Associate Professor
University of Alabama at Birmingham
Surgical Head, Pancreaticobiliary
Disease Center
UAB Hospital
Birmingham, AL

PERITONEAL

H. Richard Alexander Jr., MD, FACS
Chief Surgical Officer, Rutgers Cancer
Institute of New Jersey
Professor and Head, Surgical Oncology
Department of Surgery
Rutgers Robert Wood Johnson Medical School
New Brunswick, NJ

Brian Badgwell, MD, FACS
Professor
Department of Surgical Oncology
The University of Texas MD Anderson
Cancer Center
Houston, TX

Joel Baumgartner, MD
Associate Professor
Department of Surgery
Moores Cancer Center
UC San Diego Health
La Jolla, CA

Jeremiah (Jiz) Deneve, DO, FACS
Associate Professor
Department of Surgery
The University of Tennessee Health
Science Center
Memphis, TN

Laura Enomoto, MD, MSc, FACS
Assistant Professor
Department of Surgery
The University of Tennessee Medical Center
Knoxville, TN

Travis Grotz, MD
Assistant Professor
Department of Surgery
Mayo Clinic
Rochester, MN

Nader Hanna, MD, FACS, FSSO, FICS
Professor
Director of Clinical Operations
Division of General and Oncologic Surgery
Department of Surgery
University of Maryland School of Medicine
Baltimore, MD

Chukwuemeka Ihemelandu, MD
Associate Professor
Department of Surgery
Division of Surgical Oncology
MedStar Georgetown University Hospital
Washington, DC

Edward A. Levine, MD, FACS
Peritoneal Section Co-Chair
Professor
Associate Chair for Operations
Chief, Surgical Oncology
Wake Forest School of Medicine
Winston-Salem, NC

Gary Mann, MD
Associate Professor
Department Surgical Oncology
Roswell Park Comprehensive Cancer Center
Buffalo, NY

Harveshp Mogal, MD, MS, FACS
Director, HIPEC Program
Section Chief, Complex Abdominal Surgery
Associate Professor
University of Washington Medical Center
Seattle, WA

Maheswari Senthil, MBBS, FACS
Associate Professor and Chief
Division of Surgical Oncology
Loma Linda University Health
Loma Linda, CA

Perry Shen, MD, FACS, FSSO
Peritoneal Section Co-Chair
Professor
Associate Chair for Quality and Clinical
Outcomes
Co-Executive Director, Oncology Service Line
Department of General Surgery
Wake Forest School of Medicine
Winston-Salem, NC

Joseph Skitzki, MD, FACS
Associate Professor
Surgical Oncology
Roswell Park Comprehensive Cancer Center
Buffalo, NY

Kostantinos I. Votanopoulos, MD, PhD, FACS
Peritoneal Section Co-Chair
Professor, Surgical Oncology
Director, Wake Forest Organoid Research
Center (WFORCE)
Wake Forest School of Medicine
Winston-Salem, NC

UROTHELIAL

Piyush Agarwal, MD
Professor of Surgery and Urology
Director of Urologic Oncology Fellowship and
Bladder Cancer Program
University of Chicago
Chicago, IL

Bernard H. Bochner, MD
Attending Surgeon, Urologic Surgery Service
Sir Murray F. Brennan Chair in Surgery
Memorial Sloan Kettering Cancer Center
Professor, Department of Urology
Weill Cornell Medical College
New York, NY

Stephen A. Boorjian, MD, FACS
Carl Rosen Professor of Urology
Chair, Department of Urology
Mayo Clinic
Rochester, MN

Karim Chamie, MD, MSHS
Associate Professor
University of California Los Angeles
Los Angeles, CA

Sam Chang, MD, MBA, FACS
Professor of Urology
Vanderbilt University Medical Center
Nashville, TN

Jonathan Coleman, MD
Attending Surgeon, Urology Surgery Service
Memorial Sloan Kettering Cancer Center
Professor, Department of Urology
Weill Cornell Medical Center
New York, NY

Siamak Daneshmand, MD
Professor of Urology (Clinical Scholar)
Director of Urologic Oncology
Director of Clinical Research
Urologic Oncology Fellowship Director
USC Norris Comprehensive Cancer Center
Los Angeles, CA

Rian Dickstein, MD, FACS
Clinical Assistant Professor
University of Maryland School of Medicine
Baltimore, MD
Chief of Urology
University of Maryland Baltimore Washington
Medical Center
Glen Burnie, MD

Max Drescher, MD
Division of Urology
University of Maryland School of Medicine
Baltimore, MD

Boris Gershman, MD
Assistant Professor
Harvard Medical School
Division of Urologic Surgery
Beth Israel Deaconess Medical Center
Boston, MA

Gopal N. Gupta, MD, FACS
Professor
Department of Urology
Loyola University
Chicago, IL

Spencer T. Hart, MD
Department of Urology
Loyola University Medical Center
Maywood, IL

Ashish M. Kamat, MD, MBBS
Professor
Department of Urology, Division of Surgery
The University of Texas MD Anderson
Cancer Center
Houston, TX

Jose A. Karam, MD, FACS
Associate Professor of Urology and
Translational Molecular Pathology
The University of Texas MD Anderson
Cancer Center
Houston, TX

Wassim Kassouf, MD, CM, FRCSC
Stephen Jarslowsky Chair in Urology
Professor and Associate Chair
Department of Surgery
McGill University
Head, Urologic Oncology
Department of Surgery
McGill University Health Center
Montreal, Quebec, Canada

Zachary Klaassen, MD, MSc
Assistant Professor
Surgery, Division of Urology
Augusta University
Urologic Oncologist, Director of
Clinical Research
Division of Urology
Augusta University Medical Center
Augusta, GA

Ronald Koo , MD
Research Fellow and PhD Candidate,
Urologic Oncology
Department of Surgery, Division of Urology
McGill University
Montreal, Quebec, Canada

Shilajit Kuncu, MD
Urothelial Section Co-Chair
Professor
Chief of Urologic Oncology
Northwestern University Feinberg School of
Medicine
Chicago, IL

Patrick M. Lec, MD
Resident Physician, Urology
University of California, Los Angeles
Los Angeles, CA

Andrew T. Lenis, MD
Fellow, Urologic Oncology
Urology Service, Department of Surgery
Memorial Sloan Kettering Cancer Center
New York, NY

Seth Lerner, MD
Professor
Baylor College of Medicine
Houston, TX

Vitaly Margulis, MD, FACS
Professor, Urology
UT Southwestern Medical Center
Dallas, TX

Surena F. Matin, MD, FACS
Professor
Division of Surgery, Department of Urology
The University of Texas MD Anderson Cancer
Center
Houston, TX

Justin T. Matulay, MD
Assistant Professor
Department of Urology
Levine Cancer Institute
Atrium Health
Charlotte, NC

Andrew G. McIntosh, MD
Assistant Professor
Department of Urology
University of Oklahoma Stephenson Cancer
Center
Section Chief of Urology, Oklahoma City VA
Medical Center
Oklahoma City, OK

Matthew Mossanen, MD, MPH
Instructor of Surgery
Harvard Medical School
Urologic Oncologist
Brigham and Women's Hospital
Boston, MA

Vikram Narayan, MD
Assistant Professor
Emory University
Atlanta, GA

Neema Navai, MD
Associate Professor, Urology
The University of Texas MD Anderson Cancer
Center
Houston, TX

Vignesh T. Packiam, MD
Assistant Professor
Department of Urology
University of Iowa
Iowa City, IA

Sima Porten, MD, MPH, FACS
Associate Professor
Department of Urology
University of California San Francisco
San Francisco, CA

Mark A. Preston, MD, MPH
Assistant Professor
Harvard Medical School
Urologic Oncologist
Director of Urologic Research
Brigham and Women's Hospital
Boston, MA

Peter A. Reisz, MD
Urologic Oncology Fellow
Memorial Sloan Kettering Cancer Center
New York, NY

John Richgels, MD
Urology Resident
University of Chicago
Chicago, IL

Ragheed Saoud, MD
Urology Resident
University of Chicago
Chicago, IL

Shahrokh F. Shariat, MD
Professor and Chairman, Urology
Medical University of Vienna
Chief, Urology
Vienna General Hospital
Vienna, Austria

M. Minhaj Siddiqui, MD, FACS
Urothelial Section Co-Chair
Associate Professor
Department of Surgery, Division of Urology
University of Maryland School of Medicine
Director of Urologic Oncology and
Robotic Surgery
University of Maryland Marlene and Stewart
Greenebaum Cancer Center
Baltimore, MD

Nirmish Singla, MD, MSCS
Assistant Professor of Urology and Oncology
Director of Translational Research in
GU Oncology
The James Buchanan Brady Urological Institute
The Johns Hopkins University School of
Medicine
Baltimore, MD

Eila Skinner, MD
Professor and Chair
Department of Urology
Stanford University School of Medicine
Stanford, CA

Andrew Tracey, MD
Urologic Oncology Fellow
Memorial Sloan Kettering Cancer Center
New York, NY

Christopher J.D. Wallis, MD, PhD
Assistant Professor
Division of Urology
Department of Surgery
University of Toronto
Urologic Oncologist
Division of Urology
Department of Surgery
Mount Sinai Hospital
Toronto, Ontario, Canada

Shu Wang, MD
Research Fellow
Department of Surgery, Division of Urology
University of Maryland School of Medicine
Baltimore, MD

HEPATOBILIARY

Daniel E. Abbott, MD, FACS
Associate Professor of Surgery
University of Wisconsin
Madison, WI

Thomas A. Aloia, MD, MHCM, FACS
Vice President and Director of Oncology Services
Department of Clinical and Network Services
Institution Ascension
St. Louis, MO

Kim Bertens, MD, FACS
Assistant Professor
University of Ottawa
Section Head, Hepatobiliary Surgery
The Ottawa Hospital
Ottawa, Ontario, Canada

William C. Chapman, MD, FACS
Professor and Chief, Section of Transplantation
Chief, Division of General Surgery
Washington University in St. Louis
St. Louis, MO

Sean Cleary, MD, FACS
Professor of Surgery
Chair, Division of Hepato-Pancreatico-Biliary
Surgery
Mayo Clinic
Rochester, MN

Jordan M. Cloyd, MD, FACS
Assistant Professor, Department of Surgery
Ward Family Professor of Surgical Oncology
The Ohio State University Wexner
Medical Center
Columbus, OH

Michael D'Angelica, MD, FACS
Professor of Surgery
Weill Cornell Medical College
Attending Surgeon
Department of Hepatopancreatobiliary
Memorial Sloan Kettering Cancer Center
New York, NY

Paxton V. Dickson, MD, FACS
Associate Professor of Surgery
Division of Surgical Oncology
The University of Tennessee Health
Science Center
Memphis, TN

Vikas Dudeja, MBBS, FACS
James P. Hayes Endowed Professor
Director and Associate Professor
Division of Surgical Oncology
University of Alabama at Birmingham
Birmingham, AL

Cristina Ferrone, MD, FACS
Associate Professor of Surgery
Department of Surgery
Harvard University Medical School
Massachusetts General Hospital
Boston, MA

Richard W. Gilbert, MD, MSc
General Surgery Resident
Department of General Surgery
University of Ottawa
Ottawa, Ontario, Canada

Bhuwan Giri, MBBS
General Surgery Resident
Department of Surgery
University of Miami
Miami, FL

Michael G. House, MD, FACS, FSSO
Professor of Surgery
Chief, Division of Surgical Oncology
Indiana University School of Medicine
Indianapolis, IN

Kamram Idrees, MD, MSCI, MMHC, FACS
Associate Professor of Surgery
Chief, Division of Surgical Oncology and
Endocrine Surgery
Ingram Associate Professor of Clinical Research
Department of Surgery
Vanderbilt University
Nashville University Medical Center
Nashville, TN

William Jarnagin, MD, FACS
Chief, Department of Surgery
Memorial Sloan Kettering Cancer Center
New York, NY

Michael Kluger, MD, MPH, FACS
Associate Professor of Surgery
Department of Surgery, Division of GI and
Endocrine Surgery
Columbia University Irving Medical Center
Vagelos College of Physicians and Surgeons
New York-Presbyterian Hospital
New York, NY

Tori Lenet, MD
General Surgery Resident
University of Ottawa
Ottawa, Ontario, Canada

Shishir K. Maithel, MD, FSSO, FACS
Professor of Surgery
Scientific Director, Emory Liver and
Pancreas Center
Division of Surgical Oncology,
Department of Surgery
Emory University
Atlanta, GA

Guillaume Martel, MD, MSc, FRCSC, FACS
Associate Professor
University of Ottawa
Vered Family Chair in Hepato-Pancreato-
Biliary Research
The Ottawa Hospital
Ottawa, Ontario, Canada

Erin Maynard, MD, FACS
Associate Professor of Surgery
Associate Program Director of General
Surgery Residency
Oregon Health and Science University
Section Chief, Abdominal Organ Transplant
Portland VA Medical Center
Portland, OR

Laleh Melstrom, MD, FACS
Assistant Professor of Surgery and
Immuno-Oncology
City of Hope Comprehensive Cancer Center
Duarte, CA

Timothy M. Pawlik, MD, MPH, MTS, PhD,
FACS
Professor and Chair, Department of Surgery
The Urban Meyer III and Shelley Meyer
Chair for Cancer Research
Professor of Surgery, Oncology, and Health
Services Management and Policy
Surgeon-in-Chief
Surgery Department
The Ohio State University Wexner Medical
Center
Columbus, OH

Yana Puckett, MD, MPH, MBA, MSc
Complex General Surgical Oncology Fellow
University of Wisconsin
Madison, WI

Flavio Rocha, MD, FACS
Hepatobiliary Section Co-Chair
Associate Professor of Surgery
Hedinger Chair and Division Head of
Surgical Oncology
Physician-in-Chief, Knight Cancer Institute
Oregon Health and Science University
Portland, OR

J. Bart Rose, MD, MAS, FACS
Assistant Professor, Division of
Surgical Oncology
Director of the Pancreatobiliary Disease Center
The University of Alabama at Birmingham
Birmingham, AL

Maria C. Russell, MD, FACS
Associate Professor of Surgery
Department of Surgery
Emory University
Atlanta, GA

Shimul A. Shah, MD, MHCM, FACS
The James and Catherine Orr Endowed
Chair of Liver Transplantation
Chief, Solid Organ Transplantation
Professor of Surgery
University of Cincinnati College of Medicine
Cincinnati, OH

Paula Marincola Smith, MD, PhD
General Surgery Resident
Department of Surgery
Vanderbilt University Medical School
Nashville, TN

Rory Smoot, MD
Associate Professor
Vice-Chair, Research
Department of Surgery
Mayo Clinic
Rochester, MN

Rebecca Snyder, MD, MPH, FACS
Assistant Professor of Surgery
Division of Surgical Oncology
East Carolina University Brody School of
Medicine
Greenville, NC

Hop S. Tran Cao, MD, FACS
Associate Professor
Department of Surgical Oncology
The University of Texas MD Anderson
Cancer Center
Houston, TX

Ching-Wei Tzeng, MD, FACS
Hepatobiliary Section Co-Chair
Associate Professor
HPB Fellowship Program Director
Department of Surgical Oncology
The University of Texas MD Anderson
Cancer Center
Houston, TX

Jean-Nicolas Vauthey, MD, FACS
Professor
Chief, Hepato-Pancreato-Biliary Section
Dallas/Fort Worth Living Legend Chair for
Cancer Research
Department of Surgical Oncology
The University of Texas MD Anderson
Cancer Center
Houston, TX

Alice C. Wei, MD, MSc, FRCSC, FACS
Associate Professor of Surgery
Weill-Cornel School of Medicine
Cornell University
Associate Attending
Memorial Sloan Kettering Cancer Center
New York, NY

They say three is a charm. This book is the third volume of the American College of Surgeons Cancer Research Program's (CRP) *Operative Standards for Cancer Surgery*. This project has now, after almost 10 years, been able to cover the spectrum of surgical cancer care. It represents the culmination of a long collaboration between the Alliance for Clinical Trials in Oncology and the American College of Surgeons. The overall purpose of this project from its inception was to recognize that with any component of care, there is evidence of what is effective, but there is accompanying variability in actual practice. Bridging this gap is the challenge for care delivery programs today. The use of these guidelines, embedding them into the verification process (which has occurred over this last year), and the measurement of performance accentuates our journey toward high reliability in delivery of surgical cancer care in this country.

The first volume covered intraoperative surgical standards for breast, colon, lung, and pancreatic cancer. The second volume covered standards for cancers of the rectum, esophagus, stomach, skin (melanoma), and thyroid. This third volume covers standards for sarcoma, adrenal, neuroendocrine, peritoneal, urothelial, and hepatobiliary cancer. All three of these volumes offer recommendations on standardized techniques for optimal oncologic outcomes, which are appropriate for use in clinical trials and surgical practice. Select recommendations have also been incorporated recently into the Commission on Cancer accreditation standards.

The work overall of the editors in Volume 1 (Heidi Nelson, MD, FACS; Kelly Hunt, MD, FACS) and Volume 2 (Kelly Hunt, MD, FACS; Matthew Katz, MD, FACS) and of Matthew Katz, MD, FACS; Nirmal Veeramachaneni, MD, FACS; Susan Deming (CRP Project Manager); and Amanda Francescatti (CRP Senior Manager) in this third volume has been monumental in bringing this work forward.

The American College of Surgeons is so proud of this legacy. The effort to evaluate the operative standards will continue, with subsequent volumes and updates to existing standards based on accumulated evidence, providing an ongoing legacy of quality surgical cancer care.

David Hoyt, MD, FACS
Executive Director
American College of Surgeons

Editors and authors of the *Operative Standards for Cancer Surgery* are impressively now publishing their third volume of the manual, with ready plans to publish the fourth volume soon thereafter. It is deeply gratifying to witness the dedication and commitment of so many surgeons toward the drafting of the *Operative Standards for Cancer Surgery*. These books are testimony to the importance of quality in cancer surgery, and in that regard, the contributions of the many authors are entirely in keeping with the character and training of surgeons who give their best for patients. More than just a book, these manuals represent an authorship collaborative and a unified opinion about the critical elements of a cancer operation. Despite diverse educational training and background and perhaps even diverse technical surgical preferences, these surgeons have put aside their bias and built a new awareness about what matters most in cancer surgery.

We can agree that all things matter in the conduct of surgery and that there is no substitute for technical excellence. We have, in fact, come to realize that the quality chain is only as strong as the weakest link and patient outcomes depend on the summation of technical steps as well as on preoperative and perioperative team-based management. Indeed, emphasizing the technical aspects of optimal cancer surgery is not intended to diminish the criticality of all operative and perioperative care, but rather, the content of these manuals and subsequent research has brought to light the durable impact of cancer surgery techniques on long-term cancer survival. The content of these manuals intends only to help clarify the unique goals and quality metrics associated with cancer surgery.

The contents of these books in many regard represent a contemporary, evidence-based interpretation of cancer surgery principles. Our surgeon forefathers, such as Billroth in Germany, Handley in London, and Halsted in United States, were outspoken when it came to articulating the principles of cancer surgery. During their careers, when cancer surgery was the only cancer treatment available, the radical approaches they espoused were foundational and represented the only approaches that could achieve any hope for durable cancer outcomes. In contrast, modern cancer care now includes diverse disciplines as well as novel diagnostic and therapeutic options, many of which were not even imaginable just a few decades ago. What the authors describe in the *Operative Standards for Cancer Surgery* manuals are the modern principles that emphasize preservation of function and quality of life and adaptation of surgery to multidisciplinary treatment while at the same time acknowledging the importance of high-quality cancer surgery to long-term patient outcomes.

And finally, it must be said that the editors of these manuals have done what few others have aspired; that is, to move the pages of the book into clinical reality. There is an increasing recognition that simply publishing best practices or new knowledge does not ensure it will be implemented into routine practice. Recognizing the chasm between publication and practice, the surgeon leaders involved in the drafting of these books took the next step and turned these principles into accreditation standards. Dr. Matthew Katz and Dr. Kelly Hunt brought the lung, colon, melanoma, and breast cancer surgery critical elements to the Commission on Cancer (CoC) and under the prior leadership of Dr. Lawrence Shulman, together they operationalized the key principles into six new CoC standards. They now lead the newest cancer program within the American College of Surgeons (ACS), the Cancer Surgery Standards Program, and they are continuing with the work of implementing these standards through education, training, and the delivery of point-of-care tools such as the synoptic operative reports. Lastly, but importantly, nothing happens without the ACS staff. Amanda Francescatti, Susan Deming, and Linda Zheng all deserve a word of gratitude for their steadfast commitment to these important efforts.

Congratulations to all the contributors to these *Operative Standards for Cancer Surgery* manuals for a job well done. This work provides new insights into the conduct of surgery for the benefit of cancer patients.

Heidi Nelson, MD, FACS
Medical Director
Cancer Programs
American College of Surgeons

This volume of *Operative Standards for Cancer Surgery* represents the third in a series of evidence-based surgery manuals published through a collaboration between the American College of Surgeons (ACS) and the Alliance for Clinical Trials in Oncology.

Like the two volumes that preceded it, Volume 3 has been explicitly designed to educate surgeons and surgical trainees on the technical conduct of surgery, identify and target knowledge gaps for further study, and enhance the quality of surgical oncology as practiced in the United States. Each of these manuals describes "best practices" for the performance of technical elements of operations, which have been proven to be associated with patients' quantity and/or quality of life. To date, these standards have been used by thousands of surgeons to improve the quality of care they provide to patients with cancer.

Notably, several of the standards that have been put forth in this series have been recently adapted by the ACS Commission on Cancer (CoC) for accreditation purposes. Now, any surgeons who practices within CoC-accredited hospitals must adhere to standards 5.3 to 5.8 in the CoC manual, *Optimal Resources for Cancer Care (2020 Standards)*. These evidence-based standards describe critical elements of axillary dissection and sentinel lymph node biopsy for patients with breast cancer, wide local excision for patients with malignant melanoma, colectomy for patients with colon cancer, lung resection for patients with lung cancer, and total mesorectal excision for patients with rectal cancer. We anticipate that additional standards will go live in the future to ensure that all surgeons are conducting cancer operations in a way that benefits patients to the greatest extent possible.

Each of the sections represented in this volume was authored by a team of individuals who developed content and achieved consensus on multiple time-intensive conference calls and meetings, and we offer our sincere gratitude to each one of them. Each of these teams were expertly led by Drs. Christina Roland, Barbra S. Miller, Kaitlyn J. Kelly, Edward James Kruse, Perry Shen, Ed Levine, M. Minhaj Siddiqui, Shilajit Kundu, Flavio Rocha, and Ching-Wei Tzeng, who each deserve our profound appreciation. We are also grateful for the ongoing guidance and unwavering support of Dr. Kelly K. Hunt, director of the ACS Cancer Research Program; Dr. Heidi Nelson, medical director of ACS Cancer Programs; Dr. David Hoyt, past executive director of the ACS; and Dr. Monica Bertagnolli, group leader of the Alliance for Clinical Trials in Oncology.

And finally, we are deeply indebted to Amanda Francescatti and Susan Deming at the ACS who provided all logistical, technical, and cat-herding support for this project.

We trust that the standards contained herein will help enable all surgeons to achieve the best treatment outcomes possible on behalf of their patients.

Matthew H. G. Katz, MD, FACS
ACS CRP Cancer Care Standards Development Committee, Chair

Nirmal Veeramachaneni, MD, FACS
ACS CRP Cancer Care Standards Development Committee, Vice Chair

INTRODUCTION

When the six disease sites were selected for *Operative Standards for Cancer Surgery Volume 3*, working groups were developed, including representatives from the major professional societies for the disease sites and the Commission on Cancer. The disease site working groups determined the operative procedures that would be included and then assigned team members to each procedure, with a team leader responsible for organizing the team activities. Surgeons with expertise in health services research were assigned to each working group to serve as methodologists. The methodologists were responsible for developing a uniform process for the working groups to develop critical elements and key questions for each procedure.

METHODOLOGY FOR CRITICAL ELEMENTS

Critical elements for each procedure were developed by the working groups to include steps of the operative procedure that occur from the time of skin incision to the time of skin closure, which impact oncologic outcomes. The disease site working groups met by teleconference to choose the top four to five critical elements for each procedure for inclusion in the manual. Each step required consensus by all the members of the disease site working groups. Literature reviews were performed for each critical element and recommendations were made, including the type of data available and the grade of the recommendation. The quality of each recommendation was graded per the American College of Physicians guidelines (Table 1).

METHODOLOGY FOR KEY QUESTIONS

Key questions were identified during the process of constructing critical elements for each procedure. Key questions were areas of controversy where consensus could not be assured in order to qualify as a critical element. The methodologists determined a process for systematic review of the literature and for summarizing the findings of the working groups. It was suggested that a professional librarian be involved in the literature search whenever possible. At least two individuals were assigned to perform the literature searches and to provide a critical appraisal of the literature.

TABLE 1 Interpretation of the American College of Physicians' Guideline Grading System

Grade of Recommendation	Benefit versus Risks and Burdens	Methodological Quality of Supporting Evidence	Interpretation	Implications
Strong recommendation; high-quality evidence	Benefits clearly outweigh risks and burden or vice versa	RCTs without important limitations or overwhelming evidence from observational studies	Strong recommendation; can apply to most patients in most circumstances without reservation	For patients, most would want the recommended course of action and only a small proportion would not; a person should request discussion if the intervention was not offered. For clinicians, most patients should receive the recommended course of action. For policymakers, the recommendation can be adopted as a policy in most situations.
Strong recommendation; moderate-quality evidence	Benefits clearly outweigh risks and burden or vice versa	RCTs with important limitations (inconsistent results, methodological flaws, indirect, or imprecise) or exceptionally strong evidence from observational studies		
Strong recommendation; low-quality evidence	Benefits clearly outweigh risks and burden or vice versa	Observational studies or case series	Strong recommendation, but may change when higher-quality evidence becomes available	

Weak recommendation; high-quality evidence	Benefits closely balanced with risks and burden	RCTs without important limitations or overwhelming evidence from observational studies	Weak recommendation; best action may differ depending on circumstances or patients' or societal values	For patients, most would want the recommended course of action but some would not—a decision may depend on an individual's circumstances.
Weak recommendation; moderate-quality evidence	Benefits closely balanced with risks and burden	RCTs with important limitations (inconsistent results, methodological flaws, indirect, or imprecise) or exceptionally strong evidence from observational studies		For clinicians, different choices will be appropriate for different patients, and a management decision consistent with a patient's values, preferences, and circumstances should be reached.
Weak recommendation; low-quality evidence	Uncertainty in the estimates of benefits, risks, and burden; benefits, risks and burden may be closely balanced	Observational studies or case series	Very weak recommendation; other alternatives may be equally reasonable	For policymakers, policymaking will require substantial debate and involvement of many stakeholders.
Insufficient	Balance of benefits and risks cannot be determined	Evidence is conflicting, poor quality, or lacking	Insufficient evidence to recommend for or against routinely providing the service	For patients, decisions based on evidence from scientific studies cannot be made; for clinicians, decisions based on evidence from scientific studies cannot be made; for policymakers, decisions based on evidence from scientific studies cannot be made.

RCT = randomized, controlled trial.
Reprinted with permission from Qaseem A, Snow V, Owens DK, Shekelle P; Clinical Guidelines Committee of the American College of Physicians. The development of clinical practice guidelines and guidance statements of the American College of Physicians: Summary of methods. *Ann Intern Med*. 2010;153(3):194-199.

The general framework was to include literature from the English language by only using the PUBMED database to include literature published since 1990. Randomized trials were preferred, when available (see below).

Team members were asked to include all details of the literature review including the date of search, a list of all search terms, a list of all abstracts reviewed (including total number reviewed), all inclusion and exclusion criteria, and all literature chosen for review in detail. Consort diagrams for workflow were developed for each key question to include the number of abstracts reviewed and number of manuscripts reviewed in detail. The GRADE system (Table 2) was used to grade the level of evidence included in the detailed literature review. Summary tables were developed for each key question followed by recommendations based on the type of data and strength of available data. What follows is the process and workflow used by the disease site working group.

PROCESS AND WORKFLOW FOR KEY QUESTIONS

1) Identify key issues to address with literature review based on preliminary research and expert consensus regarding the key operative steps.
   a. Based on this preliminary review, identify key questions for which detailed evidence review will be obtained.
      i. Question should include detail about the population, the intervention, and the outcome. For example, "*in patients with T4 colorectal cancer does performing an en bloc resection reduce the risk of local recurrence*"
      ii. Each question should ideally be presented in PICO (P: population, I: intervention, C: comparator, O: outcome) format to facilitate and standardize the literature search.
2) Search the literature by using the following general strategy:
   a. MeSH terms or keyword search of search engines: PUBMED, EMBASE, Cochrane
   b. Previously published guidelines and consensus statements (e.g., National Guideline Clearinghouse: www.guideline.gov; relevant professional societies and organizations)
   c. Prior protocols from cooperative groups
      i. Obtain surgical specifications (if available) from prior cooperative group trials.
   d. Limits
      i. Publication year 1990+
      ii. English language
      iii. Type of publication
   e. Documentation
      i. Database(s) used
      ii. Search terms
      iii. Total number of hits
      iv. Number of abstracts reviewed
      v. Number of full papers reviewed
      vi. Number of papers included in the review
   f. Construct a CONSORT diagram (Fig. 1).

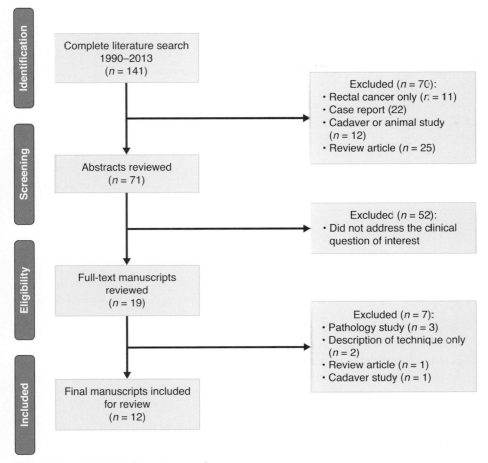

FIGURE 1   CONSORT diagram example.

3) Extract data from literature.
   a. Classify by study design (e.g., randomized controlled trial [RCT], observational [cohort, case-control, case series], systematic reviews).
      i. Was there a stated objective or hypothesis?
      ii. Population
      iii. Retrospective/prospective
      iv. Intervention
      v. Comparison
      vi. Outcome
   b. Summarize key findings.
   c. Apply exclusion.
      i. If the literature includes a large number of studies with similar results, it is reasonable to exclude poor studies from the review (e.g., sample size too small, conclusions not valid based on results, population too heterogenous

TABLE 2   Determining Quality of the Evidence

Grade	Description	Notes
++++	HIGH	Default for RCT
+++	MODERATE	
++	LOW	Default for observational studies
+	VERY LOW	

Quality is reduced by significant bias, inconsistency in the results, lack of good description of the population, intervention, control, and outcome of interest, imprecision (wide confidence intervals, may be associated with small sample sizes), publication bias (tendency to publish only desired results).

From: Grading quality of evidence and strength of recommendations. *BMJ.* 2004;328(7454):1490.

to permit interpretation of the data, duplicate data as different study, significant bias to the results not addressed). A list of excluded studies should be provided with the corresponding reason for exclusion.

   d. Assign grade of evidence for *each article*: High, Moderate, Low, or Very Low—by using the GRADE system (Table 2).

   e. Consolidate data into table form.

   f. Provide information on sample size and pertinent findings, including evaluation of the quality of evidence, and pertinent comments.

4) Generate conclusions.

   a. Group should review the document as presented by the primary reviewer(s) to ensure consensus.

5) Overall themes

   a. Pragmatic approach recognizing that resources and time are limited

      i. Targeted, not exhaustive, search of the literature but ensure balance

   b. Group members are an expert source for evaluating the validity of the recommendations.

SARCOMA CRITICAL ELEMENTS

Resection of Extremity and Trunk Soft Tissue Sarcoma

1. Pretreatment Biopsy of Soft Tissue Masses of the Extremity and Trunk

Recommendation: Pathologic subtyping of soft tissue masses suspicious for sarcoma of the extremity and trunk should be performed to facilitate planning of appropriate multimodality therapy. Histologic sampling of the tumor should generally be obtained via core needle biopsy, but an incisional biopsy should be obtained if adequate tissue cannot be acquired safely in this manner. The biopsy tract and incision should be oriented so that the entire tract (including scar, if applicable) can be excised en bloc with the tumor at the time of definitive resection.

Type of Data: Retrospective reports, case series, or case-control studies

Strength of Recommendation: Strong recommendation, moderate-quality evidence

2. Macroscopically Complete Resection of the Primary Tumor

Recommendation:

- The tumor should be resected en bloc with the entire biopsy tract to microscopically negative (R0) surgical margins. A circumferential 1- to 2-cm margin of grossly normal tissue should generally be resected to maximize the likelihood of an R0 resection. A narrower margin may be justified to preserve critical neurovascular structures, tendons, or bones that are adjacent to the tumor and that contribute significantly to limb function.
- Immediate histopathologic analysis (frozen section) should not be relied on to assess margin status intraoperatively as the differentiation between benign and malignant mesenchymal tissues is highly unreliable using currently available techniques. Further, specimen manipulation may increase the risk of tumor seeding.

Type of Data: Retrospective reports, case series, or case-control studies

Strength of Recommendation: Strong recommendation, moderate-quality evidence

3. Placement of Surgical Drains

Recommendation: Surgical drains are placed to prevent fluid accumulation in the operative bed. Drains should be used judiciously, and their entry sites should be placed as close to the incision as is feasible. This allows the percutaneous site to be included in the radiation field and excised en bloc with the specimen should reexcision be necessary or should the tumor recur.

Type of Data: Retrospective reports, case series, or case-control studies

Strength of Recommendation: Strong recommendation, high-quality evidence

Resection of Retroperitoneal and Intra-Abdominal Soft Tissue Sarcoma

1. Macroscopically Complete Resection of Primary Tumor Without Disruption of Tumor Capsule

Recommendation: Operative exposure, approach, and extent should maximize the ability to achieve a complete macroscopic (R0/R1) resection of the primary tumor without tumor rupture. Piecemeal resection is discouraged.

Type of Data: Retrospective reports, case series, or case-control studies

Strength of Recommendation: Strong recommendation, moderate-quality evidence

2. En Bloc Resection of Invaded Organs to Obtain a Complete Gross Resection

Recommendation: The degree to which retroperitoneal sarcoma invades adjacent visceral organs, muscles, major vessels, or bony structures should be estimated using preoperative cross-sectional imaging studies. Intraoperatively, structures that are directly invaded by cancer should be resected en bloc with the tumor using parenchymal-sparing, nonanatomic approaches.

Type of Data: Retrospective reports, case series, or case-control studies

Strength of Recommendation: Strong recommendation, moderate-quality evidence

ADRENAL CRITICAL ELEMENTS

Adrenalectomy Including Multivisceral Resection

1. Resection of the Primary Tumor to Microscopically Negative Margins Without Disruption of the Tumor Capsule

Recommendation: The primary objective of adrenalectomy is microscopically complete (R0) resection of the primary tumor. The tumor and the surrounding retroperitoneal fat, Gerota fascia, and peritoneum should be resected en bloc.

Type of Data: Retrospective reports, case series, or case-control studies

Strength of Recommendation: Strong recommendation, moderate-quality evidence

2. En Bloc Resection of Adjacent Organs Directly Invaded by Cancer

Recommendation: If direct invasion of an adjacent organ or muscle is suspected intraoperatively, the structure(s) should be resected en bloc with the primary adrenal tumor. Creation of an artificial plane between the primary tumor and an invaded structure should not be attempted.

Type of Data: Retrospective reports, case series, or case-control studies

Strength of Recommendation: Strong recommendation, moderate-quality evidence

Vascular Invasion

1. En Bloc Resection of Adjacent Blood Vessels Directly Involved by Primary Tumor And/Or Tumor Thrombus

Recommendation: If direct invasion of the inferior vena cava (IVC), renal vein, or renal artery by adrenal cancer is suspected intraoperatively, the vascular structure(s) should be resected en bloc with the primary adrenal tumor if technically feasible.

Type of Data: Retrospective reports, case series, or case-control studies

Strength of Recommendation: Strong recommendation, low-quality evidence

Lymphadenectomy

1. Resection of Regional Lymph Nodes Involved by Metastatic Adrenal Cancer

Recommendation: If regional lymph nodes are clinically suspected to be involved by metastatic adrenal cancer, a complete, en bloc nodal dissection of the affected lymph node basin(s) should be performed. An extended prophylactic lymphadenectomy is not recommended. If en bloc dissection is not possible, any nodal tissue that is removed separately from the primary specimen should be marked and labeled as a distinct specimen for pathologic analysis. The station(s) of origin of any involved lymph nodes should be specifically noted in the operative and pathology reports.

Type of Data: Retrospective reports, case series, or case-control studies

Strength of Recommendation: Strong recommendation, low-quality evidence

NEUROENDOCRINE CRITICAL ELEMENTS
Small Bowel Resection

1. Intraoperative Evaluation and Identification of Primary Tumor(s)

Recommendation: In patients with a small bowel neuroendocrine tumor (NET), intraoperative exploration should include assessment of the entirety of the small bowel at laparotomy. In patients with Zollinger-Ellison syndrome in whom a gastrinoma cannot be localized radiographically, the entire gastrinoma triangle should be inspected at laparotomy, and intraoperative ultrasound (IOUS) of the pancreas should be performed. If no gastrinoma can be identified using these techniques, the duodenal mucosa should be completely visualized and inspected through a lateral duodenotomy.

Type of Data: Retrospective reports, case series, or case-control studies

Strength of Recommendation: Strong recommendation, low-quality evidence

2. Regional Lymphadenectomy Along Segmental Vessels

Recommendation: Regional lymphadenectomy for jejunal and ileal small bowel NETs should include removal of all lymph nodes along the segmental vessels associated with the tumor-containing bowel segment to the level of the superior mesenteric artery and vein. For duodenal tumors treated with segmental resection or local excision, periportal and hepatic artery nodes should be sampled for lesions in D1 or D2, and proximal jejunal and adjacent retroperitoneal nodes posterior to the duodenum should be sampled for lesions in D3/D4. A minimum of eight lymph nodes should be examined for accurate pathologic staging.

Type of Data: Retrospective reports, case series, or case-control studies

Strength of Recommendation: Strong recommendation, low-quality evidence

3. Resection of the Primary Tumor

Recommendation: Full-thickness local excision is appropriate for low-grade NETs of the duodenum, including gastrinomas, that do not involve the ampulla of Vater. Lesions should be excised with a grossly negative margin of normal duodenal mucosa. For lesions of the jejunum and ileum, segmental resection is recommended, with the length of bowel to be resected dictated by the degree of lymphadenectomy.

Type of Data: Retrospective reports, case series, or case-control studies

Strength of Recommendation: Strong recommendation, low-quality evidence

Parenchyma-Preserving Pancreatectomy

1. Intraoperative Ultrasound Prior to Enucleation

Recommendation: Intraoperative ultrasound (IOUS) should be performed routinely prior to enucleation of a pancreatic neuroendocrine tumor (pNET) both to localize the tumor(s) and to evaluate the anatomic relationship between the tumor(s) and the pancreatic duct.

Type of Data: Retrospective reports, case series, or case-control studies

Strength of Recommendation: Strong recommendation, low-quality evidence

2. Resection of the Primary Tumor

Recommendation: Pancreatic neuroendocrine tumors selected for enucleation should be completely separated from adjacent normal parenchyma by careful blunt dissection. Intraoperative histopathologic analysis should be used if there is any concern for tissue invasion. For well-differentiated tumors in the body of the pancreas not amenable to enucleation, a central pancreatectomy or spleen-preserving distal pancreatectomy may be performed in order to preserve normal pancreatic parenchyma and the spleen.

Type of Data: Retrospective reports, case series, or case-control studies

Strength of Recommendation: Weak recommendation, low-quality evidence

3. Regional Lymph Node Sampling of the Peripancreatic and Celiac Lymph Nodes

Recommendation: Regional lymph node sampling of the peripancreatic and celiac lymph nodes should be considered for pNETs greater than 1.5 to 2.0 cm in size at the time of parenchyma-preserving resection.

Type of Data: Retrospective reports, case series, or case-control studies

Strength of Recommendation: Weak recommendation, low-quality evidence

PERITONEAL MALIGNANCIES CRITICAL ELEMENTS
Cytoreduction

1. Supracolic Greater Omentectomy

Recommendation: A supracolic greater omentectomy should be performed as part of all complete cytoreductive operations conducted for any peritoneal surface malignancy. In contrast, the lesser omentum should be resected only when gross tumor is identified on the structure.

Type of Data: Retrospective reports, case series, or case-control studies

Strength of Recommendation: Strong recommendation, low-quality evidence

2. Resection of Mesenteric Disease

Recommendation: The entire small intestine and mesentery should be systematically evaluated from the ligament of Treitz to the cecum. All visible mesenteric disease should be resected either by mesenteric peritonectomy or by resection of mesentery with the associated segment of bowel. Thermal ablation with high-voltage electrocautery, electrovaporization, or ultrasonic dissection may also be used to destroy mesenteric tumor nodules when complete cytoreduction cannot otherwise be safely performed.

Type of Data: Retrospective reports, case series, or case-control studies

Strength of Recommendation: Strong recommendation, low-quality evidence

3. Cytoreduction of the Diaphragm

Recommendation: Cytoreduction of disease on the peritoneal surface of the diaphragm should typically be accomplished via subdiaphragmatic peritonectomy, but full-thickness resection of the diaphragm may occasionally be required to resect cancer that invades deep into this structure.

Type of Data: Retrospective reports, case series, or case-control studies

Strength of Recommendation: Strong recommendation, low-quality evidence

4. Cytoreduction Within the Pelvis

Recommendation: If cancer is visible on the pelvic peritoneal surface, a pelvic peritonectomy should be undertaken to achieve optimal cytoreduction. Visceral and parietal peritoneum that is not grossly involved by tumor need not be excised. Resection of the rectosigmoid colon, bladder wall, ureters, ovaries, and/or uterus should be performed en bloc with the pelvic peritonectomy if these organs appear directly invaded by tumor. A bilateral oophorectomy should be performed routinely for postmenopausal patients with pelvic disease. The role of oophorectomy should be discussed preoperatively with each premenopausal patient in whom direct ovarian involvement is not identified.

Type of Data: Retrospective reports, case series, or case-control studies

Strength of Recommendation: Strong recommendation, low-quality evidence

5. Abdominal Visceral Resections

Recommendation: Fulguration of the hepatic or splenic visceral peritoneum and focal serosal resection of the stomach, small bowel, or colon with primary repair is an option for low-grade appendiceal primaries with limited serosal involvement. In cases of extensive visceral peritoneal involvement not amenable to stripping, visceral resection en bloc with involved surrounding parietal peritoneum is indicated. Parenchymal-preserving partial resections are preferred, as long as complete gross resection of all peritoneal metastasis can be achieved. Lymphadenectomy is generally unnecessary, but in the setting of a synchronous primary malignancy such as high-grade appendix, colon, or gastric cancer, standard oncologic lymphadenectomy with high ligation of the blood vessels feeding the primary tumor remains standard.

Type of Data: Retrospective reports, case series, or case-control studies

Strength of Recommendation: Strong recommendation, low-quality evidence

Drug Delivery and Safety

1. Hyperthermic Intraperitoneal Chemotherapy Following Cytoreduction

Recommendation: The decision to administer hyperthermic intraperitoneal chemotherapy (HIPEC) should be made on the basis of tumor type, patient physiology, and extent of cytoreduction. When administered, chemotherapy should be perfused following complete cytoreduction, using open or closed techniques, with close monitoring of intraperitoneal/core body temperatures, hemodynamics, and end organ function.

Type of Data: Retrospective reports, case series, or case-control studies

Strength of Recommendation: Strong recommendation, low-quality evidence

UROTHELIAL CRITICAL ELEMENTS
Endoscopic Management

1. Endoscopic Evaluation of Urethra and Bladder

Recommendation: All patients with a suspected urothelial cancer should undergo endoscopic evaluation that includes visualization of the urethra and bladder. Bimanual examination of the bladder should be performed before and after endoscopic resection to assess for tumor palpability and tumor invasion into adjacent structures. The use of white light–enhanced technologies, including photodynamic cystoscopy and narrow band imaging (NBI), should be considered to improve tumor detection. A second endoscopic evaluation performed 2 to 6 weeks following the initial resection should be performed for all high-grade TA and any T1 lesions.

Type of Data: Retrospective reports, case series, or case-control studies; prospective clinical trials

Strength of Recommendation: Strong recommendation, low-quality evidence

2. Transurethral Resection of Bladder Tumor

Recommendation: The surgeon should aim to resect the entire bladder tumor, including sampling of underlying muscle layer and tumor edges, in order to adequately stage the disease and decrease the risk of recurrence. Suspicious mucosal areas should be biopsied. In the setting of abnormal urinary biomarkers, random bladder biopsies should be considered but are otherwise unnecessary.

Type of Data: Retrospective reports, case series, or case-control studies

Strength of Recommendation: Strong recommendation, low-quality evidence

3. Endoscopic Evaluation and Treatment of Upper Tract Disease

Recommendation: When upper tract urothelial cancer is suspected, endoscopy of the upper genitourinary tract should be performed to accurately describe the anatomic location and volume of the disease involving the pelvicalyceal system and ureteral segments, as well as to obtain acceptable biopsy and cytology samples, to accurately grade and stage the tumor for surgical planning. For select patients with low-grade, noninvasive cancer, tumor ablation can adequately control disease.

Type of Data: Retrospective reports, case series, or case-control studies

Strength of Recommendation: Strong recommendation, low-quality evidence

4. Postoperative Instillation of Intravesical Chemotherapy

Recommendation: Chemotherapy (gemcitabine or mitomycin) should be instilled into the bladder within 24 hours (but ideally within 6 hours) following endoscopic resection of NMIBC.

Type of Data: Prospective clinical trials, systematic reviews, and meta-analyses

Strength of Recommendation: Strong recommendation, high-quality evidence

Partial Cystectomy

1. Intraoperative Localization of Tumor

Recommendation: All candidates for partial cystectomy should undergo a systematic intraoperative evaluation to confirm the safety and feasibility of complete tumor resection with partial cystectomy. Intraoperative evaluation may include cystoscopy, histologic confirmation, consideration for cystoscopic bladder mapping biopsies, and intraoperative palpation following bladder distention.

Type of Data: Retrospective reports, case series, or case-control studies

Strength of Recommendation: Strong recommendation, low-quality evidence

2. Resection to Adequate Margins

Recommendation: Partial cystectomy should be performed to gross resection margins of 2 cm whenever possible. Intraoperatively, the status of the resection margins should be confirmed histopathologically with frozen section analysis. Partial cystectomy should not be considered in patients in whom a gross complete resection with a negative margin cannot be anticipated or in those who carry a concurrent diagnosis of carcinoma in situ.

Type of Data: Retrospective reports, case series, or case-control studies

Strength of Recommendation: Strong recommendation, low-quality evidence

Radical Cystectomy

1. Removal of Bladder to Negative Resection Margins

Recommendation: Removal of the bladder should occur with an effort to minimize the risks of tumor spillage or positive tumor margins. Intraoperative histopathologic evaluation of the distal ureteral margin need not be performed routinely at the time of radical cystectomy in the absence of cystoscopic suspicion of tumor at the trigone or urethra. Intraoperative histopathologic evaluation of the distal urethral margin should be performed when bladder neck, prostatic (in men), or urethral invasion is suspected based on cystoscopy or when considering candidacy for orthotopic urinary diversion but is otherwise unnecessary for urethral-sparing surgery when no nearby tumor involvement is suspected.

Type of Data: Retrospective reports, case series, or case-control studies; prospective clinical trials

Strength of Recommendation: Strong recommendation, moderate-quality evidence

2. Concomitant Pelvic Organ Management in Men and Women

Recommendation: Organ preservation with organ-sparing cystectomy (OSC) is the favored approach to cystectomy for selected men and women with urothelial carcinomas T2 or less that are located away from the trigone or bladder neck and that do not involve the urethra.

Type of Data: Retrospective reports, case series, case-control studies

Strength of Recommendation: Strong recommendation, low-quality evidence

3. Pelvic Lymph Node Dissection

Recommendation: A PLND using a standard template should accompany RC for urothelial carcinoma of the bladder.

Type of Data: Retrospective reports, case series, or case-control studies; prospective clinical trials

Strength of Recommendation: Strong recommendation, moderate-quality evidence

4. Selection of a Urinary Diversion Procedure

Recommendation: Intraoperatively, the tumor extent, quality of the bowel to be used, and status of the urethra should all be evaluated to inform the final selection of a urinary diversion procedure at cystectomy.

Type of Data: Retrospective reports, case series, or case-control studies

Strength of Recommendation: Strong recommendation, low-quality evidence

Nephroureterectomy

1. Removal of Kidney and Ureter

Recommendation: Nephroureterectomy for upper tract urothelial carcinoma (UTUC) should generally include resection of the kidney and entire ureter. Segmental ureterectomy may be considered for patients with either low-grade urothelial cell carcinoma or noninvasive high-grade urothelial cell carcinoma of the upper urothelial tract.

Type of Data: Retrospective reports, case series, or case-control studies

Strength of Recommendation: Strong recommendation, low-quality evidence

2. Management of the Distal Ureter/Cuff

Recommendation: During radical nephroureterectomy, the distal ureter must be excised in its entirety, inclusive of the full-thickness intramural segment and ureteral orifice ("bladder cuff"). Open transvesical and extravesical excision approaches offer comparable oncologic efficacy. Endoscopic or minimally invasive extravesical ligation methods of cuff excision have been associated with higher intravesical recurrence rates and should not be used.

Type of Data: Retrospective reports, case series, or case-control studies; systematic reviews and meta-analyses

Strength of Recommendation: Strong recommendation, weak evidence

3. Lymphadenectomy for Upper Tract Urothelial Cancer During Definitive Resection

Recommendation: A template-based lymphadenectomy based on laterality and location of the primary tumor should be considered at the time of nephroureterectomy or segmental ureterectomy for high-risk, high-grade, or suspected high-grade UTUC.

Type of Data: Retrospective reports, case series, or case-control studies; prospective clinical trials

Strength of Recommendation: Strong recommendation, weak evidence

4. Perioperative Instillation of Intravesical Chemotherapy

Recommendation: Chemotherapy consisting of either mitomycin C or pirarubicin should be instilled into the bladder of all patients undergoing nephroureterectomy for upper tract urothelial carcinoma during or immediately following surgery.

Type of Data: Prospective clinical trials; retrospective reports, case series, or case-control studies

Strength of Recommendation: Strong recommendation, moderate-quality evidence

HEPATOBILIARY CRITICAL ELEMENTS

Liver Resection for Colorectal Liver Metastases

1. Systematic Abdominal Inspection and Intraoperative Ultrasound

Recommendation: A systematic inspection of the abdomen should be routinely performed to exclude extrahepatic cancer and assess the health of the liver at the time of operation. Systematic intraoperative ultrasound of the liver should also be routinely performed to confirm technical resectability of the tumor(s), to detect radiographically occult disease, and to confirm the operative plan.

Type of Data: Retrospective reports, case series, or case-control studies

Strength of Recommendation: Strong recommendation, low-level evidence

2. Resection of Planned Lesions to Macroscopically Negative Margins

Recommendation: All metastatic lesions planned for resection should be resected either individually or en bloc with the goal of obtaining negative macroscopic (R0/R1) parenchymal and vascular margins while simultaneously preserving maximal functional volume in the FLR. Portal lymphadenectomy should not be performed routinely. Lymphadenectomy can be considered in highly selected patients for whom there is either suspicion of or known metastatic lymphadenopathy and the goal of clearing all macroscopic disease has been established within the context of a multimodality plan.

Type of Data: Retrospective reports, case series, or case-control studies

Strength of Recommendation: Strong recommendation, medium-level evidence

Liver Resection for Hepatocellular Carcinoma

1. Laparoscopic or Open Inspection of the Abdomen and Liver

Recommendation: The liver parenchyma should be evaluated thoroughly for the presence of fibrosis and/or cirrhosis. Portal hypertension should be excluded. Inspection and/or palpation of the liver (to rule out intrahepatic metastases or multifocal disease) and peritoneal cavity is critical. Intraoperative ultrasound is recommended to evaluate and confirm the relationship of any identified lesion(s) to the vascular and biliary pedicles and to guide parenchymal transection.

Type of Data: Retrospective reports, case series, or case-control studies

Strength of Recommendation: Strong recommendation, low-quality evidence

2. All Lesions Should Be Resected to Macroscopically Negative Margins

Recommendation: All lesions should be resected either individually or en bloc in order to obtain negative margins on the parenchyma, hepatic vein (or tributaries), and Glissonian pedicle or branches while ensuring adequate FLR. Glissonian pedicle–based "anatomic" resection is preferred. When a "nonanatomic" resection technique is performed, gross margins of 1 to 2 cm should be sought. The specimen should be oriented and sent for immediate gross evaluation if concern exists for a positive margin. If the tumor is visible at the resection margin (grossly positive), re-resection of the margin should be considered if technically feasible and the volume of the FLR is sufficient. Portal lymphadenectomy is not recommended routinely, but selective lymphadenectomy should be considered in patients for whom suspicion of metastatic lymphadenopathy exists.

Type of Data: Retrospective reports, case series, or case-control studies

Strength of Recommendation: Strong recommendation, low-quality evidence

Cholangiocarcinoma

1. Resection of the Primary Tumor to Microscopically Negative Margins

Recommendation: Local excision of the bile duct alone represents inadequate oncologic surgery for patients with hilar cholangiocarcinoma. En bloc hemihepatectomy is, therefore, recommended in all operations conducted with curative intent. Resection and reconstruction of the portal vein is justified when the vein is directly involved by cancer and an R0 resection is otherwise anticipated. Resection of intrahepatic cholangiocarcinoma (ICC) consists of removal of the involved liver to microscopically negative (R0) parenchymal, biliary, and vascular margins.

Type of Data: Retrospective reports, case series, or case-control studies

Strength of Recommendation: Strong recommendation, low-quality evidence

2. Routine Portal Lymphadenectomy With Selective Sampling of Aortocaval and Retroperitoneal Nodes

Recommendation:
- For hilar cholangiocarcinoma, a complete lymphadenectomy of the basins within the hepatoduodenal ligament to resect the hilar, cystic duct, choledochal, hepatic artery, portal vein, and posterior pancreaticoduodenal lymph nodes should be routinely performed.
- For ICC, lymphadenectomy should routinely include the lymph nodes in the hepatoduodenal ligament; for tumors in the left liver, lymphadenectomy should also include the nodes at the right cardia and lesser curvature; and for tumors in the right liver, lymphadenectomy should also include the retropancreatic nodes.
- In all cases, suspicious periaortic, pericaval, superior mesenteric artery, and celiac artery lymph nodes should be sampled; if positive for metastatic cancer, resection should be aborted.

Type of Data: Retrospective reports, case series, or case-control studies

Strength of Recommendation: Strong recommendation, low-quality evidence

Gallbladder Cancer

1. Selective Staging Laparoscopy Prior to Resection of Gallbladder Cancer

Recommendation: Staging laparoscopy should be considered prior to definitive resection in selected patients in whom gallbladder cancer was identified incidentally at prior cholecystectomy. Staging laparoscopy should be performed routinely in patients with per primum gallbladder cancer to assess for radiographically occult metastatic disease prior to committing to oncologic resection. In either case, if metastatic disease is identified on exploration, resection should not be pursued.

Type of Data: Retrospective reports, case series, or case-control studies; prospective clinical trials

Strength of Recommendation: Strong recommendation, low-level evidence

2. Microscopically Complete (R0) Resection of Local Tumor

Recommendation: Resection of per primum gallbladder cancer should be performed by resection of the gallbladder en bloc with either formal IVb and V segmentectomy or wedge resection of the tumor-bearing liver. For gallbladder cancer incidentally identified in a cholecystectomy specimen, re-resection is not justified for patients with Tis and T1a disease in whom cystic duct margin is negative. For patients with T1b or greater disease, either wedge resection of the gallbladder bed or formal IVb and V segmentectomy is indicated. In all cases, a microscopically complete (R0) resection should be sought. The cystic duct margin should be sent for intraoperative assessment of involvement by carcinoma. Routine common bile duct excision should not be performed unless necessary to achieve an R0 resection.

Type of Data: Retrospective reports, case series, or case-control studies; prospective clinical trials

Strength of Recommendation: Moderate recommendation, low-quality evidence

3. Routine Portal Lymphadenectomy, With Selective Sampling of Aortocaval and Retroperitoneal Nodes

Recommendation: Lymphadenectomy comprising the nodes in the hepatoduodenal ligament (12) along the common hepatic artery (8) and behind the pancreas (13) should be routinely performed. Selective sampling of lymph nodes in the aortocaval space (16) should be performed if there is clinical suspicion. An attempt should be made to ensure three to six nodes in the specimen for staging purposes.

Type of Data: Retrospective reports, case series, or case-control studies; prospective clinical trials

Strength of Recommendation: Moderate recommendation, low-quality evidence

4. Port Site Excision Need Not Be Performed Routinely for Incidentally Discovered Gallbladder Cancer

Recommendation: Routine excision of port sites during curative reoperation for incidentally discovered gallbladder cancer does not add a survival benefit and should be avoided.

Type of Data: Retrospective reports, case series, or case-control studies

Strength of Recommendation: Strong recommendation, low-quality evidence

CONTENTS

LIST OF CONTRIBUTORS   v
FOREWORD   xvii
PREFACE   xxi
METHODOLOGY RESEARCH PROTOCOL   xxiii
SUMMARY OF CRITICAL ELEMENTS AND
    RECOMMENDATIONS   xxix

SECTION I SARCOMA   1
Introduction   2
Chapter 1: Resection of Extremity and Trunk Soft
    Tissue Sarcoma   14
Chapter 2: Resection of Retroperitoneal and Intra-abdominal
    Soft Tissue Sarcoma   40

SECTION II ADRENAL   73
Introduction   74
Chapter 3: Adrenalectomy Including Multivisceral Resection   83
Chapter 4: Vascular Invasion   103
Chapter 5: Lymphadenectomy   116

SECTION III NEUROENDOCRINE   143
Introduction   144
Chapter 6: Small Bowel Resection   156
Chapter 7: Parenchyma-Preserving Pancreatectomy   179

SECTION IV PERITONEAL
            MALIGNANCIES   215
Introduction   216
Chapter 8: Cytoreduction   223
Chapter 9: Drug Delivery and Safety   249

SECTION V UROTHELIAL   291
Introduction   292
Chapter 10: Endoscopic Management   303
Chapter 11: Partial Cystectomy   313
Chapter 12: Radical Cystectomy   319
Chapter 13: Nephroureterectomy   354

SECTION VI HEPATOBILIARY   413

Introduction   414

Chapter 14: Liver Resection for Colorectal Liver Metastases   426

Chapter 15: Liver Resection for Hepatocellular Carcinoma   433

Chapter 16: Cholangiocarcinoma   440

Chapter 17: Gallbladder Cancer   463

Index   497

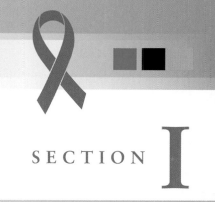

SECTION I

SARCOMA

INTRODUCTION

Soft tissue sarcomas comprise a heterogeneous family of mesenchymal malignancies that consists of greater than 60 distinct clinical entities that are associated with diversity in biologic behavior. Sarcomas can arise in virtually any anatomic location; this section focuses on cancers of the extremity, trunk, and retroperitoneum as well as gastrointestinal stromal tumors (GISTs).

Although surgical principles and approaches may be similar across the various sarcoma histologies, the site of disease and the goals of surgery as a component of multidisciplinary care vary to some degree based on the sarcoma subtype. Thus, initial diagnostics and multidisciplinary management at a sarcoma center are critical.

CLINICAL STAGING

Prior to 2017, the American Joint Committee on Cancer (AJCC) staging system for soft tissue sarcomas was based on tumor size, depth of tissue involvement, grade of the neoplasm, and extent of lymph node metastasis.[1] This system was generally simple to apply and broadly applicable to all tumors, irrespective of anatomic location. However, it was poorly prognostic in tumor sites such as head/neck and retroperitoneum, in which grade (head/neck) and tumor size (retroperitoneum) disproportionately drive prognosis relative to other staging criteria.

Recognition of this limitation led to changes the *AJCC Cancer Staging Manual*, Eighth Edition.[2] In this edition, different staging systems were described for sarcomas of the head/neck region, trunk and extremities, abdomen and thoracic visceral organs, GIST, retroperitoneum, and unusual histologies and sites. See Tables 1-1, 1-2, 1-3, and 1-4 for staging information relevant to this section.[2] Although this iteration of the *AJCC Cancer Staging Manual* is more complex than prior versions, the classification systems it describes allow for more emphasis on the unique relevance of size as it relates to specific anatomic site, the characteristic sarcoma types (diagnosis) typical for each site, and the type of tissue or organ involvement. Histologic grading based on the Fédération Nationale des Centres de Lutte Contre le Cancer methodology remains

TABLE 1-1   American Joint Committee on Cancer Staging Criteria for Soft Tissue Sarcoma of the Trunk and Extremities, Eighth Edition

TABLE 1-1A   Definition of Primary Tumor (T)

T Stage	Criteria
TX	Primary tumor cannot be assessed
T0	No evidence of primary tumor
T1	Tumor ≤5 cm in greatest dimension
T2	Tumor >5 cm and ≤10 cm in greatest dimension
T3	Tumor >10 cm and ≤15 cm in greatest dimension
T4	Tumor >15 cm in greatest dimension

TABLE 1-1B   Definition of Regional Lymph Node (N)

N Stage	Criteria
NX	Regional lymph nodes cannot be assessed
N0	No regional lymph node metastases or unknown lymph node status
N1	Regional lymph node metastasis

TABLE 1-1C   Definition of Distant Metastasis (M)

M Stage	Criteria
MX	Distant metastases cannot be assessed
M0	No distant metastasis
M1	Distant metastasis

TABLE 1-1D   Definition of Grade

Grade	Criteria
GX	Grade cannot be assessed
G1	Total differentiation, mitotic count, and necrosis score of 2 or 3
G2	Total differentiation, mitotic count, and necrosis score of 4 or 5
G3	Total differentiation, mitotic count, and necrosis score of 6, 7, or 8

TABLE 1-1E   Tumor Differentiation

Differentiation Score	Definition
1	Sarcomas closely resembling normal adult mesenchymal tissue (e.g., low-grade leiomyosarcoma)
2	Sarcomas for which histologic typing is certain (e.g., myxoid/round cell liposarcoma)
3	Embryonal and undifferentiated sarcomas, sarcomas of doubtful type, synovial sarcomas, soft tissue osteosarcoma, Ewing sarcoma/primitive neuroectodermal tumor of soft tissue

TABLE 1-1F   Mitotic Count

Mitotic Count Score	Definition
1	0–9 mitoses per 10 high-power fields
2	10–19 mitoses per 10 high-power fields
3	≥20 mitoses per 10 high-power fields

TABLE 1-1G   Tumor Necrosis

Necrosis Score	Definition
0	No necrosis
1	<50% tumor necrosis
2	≥50% tumor necrosis

Note: American Joint Committee on Cancer staging and TNM classification for soft tissue sarcoma of the trunk and extremities.[2] Used with permission of the American Joint Committee on Cancer (AJCC), Chicago, Illinois. The original and primary source for this information is the *AJCC Cancer Staging Manual*, Eighth Edition (2017) published by Springer International Publishing.

TABLE 1-1H   Prognostic Stage Groups

	T Stage	N Stage	M Stage	Grade
Stage IA	T1	N0	M0	G1, GX
Stage IB	T2, T3, T4	N0	M0	G1, GX
Stage II	T1	N0	M0	G2, G3
Stage IIIA	T2	N0	M0	G2, G3
Stage IIIB	T3, T4	N0	M0	G2, G3
Stage IV	Any T	N1	M0	Any G
	Any T	Any N	M1	Any G

TABLE 1-2   American Joint Committee on Cancer Staging Criteria for Gastric and Omental GIST, Eighth Edition

TABLE 1-2A   Definition of Primary Tumor (T)

T Stage	Criteria
TX	Primary tumor cannot be assessed
T0	No evidence of primary tumor
T1	Tumor ≤2 cm in greatest dimension
T2	Tumor >2 cm and ≤5 cm in greatest dimension
T3	Tumor >5 cm and ≤10 cm in greatest dimension
T4	Tumor >10 cm in greatest dimension

TABLE 1-2B   Definition of Regional Lymph Node (N)

N Stage	Criteria
NX	Regional lymph nodes cannot be assessed
N0	No regional lymph node metastases or unknown lymph node status
N1	Regional lymph node metastasis

TABLE 1-2C   Definition of Distant Metastasis (M)

M Stage	Criteria
MX	Distant metastases cannot be assessed
M0	No distant metastasis
M1	Distant metastasis

TABLE 1-2D   Definition of Mitotic Rate

Mitotic Rate	Criteria
Low	$\leq$5 mitoses per 5 mm^2, or per 50 high-power fields
High	>5 mitoses per 5 mm^2, or per 50 high-power fields

TABLE 1-2E   Prognostic Stage Groups

	T Stage	N Stage	M Stage	Mitotic Rate
Stage IA	T1–T2	N0	M0	Low
Stage IB	T3	N0	M0	Low
Stage II	T1–T2	N0	M0	High
Stage IIIA	T3	N0	M0	High
Stage IIIB	T4	N0	M0	High
Stage IV	Any T	N1	M0	Any rate
	Any T	Any N	M1	Any rate

Note: American Joint Committee on Cancer staging and TNM classification for gastric and omental GIST.[2] Used with permission of the American Joint Committee on Cancer (AJCC), Chicago, Illinois. The original and primary source for this information is the *AJCC Cancer Staging Manual*, Eighth Edition (2017) published by Springer International Publishing.

TABLE 1-3   American Joint Committee on Cancer Staging Criteria for Small Intestinal, Esophageal, Colorectal, Mesenteric, and Peritoneal GIST, Eighth Edition

TABLE 1-3A   Definition of Primary Tumor (T)

T Stage	Criteria
TX	Primary tumor cannot be assessed
T0	No evidence of primary tumor
T1	Tumor ≤2 cm in greatest dimension
T2	Tumor >2 cm and ≤5 cm in greatest dimension
T3	Tumor >5 cm and ≤10 cm in greatest dimension
T4	Tumor >10 cm in greatest dimension

TABLE 1-3B   Definition of Regional Lymph Node (N)

N Stage	Criteria
NX	Regional lymph nodes cannot be assessed
N0	No regional lymph node metastases or unknown lymph node status
N1	Regional lymph node metastasis

TABLE 1-3C   Definition of Distant Metastasis (M)

M Stage	Criteria
MX	Distant metastases cannot be assessed
M0	No distant metastasis
M1	Distant metastasis

TABLE 1-3D   Definition of Mitotic Rate

Mitotic Rate	Criteria
Low	≤5 mitoses per 5 mm^2, or per 50 high-power fields
High	>5 mitoses per 5 mm^2, or per 50 high-power fields

TABLE 1-3E   Prognostic Stage Groups

	T Stage	N Stage	M Stage	Mitotic Rate
Stage I	T1–T2	N0	M0	Low
Stage II	T3	N0	M0	Low
Stage IIIA	T1	N0	M0	High
	T4	N0	M0	Low
Stage II B	T2–T4	N0	M0	High
Stage IV	Any T	N1	M0	Any rate
	Any T	Any N	M1	Any rate

Note: American Joint Committee on Cancer staging and TNM classification for small intestinal, esophageal, colorectal, mesenteric, and peritoneal GIST.[2] Used with permission of the American Joint Committee on Cancer (AJCC), Chicago, Illinois. The original and primary source for this information is the *AJCC Cancer Staging Manual*, Eighth Edition (2017) published by Springer International Publishing.

TABLE 1-4   American Joint Committee on Cancer Staging Criteria for Soft Tissue Sarcoma of the Retroperitoneum, Eighth Edition

TABLE 1-4A   Definition of Primary Tumor (T)

T Stage	Criteria
TX	Primary tumor cannot be assessed
T0	No evidence of primary tumor
T1	Tumor ≤5 cm in greatest dimension
T2	Tumor >5 cm and ≤10 cm in greatest dimension
T3	Tumor >10 cm and ≤15 cm in greatest dimension
T4	Tumor >15 cm in greatest dimension

TABLE 1-4B   Definition of Regional Lymph Node (N)

N Stage	Criteria
NX	Regional lymph nodes cannot be assessed
N0	No regional lymph node metastases or unknown lymph node status
N1	Regional lymph node metastasis

TABLE 1-4C Definition of Distant Metastasis (M)

M Stage	Criteria
MX	Distant metastases cannot be assessed
M0	No distant metastasis
M1	Distant metastasis

TABLE 1-4D Definition of Grade (G)

Grade	Criteria
GX	Grade cannot be assessed
G1	Total differentiation, mitotic count, and necrosis score of 2 or 3
G2	Total differentiation, mitotic count, and necrosis score of 4 or 5
G3	Total differentiation, mitotic count, and necrosis score of 6, 7, or 8

TABLE 1-4E Tumor Differentiation

Differentiation Score	Definition
1	Sarcomas closely resembling normal adult mesenchymal tissue (e.g., low-grade leiomyosarcoma)
2	Sarcomas for which histologic typing is certain (e.g., myxoid/round cell liposarcoma)
3	Embryonal and undifferentiated sarcomas, sarcomas of doubtful type, synovial sarcomas, soft tissue osteosarcoma, Ewing sarcoma/primitive neuroectodermal tumor of soft tissue

TABLE 1-4F Mitotic Count

Mitotic Count Score	Definition
1	0–9 mitoses per 10 high-power fields
2	10–19 mitoses per 10 high-power fields
3	≥20 mitoses per 10 high-power fields

TABLE 1-4G Tumor Necrosis

Necrosis Score	Definition
0	No necrosis
1	<50% tumor necrosis
2	≥50% tumor necrosis

TABLE 1-4H   Prognostic Stage Groups

	T Stage	N Stage	M Stage	Grade
Stage IA	T1	N0	M0	GX or G1
Stage IB	T2–T4	N0	M0	GX or G1
Stage II	T1	N0	M0	G2 or G3
Stage IIIA	T2	N0	M0	G2 or G3
Stage IIIB	T3–T4	N0	M0	G2 or G3
	Any T	N1	M0	Any G
Stage IV	Any T	N1	M0	Any G
	Any T	Any N	M1	Any G

Note: American Joint Committee on Cancer staging and TNM classification for soft tissue sarcoma of the retroperitoneum.[2] Used with permission of the American Joint Committee on Cancer (AJCC), Chicago, Illinois. The original and primary source for this information is the *AJCC Cancer Staging Manual*, Eighth Edition (2017) published by Springer International Publishing.

an important component of these stage groupings.[3] Although much work remains to further refine this system within these new categories (including incorporation of histologic subtype in staging), this classification appears to be a step in the right direction, in that it recognizes and tries to respond to the diversity of tumors and their sundry clinical presentations.

MULTIDISCIPLINARY CARE

The backbone of treatment for patients with localized soft tissue sarcoma is margin-negative surgical resection with the goal of removing 1 to 2 cm of surrounding noncancerous tissue. However, both local and distant relapse are frequent events following surgery—particularly in the setting of large, high-grade tumors. This highlights the need for multimodality treatment.

Current National Comprehensive Cancer Network guidelines for treatment of soft tissue sarcoma of the extremity and trunk recommend a combination of wide resection and radiotherapy in patients with intermediate- or high-grade sarcomas of any size.[4] Amputation should be reserved for patients without a limb-sparing option, based on data from the National Cancer Institute demonstrating no difference in overall survival (OS) with amputation versus limb-sparing surgery with wide resection.[5] Surgery alone *can* be considered for patients with small (<5 cm) soft tissue sarcomas resected with widely negative (1 to 2 cm) margins. Small tumors adjacent to critical, unresectable anatomic structures, which cannot be resected to negative margins without significant attendant morbidity, should be considered for radiation therapy. Local control rates with modern multimodality therapy range from 80% to 90%.[6–8]

The evidence supporting combination radiotherapy and wide resection in this setting comes from two randomized controlled trials and a number of retrospective studies. These studies report a relative risk reduction of approximately 50% with the addition of radiotherapy relative to surgery alone and absolute reduction dependent on baseline risk.[6–8] Radiotherapy administered in the preoperative setting is associated with oncologic outcomes similar to those associated with radiotherapy administered postoperatively, but side effect profiles are dependent on timing.[9] Preoperative radiotherapy is associated with an increase in postoperative wound healing complications, whereas postoperative radiotherapy has been associated with more long-term limb dysfunction. Ultimately, the decision regarding preoperative versus postoperative radiotherapy is based on multiple factors: anatomic location, expected final margin status, anticipated wound-healing issues and reconstruction needs, and institutional preference.

Most patients with retroperitoneal sarcoma succumb to uncontrolled intraabdominal disease. Akin to the treatment approach for high-risk extremity and truncal soft tissue sarcoma, preoperative radiotherapy has been used to try to improve local control. Until recently, prospective data supporting this approach were lacking. The STRASS trial (Surgery with or without Radiation Therapy in Untreated Nonmetastatic Retroperitoneal Sarcoma; NCT01344018) was a phase 3 randomized controlled trial that compared abdominal recurrence-free survival (ARFS) rates in patients with previously untreated retroperitoneal sarcoma who underwent curative-intent surgery alone with patients who received radiotherapy prior to surgery.[10] The initial results, presented at the 2019 American Society of Clinical Oncology meeting, showed no difference in 3-year ARFS (60.4% for radiotherapy/surgery vs. 58.7% for surgery alone; $P = .954$). A post hoc subgroup analysis did demonstrate that liposarcoma histology was associated with an improved 3-year ARFS: 71.6% in the radiotherapy/surgery arm versus 60.4% in the surgery alone arm ($P = .049$), mainly in the well-differentiated subtype, but the follow-up duration was short and not a prespecified endpoint. Nevertheless, the subgroup analysis, although not conclusive or practice changing on its own, does provide some preliminary data supporting the administration of radiotherapy to patients with liposarcoma and can serve as the impetus for further studies.[10]

Although significant progress has been made in limb salvage and local control, metastasis and death remain a significant problem for patients with soft tissue sarcoma. Approximately 50% of patients with large, high-grade tumors will develop distant metastatic disease. Chemotherapy should be considered for patients with a high risk of occult distant metastases (e.g., high-grade tumors >5 cm in diameter) and for patients with certain histologies that potentially have an increased sensitivity to cytotoxic chemotherapy (i.e., synovial sarcoma). Unfortunately, the data demonstrating a consistent survival benefit for systemic chemotherapy remain somewhat controversial and debated. The Sarcoma Meta-Analysis Collaboration that included a heterogeneous group of more than 1,500 patients demonstrated a 10% improvement in recurrence-free survival (RFS) in patients who received adjuvant chemotherapy but no improvement in OS compared with active surveillance.[11] A decade later, a meta-analysis was performed that examined the efficacy of adjuvant doxorubicin-based regimens (often combined with ifosfamide), but only a small survival benefit compared with surgery alone was found ($P = .02$). However, a substantial proportion of patients who received chemotherapy experienced grades 3 and 4 toxicities, which offset the small survival benefit enjoyed by some patients. The available literature highlights an unmet need for better systemic therapies.[12,13] Regardless, systemic chemotherapy for patients at high risk of systemic relapse should be discussed in a multidisciplinary tumor board.

Imatinib mesylate (Gleevec) is a tyrosine kinase inhibitor that targets c-KIT and platelet-derived growth factor α.[14] For GIST, it can be used in the neoadjuvant, adjuvant, or metastatic settings. Although nearly 85% of GISTs are amenable to complete R0/R1 resection, almost 50% will recur. Particularly among patients with high-risk GIST, adjuvant imatinib therapy has been shown to improve both RFS and OS. The total duration of treatment is still undefined. Current standard of care in the adjuvant setting for patients with high-risk tumors is 3 years of therapy rather than only 1 year of therapy. This was shown in the Scandinavian-German trial to improve both 5-year RFS (65.6% for 3-year treatment vs. 47.9% for 1-year treatment, $P < .001$) and OS (92.0% vs. 81.7%, $P = .02$).[15] More recent studies have investigated the efficacy and safety of 5 years of adjuvant imatinib. The PERSIST-5 trial included 91 patients with intermediate- or high-risk GIST who underwent resection followed by adjuvant imatinib 400 mg/d for 5 years or until progression. The primary endpoint of this study was RFS. Although only one-half of the patients completed the 5 years of treatment, the estimated 5-year RFS was 90%, suggesting that a longer duration of adjuvant therapy might provide a durable benefit.[16] The Scandinavian Sarcoma Group is accruing patients for a multi-institutional phase 3 trial with a goal to randomize 300 patients to either 3 or 5 years of adjuvant imatinib. The primary endpoint of this study will be 5-year RFS (https://clinicaltrials.gov: NCT02413736). The anticipated study completion date is 2028.

Imatinib should be administered preoperatively for patients with large, borderline-resectable GIST, in whom up-front surgical resection to try to achieve negative margins would result in significant morbidity (such as a multivisceral resection or abdominoperineal resection). Although data guiding the appropriate timing and duration of preoperative treatment are limited, the median time to maximal response is typically 28 weeks, and response plateaus at approximately 34 weeks. Treatment beyond this time frame might not be beneficial.[17] Therefore, up to 6 months of therapy should be administered prior to considering surgical resection, with close monitoring to assess the ongoing treatment response and time to plateau.

PERIOPERATIVE CARE
Preoperative Clinical and Imaging Evaluation
Initial evaluation of a patient with newly diagnosed soft tissue mass in the trunk or extremity includes history focused on understanding its rate of growth and eliciting a history of prior trauma, which may provide information regarding risk of malignancy. Neurogenic pain is a worrisome feature. When diagnosed in the abdomen or retroperitoneum, special attention is paid to identifying patients in whom the tumor has affected appetite, resulting in nutritional compromise. Physical examination focuses

on identifying neurovascular involvement that may necessitate resection of vital structures leading to long-term impairment (e.g., femoral nerve, artery, or vein). Care should be taken to discern whether tumors are fixed to underlying structures that may need to be resected with a tumor and to identify skin changes. Arterial resections may require reconstruction by a vascular consultant, and wide resections leading to large areas of "dead space" or inability to close skin primarily often necessitate involvement by reconstructive surgery colleagues.

Preoperative workup includes cross-sectional imaging of any suspected soft tissue sarcoma. For tumors of the abdomen and retroperitoneum (including GIST), a computed tomography (CT) scan will allow for assessment of the tumor and its relationship to adjacent organs and may suggest histology (e.g., a large lipomatous lesion with septae and nodular components can be consistent with well-differentiated liposarcoma). For tumors of the extremity and trunk, magnetic resonance imaging (MRI) with and without gadolinium contrast is ideal in that it can demonstrate detailed anatomy for surgical planning and provide insight into the histologic subtype of the tumor. Lipomatous components are easily identified on T1 sequences, whereas hyperintense signals on T2 series suggest myxoid lesions. MRI can also be helpful in determining the extent of infiltrative lesions (e.g., enhancing tails extending from the dominant mass in myxofibrosarcoma).

Staging scans are generally focused on assessment of the lungs. In most instances, staging should include a CT scan of the chest, but in a subset of patients such as those with low-grade disease or a small tumor, a chest radiograph is a reasonable alternative. Dedicated imaging of the abdomen and pelvis may be appropriate for specific histologies such as myxoid/round cell liposarcoma; spinal MRI can also detect isolated metastases in high-risk tumors of this histology.

Biopsy

As soft tissue sarcomas are rare (less than 1% of cancer in adults), an accurate diagnosis can be challenging, often owing to a lack of experience with this entity by most pathologists. Percutaneous core biopsy is the preferred method to make a pathologic diagnosis and should be performed with minimal adjacent tissue contamination for extremity/trunk and retroperitoneal sarcomas. In general, sampling should be obtained from an area of the tumor that appears solid or dedifferentiated. Necrotic, cystic, or areas of benign-appearing fat are likely of low histologic yield. Percutaneous sampling with image guidance and a coaxial sheath is safe and efficacious, but coordination between the interventional radiologist and surgeon is required to minimize the risk of peritoneal tumor seeding and to minimize adjacent tissue contamination.

The biopsy pathology report should provide the precise diagnosis of the specific sarcoma subtype and the grade of the tumor. Owing to the potential morphologic overlap between sarcomas and benign mesenchymal neoplasms, as well as other malignancies (poorly differentiated carcinomas, melanoma), additional diagnostic tools such as immunohistochemistry and molecular diagnostic approaches can aid in making an accurate initial diagnosis and in subtype classification. Pathognomonic chromosomal translocations, gene amplifications, and mutations can be detected via cytogenetic analyses or next-generation sequencing and are of particular help in confirming histology. The World Health Organization classification system sets the standard for diagnostic terminology and definitions.[18] This diagnostic complexity further reinforces the value of sarcoma care at large-volume centers with sarcoma-specific multidisciplinary care teams (surgical oncology, orthopedic oncology, medical oncology, radiation therapy, pathology, radiology, nursing, and other supportive care).

For GIST, diagnosis should be achieved via endoscopic biopsy with a combination of histopathologic analysis and immunohistochemistry. Percutaneous biopsy is not used for localized disease given the risk of peritoneal seeding but may be used to confirm metastatic disease or when endoscopic biopsy is not feasible and preoperative systemic therapy for locally advanced GIST is being considered. Microscopically, GISTs are often described as spindle cell tumors (70%), with a smaller proportion being either epithelioid (20%) or mixed type (10%).[19] In 95% of cases, GISTs can be differentiated from histologically similar tumors by the expression of the antigens CD117 and DOG-1, which are tested on all tumors suspected as GIST. GISTs can be divided into high- and low-risk subtypes based on their size (>5 vs. <2 cm), tumor location (duodenum or rectum versus stomach), mitotic rate (>5 mitoses per high-power fields), presence of tumor rupture, and mutation status (i.e., deletion of KIT in exon 9).[20]

Postoperative Care and Follow-up

Early referral and incorporation of physical therapy and occupational therapy are critical to maintaining function after treatment of soft tissue sarcoma. Surveillance strategies including physical examination and cross-sectional imaging of the primary site (MRI for extremity/trunk sarcoma, CT of the abdomen and pelvis for retroperitoneal sarcoma and GIST) as well as CT of the chest to evaluate for metastatic disease are recommended every 3 to 6 months for 2 years, every 6 months until year 5, and then annually. Interval of follow-up should reflect overall risk of recurrence; patients with high-grade disease would generally be followed more closely (every 3 to 4 months over the first 2 years), and those with low-grade disease imaged every 6 months. Chest radiograph in lieu of CT may be appropriate for metastatic surveillance in a subset of patients with low-grade tumors and indolent histologies, whereas for particular histologies with higher rates of liver (e.g., leiomyosarcoma), soft tissue (e.g., myxoid/round cell liposarcoma), or bony metastases (e.g., pleomorphic liposarcoma), intermittent staging abdominal, and pelvis CT or bone scan may be appropriate.

QUALITY MEASURES

No quality metrics currently exist for soft tissue sarcoma from the Commission on Cancer.

CHAPTER 1

Resection of Extremity and Trunk Soft Tissue Sarcoma

CRITICAL ELEMENTS

- Pretreatment Biopsy of Soft Tissue Masses of the Extremity and Trunk
- Macroscopically Complete Resection of the Primary Tumor
- Placement of Surgical Drains

1. PRETREATMENT BIOPSY OF SOFT TISSUE MASSES OF THE EXTREMITY AND TRUNK

Recommendation: Pathologic subtyping of soft tissue masses suspicious for sarcoma of the extremity and trunk should be performed to facilitate planning of appropriate multimodality therapy. Histologic sampling of the tumor should generally be obtained via core needle biopsy, but an incisional biopsy should be obtained if adequate tissue cannot be acquired safely in this manner. The biopsy tract and incision should be oriented so that the entire tract (including scar, if applicable) can be excised en bloc with the tumor at the time of definitive resection.

Type of Data: Retrospective reports, case series, or case-control studies

Strength of Recommendation: Strong recommendation, moderate-quality evidence

Rationale

Tumors of the soft tissue are common, and the differential diagnosis is broad. Only a small fraction of these masses are soft tissue sarcomas, but this diagnosis must be considered prior to surgical excision of any soft tissue mass. Compared with benign lesions, soft tissue sarcomas of the extremities and trunk tend to be greater than 5 cm and located beneath the muscular fascia.[21] Definitive diagnosis requires biopsy, which is a mandatory step in the management of these malignancies. In addition to alleviating patient uncertainty and anxiety, pathologic subtyping allows for accurate staging and disease prognostication.[22] Pathologic subtype also determines, in part, the utility of adjuvant chemotherapy and radiation treatment and the appropriate extent of surgery. Excision in the absence of preoperative diagnosis may, therefore, lead to delay of appropriate delivery of multimodality therapy or may complicate definitive surgical resection.

Ideally, biopsy of suspected soft tissue sarcomas should be performed at a specialized sarcoma center and in coordination with the operating surgeon. Improper technique and poor placement may not only lead to an incorrect histologic diagnosis but may also alter the subsequent surgical plan. Studies in both the United States and Europe have shown that biopsies performed at low-volume sarcoma centers can be associated with a 20% to 40% rate of inappropriate histologic classification, and in up to 35% of cases, expert re-review of these samples led to alteration of the treatment plan.[23,24]

Biopsy of the suspected malignancy should generally be performed via percutaneous core needle biopsy. Tumors either not accessible via core needle biopsy or those that have been sampled but yielded inconclusive results may require an incisional approach. The advantages of a core needle biopsy are decreased patient morbidity, low cost, and the relative ease with which the biopsy can be performed. Palpable lesions can often be sampled in clinic, which may lead to faster diagnosis. Practitioners facile with ultrasound may use this imaging modality in their office to help target small, heterogeneous lesions or increase the accuracy of their biopsy technique.[25] In recent years, core needle biopsy has been shown to be equivalent in both sampling and ultimate diagnostic accuracy to an open or incisional biopsy technique, assuming adequate tissue can be obtained.[26,27] When a lesion is not palpable, when it is located near important neurovascular structures, or when it is heterogeneous in appearance, image guidance with either ultrasound, computed tomography, or magnetic resonance imaging may prove useful to enhance both accuracy and yield.[25,28] Image-guided biopsies should be directed to sample enhancing, solid components of the lesion.

Regardless of the biopsy method used, careful consideration must be given to the placement and orientation of the biopsy tract and incision. Owing to the implantation potential of soft tissue sarcomas and the necessity of violating the tumor capsule to complete any biopsy, resection of any previous tract (open or percutaneous core needle) en bloc with the wide resection specimen is mandatory. Otherwise, contamination of the biopsy site with microscopic tumor can theoretically increase the risk of local recurrence. This is a unique aspect of soft tissue sarcoma management that differs from requirements for adequate surgical treatment of most other cancers. Precise planning of the pretreatment biopsy is thus critically important to minimize potential tumor seeding of the biopsy scar and uninvolved muscular compartments. Specifically, the percutaneous puncture site and needle tract or incision should be placed in an area that will later be included in the surgical specimen or radiation field to mitigate the chance of local recurrence due to untreated tumor cells in the seeded tract. Incisional biopsies should be oriented longitudinally on the limbs. Once the appropriate location for biopsy has been determined, the goal is to minimize contamination of the tissues located between the biopsy site and the sarcoma. Ideally, the trajectory of the biopsy should not traverse muscular compartments that are not already involved by tumor.

Technical Aspects

When planning a percutaneous core needle biopsy under image guidance, there must be close coordination between the treating surgeon and the radiologist performing the biopsy. It should be emphasized to the radiologist that the biopsy tract should not traverse

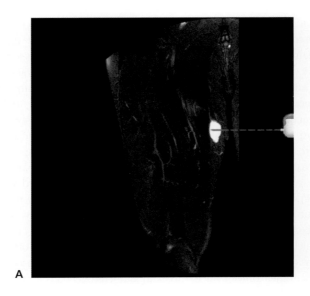

A

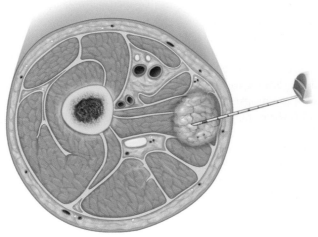

B

FIGURE 1-1   Core needle biopsy of a thigh sarcoma. Suspicious lesions should be biopsied to obtain a histologic diagnosis prior to initiating treatment or proceeding to the operating room. **A:** A core needle biopsy is advantageous as it can be performed in clinic, confers minimal morbidity, and yields sufficient tissue for a diagnosis.

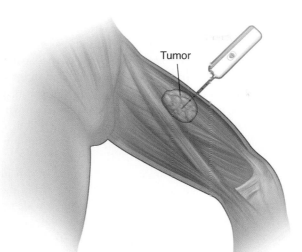

C

FIGURE 1-1 *(continued)* **B,C:** The biopsy tract should be or ented such that major neurovascular structures are avoided and so that the tract can be excised with the specimen. Use of imaging is encouraged so that the most suspicious/solid portion of the tumor is targeted.

uninvolved muscular compartments that would not be resected in any subsequent definitive surgical procedure. The location of the biopsy at the level of the skin should also be chosen to easily incorporate the biopsy tract into any future wide resection incision (Fig. 1-1).

For an open biopsy, flaps should not be created. Meticulous hemostasis is critical to minimize post-biopsy hematoma and the potential for tumor seeding.

2. MACROSCOPICALLY COMPLETE RESECTION OF THE PRIMARY TUMOR

Recommendation

- The tumor should be resected en bloc with the entire biopsy tract to microscopically negative (R0) surgical margins. A circumferential 1- to 2-cm margin of grossly normal tissue should generally be resected to maximize the likelihood of an R0 resection. A narrower margin may be justified to preserve critical neurovascular structures, tendons, or bones that are adjacent to the tumor and that contribute significantly to limb function.
- Immediate histopathologic analysis (frozen section) should not be relied on to assess margin status intraoperatively as the differentiation between benign and malignant mesenchymal tissues is highly unreliable using currently available techniques. Further, specimen manipulation may increase the risk of tumor seeding.

Type of Data: Retrospective reports, case series, or case-control studies

Strength of Recommendation: Strong recommendation, moderate-quality evidence

Rationale

Soft tissue sarcoma may occur in three distinct anatomic locations within an extremity: the skin or subcutaneous fat, the muscle or muscle fascia, or the intermuscular tissue deep to the investing fascia. In many cases, and particularly when tumors are large or deep, the mass will be adjacent to a structure important to limb function. Limb-salvage surgery should be the primary consideration for all patients with extremity and trunk sarcoma as randomized clinical trials have shown that routine amputation does not improve overall survival.[29] However, when limb salvage cannot be safely performed in a manner in which function is preserved, amputation may be more appropriate.

In developing a surgical plan, the surgeon must critically consider the anatomic presentation of the sarcoma. For superficial tumors that lie within the skin and subcutaneous fat, few critical structures are generally at risk, and a wide resection including a layer of normal tissue may be possible with little functional consequence. For large and deep soft tissue sarcomas, the tumor mass is more likely to approximate bone, neurovascular structures, or tendon, and a wide resection may not be possible without sacrifice of these critical structures.

As detailed below, management of certain histologic subtypes warrants special consideration: atypical lipomatous tumors/well-differentiated liposarcomas (ALTs), extra-abdominal desmoid tumors, dermatofibrosarcoma protuberans (DFSP), myxofibrosarcoma, and breast angiosarcomas (usually secondary to prior radiation treatment) all demonstrate unique biologic or pathologic properties that may also influence surgical decision-making.

En bloc resection of the biopsy tract

At the time of definitive surgery, the proposed wide resection incision should be designed in a way to incorporate the prior biopsy site within a fusiform ellipse. For superficial tumors confined to the skin and subcutaneous tissue, resection of the biopsy tract is typically straightforward. For deeper sarcomas, the portion of the musculature traversed with an incisional biopsy should also be resected en bloc with the underlying tumor as there is risk of tumor seeding in the tract. For tumors biopsied using a percutaneous core needle, identification of the specific trajectory of the tract through deeper soft tissues overlying the sarcoma can be technically challenging. Planning for en bloc resection of the biopsy tract requires careful assessment of imaging studies used for disease staging as well as the specific radiographic studies performed during the biopsy procedure.

Although every effort should be made to resect percutaneous core needle biopsy tracts at the time of a wide resection for sarcoma, the impact of this recommendation on local recurrence is inconclusive because the number of events in available retrospective studies is small. For example, in a series of 221 soft tissue and bone sarcomas, pathologic assessment of the biopsy tracts showed that 32% of open biopsy tracts, but only 0.8% of percutaneous core needle biopsy tracts had tumor seeding.[30] Whereas almost none of the percutaneous core needle biopsy tracts were seeded with tumor, local recurrence-free survival was much shorter for patients with biopsy tract contamination as compared with those without biopsy-site tumor seeding (mean, 11 vs. 107 months, $P < .001$). Another small retrospective study compared 36 patients who did not have their core needle biopsy tract resected with 36 patients who underwent tract resection, matching the patients for risk factors associated with local recurrence.[31] The 5-year local recurrence rates were similar: 6% in the resected group versus 8% in the nonresected group ($P = .643$).

Surgical margins

The primary goal of sarcoma surgery is to resect the tumor to microscopically negative (R0) margins. A circumferential 1- to 2-cm margin of grossly normal tissue should generally be resected to minimize the risk of a microscopically positive (R1) margin on final pathologic review.[32,33] However, resection should be tailored to minimize long-term morbidity, and narrower margins may be acceptable if resection to a wider gross margin would result in significant morbidity (Fig. 1-2).[34] If any margin is positive on final pathologic analysis (other than at bone, nerve, or major blood vessels), surgical re-resection should be strongly considered if it will not have a significant impact on functionality.

Importantly, the muscle fascia of an intramuscular sarcoma is considered an oncologic barrier and, when intact, can decrease the amount of normal tissue required to achieve a curative margin. Use of this barrier as part of the resection margin can mitigate the need to remove 1 to 2 cm of normal tissue circumferentially around the tumor and can thereby preserve function by maintaining important regional structures. This approach has been shown to achieve an acceptable rate of local control.[35]

Intraoperative frozen section

Although the overall goal of sarcoma wide resection is to obtain microscopically negative (R0) surgical margins, the role of intraoperative frozen section assessment of resection margins is limited. This is primarily owing to the high implantation potential of a soft tissue sarcoma and the possibility that intraoperative violation of the sarcoma may occur during processing of the margins, which may lead to contamination of the entire wide resection field.

Furthermore, there are technical limitations to frozen section, especially in the setting of neoadjuvant chemotherapy or radiation therapy. It is difficult to freeze fat, which would be the margin in question for a superficial sarcoma and some deeper intracompartmental tumors. It is also not possible to accurately differentiate normal adipose tissue from an ALT on frozen section. Finally, the inability to rapidly perform adjunctive stains on intraoperative frozen section can make it difficult to discern certain sarcoma histologies from posttreatment/inflammatory changes or even non-neoplastic fibroblasts with reactive changes.

Considering the above issues, intraoperative frozen section should not be relied on to assess or minimize margins. However, a pathologist who is experienced in musculoskeletal tumors should evaluate all surgical specimens to differentiate sarcoma from treatment effect or scar and to ensure proper diagnosis using the World Health Organization classification system on permanent sections.[18]

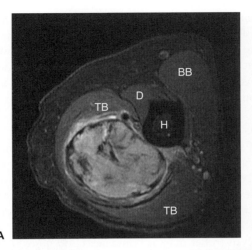

A

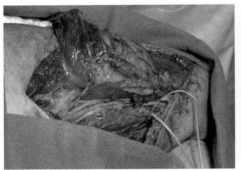

B

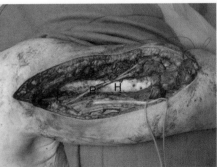

C

FIGURE 1-2   **A:** Axial image of a high-grade sarcoma located within the triceps brachii of the upper arm abutting the neurovascular bundle. BB: biceps brachii; D: deltoid; H: humerus; TB: triceps brachii. **B:** Intraoperative image of wide resection of the tumor in **A**. The tumor has been resected with a circumferential margin of normal muscle (triceps brachii). The tumor is abutting the neurovascular bundle, which has been preserved as the deep margin. **C:** Intraoperative image after wide resection of the intramuscular sarcoma. Complete resection of the tumor required en bloc removal of the triceps brachii. The neurovascular structures were preserved, and the epineural margins are seen in this image. The deep margin included the periosteum of the humerus (H). R: radial nerve.

Technical Aspects

Management of neurovascular bundles

Sarcomas generally grow in a centripetal manner, pushing aside soft tissue as they grow. They generally do not engulf surrounding structures and, instead, push neurovascular bundles aside. Tumor growth in this manner results in neurovascular bundles juxtaposed to the sarcoma and not within the sarcoma. The epineurium of critical nerves can, therefore, typically be opened, and the nerve can then be lifted away from the tumor. A similar technique can be used to free critical blood vessels from a tumor: arteriolysis will lift an artery or vascular bundle off the sarcoma and allow it to be preserved.

Because the artery and vein are often intimately associated, arteriolysis often frees the vein as well. Although resection to 1- to 2-cm gross margins is generally recommended, the delivery of adjuvant therapy (radiation and/or chemotherapy) has allowed this type of limited resection to be performed to minimize morbidity of surgery without compromising oncologic outcome.[33,34]

When the neurovascular bundle is encased in a low-grade sarcoma, bivalving the tumor to preserve major nerves and arteries may be considered if a substantial functional benefit can be anticipated. The indolent nature of low-grade lesions minimizes the risk that such a procedure would substantively increase risk of death from disease. However, this technique should be avoided in patients with an intermediate- or high-grade sarcoma. When the neurovascular bundle is encased as opposed to displaced by a high-grade tumor, sacrifice of vascular structures (often with associated nerve) is required to achieve a negative margin.

Arterial resections may mandate reconstruction, but reconstruction of veins is typically unnecessary. Although reconstruction of nerves can be performed, whether this results in return of function depends on the length of nerve resected, age of the individual, and previous adjuvant therapy. Tendon transfer and dynamic bracing can help combat the functional disability that results after nerve resection. Specific braces (ankle foot orthoses, dynamic extension splint, etc.) and specific tendon transfers will vary depending on the nerve and level that is resected.

Management of bone and tendons

It is rare for a soft tissue sarcoma to invade into bone and tendon, but tumor abutment is common. In such instances, a complete tumor resection with retention of these structures is possible and generally recommended.

In order to obtain an adequate deep margin, the periosteum of adjacent bone should be lifted with the excised tumor. This technique is performed with electrocautery and a periosteal elevator, with particular attention given to any tissue that appears to be adherent to the underlying bone (Fig. 1-2). The structure analogous to the periosteum of bone is the peritenon of tendon. This is a thin protective layer directly overlying the tendinous fibers, and it should be removed with adjacent tumor as a deep layer. If the tissue is not lifting easily or there is clear evidence of invasion into tendon or bone, then the affected tissue must be removed as part of the plan for complete en bloc resection of the mass (e.g., a partial cortical resection of bone or tendon resection).

Reconstruction of resected tissues should be considered if needed to prevent significant functional deficit or complications. The major long bones of the extremities—the femur, tibia, and humerus—invariably will require a reconstruction if excised, as the ultimate function of the limb will be compromised if not addressed. Similarly, when a bone that contributes to a major joint is removed, such as the shoulder, elbow, wrist, hip, knee, or ankle, reconstruction is necessary. "Expendable" bones in the extremities are those that are not critical to limb function, such as the clavicle, proximal and midshaft fibula, proximal radius, and distal ulna. Often, these bones may be removed without substantial consequence.

Tendons also vary in their functional importance. In the upper extremity, the rotator cuff and triceps insertion at the elbow are the most important. In the lower extremity, the abductor insertion on the greater trochanter of the femur, the quadriceps tendon and patellar tendon about the knee, and the Achilles tendon at the ankle are the most critical. Lesser tendons, such as the extensors about the wrist and ankle, the psoas tendon at the hip, the biceps tendon at the elbow, and the hamstring tendons at the knee, can often be removed with little consequence owing to anatomic redundancy. Similar to bone resection, if a critical tendon must be removed for optimal oncologic control, reconstruction with a rotational flap, free flap, or allograft should be considered in some instances to restore the sacrificed function.

Clip placement for postoperative radiation planning

Adjuvant radiotherapy plays an important role in treating patients with high-grade tumors, tumors at high risk of margin-positive resection owing to their abutment of critical anatomic structures, and tumors that are recurrent. Patients anticipated to undergo adjuvant radiotherapy should have metal clips placed in the surgical bed once the specimen has been passed off to pathology for analysis. Markers should be positioned around the perimeter of the resection cavity, as well as one placed at the center of the surgical bed, to aid in treatment planning and reproducible positioning and immobilization when the treatment is delivered in multiple fractions (Fig. 1-3). In addition, areas where gross tumor may remain or where surgical margins are close should be noted and marked with surgical clips.[36]

Indications for amputation

Limb-salvage surgery should be the primary consideration for extremity sarcomas. General indications for amputation include encasement of major neural or vascular structures, resection of which would defunctionalize the limb, and palliation for patients with metastatic/recurrent tumors that are fungating, infected, bleeding, or associated with uncontrolled pain.[37]

For sarcomas of the upper extremity, encasement of the major vascular structures; involvement of the brachial plexus; a resection that would require sacrifice of the median, radial, and ulnar nerves; or extensive soft-tissue or joint contamination are often indications for amputation.

For pelvic girdle sarcomas, the femoral neurovascular bundle, hip joint, and sciatic nerve should be carefully evaluated. If two of these three structures are involved by tumor, an external hemipelvectomy should be carefully considered. In addition, an external hemipelvectomy can be considered for soft tissue sarcomas involving multiple compartments of the proximal thigh or local recurrence of a proximal thigh or buttock tumor involving critical structures.

Indications for above-knee amputation include encasement of the popliteal vessel over a long segment and involvement of the tibial and peroneal nerve or extensive soft-tissue contamination in the setting of an inadvertent excision/biopsy. In addition, resections that would leave the foot and ankle nonfunctional are indications for a below-knee amputation.

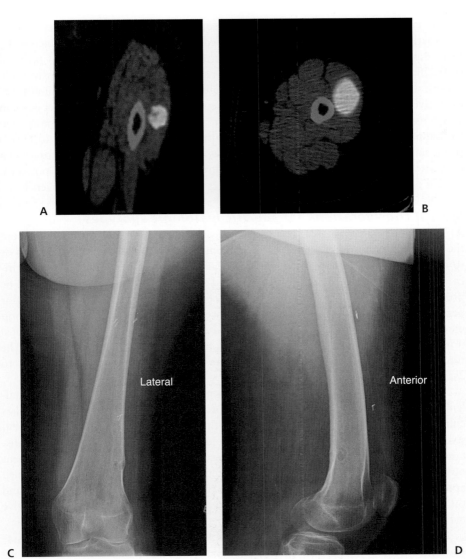

FIGURE 1-3   A,B: PET images of left thigh sarcoma. **C,D:** Postoperative radiograph demonstrating visualization of clips placed around the perimeter of the resection cavity to help the radiation oncologist target the critical areas.

Soft tissue reconstruction

The resection of large, deep sarcomas often creates a soft-tissue defect in which primary closure requires soft tissue reconstruction to prevent significant infection or wound breakdown. This may be particularly true if neoadjuvant radiation is delivered. Types of reconstruction including simple skin grafting for superficial wounds or muscle, temporary wound dressings embedded with growth factors or extracellular matrix components, or vacuum-assisted closure devices may be used to encourage granulation for delayed coverage over radiated fields or tendons. Myocutaneous defects, especially those that expose vascular structures, necessitate the use of pedicled or free flaps for limb salvage. Preoperative consultation for immediate reconstruction is critical for reconstructive planning and evaluation of patient factors to limit postoperative complications.[38] Delayed reconstruction may be indicated in select cases in which margin clearance is of concern. Vacuum-assisted closure therapy can be applied for temporary closure in select cases until pathologic evaluation is complete. This is particularly relevant for infiltrative histologies such as DFSP and myxofibrosarcoma or recurrent sarcomas. In these cases, delayed reconstruction may optimize long-term patient outcomes because margin status affects long-term risk of local recurrence.

Special considerations for specific histologic subtypes

ALTs are often encapsulated, but it may be difficult to discriminate the ALT from the surrounding normal tissue. It is not uncommon for these tumors to adhere to or to encase major neurovascular bundles. Because these tumors are low grade, critical nerves and arteries should not be resected with the tumor but instead should be preserved. Occasionally, the tumor must be bivalved in order to preserve a major peripheral nerve. For patients with ALT, observation versus re-resection is recommended for focally positive margins. When a dedifferentiated component develops, it is important to ensure the complete resection of this higher-grade component. The tumor should be resected in a manner similar to other soft tissue sarcomas to 1- to 2-cm gross margins.

Treatment of desmoid tumors of the abdominal wall and extremity/trunk is challenging and frustrating for both patients and providers. Their infiltrative nature makes complete surgical resection challenging, and their "benign" nature makes the extensive and debilitating procedures required for local control of no consequence to distant oncologic control. Currently, surgical resection is best viewed as a subsequent option rather than an initial treatment strategy. When surgical excision is deemed appropriate, the surgeon should be aware of the infiltrative nature of the lesion and the high likelihood of local recurrence even with an extensive resection to negative margins.

DFSP have a high rate of local recurrence but virtually no capacity for metastasis. However, complete excision may be challenging as this tumor can be highly infiltrative along fibrous septae. Tumor can therefore extend beyond the main mass, and occult tumor may lie outside the planned surgical field. In cosmetically sensitive areas in which tissue conservation is critical, Mohs micrographic surgery can be used to ensure clear margins.[39] At all other surgical sites, traditional resection is preferred, and well-planned surgical procedures can also be used within cosmetically sensitive areas. Sometimes, staged procedures are performed in which clear margins can be ensured by pathology with delay of the definitive closure of the surgical site. This requires a careful and coordinated choreography between surgeon and pathologist to ensure an appropriately rapid conclusion to the purposely delayed procedure.

Fibrosarcomatous transformation (fibrosarcomatous-DFSP) can occur, particularly in larger tumors, and represents morphologic progression to a higher-grade component. Importantly, fibrosarcomatous-DFSP tumors have an increased propensity for local recurrence, but more importantly, the metastatic risk becomes around 15%. DFSP with fibrosarcomatous transformation are considered high-grade soft tissue sarcomas and are treated similar to other high-grade tumors with wide resection and multimodality treatment.

Myxofibrosarcoma is a relatively hypocellular sarcoma that is most commonly low grade but has a multilobular appearance and extensive myxoid deposition. Microscopically positive margins and local recurrence are extremely common and predictable after incomplete removal.[40] These tumors can also be infiltrative along fibrous septae and can extend outside the planned field of surgical resection, especially when these tumors (and the likely related undifferentiated pleomorphic sarcoma) involve more superficial tissues.[41] Often, extension of the tumor focally to the surgical margins is only identified on subsequent permanent analysis of the specimen in which sampling can be much more extensive and histologic detail is more optimal.

Breast sarcomas are a rare group of tumors, among which angiosarcoma is one of the most common histologic subtypes. Breast angiosarcoma can arise from the breast parenchyma (primary angiosarcoma) or from the skin of the breast (secondary angiosarcoma). Distinction of these entities is critical as it guides the treatment approach based on the underlying tumor biology.

Primary angiosarcoma arises from the breast parenchyma and is typically seen in a younger population than conventional breast cancer (women aged 30 to 50 years). The standard surgical approach is a wide resection planned to obtain microscopically negative (R0) margins. In some cases, this may necessitate mastectomy and en bloc resection of skin or pectoralis muscle. Axillary lymph node surgery is not routinely indicated owing to the low risk of lymph node involvement. However, a limited lymphadenectomy should be considered if clinically or radiologically worrisome disease is present.

Secondary angiosarcoma arises from the dermis and subcutis and can develop in the setting of prior external beam radiation or chronic lymphedema (Stewart-Treves syndrome). Although rare, radiation-associated breast angiosarcoma will often present in patients with a history of breast carcinoma who underwent breast-conserving surgery and external beam radiation. These tumors can demonstrate an aggressive tumor biology and multifocality and, as a result, often require an extensive resection. A radical approach to surgical management involving a mastectomy including all skin within the radiation field has been shown to be associated with improved local-recurrence rates and disease-specific survival when compared with more conservative approaches (Fig. 1-4).[42] The radiation field is typically bounded by the clavicle cranially, rectus fascia caudally, lateral sternal border medially, and latissimus dorsi laterally. En bloc resection of pectoralis major may be required to obtain negative margins. Despite complete excision, recurrence is common in these tumors. Collaboration with plastic surgery to facilitate wound closure is paramount in order to optimize wound outcomes.

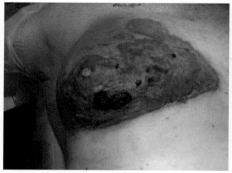
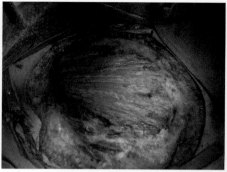

A

B

FIGURE 1-4 Management of cutaneous angiosarcoma. **A:** Intraoperative photograph of a breast angiosarcoma. **B:** Wide resection of these tumors may require mastectomy, resection of involved or overlying skin, and sometimes resection of pectoralis muscle. If the tumor is a result of prior external beam radiation, all skin and soft tissue included in the radiation field should be removed to reduce the chances of local recurrence.

3. PLACEMENT OF SURGICAL DRAINS

Recommendation: Surgical drains are placed to prevent fluid accumulation in the operative bed. Drains should be used judiciously, and their entry sites should be placed as close to the incision as is feasible. This allows the percutaneous site to be included in the radiation field and excised en bloc with the specimen should reexcision be necessary or should the tumor recur.

Type of Data: Retrospective reports, case series, or case-control studies

Strength of Recommendation: Strong recommendation, high-quality evidence

Rationale

Closed suction drains are often required to prevent hematoma and seroma formation following extremity sarcoma resection. Theoretically, tumor cells may be seeded along the drain tract. As such, an ideal drain exit site allows for easy incorporation of the tract into the radiation field plan or en bloc surgical re-resection plan if needed.

Technical Aspects

The placement of surgical drains must be strategically considered. The drains should be placed in such way that minimizes soft tissue contamination beyond the resection bed.[4] In general, drains should be oriented directly in line with the incision and within 1 to 2 cm of the incision (Fig. 1-5). Drain sites at the distal end of the incision are preferred to allow for dependent drainage. However, proximal versus distal placement is dependent on a variety of factors, including proximity of critical structures such as blood vessels and nerves, integrity of overlying soft tissue, ease of management by the patient, or avoidance of additional compartmental extension such as may occur near a joint.

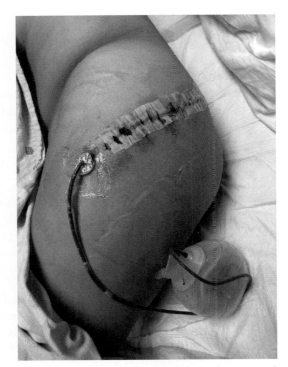

FIGURE 1-5 Representative photograph of surgical drain placement after resection of a left thigh sarcoma. Surgical drains should be used judiciously but may be helpful in cases in which the patient is at high risk of fluid accumulation after tumor resection because of large-volume residual dead space.

Sarcoma Key Question 1

In patients with clinically node-negative extremity or trunk sarcoma, does sentinel lymph node biopsy (SLNB) with or without completion lymph node dissection improve disease-free survival or overall survival (OS) compared with no SLNB?

INTRODUCTION

Metastasis of soft tissue sarcoma to regional lymph nodes is an infrequent event. The infrequency with which it is clinically observed makes investigations of the natural history and management of lymph node metastasis challenging.[43] To date, most published data that attempt to describe the incidence, impact, and treatment of regional lymph node metastasis from soft tissue sarcoma have been generated from small, retrospective, and often single-center series[43-66] or population database–based studies.[67-71]

Overall, rates of regional lymph node metastasis are 2.6% to 3.5% for patients with extremity and trunk sarcoma, with a significant proportion of patients having synchronous distant metastatic disease.[43,67] However, certain subtypes of sarcomas do have a propensity for lymphatic metastasis: rhabdomyosarcoma (incidence of 13.6%), epithelioid sarcoma (13% to 16.7%), clear cell sarcoma (16%), and vascular sarcomas (lymphangiosarcoma, angiosarcoma; 6% to 13.5%).[72-74]

The identification of regional lymph node metastasis has important staging and prognostic significance, as the presence of metastasis in lymph nodes is associated with significantly shorter survival. Indeed, nodal metastasis is classified as stage IV disease in the eighth edition of the American Joint Committee on Cancer (AJCC) staging system of truncal and extremity soft tissue sarcoma.[67,75] However, the precise association between lymphatic metastasis and survival remains controversial, and perhaps as a reflection of this, tumors with regional lymph node metastasis have been classified as both stage III and stage IV in past editions of the *AJCC Cancer Staging Manual*.[1,76] Regardless, some data do suggest that resection of isolated regional nodal disease is associated with favorable oncologic outcomes. Therefore, the clinical identification of metastatic nodes may have important surgical implications.

Although SLNB has clear proven prognostic (and possibly therapeutic) value in regional nodal staging in patients with melanoma and breast cancer, whether this procedure offers benefit for patients with soft tissue sarcoma remains poorly understood. The purpose of this work was to evaluate whether SLNB with or without completion lymph node dissection improves disease-free survival or OS of patients with clinically node-negative extremity or trunk sarcoma, compared with no SLNB.

METHODOLOGY

A systematic search of Ovid MEDLINE, Ovid Embase, Cochrane Library, Web of Science, and Scopus from January 1, 1989, to August 6, 2019, was performed. Search structures, subject headings, and keywords were tailored to each database by a medical research librarian who specializes in systematic reviews. Medical Subject Headings (MeSH) terms included "Sarcoma" and "Sentinel Lymph Node Biopsy." Title, abstract, and keyword fields were searched with a variety of search terms identifying soft tissue sarcoma and SLNB. Searches were restricted to English language and human subjects. Case reports were excluded. Multiple gray literature resources were searched for conferences, dissertations, reports, and other unpublished studies for additional relevant citations. The references of the included articles as well as later publications citing the included articles were searched. Findings are reported in accordance with the Preferred Reporting Items for Systematic Reviews and Meta-Analyses (PRISMA).[77]

The initial search yielded 569 publications (Fig. 1-6). After duplicates were removed, 311 abstracts were reviewed in detail, of which 233 were excluded because

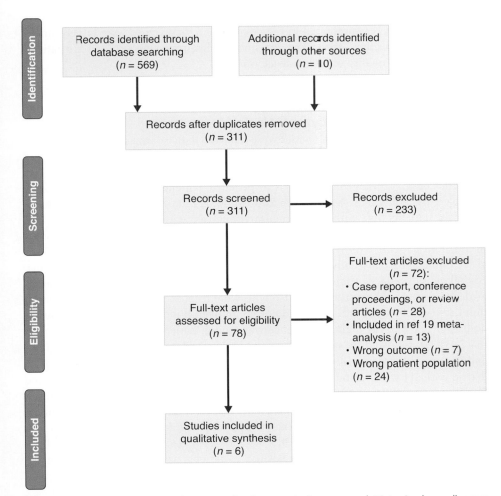

FIGURE 1-6 Preferred Reporting Items for Systematic Reviews and Meta-Analyses diagram for literature regarding use of sentinel lymph node biopsy in patients with extremity/truncal soft tissue sarcoma.

they did not address the clinical question of interest. Studies that passed the title/abstract review were retrieved for full-text review. Of these 78 studies, 72 were excluded because they were small series, already included in the meta-analysis, or included the wrong outcome or patient population. Six studies met all the criteria for inclusion in this systematic review.[55,58–61,69] Disagreements were resolved by consensus and by seeking the opinion of a third reviewer.

Data were extracted from individual studies independently by a single investigator. Each article was reviewed and assigned a quality of evidence based on the Grading of Recommendations, Assessment, Development, and Evaluation (GRADE) system.[78] The quality of the data and size of the studies precluded the ability to perform a meta-analysis.

Six studies were included in the qualitative systematic review (Table 1-5). Of these six full-text articles, there was one meta-analysis, one national registry database study, and four retrospective cohort studies. Fourteen studies of SLNB published between 2000 and 2010 were represented in the systematic review; these were largely single-institution retrospective case reports or small series, reporting on 1 to 29 patients each. Overall, the quality of the evidence was low.

FINDINGS

Incidence of Regional Lymph Node Metastasis

Rates of positive sentinel lymph nodes were reported in five of the six included studies, ranged from 4.3% to 50%, and varied across soft tissue sarcoma histologic subtypes (Table 1-6).

Alcorn et al.[55] reviewed the records of pediatric patients with soft tissue sarcoma who were treated with SLNB between 2000 and 2011 at one institution. They identified eight patients (five with rhabdomyosarcoma, two with epithelioid sarcoma, and one with synovial sarcoma) and reported an overall incidence of lymphatic metastasis of 25%; all patients with lymphatic metastasis had rhabdomyosarcoma. Andreou et al.[60] examined 62 consecutive patients who had clear cell sarcoma, synovial sarcoma, epithelioid sarcoma, or rhabdomyosarcoma and did not have clinical or radiographic evidence of regional metastatic disease who were treated with SLNB at one institution between 2002 and 2012. They reported an overall incidence of positive sentinel node(s) of 12.9%; the highest incidence was among patients with clear cell sarcoma (6/12, 50%), followed by synovial sarcoma (2/42, 4.8%), epithelioid sarcoma (0/4), and rhabdomyosarcoma (0/4). Parida et al.[61] performed a retrospective review of pediatric patients with various malignancies who underwent lymphoscintigraphy and SLNB between 2004 and 2010 at two institutions and identified 56 patients without clinical or radiographic evidence of metastatic disease who underwent SLNB. Among 23 patients with sarcoma who underwent lymphoscintigraphy and SLNB, the overall rate of positive sentinel node(s) was 4.3%. One of six (16.7%) patients had rhabdomyosarcoma; no sentinel nodes were positive in patients with epithelioid sarcoma, synovial sarcoma, clear cell sarcoma, high-grade sarcoma, Ewing sarcoma, or sarcoma not otherwise specified. Turpin et al.[62] reported positive sentinel node(s) in three of six (50%) sequential patients who had head/neck rhabdomyosarcoma and were treated with SLNB at their institution.

TABLE 1-5   Studies Included in Systematic Review of Sentinel Lymph Node Biopsy in Patients with Extremity/Truncal Soft Tissue Sarcoma

First Author, Year	Study Type	Study Period	Participants, N	Single Center?	Population Database?	Sarcoma Subtypes, n (%)	Grade of Evidence*
Alcorn,[55] 2013	Retrospective cohort	2000–2011	8	Yes	No	Rhabdomyosarcoma, 5 (62.5)	++
						Epithelioid sarcoma, 2 (25)	
						Synovial sarcoma, 1 (12.5)	
Andreou,[60] 2013	Retrospective cohort	2002–2012	62	Yes	No	Synovial sarcoma, 42 (67.7)	++
						Clear cell sarcoma, 12 (19.4)	
						Epithelioid sarcoma, 4 (6.45)	
						Rhabdomyosarcoma, 4 (6.45)	
Brady,[71] 2019	Retrospective cohort	1998–2015	1,550	No	Yes (SEER)	Fibromatous, 256 (17)	++
						Lipomatous, 107 (7)	
						Myomatous, 305 (20)	
						Synovial-like, 360 (23)	
						Ewing sarcoma, 84 (5)	
						Nerve sheath, 85 (5)	
						Granular cell and alveolar soft part sarcoma, 43 (3)	
						Epithelioid, 64 (4)	

(continued)

TABLE 1-5   **Studies Included in Systematic Review of Sentinel Lymph Node Biopsy in Patients With Extremity/Truncal Soft Tissue Sarcoma** *(continued)*

First Author, Year	Study Type	Study Period	Participants, N	Single Center?	Population Database?	Sarcoma Subtypes, n (%)	Grade of Evidence*
Parida,[61] 2012	Retrospective cohort	2004–2010	23 sarcoma	No	No (2 centers from North America)	Epithelioid sarcoma, 8 (34.8)	++
						Rhabdomyosarcoma, 6 (26.1)	
						Synovial sarcoma, 3 (13.0)	
						Clear cell sarcoma, 2 (8.7)	
						High-grade sarcoma, 2 (8.7)	
						Ewing sarcoma, 1 (4.35)	
						Sarcoma NOS, 1 (4.35)	
Turpin,[62] 2019	Retrospective cohort	Unknown	6	Yes	No	Rhabdomyosarcoma, 6 (100)	++
Wright,[63] 2012	Meta-analysis	Publication years of included studies, 2000–2010	114	No	No (meta-analysis)	Synovial, 34 (29.8)	++
						Rhabdomyosarcoma, 22 (19.3)	
						Clear cell, 17 (14.9)	
						Epithelioid, 17 (14.9)	

NOS: not otherwise specified; SEER: Surveillance, Epidemiology, and End Results.
*Grade: ++ low.

TABLE 1-6 Sentinel Lymph Node Biopsy Positivity and Outcomes in Patients with Extremity/Truncal Soft Tissue Sarcoma

First Author, Year	Sarcoma Subtypes, n (%)	Median Follow-up, mo (range)	Rate of Positive SLN (%)	Median OS, mo (range)	2-Year OS, %	5-Year OS, %	10-Year OS, %	1-Year DMFS, %	5-Year DMFS, %
Alcorn,[55] 2013	All, 8 (100)	25 (13–66)	2/8 (25)	—	—	—	—	—	—
	Rhabdomyosarcoma, 5 (62.5)	—	2/5 (40)	—	—	—	—	—	—
	Epithelioid sarcoma, 2 (25)	—	0/2 (0)	—	—	—	—	—	—
	Synovial sarcoma, 1 (12.5)	—	0/1 (0)	—	—	—	—	—	—
Andreou,[60] 2013*	All, 62 (100)	38 (1–101)	8/62 (12.9)	—	SLN neg, 84 / SLN pos, 60	SLN neg, 74 / SLN pos, 40	—	SLN neg, 80 / SLN pos, 62	SLN neg, 60 / SLN pos, 37
	Synovial sarcoma, 42 (67.7)	—	2/42 (4.8)	—	—	—	—	—	—
	Clear cell sarcoma, 12 (19.4)	—	6/12 (50)	—	—	—	—	—	—
	Epithelioid sarcoma, 4 (6.45)	—	0/4 (0)	—	—	—	—	—	—
	Rhabdomyosarcoma, 4 (6.45)	—	0/4 (0)	—	—	—	—	—	—

(continued)

TABLE 1-6 Sentinel Lymph Node Biopsy Positivity and Outcomes in Patients with Extremity/Truncal Soft Tissue Sarcoma *(continued)*

First Author, Year	Sarcoma Subtypes, n (%)	Median Follow-up, mo (range)	Rate of Positive SLN (%)	Median OS, mo (range)	2-Year OS, %	5-Year OS, %	10-Year OS, %	1-Year DMFS, %	5-Year DMFS, %
Brady,[71] 2019†	All, 1,550 (100)	77	-/315	—	—	Overall, 79 No LNS, 80 LNS, 73 SLN neg, 84 SLN pos, 49	Overall, 74 No LNS, 76 LNS, 67 SLN neg, 78 SLN pos, 41	—	—
	Synovial-like, 360 (23)	—	-/67	—	—	Overall, 84 No LNS, 83 LNS, 86 SLN neg, 84 SLN pos, 33	Overall, 76 No LNS, 76 LNS, 77 SLN neg, 84 SLN pos, 0	—	—
	Myomatous, 305 (19)	—	-/146	—	—	Overall, 55 No LNS, 48 LNS, 64 SLN neg, 79 SLN pos, 49	Overall, 49 No LNS, 42 LNS, 57 SLN neg, 71 SLN pos, 44		

Histology							
Fibromatous, 256 (17)	—	-/12	—	—	Overall, 95 No LNS, 94 LNS, 100 SLN neg, 100 SLN pos, 100	Overall, 95 No LNS, 94 LNS, 100 SLN neg, 100 SLN pos, 100	—
Lipomatous, 107 (7)	—	0/9 (0)	—	—	Overall, 98 No LNS, 97 LNS, 100 SLN neg, 100	Overall, 98 No LNS, 97 LNS, 100 SLN neg, 100	—
Nerve sheath, 85 (5)	—	0/11 (0)	—	—	Overall, 60 No LNS, 60 LNS, 55 SLN neg, 55	Overall, 54 No LNS, 54 LNS, 55 SLN neg, 55	—
Ewing sarcoma, 84 (5)	—	-/7	—	—	Overall, 72 No LNS, 73 LNS, 69 SLN neg, 71 SLN pos, 67	Overall, 72 No LNS, 73 LNS, 69 SLN neg, 71 SLN pos, 67	—

(continued)

TABLE 1-6 Sentinel Lymph Node Biopsy Positivity and Outcomes in Patients with Extremity/Truncal Soft Tissue Sarcoma (*continued*)

First Author, Year	Sarcoma Subtypes, n (%)	Median Follow-up, mo (range)	Rate of Positive SLN (%)	Median OS, mo (range)	2-Year OS, %	5-Year OS, %	10-Year OS, %	1-Year DMFS, %	5-Year DMFS, %
	Epithelioid, 64 (4)	—	-/28	—	—	Overall, 87 No LNS, 88 LNS, 83 SLN neg, 90 SLN pos, 43	Overall, 80 No LNS, 83 LNS, 69 SLN neg, 82 SLN pos, 0	—	—
	Granular cell and alveolar soft part sarcoma, 43 (3)	—	-/5	—	—	Overall, 87 No LNS, 88 LNS, 80 SLN neg, 100 SLN pos, 50	Overall, 69 No LNS, 67 LNS, 80 SLN neg, 100 SLN pos, 50	—	—
Parida,[61] 2012	All, 23 (100)	—	1/23 (4.3)	—	—	—	—	—	—
	Epithelioid sarcoma, 8 (34.8)	—	0/8 (0)	—	—	—	—	—	—
	Rhabdomyosarcoma, 6 (26.1)	—	1/6 (16.7)	—	—	—	—	—	—
	Synovial sarcoma, 3 (13.0)	—	0/3 (0)	—	—	—	—	—	—

	Clear cell sarcoma, 2 (8.7)		0/2 (0)
	High-grade sarcoma, 2 (8.7)		0/2 (0)
	Ewing sarcoma, 1 (4.35)		0/1 (0)
	Sarcoma NOS, 1 (4.35)		0/1 (0)
Turpin,[62] 2019	All, 6 (100, all rhabdomyosarcoma)	29.5 (24–81)	3/6 (50)
Wright,[63] 2012	All, 114 (100)	—	SLN neg, 48 (8–90); SLN pos, 5 (1–12) · 14/114 (12)
	Synovial, 34 (29.8)		2/34 (6)
	Rhabdomyosarcoma, 22 (19.3)		5/22 (23)
	Clear cell, 17 (14.9)		6/17 (35)
	Epithelioid, 17 (14.9)		0/17 (0)

DMFS: distant metastasis-free survival; LNS: lymph node sampling; neg: negative; OS: overall survival; pos: positive; SLN: sentinel lymph node.
*OS and DMFS pertain only to 54 patients with a minimum follow-up of 12 months.
†Not all patients underwent LNS.

The estimated percentage of sentinel node positivity from the meta-analysis by Wright et al.[63] was 17% (95% confidence interval [CI], 7% to 45%) compared with the tabulated rate of 12% (14/114). The estimated summary percentage of positive sentinel nodes decreased to 10% (95% CI, 4% to 24%) after exclusion of single-patient case reports. In this study, clear cell sarcoma was the histologic subtype with the highest rate of positive sentinel lymph nodes (6/17, 35%), followed by rhabdomyosarcoma (5/22, 23%), synovial sarcoma (2/34, 6%), and epithelioid sarcoma (0/17). Patient selection bias could affect the reported incidence rates, with potential to overestimate them depending on the threshold for performing SLNB.

Impact of Sentinel Lymph Node Biopsy on Patient Outcomes

Numerous retrospective series have reported shorter durations of OS among patients with sarcoma who have regional lymph node metastasis relative to those who do not.[44,67,68] However, the role and potential impact of SLNB on outcomes among patients with soft tissue sarcoma remains unclear, for two primary reasons. First, the accuracy of SLNB with respect to the identification of subclinical nodal disease in soft tissue sarcoma has not yet been proven. Second, typically, it has not been possible to discern whether the identification of positive sentinel lymph node(s) in patients with soft tissue sarcoma guided or altered subsequent surgical, systemic, or radiation therapies, nor has it been possible to determine whether the SLNB procedure itself—or any subsequent therapies—improved outcomes.

Of the six evaluated studies, four (Alcorn et al.,[55] Parida et al.,[61] Turpin et al.,[62] Wright et al.[63]) did not report recurrence-free survival or OS outcomes in relation to SLNB procedure (Table 1-5). Alcorn et al.[55] reported that of the two patients (of an overall eight patients in their study and with median follow-up of 25 months) who had positive sentinel node(s) (both with rhabdomyosarcoma), one died of systemic disease at 13 months of follow-up and the other was alive without evidence of disease at 45 months of follow-up. However, of the remaining six patients who had negative sentinel lymph node(s), two died of systemic disease at 26 months and 36 months follow-up. Similarly, Turpin et al.[62] reported that of the three patients (of an overall six patients with rhabdomyosarcoma in their study and with median follow-up of 29.5 months) who had positive sentinel node(s), one died of locoregional disease at 31 months follow-up, and two were alive without evidence of disease at 30 and 81 months follow-up. Of the remaining three patients, two died of disease at 24 and 26 months. It is difficult, if not impossible, to interpret these data because the number of patients evaluated in each of these studies was small, the tumor characteristics of included patients were variable (disparate histologies, tumor site, etc.) or unknown (tumor size, neoadjuvant or adjuvant therapies received), the subsequent treatments administered were unknown, and there was no comparison between patients who had negative and positive sentinel node(s) of either recurrence-free survival or OS.

The remaining three studies (Andreou et al.,[60] Brady et al.,[71] and Wright et al.[63]) reported poorer OS among patients with positive sentinel node(s). Andreou et al.[60] reported trends toward lower 2- and 5-year OS and lower 1- and 5-year distant metastasis-free survival in patients who had positive sentinel node(s) compared with those with negative sentinel node(s). Brady et al.[71] examined rates of lymph node sampling and lymph node involvement in soft tissue sarcoma using the Surveillance, Epidemiology, and End Results registry. Lymph node sampling was performed in 14% of patients overall, and those with one or more positive sentinel nodes had poorer 5- and 10-year OS compared to those with negative sentinel nodes. Lymph node sampling was not performed at equal rates across soft tissue sarcoma histologies: the lymph node sampling was performed most commonly for patients with myomatous (48%), synovial-like (19%), and epithelioid (44%) histologies.

In their meta-analysis, Wright et al.[63] reported that patients with one or more positive sentinel nodes had a shorter median OS duration compared with those with negative sentinel nodes (5 vs. 48 months) and had higher estimated event rates with median difference in locoregional recurrence of 12 (95% CI, −14 to 54), distant recurrence of 42 (95% CI, −4 to 80), any recurrence of 56 (95% CI, −8 to 86), and death of 43 (95% CI, 3 to 85). However, the 95% CIs for all differences in estimated event rates were wide, with only death rates differing significantly between groups.

Completion Lymph Node Dissection after Positive Sentinel Lymph Node Biopsy

There is insufficient data from the six evaluated studies to address the utility and impact of completion lymph node dissection following positive SLNB. In both Alcorn et al.[55] and Brady et al.,[71] it is unknown what, if any, subsequent regional or systemic treatment was received by patients with positive SLNB. Management of positive SLNB was heterogeneous and incompletely described in the four other included studies.[60–63]

CONCLUSION

The role of SLNB in patients with soft tissue sarcoma remains unclear. Knowledge of the true incidence of regional lymph node metastasis across the disparate soft tissue sarcoma subtypes and the impact of surgical resection of lymphatic metastases is limited and has been informed by either small, single-center, retrospective series or population-based database studies. Further, the literature describing the impact of regional nodal staging and management on patient outcomes is significantly confounded by heterogeneity with respect to patients evaluated and the clinical practices used to treat them.

Evaluation of the regional lymph node basin in highly selected patients at particular risk of regional lymph node metastasis—with ultrasound, SLNB, and possibly completion nodal dissection—may be considered as a means to diagnose occult metastatic disease and improve prognostication. However, ultimately, multicenter prospective studies are needed to answer the following questions: (1) What is the true incidence of regional lymph node metastasis in soft tissue sarcoma? (2) Does SLNB offer a benefit for patients with clinically occult regional lymph node metastasis?

CHAPTER 2

Resection of Retroperitoneal and Intra-Abdominal Soft Tissue Sarcoma

CRITICAL ELEMENTS

- Macroscopically Complete Resection of Primary Tumor without Disruption of Tumor Capsule
- En Bloc Resection of Invaded Organs to Obtain a Complete Gross Resection

1. MACROSCOPICALLY COMPLETE RESECTION OF PRIMARY TUMOR WITHOUT DISRUPTION OF TUMOR CAPSULE

Recommendation: Operative exposure, approach, and extent should maximize the ability to achieve a complete macroscopic (R0/R1) resection of the primary tumor without tumor rupture. Piecemeal resection is discouraged.

Type of Data: Retrospective reports, case series, or case-control studies

Strength of Recommendation: Strong recommendation, moderate-quality evidence

Rationale

A macroscopically complete (R0/R1) resection is the minimum standard of care for patients with retroperitoneal sarcoma and/or visceral sarcomas of the gastrointestinal tract.[4,79] Surgery should include resection of the tumor en bloc with any adjacent structures that are directly invaded by tumor. Because the median size of primary retroperitoneal sarcoma on diagnosis is 20 cm, these tumors are typically located near critical anatomy, and a multivisceral resection may be necessary to remove them. Because the best chance for a potentially curative operation is at the time of initial presentation, it is increasingly appreciated that patient outcomes are optimized by multidisciplinary evaluation with surgical expertise at a high-volume sarcoma treatment center.[80-82]

Although the extent of resection remains a topic of debate among experts, the critical technical principle of surgery for retroperitoneal sarcoma is the resection of the primary tumor without disruption of the tumor capsule. Tumor rupture is a key prognostic factor for both retroperitoneal sarcoma and gastrointestinal stromal tumors (GISTs), as it may result in dissemination of tumor cells throughout the retroperitoneum/peritoneum and may lead to increased risk of recurrence. Outcomes following tumor rupture in patients with primary retroperitoneal sarcoma are comparable to patients with gross residual disease (R2 resection).[83] Importantly, tumor rupture is an independent risk factor for both local recurrence and short overall survival.[80,83] In addition to tumor size, mitotic count, and anatomic location, tumor rupture is a significant prognostic factor for patients with GIST, and these patients are automatically considered to be at high risk in the modified National Institutes of Health Risk Classification.[15] Multiple studies report tumor rupture as an independent predictor of worse outcomes in patients with GIST.[84-89]

Definitions of tumor rupture for GIST are generally applicable to retroperitoneal sarcoma.[90] Iatrogenic causes include tumor fracture from piecemeal resection, tumor manipulation, or incisional biopsy—the last of which is rarely indicated for this reason. Instead, the current standard approach for biopsy includes percutaneous, image-guided biopsy, which has been found to be safe for retroperitoneal sarcoma.[91,92]

Technical Aspects

Avoidance of tumor rupture due to intraoperative manipulation begins with the appropriate incision to optimize exposure.[93] The choice of incision is guided by the size and location of the tumor as well as the surgeon's experience. One standard incision is a midline laparotomy, as it provides access to the retroperitoneum after mobilization of the ipsilateral colon. In cases in which access to the spine and/or central vascular structures may be challenging, a transverse or an oblique extension from the midline may facilitate visualization; an inguinal counterincision may be required for tumors that extend into the groin. Furthermore, exposure to the retroperitoneum is enhanced with lateral positioning on a bean bag. A thoracoabdominal incision or a modified Makuuchi incision[94] is the other option that can provide optimal access and visualization to tumors in the upper quadrants and can facilitate access to the diaphragm for en bloc resection and repair. In addition, incisions can be considered for smaller low-grade tumors in the lower retroperitoneum and pelvis that provide the advantage of extraperitoneal access (Gibson incision). With the patient in a lateral decubitus position, a transverse flank incision allows access to the cranial pelvis including the psoas muscle and iliac vessels (Fig. 1-7). This incision can be extended inferomedially to the anterior cranial iliac spine to provide further exposure of the deeper pelvis.

As piecemeal resection has been shown to be an independent predictor of local recurrence, sarcomatosis, and short overall survival,[95] transection of the tumor should only be considered in rare circumstances to facilitate complete resection. For example, a low-grade tumor involving the sciatic notch and growing in a dumbbell shape out of the pelvis might require transection in a controlled manner to limit tumor spillage while sparing the sciatic nerve.

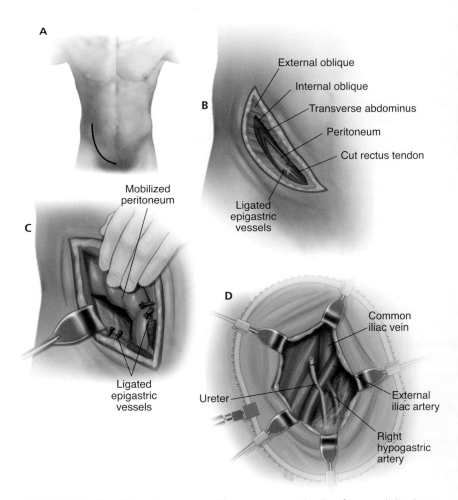

FIGURE 1-7   The Gibson incision provides exposure to the iliac fossa and distal one-third of the ureter. **A:** The incision is placed 2 cm medially to the anterior superior iliac spine, sweeping inferomedially to 1 cm above the inguinal ligament and stopping laterally to the midline. **B:** After skin incision, the external oblique aponeurosis is opened parallel to the muscular fibers, and the external oblique muscle is split with blunt dissection. The internal oblique and transversus abdominus aponeuroses and muscles are treated similarly. Maximal exposure requires division of the lateral border of the rectus muscle or dissection of its tendinous attachment from the pubic symphysis as well as ligation of the caudal epigastric vessels. **C:** The structures of the iliac fossa are visualized after careful dissection of the peritoneum off of the lateral pelvic sidewall. **D:** A Bookwalter retractor has been placed to maintain wide visualization of the iliac fossa. Here, the iliac artery and vein as well as the dome of the bladder and insertion of the ureter may be accessed by the surgeon.

2. EN BLOC RESECTION OF INVADED ORGANS TO OBTAIN A COMPLETE GROSS RESECTION

Recommendation: The degree to which retroperitoneal sarcoma invades adjacent visceral organs, muscles, major vessels, or bony structures should be estimated using preoperative cross-sectional imaging studies. Intraoperatively, structures that are directly invaded by cancer should be resected en bloc with the tumor using parenchymal-sparing, nonanatomic approaches.

Type of Data: Retrospective reports, case series, or case-control studies

Strength of Recommendation: Strong recommendation, moderate-quality evidence

Rationale

In patients with retroperitoneal sarcoma, surgical planning requires the expertise of a dedicated multidisciplinary team and consultation of other surgical services (vascular, orthopedic, urology) as needed. Macroscopically complete (R0/R1) resection is the most important treatment-related determinant of survival,[83] and multivisceral resection to include anatomic structures that are directly invaded by cancer should be used as needed to achieve this goal. Whether extended resection of adjacent organs that abut the tumor but are not directly invaded by it is associated with improved outcomes remains controversial.

Planned incomplete (R2) resection is not routinely offered to patients with retroperitoneal sarcoma given that outcomes are poor. However, in selected cases, R2 resection may be indicated for symptom palliation following multidisciplinary evaluation. Benefits of such intervention should be balanced with anticipated surgical morbidity, evaluation of tumor biology, patient comorbidities, performance status, and goals of care prior to surgery.[96]

Similar to extremity soft tissue sarcoma, retroperitoneal sarcoma should ideally be resected with a circumferential margin of normal tissue to maximize the chances of durable local control. For retroperitoneal sarcoma, the tissues at the "margins" of the tumor typically include adjacent anatomic structures and viscera.

In a significant number of cases, retroperitoneal or preperitoneal organs are directly invaded by cancer and therefore must be resected en bloc with the tumor to obtain a macroscopically complete (R0/R1) resection (Fig. 1-8). This may be assumed intraoperatively when an intact, easily transected adventitial or fascia plane is not retained between the tumor and organ. The most commonly resected organs are kidney, colon, and psoas muscle.[80] Nephrectomy should be performed en bloc with the tumor and the perinephric fat if removal of the intact kidney capsule would not allow for complete gross resection. Renal vessels should be divided at their origin. Resection of the colon and colonic mesentery is often needed to avoid exposure of the anterior aspect of the tumor if the anterior leaflet of the mesentery cannot be easily separated from the mesenteric vessels.

Resection of adjacent anatomic structures when they are not directly invaded by cancer must be considered carefully in the context of the anticipated associated morbidity.

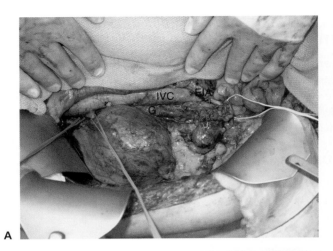

A

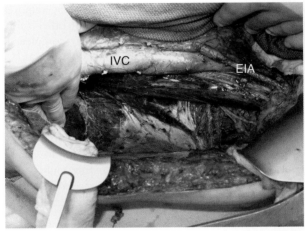

B

FIGURE 1-8 Surgery for a retroperitoneal liposarcoma requires resection of the tumor and all involved adjacent structures. **A:** The liposarcoma is seen in situ, located just lateral to the inferior vena cava (IVC). The yellow vessel loop encircles the ureter. The red and blue vessel loops encircle the right renal artery and vein, respectively. EIA: external iliac artery; G: gonadal vein. **B:** The tumor has been resected en bloc with the right kidney, renal vessels, gonadal vein, ureter, adjacent retroperitoneal fat, and muscular fascia.

(See Sarcoma Key Question 2.) Common examples include right-sided retroperitoneal sarcoma adjacent to the duodenum and head of the pancreas, left-sided retroperitoneal sarcoma adjacent to the tail of the pancreas and duodenojejunal junction, and tumors adjacent to the central abdominal vessels. In general, critical anatomic structures close to retroperitoneal sarcoma should be dissected under their adventitia/perineurium/periosteum to maximize margins.

Technical Aspects

A formal lymphadenectomy is not required for most retroperitoneal sarcomas. Non-anatomic resections of invaded organs, such as partial colectomy, wedge resection of the liver, or partial cystectomy, should be performed when feasible. Partial resection of the wall of the lateral wall of the second portion of the duodenum with duodenojejunostomy for reconstruction should be routine if the ampulla can be preserved. En bloc splenectomy and distal pancreatectomy are sometimes needed for tumors extending into the left upper quadrant.

Retroperitoneal sarcoma can extend into the chest through the diaphragm, into the anterior thigh through the femoral canal, into the gluteal compartment through the sciatic notch, into the medial thigh from the obturator foramen, or into the scrotum from the inguinal canal. Retroperitoneal sarcoma extending outside the abdomen should not be considered unresectable and can be managed with tailored resections with the appropriate surgical expertise.[4,5]

Psoas resection

If the psoas muscle is involved, it should be partially or completely resected. The femoral nerve and its roots should be identified and preserved when feasible but can be sacrificed with reasonable long-term outcomes if required for complete resection.[97] Full-thickness involvement of abdominal wall musculature including transversalis, internal, and/or external oblique is uncommon. However, partial abdominal wall resections with reconstruction should be performed liberally to avoid a positive soft tissue margin.

Management of neurovascular and bony structures

Direct invasion of the iliac vessels is not an absolute contraindication for surgery. Resection and reconstruction should be performed as needed to facilitate macroscopically compete resection. Similarly, direct extension of the tumor into ribs, vertebral bodies, vertebral transverse processes, and iliac wing can be managed with site-tailored resections.

Consideration of specific histologies

An important factor to consider when planning surgery for retroperitoneal sarcoma is tumor histology. Specifically, liposarcoma is associated with a high rate of local recurrence. In liposarcoma resections, all retroperitoneal fat from the diaphragm to the pelvis should be removed en bloc with the tumor with the aim of minimizing marginal involvement (Fig. 1-8). This approach also aids in the detection of tumor recurrence with postoperative surveillance imaging. Resection of the psoas fascia muscle should be performed routinely en bloc with the tumor mass, whereas the extent of psoas muscle resection should be considered in cases of direct invasion. Retroperitoneal sarcoma arising primarily from nerves (malignant peripheral nerve sheath tumor) or vessels (leiomyosarcoma) are characterized by a high metastatic risk. They should be resected en bloc with the structure of origin with negative margins, and multivisceral resection should be used if adjacent organs are invaded (Fig. 1-9). With malignant peripheral nerve sheath tumor and leiomyosarcoma,

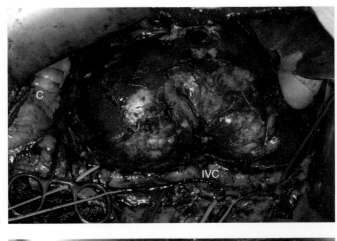

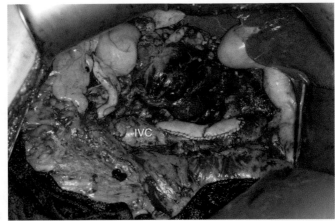

FIGURE 1-9   Retroperitoneal sarcoma involving the inferior vena cava (IVC). **A:** A large retroperitoneal sarcoma in situ. The most cranial aspect of the tumor is adherent to the anterior surface of the IVC. The colon (C) has been mobilized caudal off of the anterior surface of the tumor. **B:** The tumor has been resected en bloc with the anterior surface of the IVC. This was repaired with a patch, and the patient was placed on aspirin postoperatively.

frozen sections of the nerve or vein margins might be considered. In solitary fibrous tumor, a limited approach is acceptable, as these tumors have a low risk of local recurrence after complete resection.[6]

Gastrointestinal stromal tumors

Primary localized GIST should be resected to macroscopically negative margins with an intact tumor pseudocapsule. Usually, a 1- to 2-cm grossly negative bowel margin is adequate to obtain an R0 resection.[98] Multivisceral resection should be performed to achieve negative margins and limit tumor rupture.

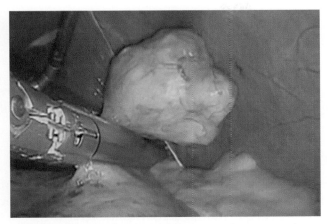

FIGURE 1-10 Small gastrointestinal stromal tumors can be resected laparoscopically. Care must be taken not to rupture the tumor, and conversion to an open procedure should be considered if the tumor requires direct manipulation to achieve proper visualization.

Laparoscopic resection of a GIST should be considered for small tumors amenable to this approach (Fig. 1-10). It should be noted that GISTs tend to be very friable, and care should be taken to avoid direct manipulation of the tumor. Rather, the adjacent bowel should be primarily handled to avoid tumor shedding. In addition, following laparoscopic resection, the GIST should be removed with an extraction bag.

Desmoid tumors

Desmoid tumors arising from the mesentery are particularly challenging. Multimodality management is critical for optimal outcomes.[99] In the abdomen and retroperitoneum, involvement of central mesenteric vessels often precludes surgical resection. After multidisciplinary evaluation, if surgical resection is deemed appropriate, careful dissection of the mesenteric vessels with preservation of major trunks not directly encased/invaded by the tumor is critical for bowel preservation, as there is a significant risk of short-gut syndrome with large tumors. Similar to extremity and trunk soft tissue sarcomas, the surgical goal is R0 resection, although R1 margins are acceptable if necessary to limit surgical morbidity.

Sarcoma Key Question 2

In patients with primary retroperitoneal sarcoma, does extended resection improve locoregional disease control compared with macroscopically complete resection?

INTRODUCTION

Complete surgical resection to grossly negative margins is the standard of care for patients with localized retroperitoneal sarcoma. However, local recurrence after resection is common: Up to 45% of patients develop a local recurrence at 10 years.[100] This high rate of recurrence is due in part to the ill-defined anatomic compartment within which the tumors are located and the close proximity of the tumors to vital structures and visceral organs as well as their typically large size. Together, these factors often make it difficult to achieve widely negative margins at surgery. Recently, histologic subtype has emerged as another—and potentially the most important—risk factor for local recurrence.[100,101]

Strategies have been proposed to reduce the likelihood of local recurrence. Data from a phase 3 study of preoperative radiotherapy plus surgery versus surgery alone for patients with retroperitoneal sarcoma (STRASS, EORTC 62092) presented at the American Society of Clinical Oncology 2019 annual meeting demonstrated no difference in abdominal recurrence-free survival across all histologies, although there was a potential benefit associated with radiation that was observed in patients with well-differentiated liposarcoma.

Extended resection—complete resection of the tumor en bloc with systematic removal of adjacent, grossly uninvolved organs (so-called compartmental resection)—has been proposed as another means to reduce local recurrence, but its benefits have been debated.[102,103] The purpose of this work was to determine whether extended resection was associated with improved locoregional disease control compared with macroscopically complete resection in patients with primary retroperitoneal sarcoma.

METHODOLOGY

A systematic search in Ovid MEDLINE, Ovid Embase, Cochrane Library, Web of Science, and Scopus from January 1, 1989, to July 26, 2019, was performed. Search structures, subject headings, and keywords were tailored to each database by a medical research librarian specializing in systematic reviews. Medical Subject Headings (MeSH) terms included "Retroperitoneal Neoplasms," "Sarcoma," and "Margins of Excision." Title, abstract, and keyword fields were searched with a variety of search terms identifying retroperitoneal sarcoma and resection. Searches were restricted to English language and human subjects. Searches were not restricted by study design, but case reports (<20 patients) were excluded. Multiple gray literature resources were searched for conferences, dissertations, reports, and other unpublished studies for additional relevant citations. The references of the included articles as well as later publications citing the included articles were searched. Findings are reported in accordance with the Preferred Reporting Items for Systematic Reviews and Meta-Analyses (PRISMA).[78]

The initial search yielded 3,284 publications (Fig. 1-11). After the initial search, the titles and abstracts of the articles were independently screened by two principal investigators to identify potentially relevant studies. Multiple reports of the same study were identified and linked and then excluded if duplicated or not relevant. Reports that described different findings from the same study were combined, and papers that reported results that had already been published were excluded. Studies that passed

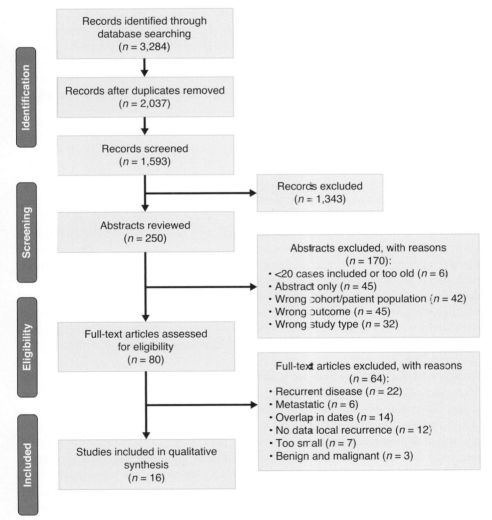

FIGURE 1-11 Preferred Reporting Items for Systematic Reviews and Meta-Analyses diagram for literature regarding primary retroperitoneal sarcoma and resection.

the title/abstract review were retrieved for full-text review. The remaining full-text articles were independently screened by the two investigators. Disagreements were resolved by consensus and by seeking the opinion of a third reviewer.

Two hundred fifty unique articles were retrieved for review. One hundred seventy abstracts were excluded because the study did not address the clinical question of interest. Thus, 80 full-text articles were reviewed independently by both investigators. Of these 80 articles, 64 were excluded because they either included both primary and recurrent/metastatic retroperitoneal sarcoma, did not have granular data on local recurrence, or were overlapping studies from the same institution; the final 16 studies met all the criteria for inclusion in this systematic review.[83,100,104–117]

Data were extracted from individual studies independently by a single investigator. Each article was reviewed and assigned a quality of evidence based on the Grading of Recommendations, Assessment, Development, and Evaluation (GRADE) system.[78] The quality of the data and size of the studies precluded the ability to perform a meta-analysis.

Sixteen studies were included in the qualitative systematic review (Table 1-7). No randomized studies compared local recurrence in patients with primary retroperitoneal sarcoma following treatment with extended resection versus macroscopically complete resection. All of the included studies were retrospective cohort studies describing an institution's surgical experience with retroperitoneal sarcoma. Overall, the quality of the evidence was low.

FINDINGS

Definition of Extent of Surgical Resection

Nine studies defined the extent of surgical resection in the methods (Table 1-7). Two studies clearly defined complete compartmental resection as "systematic resection of uninvolved organs to obtain rim of normal surrounding tissue."[83,107] The remaining seven studies had variable terminology regarding the extent of resection, describing it as "total gross excision,"[100] "remove the tumor with adjacent organs when not dissectible or when organs are macroscopically infiltrated,"[113] or "complete removal of adjacent infiltrated organs when necessary."[111] How infiltration was defined intraoperatively was not identified, and it was often left to the discretion of the operating surgeon. Seven studies did not discuss surgical technique at all in the methods.

Impact of Extent of Surgery on Multivisceral Resection

Multivisceral resection is often required for complete resection of retroperitoneal sarcoma. Given that extended resection (complete compartment resection) is defined as systematic resection of *uninvolved* organs to obtain a rim of normal surrounding tissue, this would at least theoretically result in an increase in the proportion of multivisceral resections relative to that in patients who had undergone macroscopically complete resection. In the studies included (Table 1-8), 66.5% (interquartile range [IQR], 54.53 to 80.03) of patients had undergone multivisceral resection. In the two studies that defined complete compartmental resection,[83,107] multivisceral resection was performed in the same proportion of patients undergoing compartmental resection (32% and 30.3%) as those having a macroscopically complete resection (35% and 31.2%).

TABLE 1-7 Studies Included in Systematic Review of Primary Retroperitoneal Sarcoma and Resection

First Author, Institution, Years	Number of Patients and Sarcoma Subtypes, n (%)	Median Tumor Size, cm (range)	Tumor Grade, n (%)	Completeness of Resection, n (%)	Type of Resection, Definition	Grade of Evidence*
Bonvalot,[83] Institut Gustave-Roussy, Centre Leon Berard, Institut Bergonie, France, 1985–2005	N = 382 Well-differentiated liposarcoma, 106 (28) Myxoid or undifferentiated liposarcoma, 84 (22) Leiomyosarcoma, 68 (18) Malignant histiofibrosarcoma, 34 (9) Others, 90 (23)	18 (3–60)	Low, 123 (32) Int, 129 (34) High, 112 (29.5) GX, 18 (4.5)	R0, 176 (47) R1, 103 (26) R2, 38 (10) RX, 57 (15)	1. Complete compartmental resection: systematic resection of uninvolved organs to obtain rim of normal surrounding tissue; typically colon in front, kidney within, and psoas at the back 2. Simple complete: shelling out tumor alone 3. Contiguously involved organ resection: resecting macroscopically involved organs	++
Ikoma,[104] MD Anderson Cancer Center, 1995–2011	N = 83 Well-differentiated liposarcoma, 83 (100)	54% >30	Low, 83 (100)	R0/R1, 76 (92) R2, 7 (8)	NA	++
Ito,[105] Brigham and Women's Hospital, 1990–2006	N = 20 Leiomyosarcoma, 20 (100)	9.3 (4–23)	Low, 2 (10) Int, 7 (35) High, 10 (50)	R0/R1, 19 (95) R2, 1 (5)	NA	++

(continued)

TABLE 1-7 Studies Included in Systematic Review of Primary Retroperitoneal Sarcoma and Resection (continued)

First Author, Institution, Years	Number of Patients and Sarcoma Subtypes, n (%)	Median Tumor Size, cm (range)	Tumor Grade, n (%)	Completeness of Resection, n (%)	Type of Resection, Definition	Grade of Evidence*
Keung,[106] Brigham and Women's Hospital, 1998–2008	N = 119 Dedifferentiated liposarcoma, 119 (100)	20.5 (0.8–75)	Int, 63 (53) High, 33 (28) GX, 23 (19)	R0/R1, 95 (79.8) R2, 13 (10.9) RX, 11 (9.2)	NA	++
Li,[107] Shijitan Hospital of Capital Medical University, 1980–2005	N = 231 Liposarcoma, 93 (40.3) Neurinoma, 41 (17.7) MFH, 46 (19.9) Other, 53 (22.1)	16 (3–65)	Low, 90 (39) Int, 82 (35.5) High, 59 (25.5)	R0, 109 (47.2) R1, 69 (29.9) R2, 53 (22.9)	1. Complete compartmental resection: systematic resection of uninvolved organs to obtain rim of normal surrounding tissue 2. Simple complete: shelling out tumor alone 3. Contiguously involved organ resection: resecting macroscopically involved organs	++
Molina,[108] Massachusetts General Hospital, 1991–2013	N = 41 Well-differentiated liposarcoma, 13 (31.7) Dedifferentiated liposarcoma, 26 (63.4) Myxoid, 1 (2.4) NOS, 1 (2.4)	19.5 (15–31.8)	Low, 10 (24.4) Int, 17 (41.5) High, 14 (34.2)	R0, 15 (37.6) R1, 26 (63.4)	Complete resection without fragmentation	++

Study	N, Histology (%)	Median follow-up (range)	Grade (%)	Margins (%)	Surgical approach	
Mussi,[109] Institut Clinico Humaintas, 1996–2008	N = 77 Liposarcoma, 30 (39) Leiomyosarcoma, 20 (26) Other, 27 (35)	17 (3–91)	Low, 25 (32.5) Int, 21 (27.3) High, 31 (40.2)	R0/R1, 68 (88.3)	1. Multivisceral resection in all primary cases even when gross infiltration was not recognized 2. Simple: tumor alone or with omentum 3. Associated visceral resection: at least 1 adjacent organ	++
Neuhaus,[110] Royal Marsden Hospital, 1990–2003	N = 72 Well-differentiated or dedifferentiated liposarcoma, 61 (85) Myxoid or round cell, 9 (13) Pleomorphic, 2 (3)	30 (11–60)	Low, 41 (57) High, 31 (43)	R0/R1, 63 (88)	NA	++
Pacelli,[111] Instituto di Clinical Chirurgica, 1984–2003	N = 73 Liposarcoma, 27 (37) Leiomyosarcoma, 18 (25) Dedifferentiated liposarcoma, 4 (5) Other, 24 (33)	17.2	Low, 47 (64) High, 26 (36)	R0, 40 (55) R1, 11 (15)	Complete resection with adjacent infiltrated organs when necessary; "often possible to mobilize the colon frontward"	++

(continued)

TABLE 1-7 Studies Included in Systematic Review of Primary Retroperitoneal Sarcoma and Resection *(continued)*

First Author, Institution, Years	Number of Patients and Sarcoma Subtypes, n (%)	Median Tumor Size, cm (range)	Tumor Grade, n (%)	Completeness of Resection, n (%)	Type of Resection, Definition	Grade of Evidence*
Rhu,[112] Samsung Medical Center, 2000–2015	N = 79 Well-differentiated liposarcoma, 31 (39.2) Dedifferentiated liposarcoma, 42 (53.2) Myxoid/round cell, 4 (5.1) Pleomorphic, 2 (2.5)	Mean, 24.24 ± 10.83 (7–60)	Low, 33 (44.6) Int, 28 (37.8) High, 13 (17.6) GX, 5 (6.3)	Positive, 20 (25.3) Unknown, 59 (74.7)	Not defined	++
Rossi,[113] University of Padova, 1989–2010	N = 43 Liposarcoma, 24 (56) Leiomyosarcoma, 10 (23) Other, 9 (21)	15	Low, 19 (44.2) Int, 9 (20.9) High, 15 (34.9)	R0, 11 (25.6) R1, 29 (67.4) R2, 3 (7)	Remove tumor with adjacent organs when not dissectible or when organs are macroscopically infiltrated. Clinically uninvolved but adjacent organs were not resected.	++
Schwartz,[114] USSC, 2000–2016	N = 571 Leiomyosarcoma, 162 (28) Liposarcoma, 196 (34) Sarcoma NOS, 26 (5) Other, 187 (3)	<10, 201 (35) 10–20 cm, 217 (38) >20 cm, 145 (25)	Low, 131 (23) High, 326 (57)	R0, 328 (57) R1, 184 (32) R2, 45 (8)	NA	++

Study	Histology			++
Smith,[115] Royal Marsden, 2005–2014	N = 362 Well-differentiated liposarcoma, 83 (22.9) Dedifferentiated liposarcoma, 150 (41.4) Leiomyosarcoma, 71 (19.6) Solitary fibrous tumor, 16 (4.4) Pleomorphic sarcoma, 10 (2.8) MPNST, 5 (1.4) Other, 27 (7.5)	24 (3–60)	Low, 100 (27.6) Int, 148 (40.9) High, 77 (21.3) GX, 37 (10.2)	R0/R1, 348 (96.1)	1. "Remove all macroscopic disease with contiguous organs if macroscopic involvement of non-vital adjacent organs to minimize microscopically positive margins." 2. Marginal excision along IVC, aorta, femoral nerve, duodenum, pancreatic head	++
Snow,[116] Peter MacCallum, 2008–2016	N = 88 Well-differentiated liposarcoma, 17 (19) Dedifferentiated liposarcoma, 29 (33) Leiomyosarcoma, 17 (19) Pleomorphic sarcoma, 7 (8) Solitary fibrous tumor, 8 (9) Other, 10 (11)	14 (20–400)	Low, 29 (33) Int, 29 (33) High, 24 (27) GX, 6 (7)	R0/R1, 83 (94)	NA	++

(continued)

TABLE 1-7 Studies Included in Systematic Review of Primary Retroperitoneal Sarcoma and Resection *(continued)*

First Author, Institution, Years	Number of Patients and Sarcoma Subtypes, n (%)	Median Tumor Size, cm (range)	Tumor Grade, n (%)	Completeness of Resection, n (%)	Type of Resection, Definition	Grade of Evidence*
Tan,[100] Memorial Sloan Kettering Cancer Center, 1982–2010	N = 675 Well-differentiated and myxoid liposarcoma, 186 (28) Dedifferentiated, round cell, and pleomorphic liposarcoma, 213 (32) Low-grade leiomyosarcoma, 18 (3) High-grade leiomyosarcoma, 132 (20) Solitary fibrous tumor, 33 (5) MPNST, 23 (3) Translocation-associated and other, 34 (5) NOS, 35 (5)	17 (2–139)	Low, 242 (36) High, 431 (64)	R0, 337 (50) R1, 237 (35) R2, 58 (9)	Total gross excision	++
Zhao,[117] General Hospital of Chinese People's Liberation Army, 2000–2007	N = 71 Well-differentiated liposarcoma, 37 (52) Dedifferentiated liposarcoma, 17 (24) Myxoid, 12 (17) Pleomorphic, 5 (7)	21.78 (± 12.07), mean	Low, 42 (59) High, 29 (41)	R0, 39 (54.9) R1, 22 (31) R2, 10 (14.1)	R0: clean margins defined by surgeon and pathologist R1: complete tumor resection with positive margins or opening of pseudocapsule R2: residual macroscopic tumor	++

GX: grade unknown; Int: intermediate; IVC: inferior vena cava; MFH: malignant fibrous histiocytoma; MPNST: malignant peripheral nerve sheath tumor; NA: not available; NOS: not otherwise specified; R0: negative microscopic margin; R1: positive microscopic margin; R2: gross incomplete resection; RX: resection margin unknown.
*Grade: ++ low.

TABLE 1-8 Outcomes of Studies Included in Systematic Review of Primary Retroperitoneal Sarcoma and Resection

First Author, Institution, Years	Median Follow-up (range)	XRT, n (%)	Multivisceral Resection, n (%)	Number Organs Resected	Local Recurrence	MVA (HR) for Local Recurrence: Margin, Surgery Type, or Number of Organs Resected
Bonvalot,[83] Institut Gustave-Roussy, Centre Leon Berard, Institut Bergonie, France, 1985–2005	4.4 y (1–18)	IORT: 18 (4.7) XRT: 121 (31.6)	Simple, 65 (17) Compartmental, 120 (32) Contiguously resected organ, 130 (35) Gross residual, 38 (10) Re-excision, 21 (6)	250 (65%) at least 1 organ resected	Local recurrence, 134 (47%) LRFS 1 y, 13% 3 y, 37% 5 y, 49%	Compartmental: 1 Simple: 1.99 (1.03–3.84), 0.04 Contiguous: 2.17 (1.19–3.94), 0.01 R0: 1 R1: 1.88 (1.18–2.98), 0.008 R2: 2.14 (1.28–3.57), 0.003
Ikoma,[104] MD Anderson Cancer Center, 1995–2011	7.3 y (1.5–19.8)	NA	38 (46)	Median, 2 (1–5)	Local recurrence, 44 (58%) 5-y local recurrence rate, 38% Median time to recurrence, 2.8 y in those that recurred	Concomitant organ resection: No: 1 Yes: 1.022 (0.537–1.946), 0.946
Ito,[105] Brigham and Women's Hospital, 1990–2006	41 mo (2–176)	IORT: 1 (5) XRT: 8 (40)	14 (70)	NA	Local-only recurrence, 3 (16%)	NA
Keung,[106] Brigham and Women's Hospital, 1998–2008	74.1 mo (0.9–184.9)	NA	112 (94.1)	Median, 2	Median LRFS, 23.9 (range, 19.5–28.3) mo in R0/R1	Number of organs, not significant (HR not given) Margins not in MVA

(continued)

TABLE 1-8 Outcomes of Studies Included in Systematic Review of Primary Retroperitoneal Sarcoma and Resection *(continued)*

First Author, Institution, Years	Median Follow-up (range)	XRT, n (%)	Multivisceral Resection, n (%)	Number Organs Resected	Local Recurrence	MVA (HR) for Local Recurrence: Margin, Surgery Type, or Number of Organs Resected
Li,[107] Shijitan Hospital of Capital Medical University, 1980–2005	35 mo (1–221)	NA	Simple, 36 (15.6) Compartmental, 70 (30.3) Contiguously resected organ, 72 (31.2) Gross residual, 53 (22.9)	NA	Local recurrence, 88 (38%) Median time to recurrence, 41 (range, 1–221) mo	Type of surgery not significant: HR not listed R0: 1 R1: 1.769 (1.162–2.694), 0.008 R2: 1.690 (1.089–2.625), 0.019
Molina,[108] Massachusetts General Hospital, 1991–2013	74.5 mo (31.9–97.7)	27 (65.8)	22 (53.7)	Median, 2 (IQR, 1–3)	Local recurrence, 7 (17%)	Competing risks univariate, number of organs: <3: 1 >3: 1.34 (0.28–6.54), 0.7161 R0: 1 R1: 0.24 (0.03–1.81), 0.1652 No multivariate
Mussi,[109] Institut Clinico Humaintas, 1996–2008	17.5 mo	23 (29)	51 (66)	Mean, 1.9/patient	5-y RFS, 52%	Simple resection: 0.989 (0.49–3.578), 0.355 vs. associated viscera resection (1)

Study						
Neuhaus,[110] Royal Marsden Hospital, 1990–2003	26 mo (12–151)	NA	42 (57)	17 (24) >1 organ resected	24 (41%) of 58 with 5-y follow-up data recurred Median time to recurrence, 39 (range, 25–53) mo	"Contiguous organ resection not related to increased risk of local recurrence"; not in table R0/R1: 0.18 (0.07–0.48), 0.001
Pacelli,[111] Instituto di Clinical Chirurgica, 1984–2003	Mean, 46.2 ± 44.1 mo	4 (5)	40/51 (78)	NA	Local recurrence, 19 (37.2%) at mean 14.1 ± 12.1 mo	Not done for local recurrence
Rhu,[112] Samsung Medical Center, 2000–2015	NA	45 (57)	Simple, 9 (11.3) Contiguously resected organs, 2 (2.5) Radical, 68 (86.1)	1 organ, 34 (43) 2 organs, 22 (27.8) ≥3 organs, 14 (17.8) Mean, 1.9/patient	LRFS: 1 y, 70.4% 3 y, 56.3% 5 y, 44.6%	<3 organs: 1 >3: 1.128 (0.421–3.026), 0.081 Margin: not included in MVA because not significant univariate
Rossi,[113] University of Padova, 1989–2010	49 mo (IQR, 19–103)	NA	21 (48.8)	Median, 2 (IQR 1–3)	Local recurrence, 11 (25.5%)	Only histiotype significant (no HR given)
Schwartz,[114] USSC, 2000–2016	30.6 mo (IQR, 11.2–60.4)	146 (27)	431 (75)	1–2 organs, 315 (55) 3–4 organs, 82 (14) ≥5 organs, 34 (6)	Median LRFS, 25.4 (range, 14.6–36.2)	NA
Smith,[115] Royal Marsden, 2005–2014	26 mo (1–117)	18 (5.6)	292 (80.7)	2 (0–6)	3-y LRFS: WDLPS, 98% DDLPS, 56.7% LMS, 80%	MVA organs resected 0: 1 1: 0.98 (0.48–1.98), 0.944 2: 1.30 (0.63–2.67), 0.484 3: 1.52 (0.74–3.13), 0.259

(continued)

TABLE 1-8 Outcomes of Studies Included in Systematic Review of Primary Retroperitoneal Sarcoma and Resection (continued)

First Author, Institution, Years	Median Follow-up (range)	XRT, n (%)	Multivisceral Resection, n (%)	Number Organs Resected	Local Recurrence	MVA (HR) for Local Recurrence: Margin, Surgery Type, or Number of Organs Resected
Snow,[116] Peter MacCallum, 2008–2016	36 mo	63 (72)	60 (67)	Median, 1 1 organ, 26 (29) 2 organs, 17 (19) 3 organs, 15 (17) 4+ organs, 3(3)	5-y LRFS, 65% (range, 52–80)	0: 1 1: 1.1 (0.4–3.2), 0.65 2+: 0.72 (0.22–2.4) R2: 1 R0/R1: 0.14 (0.041–0.51), 0.001
Tan,[100] Memorial Sloan Kettering Cancer Center, 1982–2010	3.3 y; 7.5 y for survivors	54 (8)	391 (58)	1 organ, 207 (31) 2 organs, 112 (16) 3 organs, 39 (6) 4 organs, 18 (3) ≥5 organs, 15 (2)	Local recurrence, 218 (38%) 5-y LRFS, 39% 10-y LRFS, 45%	Number of organs resected: < 3: 1 ≥3: 1.0 (0.7–1.6), 0.86
Zhao,[117] General Hospital of Chinese People's Liberation Army, 2000–2007	NA	20 (28)	22 (31)	NA	59/61 R0/R1 (96.7%) recurred Median time to local recurrence, 21 mo LRFS: 1 y, 77% 3 y, 29.8% 5 y, 19.7%	Organ resection not significant on univariate (not included in MVA)

DDLPS: dedifferentiated liposarcoma; HR: hazard ratio; IORT: intraoperative radiation therapy; IQR: interquartile range; LMS: leiomyosarcoma; LRFS: local recurrence-free survival; MVA: multivariate analysis; NA: not available; R0: negative microscopic margin; R1: positive microscopic margin; R2: gross incomplete resection; RFS: recurrence-free survival; WDLPS: well-differentiated liposarcoma; XRT: radiation therapy.

The median number of organs resected for most series was two (range, 1 to 5), but this was inconsistently reported. The kidney and colon were the most commonly resected organs in most series.

Impact of Extent of Surgery on Local Recurrence

Method of reporting on local recurrence was inconsistent across studies (Table 1-8). Ten studies[83,100,104,105,107,108,110,111,113,117] reported absolute local recurrence. In these studies, a median of 38% (IQR, 23.38 to 49.75) of patients developed a local recurrence during the study period (median follow-up, 39.6 [IQR, 26 to 74.3] months). Seven studies[104,106,107,110,111,114,117] reported a median local-recurrence–free survival of 25.4 (IQR, 21 to 67.2) months, and seven studies[83 100,104,109,112,116,117] reported the percentage of patients who experienced recurrence at 5 years (median, 48%; IQR, 21 to 67.2 months). It should be noted that there was significant heterogeneity in the histologies included in the studies, which would have a significant impact on local recurrence risk.

Association between Margins, Extended Resection, Multivisceral Resection, and Local Recurrence

There was significant heterogeneity in the variables included in multivariate analyses (Table 1-8). In general, patients who underwent macroscopically complete resection (R0/R1) were less likely to experience recurrence than those who had residual disease (R2).[83,107,108,110,116] Of the two studies that defined extended resection/complete compartmental resection, the study by Bonvalot et al.[83] demonstrated increased local recurrence with noncompartmental resection, whereas the study by Li et al.[107] did not demonstrate any association between the type of surgery and local recurrence. Ten studies included multivisceral resection in multivariate modeling.[100,104,106,108–110,112,115–117] There was no association between local recurrence and number of organs resected in any of these studies.

CONCLUSION

Complete macroscopic resection remains the only potentially curative treatment of retroperitoneal sarcoma. Although numerous studies have described extended resection for the treatment of primary retroperitoneal sarcoma, the lack of standardization in the definition of extended resection limits the ability to draw conclusions from these studies. Among studies that have clearly defined extended resection as complete compartmental surgery, there appears to be no difference in the incidence of multivisceral resection or number of organs resected by extended resection relative to complete macroscopic resection. In addition, although there was a significant and heterogeneous number of histologies included across all studies, which likely affects local recurrence rates, local recurrence rates for retroperitoneal sarcoma were high across all studies. Future studies should clearly define extended resection, stratify data by histology, and consistently report local recurrence metrics to allow for cross-institutional comparisons. At present, it is impossible to support the routine removal of uninvolved adjacent organs for patients with retroperitoneal sarcoma.

REFERENCES

1. Edge SB, Byrd DR, Compton CC, Fritz AG, Greene FL, Trotti A, eds. *AJCC Cancer Staging Manual*. 7th ed. Springer; 2010.
2. Amin MB, Edge SB, Green FL, et al, eds. *AJCC Cancer Staging Manual*. 8th ed. Springer; 2017.
3. Guillou L, Coindre JM, Bonichon F, et al. Comparative study of the National Cancer Institute and French Federation of Cancer Centers Sarcoma Group grading systems in a population of 410 adult patients with soft tissue sarcoma. *J Clin Oncol*. 1997;15(1):350-362. doi:10.1200/JCO.1997.15.1.350
4. National Comprehensive Cancer Network. NCCN Clinical Practice Guidelines in Oncology: soft tissue sarcoma. Updated February 2021. Accessed February 21, 2022. https://www.nccn.org/professionals/physician_gls/pdf/sarcoma.pdf
5. Rosenberg SA, Tepper J, Glatstein E, et al. The treatment of soft-tissue sarcomas of the extremities: prospective randomized evaluations of (1) limb-sparing surgery plus radiation therapy compared with amputation and (2) the role of adjuvant chemotherapy. *Ann Surg*. 1982;196(3):305-315. doi:10.1097/00000658-198209000-00009
6. Yang JC, Chang AE, Baker AR, et al. Randomized prospective study of the benefit of adjuvant radiation therapy in the treatment of soft tissue sarcomas of the extremity. *J Clin Oncol*. 1998;16(1):197-203. doi:10.1200/JCO.1998.16.1.197
7. Beane JD, Yang JC, White D, Steinberg SM, Rosenberg SA, Rudloff U. Efficacy of adjuvant radiation therapy in the treatment of soft tissue sarcoma of the extremity: 20-year follow-up of a randomized prospective trial. *Ann Surg Oncol*. 2014;21(8):2484-2489. doi:10.1245/s10434-014-3732-4
8. Pisters PW, Harrison LB, Leung DH, Woodruff JM, Casper ES, Brennan MF. Long-term results of a prospective randomized trial of adjuvant brachytherapy in soft tissue sarcoma. *J Clin Oncol*. 1996;14(3):859-868. doi:10.1200/JCO.1996.14.3.859
9. O'Sullivan B, Davis AM, Turcotte R, et al. Preoperative versus postoperative radiotherapy in soft-tissue sarcoma of the limbs: a randomised trial. *Lancet*. 2002;359(9325):2235-2241. doi:10.1016/S0140-6736(02)09292-9
10. Bonvalot S, Gronchi A, Le Péchoux C, et al. Preoperative radiotherapy plus surgery versus surgery alone for patients with primary retroperitoneal sarcoma (EORTC-62092: STRASS): a multicentre, open-label, randomised, phase 3 trial. *Lancet Oncol*. 2020;21(10):1366-1377. doi:10.1016/S1470-2045(20)30446-0
11. Adjuvant chemotherapy for localised resectable soft-tissue sarcoma of adults: a meta-analysis of individual data. *Lancet*. 1997;350(9092):1647-1654.
12. Woll P, Reichardt P, Le Cesne A, et al. Adjuvant chemotherapy with doxorubicin, ifosfamide, and lenograstim for resected soft-tissue sarcoma (EORTC 62931): a multicentre randomised controlled trial. *Lancet Oncol*. 2012;13(10):1045-1054. doi:10.1016/S1470-2045(12)70346-7
13. Italiano A, Delva F, Mathoulin-Pelissier S, et al. Effect of adjuvant chemotherapy on survival in FNCLCC grade 3 soft tissue sarcomas: a multivariate analysis of the French Sarcoma Group Database. *Ann Oncol*. 2010;21(12):2436-2441. doi:10.1093/annonc/mdq238
14. Druker B, Tamura S, Buchdunger E, et al. Effects of a selective inhibitor of the Abl tyrosine kinase on the growth of Bcr-Abl positive cells. *Nat Med*. 1996;2(5):561-566. doi:10.1038/nm0596-561
15. Joensuu H, Eriksson M, Sundby Hall K, et al. One vs three years of adjuvant imatinib for operable gastrointestinal stromal tumor: a randomized trial. *JAMA*. 2012;307(12):1265-1272. doi:10.1001/jama.2012.347
16. Raut C, Espat N, Maki R, et al. Efficacy and tolerability of 5-year adjuvant imatinib treatment for patients with resected intermediate- or high-risk primary gastrointestinal stromal tumor: the PERSIST-5 clinical trial. *JAMA Oncol*. 2018;4(12):e184060. doi:10.1001/jamaoncol.2018.4060
17. Tirumani S, Shinagare A, Jagannathan J, Krajewski K, Ramaiya N, Raut C. Radiologic assessment of earliest, best, and plateau response of gastrointestinal stromal tumors to neoadjuvant imatinib prior to successful surgical resection. *Eur J Surg Oncol*. 2014;40(4):420-428. doi:10.1016/j.ejso.2013.10.021
18. Fletcher CD, Bridge JA, Hogendoorn PC, Mertens F, eds. *WHO Classification of Tumours of Soft Tissue and Bone*. 4th ed. IARC Press; 2013.
19. Kindblom L, Remotti H, Aldenborg F, Meis-Kindblom J. Gastrointestinal pacemaker cell tumor (GIPACT): gastrointestinal stromal tumors show phenotypic characteristics of the interstitial cells of Cajal. *Am J Pathol*. 1998;152(5):1259-1269.
20. Miettinen M, Lasota J. Gastrointestinal stromal tumors: pathology and prognosis at different sites. *Semin Diagn Pathol*. 2006;23(2):70-83. doi:10.1053/j.semdp.2006.09.001
21. Rydholm A, Berg NO. Size, site and clinical incidence of lipoma. Factors in the differential diagnosis of lipoma and sarcoma. *Acta Orthop Scand*. 1983;54(6):929-934. doi:10.3109/17453678308992936

22. Tuttle R, Kane JM III. Biopsy techniques for soft tissue and bowel sarcomas. *J Surg Oncol.* 2015;111(5):504-512. doi:10.1002/jso.23870

23. Mankin HJ, Mankin CJ, Simon MA. The hazards of the biopsy, revisited. Members of the Musculoskeletal Tumor Society. *J Bone Joint Surg Am.* 1996;78(5):656-663. doi:10.2106/00004623-199605000-00004

24. Ray-Coquard I, Montesco MC, Coindre JM, et al. Sarcoma: concordance between initial diagnosis and centralized expert review in a population-based study within three European regions. *Ann Oncol.* 2012;23(9):2442-2449. doi:10.1093/annonc/mdr610

25. López JI, Del Cura JL, Zabala R, Bilbao FJ. Usefulness and limitations of ultrasound-guided core biopsy in the diagnosis of musculoskeletal tumors. *APMIS.* 2005;113(5):353-360. doi:10.1111/j.1600-0463.2005.apm_113507.x

26. Heslin MJ, Lewis JJ, Woodruff JM, Brennan MF. Core needle biopsy for diagnosis of extremity soft tissue sarcoma. *Ann Surg Oncol.* 1997;4(5):425-431. doi:10.1007/BF02305557

27. Strauss DC, Qureshi YA, Hayes AJ, Thway K, Fisher C, Thomas JM. The role of core needle biopsy in the diagnosis of suspected soft tissue tumours. *J Surg Oncol.* 2010;102(5):523-529. doi:10.1002/jso.21600

28. Dupuy DE, Rosenberg AE, Punyaratabandhu T, Tan MH, Mankin HJ. Accuracy of CT-guided needle biopsy of musculoskeletal neoplasms. *AJR Am J Roentgenol.* 1998;171(3):759-762. doi:10.2214/ajr.171.3.ajronline_171_3_001

29. Rosenberg SA, Kent H, Costa J, et al. Prospective randomized evaluation of the role of limb-sparing surgery, radiation therapy, and adjuvant chemoimmunotherapy in the treatment of adult soft-tissue sarcomas. *Surgery.* 1978;84(1):62-69.

30. Barrientos-Ruiz I, Ortiz-Cruz EJ, Serrano-Montilla J, Bernabeu-Taboada D, Pozo-Kreilinger JJ. Are biopsy tracts a concern for seeding and local recurrence in sarcomas? *Clin Orthop Relat Res.* 2017;475(2):511-518. doi:10.1007/s11999-016-5090-y

31. Siddiqi MA, Kim HS, Jede F, Han I. Association of core needle biopsy tract resection with local recurrence in extremity soft tissue sarcoma. *Skeletal Radiol.* 2017;46(4):507-512. doi:10.1007/s00256-017-2579-8

32. Kandel R, Coakley N, Werier J, Engel J, Ghert M, Verma S. Surgical margins and handling of soft-tissue sarcoma in extremities: a clinical practice guideline. *Curr Oncol.* 2013;20(3):e247-e254. doi:10.3747/co.20.1308

33. King DM, Hackbarth DA, Kirkpatrick A. Extremity soft tissue sarcoma resections: how wide do you need to be? *Clin Orthop Relat Res.* 2012;470(3):692-699. doi:10.1007/s11999-011-2167-5

34. Li X, Moretti VM, Ashana AO, Lackman RD. Impact of close surgical margin on local recurrence and survival in osteosarcoma. *Int Orthop.* 2012;36(1):131-137. doi:10.1007/s00264-011-1230-x

35. Kawaguchi N, Ahmed AR, Matsumoto S, Manabe J, Matsushita Y. The concept of curative margin in surgery for bone and soft tissue sarcoma. *Clin Orthop Relat Res.* 2004;(419):165-172. doi:10.1097/00003086-200402000-00027

36. Swinscoe JA, Dickie CI, Ireland RH. Immobilization and image-guidance methods for radiation therapy of limb extremity soft tissue sarcomas: results of a multi-institutional survey. *Med Dosim.* 2018;43(4):377-382. doi:10.1016/j.meddos.2017.12.003

37. Erstad DJ, Ready J, Abraham J, et al. Amputation for extremity sarcoma: contemporary indications and outcomes. *Ann Surg Oncol.* 2018;25(2):394-403. doi:10.1245/s10434-017-6240-5

38. Slump J, Bastiaannet E, Halka A, et al. Risk factors for postoperative wound complications after extremity soft tissue sarcoma resection: a systematic review and meta-analyses. *J Plast Reconstr Aesthet Surg.* 2019;72(9):1449-1464. doi:10.1016/j.bjps.2019.05.041

39. Mullen JT. Dermatofibrosarcoma protuberans: wide local excision versus Mohs micrographic surgery. *Surg Oncol Clin N Am.* 2016;25(4):827-839. doi:10.1016/j.soc.2016.05.011

40. Roland CL, Wang W-L, Lazar AJ, Torres KE. Myxofibrosarcoma. *Surg Oncol Clin N Am.* 2016;25(4):775-788. doi:10.1016/j.soc.2016.05.008

41. Fanburg-Smith JC, Spiro IJ, Katapuram SV, Mankin HJ, Rosenberg AE. Infiltrative subcutaneous malignant fibrous histiocytoma: a comparative study with deep malignant fibrous histiocytoma and an observation of biologic behavior. *Ann Diagn Pathol.* 1999;3(1):1-10. doi:10.1016/s1092-9134(99)80003-3

42. Li GZ, Fairweather M, Wang J, Orgill DP, Bertagnolli MM, Raut CP. Cutaneous radiation-associated breast angiosarcoma: radicality of surgery impacts survival. *Ann Surg.* 2017;265(4):814-820. doi:10.1097/SLA.0000000000001753

43. Fong Y, Coit DG, Woodruff JM, Brennan MF. Lymph node metastasis from soft tissue sarcoma in adults. Analysis of data from a prospective database of 1772 sarcoma patients. *Ann Surg.* 1993;217(1):72-77. doi:10.1097/00000658-199301000-00012

44. Behranwala KA, A'Hern R, Omar AM, Thomas JM. Prognosis of lymph node metastasis in soft tissue sarcoma. *Ann Surg Oncol.* 2004;11(7):714-719. doi:10.1245/ASO.2004.04.027

45. Nishida Y, Yamada Y, Tsukushi S, Shibata S, Ishiguro N. Sentinel lymph node biopsy reveals a positive popliteal node in clear cell sarcoma. *Anticancer Res.* 2005;25(6C):4413-4416.

46. van Akkooi ACJ, Verhoef C, van Geel AN, Kliffen M, Eggermont AMM, de Wilt JHW. Sentinel node biopsy for clear cell sarcoma. *Eur J Surg Oncol.* 2006;32(9):996-999. doi:10.1016/j.ejso.2006.03.044

47. Gow KW, Rapkin LB, Olson TA, Durham MM, Wyly B, Shehata BM. Sentinel lymph node biopsy in the pediatric population. *J Pediatr Surg.* 2008;43(12):2193-2198. doi:10.1016/j.jpedsurg.2008.08.063

48. Kayton ML, Delgado R, Busam K, et al. Experience with 31 sentinel lymph node biopsies for sarcomas and carcinomas in pediatric patients. *Cancer.* 2008;112(9):2052-2059. doi:10.1002/cncr.23403

49. Swing DC Jr, Geisinger KR. Sentinel lymph node mapping for alveolar rhabdomyosarcoma. *AJSP: Rev Rep.* 2008;13(3):119-121. doi:10.1097/PCR.0b013e31817ae05f

50. Tunn P-U, Andreou D, Illing H, Fleige B, Dresel S, Schlag P. Sentinel node biopsy in synovial sarcoma. *Eur J Surg Oncol.* 2008;34(6):704-707. doi:10.1016/j.ejso.2007.07.014

51. Dall'Igna P, De Corti F, Alaggio R, Cecchetto G. Sentinel node biopsy in pediatric patients: the experience in a single institution. *Eur J Pediatr Surg.* 2014;24(6):482-487. doi:10.1055/s-0034-1396422

52. Seal A, Tse R, Wehrli B, Hammond A, Temple CL. Sentinel node biopsy as an adjunct to limb salvage surgery for epithelioid sarcoma of the hand. *World J Surg Oncol.* 2005;3(1):41. doi:10.1186/1477-7819-3-41

53. Albores-Zúñiga O, Padilla-Rosciano A, Martínez-Said H, Cuéllar-Hubbe M, Ramírez-Bollas J. Clear cell sarcoma and sentinel lymph node biopsy. Case report and literature review. Article in Spanish. *Cir Cir.* 2006;74(2):121-125.

54. Kayton ML, Meyers P, Wexler LH, Gerald WL, LaQuaglia MP. Clinical presentation, treatment, and outcome of alveolar soft part sarcoma in children, adolescents, and young adults. *J Pediatr Surg.* 2006;41(1):187-193. doi:10.1016/j.jpedsurg.2005.10.023

55. Alcorn KM, Deans KJ, Congeni A, et al. Sentinel lymph node biopsy in pediatric soft tissue sarcoma patients: utility and concordance with imaging. *J Pediatr Surg.* 2013;48(9):1903-1906. doi:10.1016/j.jpedsurg.2013.04.013

56. Fantini F, Monari P, Bassissi S, Maiorana A, Cesinaro A. Sentinel lymph node biopsy in clear cell sarcoma. *J Eur Acad Dermatol Venereol.* 2007;21(9):1271-1272. doi:10.1111/j.1468-3083.2007.02164.x

57. Picciotto F, Zaccagna A, DeRosa G, et al. Clear cell sarcoma (malignant melanoma of soft parts) and sentinel lymph node biopsy. *Eur J Dermatol.* 2005;15(1):46-48.

58. Riad S, Griffin AM, Liberman B, et al. Lymph node metastasis in soft tissue sarcoma in an extremity. *Clin Orthop Relat Res.* 2004;426:129-134. doi:10.1097/01.blo.0000141660.05125.46

59. Pradhan A, Grimer R, Abudu A, et al. Epithelioid sarcomas: how important is loco-regional control? *Eur J Surg Oncol.* 2017;43(9):1746-1752. doi:10.1016/j.ejso.2017.07.002

60. Andreou D, Boldt H, Werner M, Hamann C, Pink D, Tunn P-U. Sentinel node biopsy in soft tissue sarcoma subtypes with a high propensity for regional lymphatic spread—results of a large prospective trial. *Ann Oncol.* 2013;24(5):1400-1405. doi:10.1093/annonc/mds650

61. Parida L, Morrisson GT, Shammas A, et al. Role of lymphoscintigraphy and sentinel lymph node biopsy in the management of pediatric melanoma and sarcoma. *Pediatr Surg Int.* 2012;28(6):571-578. doi:10.1007/s00383-012-3066-x

62. Turpin B, Pressey JG, Nagarajan R, et al. Sentinel lymph node biopsy in head and neck rhabdomyosarcoma. *Pediatr Blood Cancer.* 2019;66(3):e27532. doi:10.1002/pbc.27532

63. Wright S, Armeson K, Hill EG, et al. The role of sentinel lymph node biopsy in select sarcoma patients: a meta-analysis. *Am J Surg.* 2012;204(4):428-433. doi:10.1016/j.amjsurg.2011.12.019

64. Neville HL, Andrassy RJ, Lally KP, Corpron C, Ross MI. Lymphatic mapping with sentinel node biopsy in pediatric patients. *J Pediatr Surg.* 2000;35(6):961-964. doi:10.1053/jpsu.2000.6936

65. McMulkin H, Yanchar N, Fernandez C, Giacomantonio C. Sentinel lymph node mapping and biopsy: a potentially valuable tool in the management of childhood extremity rhabdomyosarcoma. *Pediatr Surg Int.* 2003;19(6):453-456. doi:10.1007/s00383-003-0956-y

66. Al-Refaie WB, Ali MW, Chu DZ, Paz IB, Blair SL. Clear cell sarcoma in the era of sentinel lymph node mapping. *J Surg Oncol.* 2004;87(3):126-129. doi:10.1002/jso.20096

67. Keung EZ, Chiang Y-J, Voss RK, et al. Defining the incidence and clinical significance of lymph node metastasis in soft tissue sarcoma. *Eur J Surg Oncol.* 2018;44(1):170-177. doi:10.1016/j.ejso.2017.11.014

68. Johannesmeyer D, Smith V, Cole DJ, Esnaola NF, Camp ER. The impact of lymph node disease in extremity soft-tissue sarcomas: a population-based analysis. *Am J Surg.* 2013;206(3):289-295. doi:10.1016/j.amjsurg.2012.10.043

69. Ecker BL, Peters MG, McMillan MT, et al. Implications of lymph node evaluation in the management of resectable soft tissue sarcoma. *Ann Surg Oncol.* 2017;24(2):425-433. doi:10.1245 /s10434-016-5641-1

70. Sherman KL, Kinnier CV, Farina DA, et al. Examination of national lymph node evaluation practices for adult extremity soft tissue sarcoma. *J Surg Oncol.* 2014;110(6):682-688. doi:10.1002/jso.23687

71. Brady A-C, Picado O, Tashiro J, Sola JE, Perez EA. Lymph node sampling and survival in child and adolescent extremity soft tissue sarcoma. *J Surg Res.* 2019;241:205-214. doi:10.1016/j.jss .2019.03.030

72. Blazer DG III, Sabel MS, Sondak VK. Is there a role for sentinel lymph node biopsy in the management of sarcoma? *Surg Oncol.* 2003;12(3):201-206. doi:10.1016/s0960-7404(03)00030-6

73. Skinner KA, Eilber FR. Soft tissue sarcoma nodal metastases: biologic significance and therapeutic considerations. *Surg Oncol Clin N Am.* 1996;5(1):121-127. doi:10.1016/S1055-3207(18)30408-3

74. Mazeron JJ, Suit HD. Lymph nodes as sites of metastases from sarcomas of soft tissue. *Cancer.* 1987;60(8):1800-1808. doi:10.1002/1097-0142(19871015)60:8<1800::aid-cncr2820600822>3 .0.co;2-n

75. Yoon SS, Maki RG, Asare EA, et al. Soft tissue sarcoma of the trunk and extremities. In: Amin MB, Edge SB, Green FL, et al, eds. *AJCC Cancer Staging Manual.* 8th ed. Springer; 2017:507-516.

76. Green F, Page D, Fleming I, et al. *AJCC Cancer Staging Manual.* 6th ed. Springer; 2002.

77. Moher D, Liberati A, Tetzlaff J, Altman DG; PRISMA Group. Preferred reporting items for systematic reviews and meta-analyses: the PRISMA statement. *PloS Med.* 2009;6(7):e1000097. doi:10.1371/journal.pmed.1000097

78. Balshem H, Helfand M, Schünemann HJ, et al. GRADE guidelines: 3. Rating the quality of evidence. *J Clin Epidemiol.* 2011;64(4):401-406. doi:10.1016/j. clinepi.2010.07.015

79. Trans-Atlantic RPS Working Group. Management of primary retroperitoneal sarcoma (RPS) in the adult: a consensus approach from the Trans-Atlantic RPS Working Group. *Ann Surg Oncol.* 2015;22(1):256-263. doi:10.1245/s10434-014-3965-2

80. Gronchi A, Strauss DC, Miceli R, et al. Variability in patterns of recurrence after resection of primary retroperitoneal sarcoma (RPS): a report on 1007 patients from the multi-institutional collaborative RPS working group. *Ann Surg.* 2016;263(5):1002-1009. doi:10.1097/SLA .0000000000001447

81. Keung EZ, Chiang Y-J, Cormier JN, et al. Treatment at low-volume hospitals is associated with reduced short-term and long-term outcomes for patients with retroperitoneal sarcoma. *Cancer.* 2018;124(23):4495-4503. doi:10.1002/cncr.31699

82. Blay J-Y, Honoré C, Stoeckle E, et al. Surgery in reference centers improves survival of sarcoma patients: a nationwide study. *Ann Oncol.* 2019;30(7):1143-1153. doi:10.1093/annonc/mdz124

83. Bonvalot S, Rivoire M, Castaing M, et al. Primary retroperitoneal sarcomas: a multivariate analysis of surgical factors associated with local control. *J Clin Oncol.* 2009;27(1):31-37. doi:10.1200/JCO.2008.18.0802

84. Rutkowski P, Nowecki ZI, Michej W, et al. Risk criteria and prognostic factors for predicting recurrences after resection of primary gastrointestinal stromal tumor. *Ann Surg Oncol.* 2007;14(7):2018-2027. doi:10.1245/s10434-007-9377-9

85. Joensuu H, Vehtari A, Riihimaki J, et al. Risk of recurrence of gastrointestinal stromal tumour after surgery: an analysis of pooled population-based cohorts. *Lancet Oncol.* 2012;13(3):265-274. doi:10.1016/S1470-2045(11)70299-6

86. Yanagimoto Y, Takahashi T, Muguruma K, et al. Re-appraisal of risk classifications for primary gastrointestinal stromal tumors (GISTs) after complete resection: indications for adjuvant therapy. *Gastric Cancer.* 2015;18(2):426-433. doi:10.1007/s10120-014-0386-7

87. Hølmebakk T, Bjerkehagen B, Boye K, Bruland Ø, Stoldt S, Sundby Hall K. Definition and clinical significance of tumour rupture in gastrointestinal stromal tumours of the small intestine. *Br J Surg.* 2016;103(6):684-691. doi:10.1002/bjs.10104

88. Hølmebakk T, Hompland I, Bjerkehagen B, et al. Recurrence-free survival after resection of gastric gastrointestinal stromal tumors classified according to a strict definition of tumor rupture: a population-based study. *Ann Surg Oncol.* 2018;25(5):1133-1139. doi:10.1245/s10434-018-6353-5

89. Nishida T, Cho H, Hirota S, et al. Clinicopathological features and prognosis of primary gists with tumor rupture in the real world. *Ann Surg Oncol.* 2018;25(7):1961-1969. doi:10.1245 /s10434-018-6505-7

90. Nishida T, Hølmebakk T, Raut CP, Rutkowski P. Defining tumor rupture in gastrointestinal stromal tumor. *Ann Surg Oncol.* 2019;26(6):1669-1675. doi:10.1245/s10434-019-07297-9

91. Wilkinson MJ, Martin JL, Khan AA, Hayes AJ, Thomas JM, Strauss DC. Percutaneous core needle biopsy in retroperitoneal sarcomas does not influence local recurrence or overall survival. *Ann Surg Oncol.* 2015;22(3):853-858. doi:10.1245/s10434-014-4059-x

92. Berger-Richardson D, Swallow CJ. Needle tract seeding after percutaneous biopsy of sarcoma: risk/benefit considerations. *Cancer.* 2017;123(4):560-567. doi:10.1002/cncr.30370

93. Bonvalot S, Raut CP, Pollock RE, et al. Technical considerations in surgery for retroperitoneal sarcomas: position paper from E-Surge, a master class in sarcoma surgery, and EORTC-STBSG. *Ann Surg Oncol.* 2012;19(9):2981-2991. doi:10.1245/s10434-012-2342-2

94. Chang SB, Palavecino M, Wray CJ, Kishi Y, Pisters PWT, Vauthey J-N. Modified Makuuchi incision for foregut procedures. *Arch Surg.* 2010;145(3):281-284. doi:10.1001/archsurg.2010.7

95. Toulmonde M, Bonvalot S, Méeus P, et al. Retroperitoneal sarcomas: patterns of care at diagnosis, prognostic factors and focus on main histological subtypes: a multicenter analysis of the French Sarcoma Group. *Ann Oncol.* 2014;25(3):735-742. doi:10.1093/annonc/mdt577

96. Zerhouni S, Van Coevorden F, Swallow CJ. The role and outcomes of palliative surgery for retroperitoneal sarcoma. *J Surg Oncol.* 2018;117(1):105-110. doi:10.1002/jso.24934

97. Callegaro D, Miceli R, Brunelli C, et al. Long-term morbidity after multivisceral resection for retroperitoneal sarcoma. *Br J Surg.* 2015;102(9):1079-1087. doi:10.1002/bjs.9829

98. McCarter MD, Antonescu CR, Ballman KV, et al. Microscopically positive margins for primary gastrointestinal stromal tumors: analysis of risk factors and tumor recurrence. *J Am Coll Surg.* 2012;215(1):53-60. doi:10.1016/j.jamcollsurg.2012.05.008

99. Kasper B, Baumgarten C, Garcia J, et al. An update on the management of sporadic desmoid-type fibromatosis: a European Consensus Initiative between Sarcoma Patients EuroNet (SPAEN) and European Organization for Research and Treatment of Cancer (EORTC)/Soft Tissue and Bone Sarcoma Group (STBSG). *Ann Oncol.* 2017;28(10):2399-2408. doi:10.1093/annonc/mdx323

100. Tan MC, Brennan MF, Kuk D, et al. Histology-based classification predicts pattern of recurrence and improves risk stratification in primary retroperitoneal sarcoma. *Ann Surg.* 2016;263(3):593-600. doi:10.1097/SLA.0000000000001149

101. Gronchi A, Miceli R, Allard MA, et al. Personalizing the approach to retroperitoneal soft tissue sarcoma: histology-specific patterns of failure and postrelapse outcome after primary extended resection. *Ann Surg Oncol.* 2015;22(5):1447-1454. doi:10.1245/s10434-014-4130-7

102. Pisters PW. Resection of some—but not all—clinically uninvolved adjacent viscera as part of surgery for retroperitoneal soft tissue sarcomas. *J Clin Oncol.* 2009;27(1):6-8. doi:10.1200/JCO .2008.18.7138

103. Crago AM. Extended surgical resection and histology in retroperitoneal sarcoma. *Ann Surg Oncol.* 2015;22(5):1401-1403. doi:10.1245/s10434-014-4135-2

104. Ikoma N, Roland CL, Torres KE, et al. Concomitant organ resection does not improve outcomes in primary retroperitoneal well-differentiated liposarcoma: a retrospective cohort study at a major sarcoma center. *J Surg Oncol.* 2018;117(6):1188-1194. doi:10.1002/jso.24951

105. Ito H, Hornick JL, Bertagnolli MM, et al. Leiomyosarcoma of the inferior vena cava: survival after aggressive management. *Ann Surg Oncol.* 2007;14(12):3534-3541. doi:10.1245/s10434 -007-9552-z

106. Keung EZ, Hornick JL, Bertagnolli MM, Baldini EH, Raut CP. Predictors of outcomes in patients with primary retroperitoneal dedifferentiated liposarcoma undergoing surgery. *J Am Coll Surg.* 2014;218(2):206-217. doi:10.1016/j.jamcollsurg.2013.10.009

107. Li B, Luo C-H, Zheng W. Risk factors for recurrence and survival in patients with primary retroperitoneal tumors. *J BUON.* 2013;18(3):782-787.

108. Molina G, Hull MA, Chen Y-L, et al. Preoperative radiation therapy combined with radical surgical resection is associated with a lower rate of local recurrence when treating unifocal, primary retroperitoneal liposarcoma. *J Surg Oncol.* 2016;114(7):814-820. doi:10.1002/jso.24427

109. Mussi C, Colombo P, Bertuzzi A, et al. Retroperitoneal sarcoma: is it time to change the surgical policy? *Ann Surg Oncol.* 2011;18(8):2136-2142. doi:10.1245/s10434-011-1742-z

110. Neuhaus SJ, Barry P, Clark MA, Hayes AJ, Fisher C, Thomas JM. Surgical management of primary and recurrent retroperitoneal liposarcoma. *Br J Surg.* 2005;92(2):246-252. doi:10.1002 /bjs.4802

111. Pacelli F, Tortorelli AP, Rosa F, et al. Retroperitoneal soft tissue sarcoma: prognostic factors and therapeutic approaches. *Tumori.* 2008;94(4):497-504.

112. Rhu J, Cho CW, Lee KW, et al. Radical nephrectomy for primary retroperitoneal liposarcoma near the kidney has a beneficial effect on disease-free survival. *World J Surg.* 2018;42(1):254-262. doi:10.1007/s00268-017-4157-6

113. Rossi CR, Varotto A, Pasquali S, et al. Patient outcome after complete surgery for retroperitoneal sarcoma. *Anticancer Res.* 2013;33(9):4081-4087.
114. Schwartz PB, Vande Walle K, Winslow ER, et al. Predictors of disease-free and overall survival in retroperitoneal sarcomas: a modern 16-year multi-institutional study from the United States Sarcoma Collaboration (USSC). *Sarcoma.* 2019;2019:5395131.
115. Smith HG, Panchalingam D, Hannay JA, et al. Outcome following resection of retroperitoneal sarcoma. *Br J Surg.* 2015;102(13):1698-1709. doi:10.1002/bjs.9934
116. Snow HA, Hitchen TX, Head J, et al. Treatment of patients with primary retroperitoneal sarcoma: predictors of outcome from an Australian specialist sarcoma centre. *ANZ J Surg.* 2018;88(11):1151-1157. doi:10.1111/ans.14842
117. Zhao X, Li P, Huang X, Chen L, Liu N, She Y. Prognostic factors predicting the postoperative survival period following treatment for primary retroperitoneal liposarcoma. *Chin Med J (Engl).* 2015;128(1):85-90. doi:10.4103/0366-6999.147822

Synoptic Operative Report: Extremity Sarcoma

Date of procedure _____   Surgeon(s) _____

_____

Preoperative biopsy

☐ Core biopsy
☐ Incisional biopsy
☐ Excisional biopsy
☐ None

Operative intent

☐ Curative
☐ Palliative

Management of adjacent tissues:
Select those resected

☐ En bloc
☐ Bone
☐ Muscle
☐ Nerve
☐ Periosteum
☐ Artery
☐ Vein
☐ Lymph node
☐ Other

Surgeon intraoperative
   assessment of margins

☐ R0
☐ R1
☐ R2

Synoptic Operative Report: Retroperitoneal Sarcoma

Date of procedure _____   Surgeon(s) _____

_____

Operative Intent	☐ Curative
	☐ Palliative
Preoperative biopsy	☐ Yes
	☐ No

Management of adjacent organs and describe if macroscopically involved or part of planned extended resection

☐ Abdominal wall
☐ Adrenal
☐ Bladder
☐ Coccyx/Sacrum
☐ Colon
☐ Gallbladder
☐ Kidney
☐ Liver
☐ Muscle
☐ Omentum
☐ Ovary
☐ Pancreas
☐ Prostate/Seminal vesicle
☐ Spleen
☐ Artery
☐ Vein
☐ Nerve
☐ Rib
☐ Rectum
☐ Small bowel
☐ Stomach
☐ Vagina
☐ Ureter
☐ Uterus
☐ Not examined
☐ Other

Synoptic Operative Report: Retroperitoneal Sarcoma

Date of procedure _____   Surgeon(s) _____

_____

Surgeon intraoperative assessment
of extent of resection

☐ R0/R1
Extended resection?
☐ Yes
☐ No
☐ R2

COMMENTARY: SARCOMA SECTION

Fritz C. Eilber, MD
Director, UCLA JCCC Sarcoma Program
Professor of Surgery
Professor of Molecular Pharmacology
UCLA Division of Surgical Oncology

There are two common types of surgical and/or management errors that unfortunately occur frequently with soft tissue sarcomas. Each of these highlights many of the important points made by the authors in the *Operative Standards for Cancer Surgery*, Volume 3.

The first and most well-known error is underestimating the aggressiveness of soft tissue tumors. This has been emphasized in the literature and surgical oncology teaching and is illustrated by this example. A presumed benign extremity tumor is resected through a horizontal incision with no preoperative imaging or tissue diagnosis, no drain is placed, and the patient gets a postoperative hematoma. Final pathology demonstrates a high-grade sarcoma with diffusely positive margins. A potentially curable patient is now in a limb-threatening and life-threatening situation. As highlighted by the authors, this can be avoided by appropriate preoperative workup which includes cross-sectional imaging and a core needle biopsy. Cross-sectional imaging with computed tomography (CT) or magnetic resonance imaging (MRI) is critical. An ultrasound is insufficient preoperative imaging. In most cases, an image-guided core needle biopsy should be obtained for tissue diagnosis. Image guidance (ultrasound or CT) by an experienced musculoskeletal or interventional radiologist is the optimal method to obtain an accurate pathologic diagnosis. Image guidance allows avoidance of neurovascular structures and, importantly, allows for targeting of areas within these often heterogeneous tumors. Although a core needle biopsy can occasionally be done safely in clinic without image guidance, it is far from optimal and carries unnecessary risks. Incisional or operative biopsies should be avoided and can significantly complicate surgical and oncologic management. Although an operative biopsy should be considered to seed the area of the surgical scar, the concern about seeding with core needle biopsies is overstated and basically a nonissue except for select histologic subtypes (chordoma, chondrosarcoma, etc.). Regardless, the importance of knowing the histologic subtype of sarcoma far outweighs any theoretic seeding risk.

The second error is when a patient undergoes an unnecessarily radical or morbid operation for either a nonaggressive or an aggressive sarcoma that would have benefited from preoperative therapy. Unfortunately, this is seen as frequently as the first, more well-known error. As stated by the authors in the *Operative Standards for Cancer Surgery*, Volume 3, "The goals of surgery as a component of multidisciplinary care vary to some degree based on the sarcoma subtype." I would even go a step further and state that surgery as a component of multidisciplinary care depends 100% on the sarcoma subtype. Surgical resection for a high-grade leiomyosarcoma abutting the neurovascular bundle is completely different than that for well-differentiated liposarcoma. An extraosseous Ewing sarcoma (primitive neuroectodermal tumor) needs preoperative chemotherapy, and a desmoid does not even necessarily need surgery at all. As the authors most appropriately state, "Initial diagnostics and multidisciplinary management at a sarcoma center are critical." Presentation of each patient's case in the context of a multidisciplinary sarcoma conference is the standard of care. Treatment decisions, including the extent of surgical resection, should be evaluated on an individual patient basis in the setting of an experienced multidisciplinary sarcoma program. Although broadly true for all malignancies, this is particularly critical for sarcoma as they are so rare and have such a broad range of histologic subtypes with similarly broad clinical behaviors.

Finally, sarcomas are mesenchymal malignancies and rarely, if ever, metastasize to regional lymph nodes. As the authors point out, there are a few histologic subtypes that occasionally can develop nodal spread; however, beyond occasionally performing as sentinel lymph node biopsy in these select subtypes, there is no role for nodal dissection in sarcoma surgery. Because of this, these mesenchymal malignancies have historically fit poorly into the American Joint Committee on Cancer (AJCC) Tumor Node Metastasis (TNM) staging system. To address this, the original prognostic models, or nomograms, were developed for soft tissue sarcoma and provide an individual patient outcome prediction rather than an often broad range of outcomes for a particular AJCC stage. Nomograms for soft tissue sarcoma are widely available based on site of primary disease and histology subtype and can help the physician and patient risk stratify the disease.

In summary, the authors highlight the important points in the evaluation, workup, and care of sarcoma patients. Understanding such standards for cancer surgery is critical in avoiding unnecessary and avoidable errors in oncologic patient care.

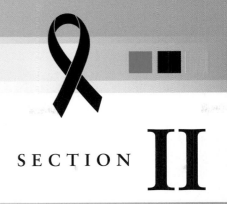

SECTION **II**

ADRENAL

INTRODUCTION

The two most common primary malignancies of the adrenal gland include adreno-cortical carcinoma (ACC), arising from the adrenal cortex, and malignant pheochromocytoma, arising from the adrenal medulla. Both cancers are extremely rare, with estimated incidences of 0.5 to 2 and 2 to 8 cases per million people each year, respectively.[1-4] In most cases, ACC is sporadic, follows a bimodal age distribution with peaks in childhood and the fourth and fifth decades of life, and represents 2% of all adrenal incidentalomas.

ACC is associated with a number of genetic mutations and is part of a number of hereditary syndromes such as Li-Fraumeni syndrome, Beckwith-Wiedemann syndrome, multiple endocrine neoplasia 1 syndrome, congenital adrenal hyperplasia, Lynch syndrome, familial polyposis coli, neurofibromatosis type 1 (NF-1), and Carney complex.[5-7] The highest prevalence of ACC is found in southern Brazil and is due to a significant prevalence in the population of germline TP53 mutations (Li-Fraumeni syndrome).[4,8,9]

Pheochromocytomas are catecholamine-secreting neuroendocrine tumors arising from chromaffin cells in the adrenal medulla.[10] Paragangliomas are extra-adrenal catecholamine-secreting tumors. The incidence of pheochromocytoma increases to 0.5% in patients with hypertension and can be as high as 4% in patients with adrenal incidentalomas.[3,10-12] Up to 30% of pheochromocytomas are associated with a variety of inherited conditions including multiple endocrine neoplasia type 2 syndrome, von Hippel-Lindau syndrome, NF-1, and hereditary paraganglioma syndromes due to succinate dehydrogenase mutations.[13,14] A minority of pheochromocytomas (10% to 17%) are clinically malignant; however, the incidence is higher than previously thought,[15-18] and all pheochromocytomas have the potential to be malignant according to the *World Health Organization Classification of Tumours of Endocrine Organs*.[17] In sporadic pheochromocytomas, less than 10% of tumors are malignant; however, in patients with mutations of the succinate dehydrogenase-B gene and tumors originating in extra-adrenal locations (paragangliomas), 30% to 50% may be malignant.[10]

This section will concentrate on the surgical management of ACC and malignant pheochromocytoma and will exclude paragangliomas.

CLINICAL STAGING

ACC is a rare and aggressive disease with a 5-year overall survival ranging from 39% to 55% after surgical resection performed with curative intent.[15,19-23] The majority of patients are diagnosed at an advanced stage, with approximately one-half having metastatic disease at diagnosis. Surgery is generally not pursued in these patients, and 5-year overall survival in patients with stage IV disease is reported to be 10%.[23] Systemic therapy has limited success, and surgery remains the only potentially curative treatment option for ACC.[23] Disease stage and margin-free resection are the most important prognostic factors in patients having undergone resection of ACC. The two most commonly used staging systems for ACC are those from the American Joint Committee on Cancer (AJCC)[24] and the European Network for the Study of Adrenal Tumors (Table 2-1).[23]

Currently, there is no staging system for malignant pheochromocytoma.

TABLE 2-1 American Joint Committee on Cancer Seventh/Eighth Editions and European Network for the Study of Adrenal Tumor Staging Systems

TABLE 2-1A AJCC Seventh/Eighth Editions and ENSAT Tumor (T) Stage Systems

Stage	AJCC Seventh/Eighth Editions	ENSAT
T1	Size ≤5 cm No extra-adrenal extension	Size ≤5 cm
T2	Size >5 cm No extra-adrenal extension	Size >5 cm
T3	Any size Extension into periadrenal fat	Infiltration into surrounding tissue
T4	Any size Extension into nearby tissues or organs (e.g., kidney, spleen, pancreas, liver, diaphragm, aorta, vena cava)	Invasion into adjacent organs or venous tumor thrombus in vena cava or renal vein

TABLE 2-1B AJCC and ENSAT Staging Classification

Stage	Description
I	T1, N0, M0
II	T2, N0, M0
III	T1–T2, N1, M0 T3–T4, N0–N1, M0
IV	T1–T4, N0-N1, M1

M0: no distant metastases; M1: presence of distant metastases; N0: no positive lymph node; N1: positive lymph node. *Note:* American Joint Committee on Cancer staging and TNM classification for adrenal cancer.[25] Used with permission of the American Joint Committee on Cancer (AJCC), Chicago, Illinois. The original and primary source for this information is the *AJCC Cancer Staging Manual*, Eighth Edition (2017) published by Springer International Publishing

MULTIDISCIPLINARY CARE

A multidisciplinary approach is crucial for optimal management of patients with ACC or malignant pheochromocytoma. Every case of suspected ACC or malignant pheochromocytoma should be discussed in detail with a panel of experts at the time of the initial diagnosis and routinely during follow-up to re-evaluate disease status and prognosis and to consider all diagnostic and treatment modalities available, including clinical trials. These panels should include at a minimum the following specialties: endocrinology, oncology, pathology, radiology, and surgery. In addition, successful management of these patients usually involves access to adrenal-specific expertise in interventional radiology, radiation oncology, nuclear medicine, genetics, and palliative care teams.[23]

Given the rarity of the disease, screening of the general population for ACC is not recommended. However, it is recommended that any patient diagnosed with ACC undergo genetic testing for germline mutations. The strongest evidence for genetic testing recommendations is for mutations of the TP53 gene (Li-Fraumeni syndrome)[6,26,27] and the mismatch repair genes MSH and MLH (Lynch syndrome).[9,23] Tissue obtained from the tumor can also be tested to identify somatic mutations which may guide personalized therapies. This is especially helpful when standard first- and second-line treatments have failed.

Genetic testing for germline mutations should be strongly considered in all patients diagnosed with pheochromocytoma. The operative procedure may be altered by the results of genetic testing, and are thus ideally reviewed prior to surgery. A panel of tests is commercially available for this purpose.[10,28]

Treatments for patients with ACC may include systemic or local therapeutic options. Timing of each (adjuvant, neoadjuvant, definitive, palliative) depends on the stage and extent of disease. Strategies for local control of disease can include surgery, radiofrequency ablation, cryotherapy, microwave ablation, external- or single-beam radiotherapy, and liver-directed therapies.

PERIOPERATIVE CARE

Every patient with an adrenal tumor should undergo careful evaluation with a detailed history and physical examination, accompanied by thorough endocrine biochemical testing and imaging using adrenal-specific protocols, as these are essential components to establish the origin of the tumor (cortex vs. medulla vs. other primary malignancy metastatic to the adrenal gland).[10,23] Table 2-2 summarizes the typical biochemical and imaging evaluation pursued in patients found to have an adrenal mass. ACC should be suspected in any patient with rapid development of signs and symptoms of Cushing syndrome[29] (muscle weakness, hypokalemia, muscle wasting, and constitutional symptoms) and/or a large retroperitoneal mass, although nearly one-half of patients will have no hormone excess, and ACCs smaller than 4 cm have been reported.[30] Signs and symptoms of sex steroid excess, including hirsutism or virilization in women or recent onset of gynecomastia in men, should also be elicited from the patient and are strong indicators of androgen- or estrogen-producing ACCs.[30,31] Any evidence of excess or autonomous secretion of more than one adrenal hormone should also raise suspicion of ACC.[23,30–32] Aldosterone-secreting ACCs are rare and can be accompanied by severe hypokalemia or autonomous cortisol secretion.[33] Furthermore, aldosterone-secreting ACCs are larger than most benign aldosteronomas but smaller than the average ACC.

A comprehensive biochemical analysis is not only crucial to diagnose hormone excess, but also aids in postoperative surveillance given hormone levels can be used as

TABLE 2-2   Diagnostic Evaluation for Patients with Suspected or Known Primary Adrenal Malignancy

Diagnostic Evaluation

Hormonal Workup

Glucocorticoid excess Sex steroids and steroid precursors Mineralocorticoid excess Catecholamine excess	• 1-mg dexamethasone suppression test − Alternatively, late-night salivary cortisol or serum bedtime cortisol • 24-h urine cortisol if overt clinical signs of cortisol excess to quantify degree of excess • Basal plasma ACTH • DHEA-S • 17-hydroxyprogesterone • Androstenedione • Testosterone (only in women) • 17-beta-estradiol (only in men and postmenopausal women) • 11-deoxycortisol • Potassium • Aldosterone • Renin • Fractionated plasma metanephrines and normetanephrines or 24-h urine

Imaging

	• Adrenal protocol CT or MRI of abdomen and pelvis • Chest CT if adrenal mass is indeterminate or malignant • ±FDG or DOTATATE PET/CT (DOTATATE if suspected pheochromocytoma) • Bone or brain imaging (if suspected skeletal or brain metastases)

Adrenal Biopsy

	• Not recommended in general unless mass is suspected to be a metastasis from a primary tumor of nonadrenal origin and no other suitable metastatic site can be biopsied to guide systemic treatment • Patients with possible adrenal lymphoma (often bilateral), those unfit for surgery from a medical standpoint, or those with unresectable disease when histopathologic proof is required to inform oncologic management

ACTH: adrenocorticotropic hormone; DHEA-S: dehydroepiandrosterone sulfate; FDG: ^{18}F-fluoro-2-deoxy-D-glucose.

markers of tumor recurrence.[23,32] Cortisol-secreting ACCs are associated with worse outcomes.[29] If hypercortisolism is present, it is important to prove adrenocorticotropic hormone independence. Finally, conventional computed tomography (CT) imaging cannot fully discriminate ACC from pheochromocytoma as both tumors are usually categorized as indeterminate according to CT criteria, but biochemistry or specialized imaging should distinguish between the two in almost all cases.

ACCs are usually large (7 to 10 cm on average), heterogeneous, and characterized by low lipid content with slower washout of contrast due to increased neovascularization. Careful evaluation of the tumor and the surrounding tissues for evidence of local invasion or locoregional nodal metastases as well as distant metastases is crucial to inform the overall treatment strategy, facilitate surgical planning when indicated, and predict long-term outcome. Imaging of the chest, abdomen, and pelvis should be obtained prior to initiation of any treatment for ACC or malignant pheochromocytoma. Lung and liver metastases are most common. Bone metastases are not uncommon. Brain metastases from ACC are rare, usually occurring more than 10 years after diagnosis.[23]

CT, magnetic resonance imaging (MRI), and ^{18}F-fluoro-2-deoxy-D-glucose positron emission tomography (FDG-PET) aid in differentiating benign from potentially malignant adrenal tumors. However, no single imaging method can definitively prove the diagnosis of ACC. CT and MRI criteria are optimized to identify benign lesions and are useful as tools to exclude adrenal malignancy.[34–38] Key to treatment of adrenal masses is that if an adrenal mass is categorized as indeterminate by imaging characteristics (and pheochromocytoma and other nonadrenal etiologies have been ruled out), the mass should be treated as if it is ACC until proven by final pathology. This affects surgical planning and conduct of the operation (if pursued), as the critical elements of adrenalectomy for ACC are different from those for benign adrenal disorders.

FDG-PET/CT may be used as a complementary imaging modality to further characterize an adrenal mass that falls in the indeterminate category after adrenal protocol CT or MRI. In addition, FDG-PET/CT may be used to detect extra-adrenal metastatic disease and nodal involvement.[34–37] MRI is preferred for evaluation of liver metastases and will often detect more than those identified via CT. MRI is also useful to understand the potential for vascular invasion by the tumor and presence and extent of intravenous tumor thrombus, given that CT is less specific in this regard. Recently, ^{68}Ga-DOTATATE-PET/CT has emerged and has greater sensitivity for the extent of disease when assessing neuroendocrine tumors, including pheochromocytoma.[37–39] The sensitivity for identifying metastatic disease is superior to other imaging modalities, except for within the liver, for which MRI remains superior.

Biopsy of an adrenal mass is to be avoided in general and should never be pursued before ruling out either resectable ACC or pheochromocytoma. Differentiation of benign from malignant adrenocortical tumors via biopsy is challenging; may lead to misdiagnosis; and may result in hemorrhage, tumor seeding of the needle tract,[40–43] and hypertensive crisis if the tumor is a pheochromocytoma.[44] Specific indications for biopsy might include concern for metastasis to the adrenal gland (although often unnecessary if it is the only site of disease because resection is often pursued), infectious etiologies, lymphoma, need for tissue diagnosis to proceed with neoadjuvant chemotherapy, or patients who are not candidates for surgery. Often, other sites of disease are more amenable to biopsy in patients with ACC with metastatic disease.[40,45]

Given the aggressive nature of ACC, the decision to proceed with surgery should be made only if complete resection of the tumor is anticipated.[23,41] Open adrenalectomy with multivisceral resection, vascular reconstruction, and/or lymphadenectomy when indicated remains the preferred surgical approach for any known or suspected ACC.[23,41,46,47] Neoadjuvant chemotherapy for ACC may increase the chance of R0 resection; R1 resections are associated with worse outcomes.[48] Cytoreductive or R2 resections for ACC and malignant pheochromocytoma are to be avoided because they are associated with high rates of progression and limited to no durable improvement in overall survival. In highly selected situations, there may be some benefit in controlling severe hormone excess or preservation of a vital structure.[20,23,41]

There is now sufficient evidence to suggest that adrenalectomy performed by a high-volume surgeon is associated with shorter length of hospital stay and fewer complications.[49–51] In addition, the creation of national centers for adrenal surgery improved disease-free survival in the Netherlands.[2,52] The complexity of surgery for ACC and malignant pheochromocytoma requires expertise in both adrenal and oncologic surgery. Furthermore, owing to the complexity of some operations, involvement of surgeons with complementary expertise (e.g., endocrine, vascular, hepatobiliary, urologic, cardiothoracic, transplant) may be required.[23] To ensure that the pathologist can judge the completeness of surgery, any fragmentation or morcellation of the tumor is to be avoided. Use of synoptic operative and pathology reports is recommended and useful for downstream management (see Synoptic Operative Reports at the end of this section). Suggested components for the synoptic operative report can be found at the end of this section. The College of American Pathologists has developed a synoptic pathology report. In addition to the included metrics, inclusion of additional information regarding number of tumor sections examined, specimen integrity (capsular disruption, tumor fragmentation), site(s) of lymph node(s) removed, and ratio of positive to total number of lymph nodes removed by site can further optimize the clinical utility of the report. Microsatellite instability status and presence of mutations may also be helpful.

Preoperative excess hormone secretion can be treated in partnership with an endocrinologist using various medications (Table 2-3).[45] In consultation with an endocrinologist, intraoperative and postoperative glucocorticoid replacement is often recommended, preferably with hydrocortisone, in all patients with overt Cushing syndrome. In those with evidence of possible or mild autonomous cortisol secretion (post-dexamethasone cortisol $\geq$50 to 140 nmol/L or $\geq$1.8 to 5 µg/dL),[53,54] steroid administration may be held and postoperative testing of the hypothalamic-pituitary-adrenal axis may be performed at the direction of an endocrinologist. Postoperatively, the dose of glucocorticoid should be tapered on an individualized basis.[23,41,45,53,54]

For patients with malignant pheochromocytoma, preoperative alpha-blockade alone or in combination with beta-blockade, depending on the clinical scenario, is recommended to prevent perioperative cardiovascular, renal, and/or neurologic complications (Table 2-4).[10] Selective alpha-blockers have become more popular in recent years as phenoxybenzamine has become less available and more expensive.[55–57] Calcium channel blockers such as nicardipine can be prescribed in addition to alpha-blockers in patients with difficult-to-control hypertension or alone in those with minimal to no hypertension who may not tolerate the effects of alpha-blockade.[10] It is in rare circumstances that calcium channel blockers should be considered as the

TABLE 2-3   Medications to Control Adrenal Hormone Excess

Type of Medication	Medication	Mechanism of Action	Starting Dose	Notes
Cortisol (first line)	Metyrapone	Inhibits 11-beta-hydroxylase	250 mg every 4 h; not to exceed 6 g/d	First choice for moderate to severe cortisol excess. Monitor cortisol and 11-deoxycortisol levels.
Cortisol (alternative)	Ketoconazole	Inhibits 11-beta-hydroxylase, 17-hydroxylase, and 17,20-lyase	200 mg daily; goal, 600–800 mg daily	Not effective for moderate to severe HC
Cortisol (alternative)	Mifepristone	Cortisol receptor blocker	300 mg daily; maximum 1,200 mg daily	Cannot use cortisol level to monitor effect as receptor blockade leads to rise in cortisol. Monitor by symptoms and glucose levels.
Cortisol (alternative)	Etomidate	Inhibits 11-beta-hydroxylase	0.04 mg/kg/h intravenous	Requires ICU monitoring
Cortisol (alternative)	Mitotane	Inhibits cholesterol side-chain cleavage enzyme, 11-beta-hydroxylase, 18-hydroxylase, and 3β-hydroxysteroid dehydrogenase	1 g twice daily	Ineffective for moderate to severe cortisol excess; adrenolytic; requires steroid replacement in those without hormone excess; derivative of insecticide DDT
Cortisol (alternative)	Osilodrostat	Inhibits 11-β-hydroxylase and aldosterone synthase	2 mg twice daily	Monitor cortisol level; titrate slowly.
Aldosterone	Spironolactone	MR antagonist	25 mg daily	Counteracts mineralocorticoid effect of excess cortisol and hypokalemia in severe cases
	Eplerenone	MR antagonist	50 mg daily	
	Amiloride	Antikaliuretic diuretic	5 mg daily	
Androgens	Spironolactone	Blocks androgen receptor	25 mg daily	Monitor potassium level and volume status.
Estrogens (males)	Anastrozole	Aromatase inhibitor	1 mg daily	Assess thromboembolic risk.

DDT: dichloro-diphenyl-trichloroethane; HC: hypercortisolism; ICU: intensive care unit; MR: mineralocorticoid receptor.

TABLE 2-4   Common Medications for Preoperative Blockade of Pheochromocytoma

Medication	Description
Phenoxybenzamine	• Irreversible nonselective alpha-antagonist with a half-life of 24 h • Start at least 10–14 d before surgery, 10 mg b.i.d. to t.i.d. and titrate to effect • Once alpha-blockade is established, beta receptor blockers can be used to treat reflex tachycardia unresponsive to fluid administration. • Can result in longer periods of postoperative hypotension owing to long half-life compared with other alpha-blockers • May be difficult to obtain from pharmacies; prohibitively expensive when not covered by insurance
Doxazosin, prazosin, terazosin	• Competitive antagonists of alpha-1 adrenergic receptors with minimal alpha-2 receptor effects • Start at least 10–14 d before surgery and titrate to effect. • Generally shorter half-lives, less reflex tachycardia, and lower incidence of postoperative hypotension compared with phenoxybenzamine • Incidence and duration of intraoperative hypertensive episodes can be significantly greater compared with phenoxybenzamine • Greater availability, generally more affordable and more likely to be covered by insurance compared with phenoxybenzamine
Calcium channel blockers	• Blocks norepinephrine-mediated calcium influx in smooth muscles leading to arterial vasodilation • Can be combined with alpha-blockers when necessary (starting doses: nifedipine, 30 mg/d; nicardipine, 20 mg t.i.d., or 30 mg b.i.d. if sustained release; amlodipine, 5 mg/d) • Incidence and duration of intraoperative hypertensive episodes can be significantly greater compared with phenoxybenzamine. • Useful in patients with no or minimal preoperative hypertension or in patients who cannot tolerate alpha-blockade and can be used in combination with other antihypertensives
Metyrosine	• Rarely used; usually reserved for patients with highly active pheochromocytomas who cannot tolerate alpha-blockers or have hypertension refractory to alpha receptor, beta receptor blockers, and calcium channel blockers • Tyrosine hydroxylase inhibitor limiting production of catecholamines • Start 250 mg p.o. q.i.d. Increase by 250–500 mg total daily up to 4 g/d maximum. • Decreases cardiovascular specific complications (i.e., arrhythmias) and intraoperative hemodynamic variability • Delayed onset of effect until existing/stored catecholamines have been released. • Side effects may include somnolence, depression, and galactorrhea. • Expensive, can be difficult to obtain from pharmacies (including hospital based)

b.i.d.: twice a day; p.o.: by mouth; q.i.d.: four times a day; t.i.d.: three times a day.

sole first-line therapy. This decision should be made by someone highly experienced in managing and operating on patients with pheochromocytoma. Preoperative alpha-adrenergic receptor blockade, always started prior to any beta-blockade, is usually initiated at least 7 to 14 days, if not longer, before the scheduled operation to allow adequate time to optimize blood pressure and heart rate and expand intravascular volume. Treatment includes liberalizing sodium in the diet and fluid intake, depending on comorbidities.

Postoperatively, although adjuvant therapy with mitotane is considered in all patients with ACC, it is specifically recommended in those perceived to be at a high risk of recurrence. First-line chemotherapy, in addition to mitotane, for those with residual disease or who develop metastases includes etoposide, doxorubicin, and cisplatin. Adjuvant radiation therapy can be considered in addition to mitotane therapy on an individual basis.[7,23,41,45] The decision for reoperative surgery in patients with recurrent ACC is complex, based on multiple factors, and if pursued should be done with caution given the high rate of re-recurrence and often short duration of benefit.[58]

In patients with metastatic pheochromocytoma, surgery may be carefully considered on an individual basis, as benefit can be gained with surgery[59]; however, tumor debulking alone should be viewed with caution as this has not been associated with long-term clinically significant biochemical response in some studies.[60] For those patients diagnosed with an unresectable malignant pheochromocytoma or evidence of metastatic disease not amenable to local therapy, treatment with iodine ^{131}I metaiodobenzylguanidine (also known as iobenguane ^{131}I)[61] or lutetium ^{177}Lu DOTATATE[62] may be considered.

QUALITY MEASURES

Formalized quality measures for rare cancers can be difficult to develop owing to the scarcity of data, and ACC and malignant pheochromocytoma are not exceptions. Although there are various guidelines that provide best-management approaches for ACC, the only factors associated with better outcomes have been guideline-centered care, R0 resection of the tumor, and treatment at referral centers with multidisciplinary teams comprising specialists in multiple fields with expertise in the management of adrenal disorders. In light of this, the greatest quality measure for these patients may ultimately be referral to large multidisciplinary centers.

CHAPTER 3

Adrenalectomy Including Multivisceral Resection

CRITICAL ELEMENTS

- Resection of the Primary Tumor to Microscopically Negative Margins without Disruption of the Tumor Capsule
- En Bloc Resection of Adjacent Organs Directly Invaded by Cancer

1. RESECTION OF THE PRIMARY TUMOR TO MICROSCOPICALLY NEGATIVE MARGINS WITHOUT DISRUPTION OF THE TUMOR CAPSULE

Recommendation: The primary objective of adrenalectomy is microscopically complete (R0) resection of the primary tumor. The tumor and the surrounding retroperitoneal fat, Gerota fascia, and peritoneum should be resected en bloc.

Type of Data: Retrospective reports, case series, or case-control studies

Strength of Recommendation: Strong recommendation, moderate-quality evidence

Rationale

Surgery is the primary treatment modality for nonmetastatic, technically resectable *adrenocortical carcinoma* (ACC).[23,63,64] In highly selected cases, often after chemotherapy, some primary tumors may be resected in patients with synchronous metastatic disease (see Adrenal Key Question 2).[48,65,66] At surgery, microscopically complete (R0) resection of the primary tumor, along with any regional lymph nodes, organs, or blood vessels involved by cancer—without disruption of the tumor capsule—is critical.

Incomplete resection of cancer that has invaded through the capsule into the periadrenal fat or has spilled via disruption of the tumor capsule at surgery can lead to local recurrence and peritoneal carcinomatosis. Multiple studies have reported that microscopically or macroscopically incomplete (R1 or R2) resection as well as older age, high tumor grade, distant metastasis, the use of a laparoscopic approach, micro- and macroscopic lymphovascular invasion, cortisol production, and the need for resection of contiguous organs or vascular structures at surgery are all associated with cancer recurrence and shorter overall survival.[20,47,64,67–72] In one study, the 5-year survival rate was 50.4% after R0 resection, 23.2% after R1 resection, and 10.8% after R2 resection. The median survival duration after R0 resection was 51.2 months versus 7.0 months after a margin-positive resection.[20] These data emphasize the critical need for an R0 resection at surgery.

Wide, en bloc resection of the tumor and the surrounding retroperitoneal fat, Gerota fascia, and peritoneum is advised at the time of adrenalectomy for ACC. Microscopic periadrenal invasion by cancer cells has been reported in up to 25% of cases in which invasion is not anticipated on the basis of either preoperative imaging or intraoperative findings.[47] Limited resection of the gland without surrounding fat may therefore leave microscopic disease in situ following resection. Furthermore, it may affect the delivery of subsequent stage-specific therapy, as invasion of the periadrenal fat indicates stage III disease for which adjuvant therapy is recommended.[47]

For pheochromocytoma, radicality of resection is equally as important as it is for ACC. In patients with pheochromocytoma, inadvertent surgical disruption of the capsule of the tumor may result in pheochromocytomatosis. This phenomenon is increasingly identified in the era of laparoscopic surgery, is characterized by dissemination of adrenal medullary cells throughout the abdomen, and is similar to the peritoneal carcinomatosis that is associated with ACC.

At adrenalectomy, any indeterminate mass of adrenocortical origin should be treated by the surgeon as malignant. The following technical strategies should be used to increase the likelihood of an R0 resection.

Technical Aspects

The anatomic location of the adrenal glands dictates the technical approach necessary to achieve an R0 resection. Both adrenal glands are located in the retroperitoneum and are surrounded by Gerota fascia and retroperitoneal adipose tissue. An appropriate incision must allow adequate access to the tumor (Fig. 2-1). Classically, a wide subcostal incision, with or without cranial extension, provides ample access to a right or left adrenal tumor. Vertical midline, flank, Makuuchi,[73] and thoracoabdominal incisions are also appropriate, and each has unique advantages and disadvantages. Thoracoabdominal incisions are rarely required but may be helpful for reoperative cases or cases in which a large, invasive tumor extends into the thoracic cavity.

Exploration of the peritoneal cavity is performed to ensure the absence of peritoneal or visceral metastases. The liver is released from its attachments to the level of the diaphragm. Intraoperative ultrasound may be performed to reevaluate the liver for metastatic disease; to evaluate the major vasculature for evidence of direct invasion or intravascular thrombus; and to evaluate the liver, kidneys, and pancreas for evidence of direct invasion. In all cases, direct visualization of the tumor should be avoided when possible, and the tumor should be handled as little as possible in order to minimize the possibility of capsule disruption.

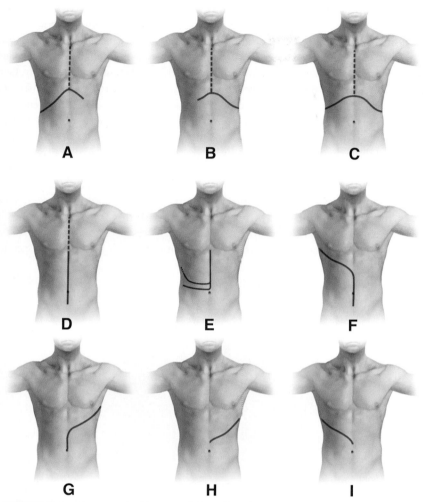

FIGURE 2-1   Common incisions used for adrenalectomy, dependent on patient and tumor characteristics and need for vascular access. **A,B:** Subcostal. **C:** Bilateral subcostal. **D:** Midline. **E:** Makuuchi—two options, the more cranial horizontal line allowing for extension between the ribs if desired. **F,G:** Thoracoabdominal. **H,I:** Flank extending between ribs. *Dashed line* indicates possible extension of incision.

Right adrenalectomy

For right adrenalectomy, mobilization of the right colon, hepatic flexure, and transverse colon is dictated by the extent of the tumor. In most cases, mobilization of the hepatic flexure to the inferior vena cava (IVC) and aorta followed by a Kocher maneuver suffices to gain access to the cranial aspect of the kidney and renal hilum. The right lobe of the liver is mobilized, releasing the triangular and coronary ligaments. Mobilization of the left lobe is also helpful, as this allows the liver to rotate about the vena cava.

Resection of the adrenal mass should include a wide, en bloc resection of the retroperito-neal fat surrounding the gland (Fig. 2-2A). Shelling out the gland from the periadrenal and perirenal fat should be avoided. Attempting to create a plane where none exists between the tumor and adjacent organ (liver, kidney, vena cava, etc.) should likewise be avoided as shedding of tumor cells may lead to tumor bed and peritoneal recurrence. Similarly, Gerota fascia and the posterior parietal peritoneum should be resected en bloc; these structures represent the anterior surgical margin unless the tumor invades the posterior liver.

The fat caudal to the adrenal gland and tumor overlying the cranial half of the kid-ney and the renal hilum should be dissected and mobilized cranially to provide a cau-dal margin. Similarly, dissection laterally to the abdominal sidewall, cranially along the diaphragm, and posteriorly to the musculature should be performed to achieve wide margins around the tumor. Dissection over the anterior aspect of the vena cava from left to right allows for preservation of as much soft tissue adjacent to the medial aspect of the adrenal gland and tumor. Dissection posterior to the IVC should also strive to reach the medial aspect of the vena cava to resect adjacent soft tissue and lymphatic channels. There are few, if any, lymph nodes in this area of the dissection.

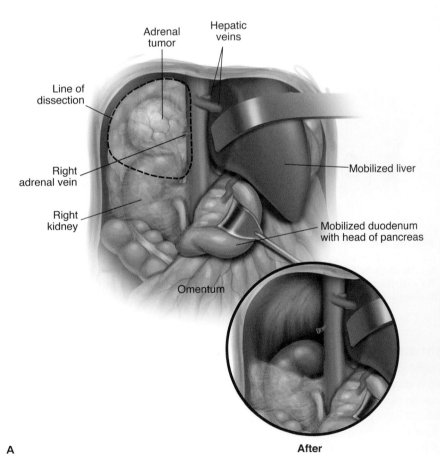

A   **After**

FIGURE 2-2   Exposure and line of dissection for right (**A**)

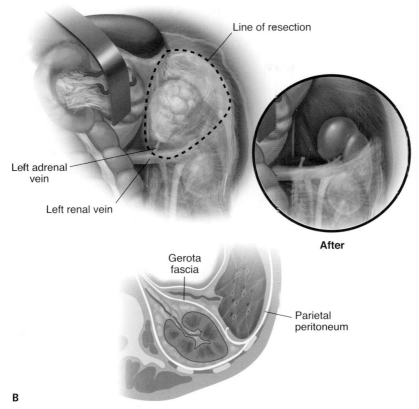

Line of resection

Left adrenal vein

Left renal vein

After

Gerota fascia

Parietal peritoneum

B

FIGURE 2-2 *(continued)* and left (**B**) adrenalectomy. The periadrenal fat and Gerota fascia should be included with the tumor to provide ample margins.

There are two particular areas of concern on the right side with respect to resection margins. The first is the medial aspect of the gland where it abuts the IVC. The right adrenal vein is usually quite short. Typically, there is little, if any, tissue between the adrenal gland and IVC. To achieve a complete resection, the entire posterolateral aspect of the IVC must therefore be skeletonized, and exquisite care must be taken to ensure a complete resection in this area. Further, although the IVC is not frequently invaded directly, tumor thrombus may enter the lumen of the vena cava, typically via the adrenal vein orifice, mandating resection of a portion of the vena cava wall at the adrenal vein orifice, tumor thrombectomy, and closure or reconstruction of the venorrhaphy. (See Chapter 4.) A second area of concern on the right side is the caudal aspect of the gland that may extend to and/or involve the kidney or vasculature of the renal hilum. Owing to concern for potential injury to the renal hilum, a small portion of adrenal tissue might inadvertently be left near the renal hilum if not carefully and completely dissected.

Left adrenalectomy

Left adrenalectomy is performed in a similar fashion (Fig. 2-2B). A left medial visceral rotation, leaving the kidney in place, is performed. The lesser sac need not be entered unless imaging and intraoperative findings suggest the need for distal pancreatectomy.

Unlike the case with tumors on the right, there is no well-defined peritoneal lining overlying the anterior aspect of the left adrenal gland, and mobilization of soft tissue on the surface of the gland with the pancreas and splenic vessels must be carefully avoided as the spleen and pancreas are mobilized medially. Gerota fascia in this area is often thin after mobilizing the spleen and pancreas, allowing visualization of the adrenal gland through a thin film of extra-adrenal tissue. Dissection along the antero-lateral aspect of the left side of the aorta will allow identification of an optimal plane to release soft tissue from the anterior and lateral aorta toward the medial border of the adrenal gland. Thickened ganglion tissue, lymph nodes from around the celiac axis and superior mesenteric artery, and enlarged lymphatic channels that can result in a significant leak if not properly ligated are often encountered. (See Chapter 5.)

The medial aspect of the left adrenal gland abuts the body of the pancreas and the splenic vessels. Typically, the pancreas and left adrenal gland are separated by the anterior aspect of Gerota fascia, a thin plane of tissue less robust than the parietal peritoneum on the right. The caudal tip of the left adrenal gland often extends more caudally toward the left renal hilum than on the right. Thus, care must be taken in this area to completely excise the gland without injuring the renal hilar structures. As on the right side, ACCs on the left may present with evidence of venous tumor thrombus involving the left adrenal vein, communicating vein to the phrenic vein, left renal vein, and IVC. (See Chapter 4.)

2. EN BLOC RESECTION OF ADJACENT ORGANS DIRECTLY INVADED BY CANCER

Recommendation: If direct invasion of an adjacent organ or muscle is suspected intraoperatively, the structure(s) should be resected en bloc with the primary adrenal tumor. Creation of an artificial plane between the primary tumor and an invaded structure should not be attempted.

Type of Data: Retrospective reports, case series, or case-control studies

Strength of Recommendation: Strong recommendation, moderate-quality evidence

Rationale
Extra-adrenal invasion of adjacent organs by ACC is common. The rate of multiorgan resection at the time of adrenalectomy is as high as 40% in some series. The most commonly resected organs are the kidney (56%), liver (28%), spleen (24%), and pancreas (16%). A study of 167 patients demonstrated that as long as resection margins were negative, adrenalectomy with en bloc resection of involved adjacent organs was associated with nearly identical disease-free and overall survival durations as resection of tumors that did not invade adjacent organs.[74] This is the most convincing evidence to date that en bloc resection of adjacent organs is appropriate as long as negative margins can be achieved. In contrast, en bloc resection of organs not directly invaded by ACC does not prolong time to recurrence or survival.

Malignant pheochromocytomas may also invade adjacent organs but do so less often than ACC. The approach used to resect an invasive malignant pheochromocytoma should be similar to that used to resect ACC.

Technical Aspects

Careful review of preoperative imaging is essential to allow for appropriate surgical planning and promote effective intraoperative decision-making. Intraoperatively, if a tissue plane is not readily apparent between the tumor and adjacent organs, the surgeon should be prepared to remove the organ or a portion of the organ en bloc with the tumor.

Resection of invasive ACC is often more straightforward on the left compared with the right. The surrounding organs often necessitating en bloc resection on the left include the spleen, kidney, body and tail of the pancreas, and diaphragm.

Resection of a large, invasive ACC on the right side can be more problematic owing to the possibility of invasion of the posterior aspect of the liver, IVC, and/or diaphragm. Because the right adrenal gland is normally intimately associated with the posterior aspect of the liver, it may not be possible to determine with certainty if there is invasion into the liver on preoperative imaging; thus, the surgeon must be prepared to perform liver resection or IVC resection with reconstruction even if no definite evidence of invasion is identified preoperatively. If adherence to, or minimal invasion of, the liver is noted intraoperatively, a thin rim of liver can be resected en bloc with the tumor in a nonanatomic fashion to negative margins. Intraoperative ultrasound may assist with this evaluation. If gross invasion of the liver not amenable to nonanatomic liver resection is noted, the decision should be made early as to whether the liver will be divided before or after mobilization of the adrenal gland; early mobilization and division of the right lobe of the liver can facilitate resection of very large right ACCs invading or adherent to the right liver.

The diaphragm is usually easily managed if a portion requires resection to achieve negative cranial margins. Partial resection of the diaphragm may also facilitate the dissection along the supra- and retrohepatic vena cava. Standard methods for reconstruction should be used.

Management of the kidney and its hilum will vary dependent on the situation. Direct invasion of the renal vein distal to the gonadal vein affords the opportunity for local resection with or without reconstruction, as drainage may be sufficient through the gonadal vein alone. Involvement of the perirenal fat should not necessitate nephrectomy if there is no clear involvement of the renal parenchyma. If the parenchyma does appear to be involved, a portion of it may be excised to a negative margin, preserving as much kidney parenchyma as possible (Fig. 2-3).

Partial or total nephrectomy may be necessary depending on the degree of involvement by the tumor. Importantly, if preoperative imaging is suggestive of the need for nephrectomy, neoadjuvant chemotherapy may be warranted in selected situations given that first-line chemotherapy for ACC (etoposide, doxorubicin, cisplatin plus mitotane) is nephrotoxic. Assessment of bilateral contribution to renal function via nuclear scintigraphy prior to nephrectomy should also be considered for the purposes of preoperative planning, patient counseling, and postoperative management.

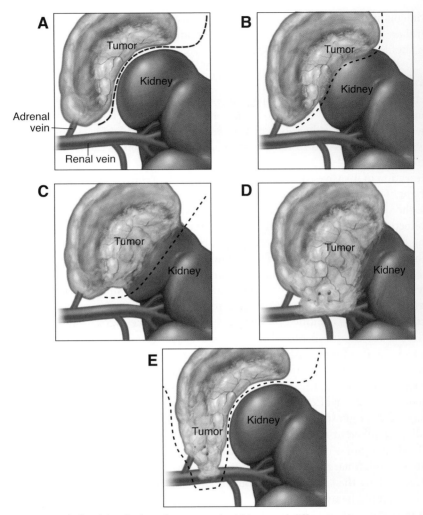

FIGURE 2-3 Relationship of adrenal tumor to the kidney and differences in management. The renal vein overlies the renal artery in this figure and is hidden from view. **A:** No adherence or invasion with standard resection including periadrenal fat dissected off of the kidney. **B:** Adherence of tumor to the perirenal fat or external renal capsule without renal invasion managed by dissection beneath the renal capsule to obtain negative margins and preserve renal parenchyma. **C:** Limited direct invasion of renal parenchyma by tumor and without involvement of renal hilar vasculature necessitating partial or total nephrectomy. **D:** Direct invasion of renal parenchyma including renal vasculature not amenable to partial nephrectomy or vascular reconstruction. **E:** Isolated renal vein invasion without invasion of renal parenchyma potentially amenable to renal vein ligation and preservation of venous outflow through the gonadal vein, a duplicate vein, or venous reconstruction.

Adrenal Key Question 1

In patients with stage I/II adrenocortical carcinoma (ACC), is minimally invasive adrenalectomy associated with similar rates of R0 resection, 5-year disease-free survival, and overall survival compared with open adrenalectomy?

INTRODUCTION

ACC is an aggressive malignancy. A microscopically complete (R0) resection with or without additional adjuvant therapy offers patients the best chance for cure.[20,23,41,67,75–77] The goal of adrenalectomy is complete en bloc resection of the primary tumor, other involved organs or structures, and any clinically involved regional lymph nodes. General consensus exists that ACCs should be resected using an open surgical technique when tumors are large, locally invasive into surrounding organs or major vessels (T4) or are associated with clinically evident regional lymphadenopathy (N1). However, controversy exists with respect to the role of minimally invasive surgery, particularly for tumors that are less than 6 cm in diameter and appear to be confined to the adrenal gland (stage I/II tumors).[23,41]

Concerns regarding the use of minimally invasive adrenalectomy for ACC relate to a perceived inability to perform the oncologically critical elements of the operation using minimally invasive surgery and the greater potential for tumor rupture and/or margin-positive resection. Ultimately, there is concern for early local disease recurrence, peritoneal carcinomatosis, and decreased overall survival relative to the risk with open surgery. ACCs tend to be fragile tumors with a thin capsule. In stage I and stage II tumors, microscopic disruption of the capsule and spread of tumor cells into the retroperitoneum or peritoneum can lead to local recurrence and/or peritoneal carcinomatosis even without gross tumor rupture. A high priority must be placed on avoiding capsule disruption, intraoperative tumor spillage, and positive surgical margins (R1 or R2). The purpose of this work was to evaluate whether minimally invasive adrenalectomy is associated with similar rates of R0 resection, 5-year disease-free survival, and overall survival in patients with stage I/II ACC compared with open adrenalectomy.

METHODOLOGY

A systematic search of PubMed was performed from 1990 to 2019 beginning in January, 2018. The final search was performed on September 15, 2019. Medical Subject Headings (MeSH) terms included "Adrenalectomy," "Adrenocortical Carcinoma," "Laparoscopic," "Minimally Invasive," "Retroperitoneoscopic," or "Robotic." Searches were restricted to English language and human subjects. Findings are reported in accordance with the Preferred Reporting Items for Systematic Reviews and Meta-Analyses (PRISMA).[78]

The initial search yielded 190 articles (Fig. 2-4), after which 126 articles were excluded. Reasons for exclusion included 5 studies reporting malignancies of nonadrenal origin and 12 studies reporting benign adrenal disease. Twenty-three studies could not be found in English, and 27 studies involved animals. Other reasons for exclusion

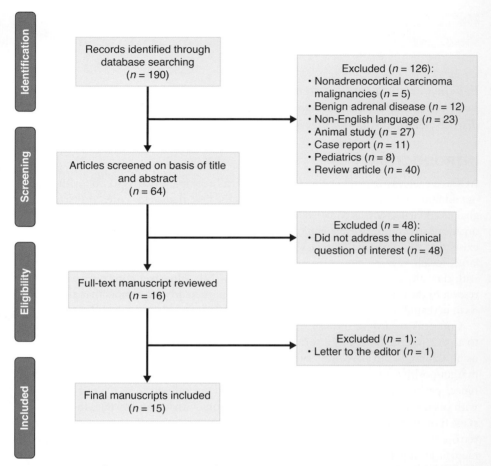

FIGURE 2-4   Preferred Reporting Items for Systematic Reviews and Meta-Analyses diagram for literature regarding whether minimally invasive adrenalectomy in patients with stage I/II adrenocortical carcinoma is associated with similar rates of R0 resection, 5-year disease-free survival, and overall survival compared with open adrenalectomy.

included reports focusing on the pediatric population (8) or case reports (11). Forty review articles were also excluded. The remaining 64 abstracts were reviewed with an additional 48 excluded due to not addressing the clinical question of interest. Sixteen full-text manuscripts were fully reviewed. One letter to the editor was excluded; thus, 15 studies ultimately met all criteria for inclusion in the systematic review.[47,79–92]

Data were extracted from individual studies by the writing group. Each article was reviewed and assigned a quality of evidence based on the Grading of Recommendations, Assessment, Development, and Evaluation (GRADE) system.[93] The quality of the data and size of the studies precluded the ability to perform a meta-analysis.

Fifteen studies were included in the qualitative systematic review (Table 2-5). All studies were retrospective and nonrandomized. Data for included studies were collected single institutions, multiple institutions, or national databases or registries. The overall quality ranged from low to moderate.

TABLE 2-5 Selected Studies Comparing Laparoscopic and Open Approaches to Adrenalectomy for Adrenocortical Carcinoma

Author, Year	Data Source	Study Patients, N	Cases, n LA/OA	Median Tumor Size, cm LA/OA	AJCC or ENSAT Stage, % LA/OA	Tumor Rupture, % LA/OA	+ Margin, % LA/OA	Overall Survival, mo LA/OA	Recurrence, mo LA/OA	Grade of Evidence*	Comments
Brix et al.,[94] 2010	German ACC registry	152	35/117	6.2/8.0 $P = .001$	ENSAT III 89/68 $P = .001$	9/15 $P = .4$	6/12 $P = .45$	NR $P = .55$	Any site $P = .82$	+++	12/35 LA converted to OA (final coding of approach in this situation not stated)
Cooper et al.,[95] 2013	Institutional	92	46/46	8.0/12.3 $P = <.0001$	AJCC T1, T2 63/56 $P = .1$	NR	28.3/8.7 $P = .01$	Median 54/110 $P = .07$	Median RFS 11/20 $P = .005$	++	Peritoneal recurrence 54%/19%; $P = .006$ R2 resections excluded in data calculations
Donatini et al.,[96] 2014	Institutional	34	13/21	5.5/6.8 $P = .112$	All ENSAT I, II	Excluded	Excluded	% survival at 5 y: 85/81 $P = .634$	5-y LA = 31% OA = 24% $P = .655$	++	Stage I, II ENSAT only No differences in 5-y recurrence or survival R1, R2 resections not included in data

(continued)

TABLE 2-5 Selected Studies Comparing Laparoscopic and Open Approaches to Adrenalectomy for Adrenocortical Carcinoma (continued)

Author, Year	Data Source	Study Patients, N	Cases, n LA/OA	Median Tumor Size, cm LA/OA	AJCC or ENSAT Stage, % LA/OA	Tumor Rupture, % LA/OA	+ Margin, % LA/OA	Overall Survival, mo LA/OA	Recurrence, mo LA/OA	Grade of Evidence*	Comments
Fosså et al.,[79] 2013	Institutional	32	17/15	8.0/13.0 $P = .002$	ENSAT I, II 76/46 $P = .06$	29/13	29/20 $P = 1.0$	Median 103.6/36.5 $P = .22$	Median PFS 15.2/8.1 $P = .06$	++	ENSAT stage I, II 12% conversion from LA to OA Pattern of recurrence similar LA vs. OA
Gonzalez et al.,[80] 2005	Institutional	160	6/154	6.0/13.0 $P = .0003$	AJCC I, II 100/64	16/1.3	R1 status NR	LA = NR OA = 43	LA = NR OA = 13	++	Multivisceral resection in 35.9% OA Peritoneal carcinomatosis as initial site of recurrence, 83% LA vs. 8% OA; $P = .0001$ Tumors ≤6 cm, 66.6% OA, no recurrence at 21 mo. 5/5 LA ≤6 cm recurred, 1 rupture, 4/5 died (mean 12-mo survival)

Study	Type	N								Comments
Huynh et al.,[81] 2016	NCDB	423	137/286 8.0/12.7 P < .001	ENSAT I, II 69.3/57.1	NR	15% vs. 18% overall (see comments)	NR	Data not captured by NCDB	++	Higher + margin rate in T3 subgroup LA, 54.7% vs. OA, 21.7% P = .0009 Low-grade evidence due to lack of certain data fields and confounding variables
Leboulleux et al.,[82] 2010	Institutional	61	6/55 6.9/13.7 P = .006	ENSAT I, II 83/52	NR	NR	Survival after development of peritoneal carcinomatosis: 5/38 P = NR	2-y RFS any site 66%/28% P = .07	++	Surgical approach the only factor associated with development of peritoneal carcinomatosis Peritoneal carcinomatosis in 4/6 LA, 11/55 OA; P = .016
Lee et al.,[97] 2017	Multi-institutional	201	47/154 5.5/10.9 P = .001	AJCC T1, T2 75/44 P = .001	AJCC T1, T2 12.2/9.4 P = .612	27.5/28 P = .953	Median 91/53.9 P = .289	Median DFS 14.3/9.8 P = .174	++	LA to OA conversion, 19% Recurrence LA/OA, 48.9%/64.1% P = .07 (all recurrence sites, all stages)

(continued)

TABLE 2-5 Selected Studies Comparing Laparoscopic and Open Approaches to Adrenalectomy for Adrenocortical Carcinoma (continued)

Author, Year	Data Source	Study Patients, N	Cases, n LA/OA	Median Tumor Size, cm LA/OA	AJCC or ENSAT Stage, % LA/OA	Tumor Rupture, % LA/OA	+ Margin, % LA/OA	Overall Survival, mo LA/OA	Recurrence, mo LA/OA	Grade of Evidence*	Comments
Lombardi et al.,[83] 2012	Multi-institutional	156	30/126	7.7/9.0 (mean) $P=.147$	All ENSAT I, II	Excluded	Excluded	Median 108/60 $P=.2$	Median RFS 72/48 $P=.120$	++	More LA patients had incidentalomas.
Miller et al.,[84] 2010	Institutional	88	17/71	6.0/10.1 $P=NR$	ENSAT I, II 70/50	50/18 + margin or tumor rupture combined $P=.01$	50/18 + margin or tumor rupture combined	NR	Local recurrence: 9.6/19.2 $P<.005$	++	+ margin and tumor rupture greater in LA group despite smaller, less invasive tumors, lower-stage tumors
Miller et al.,[47] 2012	Institutional	156	46/110	7.4/12.0 $P=NR$	ENSAT I, II 72/50	30/16 + margin or tumor rupture combined $P=.04$	30/16 + margin or tumor rupture combined	Stage II only 51/103 $P=.002$	17.6/52.9 $P=.001$	++	Overall survival longer for OA stage II; Time to recurrence shorter in LA patients, including R0-only resections; $P=.002$; Initial resection at study center in 15%

Study											Comments
Mir et al.,[85] 2013	Institutional	44	18/26	7.0/13.0 P = .001	AJCC I, II 82/35 P = NR	NR	39/38 P = NS	2-y overall survival 58%/54% P = .6	39%/60% at 2 y P = .7 Risk adjusted for stage: P = .09	++	Included stage IV patients OA group with larger tumors, higher stage Cancer-specific deaths, 59%/73%; P = .361
Porpiglia et al.,[86] 2010	Institutional	43	18/25	9.0/10.5 P = .39	All ENSAT I, II	Excluded	Excluded	NR	Median RFS 23/18 P = .8	++	Resection performed at center in 23% LA to OA conversions excluded R1, R2 resections excluded No stage III patients
Wu et al.,[87] 2018	Institutional	44	21/23	5.8/6.9 P = NR	All ENSAT I, II	1 LA converted to OA owing to rupture	NR	5-y overall survival 47% vs. 43% P = .635	5-y RFS 39/36 P = .8	++	Surgical margin status not assessed
Zheng et al.,[88] 2018	Institutional	42	20/22	6.3/10.1 P = .001	ENSAT I, II 80/60	Excluded	Excluded	NR	3-y RFS 23.5% vs. 21.4% P = .6	++	OA patients with significantly larger tumors than LA R1, R2 resections not included in data calculations (only R0 resections)

ACC: adrenocortical carcinoma; AJCC: American Joint Committee on Cancer; DFS: disease-free survival; ENSAT: European Network for the Study of Adrenal Tumors; LA: laparoscopic adrenalectomy; NCDB: National Cancer Database; NR: not reported; NS: nonsignificant; OA: open adrenalectomy; PFS: progression-free survival; RFS: recurrence-free survival.
*Grade: ++ low; +++ moderate.

Given the rarity of ACC[98] and uncertainty in preoperative diagnosis of ACC in indeterminate adrenal nodules, no randomized controlled trials have been performed that compare open adrenalectomy with any minimally invasive approach (laparoscopic transabdominal, retroperitoneoscopic, or robot assisted). However, numerous studies have compared these approaches retrospectively. All previously reported studies and conclusions are limited by the retrospective design, relatively limited sample size, and inherent selection bias.

FINDINGS

Early case reports and small case series reporting outcomes associated with a laparoscopic approach for resection of ACC noted port-site and tumor bed recurrences.[89,90,99] Additional studies comparing laparoscopic and open approaches followed; some analyses reported a higher rate of tumor capsule penetration/rupture and tumor spill–related carcinomatosis with laparoscopic adrenalectomy compared with open adrenalectomy.[80,82,84] However, other studies have challenged this finding, reporting that a laparoscopic approach can achieve equivalent oncologic outcomes in patients with stage I or II ACC.[79,85,91,94,96,97] These disparate conclusions have led to different recommendations from medical and surgical societies whose members treat and study patients with ACC. For example, the American Association of Endocrine Surgeons and the American Association of Clinical Endocrinologists[75] have recommended open adrenalectomy for known or suspected ACC. In contrast, the European Society of Endocrinology, in collaboration with the European Network for the Study of Adrenal Tumors (ENSAT) and the European Society of Endocrine Surgeons, has endorsed laparoscopic adrenalectomy as a potential option for indeterminate adrenal tumors less than 6 cm in size that are neither clearly malignant nor highly suspicious for malignancy.[23,41]

Several institutions treating a high volume of ACC patients have retrospectively examined their data regarding the use of minimally invasive adrenalectomy. As a follow-up to a previously reported study[84] that suggested the inferiority of laparoscopic relative to open adrenalectomy, Miller et al.[47] examined 156 patients, 46 of whom underwent laparoscopic adrenalectomy and 110 of whom underwent open adrenalectomy. Thirty percent of patients treated laparoscopically had positive margins or intraoperative tumor spill compared with 16% in the open group ($P = .04$). Importantly, in approximately 25% of patients found to have invasion of the periadrenal fat on final pathology (stage III), invasion was neither appreciated preoperatively nor intraoperatively by either the radiologist or surgeon—a finding that suggests differentiating between stage II and stage III tumors cannot be done confidently and that has implications if used to select a minimally invasive versus open approach. Time to peritoneal recurrence was shorter in patients treated laparoscopically, and the overall survival of ENSAT stage I and stage II patients treated with an open approach was longer compared with that of patients who underwent laparoscopic adrenalectomy ($P = .002$).

Gonzalez et al.[80] compared outcomes of 115 patients who underwent open adrenalectomy with outcomes of 6 who underwent laparoscopic adrenalectomy. All 6 patients treated with laparoscopic adrenalectomy experienced cancer recurrence, 5 of whom had peritoneal carcinomatosis (83%). In contrast, only 35% of those treated with open adrenalectomy experienced local recurrence, and only 8% were diagnosed with peritoneal recurrence (open vs. laparoscopic resection, Fisher exact test; P = .0001). Similarly, Leboulleux et al.[82] reported an increased risk of peritoneal carcinomatosis after laparoscopic adrenalectomy (67%) compared with open adrenalectomy (27%) (P = .016). The surgical approach used was the only factor identified to account for this difference. In both studies, concern was raised for the possible confounding effect of surgeon experience with laparoscopic surgery.

Cooper et al.[95] examined recurrence and survival patterns among 92 patients with American Joint Committee on Cancer (AJCC) stage I and stage II ACC treated with laparoscopic (n = 46) or open (n = 46) adrenalectomy. Patients treated with laparoscopic adrenalectomy had a higher rate of positive margins compared with patients who underwent open adrenalectomy (28% vs. 8.7%; P = .01). Furthermore, when adjusted for T-score, the median recurrence-free survival (11 vs. 20 months; P < .0001) and overall survival (54 vs. 110 months; P < .0001) durations of patients who underwent laparoscopic surgery were significantly shorter than that of patients who underwent open surgery. Peritoneal recurrence was significantly more common among patients who underwent laparoscopic adrenalectomy (54% vs. 19%; P = .006). Several other studies have similarly demonstrated a higher rate of tumor rupture, local recurrence, and peritoneal carcinomatosis among patients treated using a minimally invasive approach.[87,88,92] Whereas another study by Huynh et al.[81] reported no difference in margin positivity rates among patients with ENSAT stage I/II tumors treated with laparoscopic or open adrenalectomy, a significantly higher rate of positive margins was found among patients with ENSAT stage III tumors.

Other authors, however, have reported equivalent rates of positive margins, capsular penetration/rupture, and tumor spill. Durations of recurrence-free and overall survival in these studies have also been similar when comparing minimally invasive and open surgical approaches. For example, Lee et al[97] included retrospective data from 13 tertiary care centers in an analysis of 201 patients, 47 of whom underwent laparoscopic adrenalectomy and 154 of whom underwent open adrenalectomy. There was no difference in intraoperative tumor rupture (P = .612) or R0 resection (P = .953) between the groups. They found no significant difference in overall (P = .289) or disease-free survival (P = .174). Sgourakis et al.[91] conducted a meta-analysis of patients with ENSAT stage I or stage II tumors who underwent open or laparoscopic adrenalectomy between 1992 and 2014. No significant differences in 2-, 3-, 4-, or 5-year survival rates were identified between groups. Surgical complications and R0 resection were not significantly different between groups. Other single-institution series from high-volume centers have similarly reported no differences in tumor rupture, disease-specific survival, or overall 5-year survival.[79,85,94,96] Given that all these data were retrospectively generated from small numbers of nonrandomized patients treated with heterogeneous surgical techniques, it is challenging to extrapolate existing data into a set of general principles.

Lombardi et al.[83] conducted a multi-institutional study of 156 patients with ENSAT I/II ACC who underwent R0 adrenalectomy, 30 of whom were treated laparoscopically and 126 of whom were treated with an open approach. No differences in the rates of 5-year disease-free (38% vs. 58%; P = not significant [NS, P > .05]) or 5-year overall survival (48% vs. 67%; P = NS) were identified. Porpiglia et al.[86] examined 43 patients with ENSAT I/II tumors who underwent R0 resection (R1 and R2 excluded from analysis), 18 of whom had a laparoscopic operation and 25 of whom had an open operation. Patients converted from laparoscopic to open resections were not included in the analysis. The median recurrence-free survival of patients treated with open surgery was 18 versus 23 months in patients treated laparoscopically ($P = .8$). There was no significant difference between the median durations of recurrence-free survival. The results from both studies are biased by the fact that R1 and R2 resections and those with tumor rupture were not included—clearly an idealized situation, given that surgeons cannot prospectively determine who will undergo an R1 or R2 resection or in which patients the tumor capsule will be breached.

Because R0 resection provides the best chance of cure for patients with ACC,[20,23,41,67,75–77] the importance of surgical technique is paramount irrespective of the approach used to access the retroperitoneum. Extrapolation of data generated in studies of other malignancies to ACC, with specific regard to minimally invasive resection, is difficult for several reasons: ACC is a very aggressive cancer; tumors often have a soft, delicate, friable, easily penetrable tumor capsule; and tumors are located deep within the upper retroperitoneum, making access to the tumor more difficult and working space more limited. Furthermore, most surgeons resect few ACCs in their career and may not be familiar with the nuances of evaluation and management of the disease or the critical elements to be performed during adrenalectomy for cancer. It is therefore possible that equivalent outcomes observed in many comparisons of the various operative approaches are artifacts of limited preoperative evaluation, poor oncologic technique, and heterogeneous medical/oncologic management over the course of the disease.

Obvious limitations are common to many trials listed in Table 2-5, such as the small numbers of patients they include and the bias associated with selection of those patients for surgery. Other less obvious limitations also exist. First, most of these studies focused on endpoints—such as overall survival—that are confounded by variables other than surgical technique; comparisons of operative approaches should instead focus on differences in tumor bed recurrence and rates of peritoneal disease. Similarly, heterogeneity of evaluation, inconsistency with respect to the performance of the critical elements of adrenalectomy, and variation in long-term treatment significantly limit the ability to detect any potential impact of surgical technique on outcome. Furthermore, conversion of a case begun using a minimally invasive approach to an open approach often occurs at a time when key oncologic principles have been violated; inclusion of these cases in the datasets, as occurred in many of these studies, can lead to generation of inaccurate conclusions. Pathologic examination of the specimen may be compromised after laparoscopic resection if the tumor has been morcellated or crushed to facilitate extraction. Morcellation inhibits the ability of the pathologist to perform a full assessment of the tumor and periadrenal soft tissue, and it affects reporting of margins, stage, and long-term outcomes. Whether morcellation was performed is not reliably reported. The impact of tumor grade and peritumoral or large vessel invasion on survival was not studied in most of these analyses. And, in almost all studies, large tumors were more frequently removed using an open approach, often as part of multivisceral resection. It is well known that patients with higher-stage tumors fare worse than those with lower-stage tumors. Finally, removal of stage I and stage II tumors, especially those amenable to a minimally invasive approach according to guidelines (now set at <6 cm),[41] should rarely be associated with tumor rupture and positive margins. However, in series that specifically evaluated subgroups of patients with stage I and stage II tumors, significantly higher rates were reported among patients treated with minimally invasive surgery (Table 2-5). It should be noted that the recommendations stating what tumors should be treated with minimally invasive resection decreased from less than 8 to 10 cm[41,96] to less than 6 cm.[23,41] However, no reasoning or data leading to the change in recommendation was provided. In summary, despite the appearance of equivalence of operative approach in many of the evaluated studies, multiple confounding factors should be taken into consideration when reviewing the available literature.

Ultimately, a concerted effort should be made to accurately determine the likelihood of ACC prior to proceeding with surgery for an adrenal mass. Some characteristics to be included in this assessment are tumor size, capsular integrity and invasion of the periadrenal fat or adjacent organs, excess hormone production (e.g., cortisol, androgens), tumor heterogeneity, and other imaging characteristics as demonstrated on high-quality adrenal-protocol CT scan. For indeterminate adrenal masses in which malignancy is in the differential, ^{18}F-fluoro-2-deoxy-D-glucose positron emission tomography/computed tomography (FDG-PET/CT) scan can be considered to aid in this assessment. None of these are perfectly predictive of ACC, but they can be used to improve risk stratification for each patient. When ACC is part of the differential diagnosis, the approach that has the highest likelihood of allowing the surgeon to carry out the oncologically critical elements of adrenalectomy should be pursued. With the exception of surgeons highly experienced in treating both benign adrenal tumors and ACC at high-volume referral centers, resection of indeterminate adrenal masses should most often be undertaken as an open operation. Should the experienced ACC surgeon be able to carry out all aspects of the described critical elements for resection of ACC and provide acceptable oncologic outcomes from a surgical standpoint (rate of capsular disruption, margin status, other standard surgical outcome measures equal to those of an open approach for similar size and stage tumors according to benchmarks from experienced groups), either a laparoscopic or an open approach in appropriately and carefully selected patients after thorough preoperative evaluation and careful review of the imaging may be reasonable. Advantages and disadvantages of the two approaches are outlined in Table 2-6. An open approach is generally recommended from an oncologic standpoint.

In summary, some studies examined herein revealed no significant differences in overall 5-year survival or disease-free survival according to operative approach. Other studies reviewed revealed increased rates of capsular disruption, positive margins, local and peritoneal recurrence, and decreased overall survival with a minimally invasive approach. All evaluated studies are limited by their retrospective design, referral bias, selection bias, and other less obvious limitations, and most are underpowered owing to the rarity of the disease. Furthermore, the quality of the conclusions generated in these studies is in question because of the likelihood that, in many cases, the oncologically critical portions of the procedures reported were conducted in a manner inconsistent with the recommendations described in this body of work.

TABLE 2-6   Advantages and Disadvantages of Open and Laparoscopic Approaches for Adrenalectomy

Approach	Advantages	Disadvantages
Open adrenalectomy (recommended default approach for known or suspected ACC)	Improved surgical exposure Not limited by constrained working space (e.g., retroperitoneoscopic method, BMI, hepatomegaly) Allows for gentle tumor retraction and tactile sensation Easier to resect the periadrenal/perinephric fat tissue en bloc Low risk of tumor rupture when delivering the specimen out of the wound	Increased pain Longer hospital stay Increased wound complications (infection, hernia)
Minimally invasive adrenalectomy	Decreased pain Shorter hospital stay Faster return to work Fewer wound complications	Need to extract tumor intact, thus limited by the small size of the incision Decreased tactile sensation Increased focal pressure on the tumor (force/area) from laparoscopic instruments used for exposure and dissection Constrained working space Diminished ability for multivisceral resection, examination of lymph nodes, and performance of lymphadenectomy

ACC: adrenocortical carcinoma; BMI: body mass index.

CONCLUSION

The strength of the data from the available studies limits the ability to generate a firm recommendation regarding the equivalence of a laparoscopic or minimally invasive compared with open approach for resection of stage I or II ACC. In most cases, completion of the critical elements of adrenalectomy for cancer will be best facilitated by an open approach. This is especially true for surgeons performing limited numbers of adrenalectomies and/or with limited experience in treating patients with ACC. It may be that a laparoscopic or minimally invasive approach is reasonable for carefully selected patients with suspected small ACC (<6 cm) and favorable tumor anatomy when the individual surgeon has considerable experience with both minimally invasive adrenalectomy and surgical resection of ACC and produces acceptable oncologic outcomes from a surgical standpoint. Ultimately, the surgeon must ensure that all critical technical elements of adrenalectomy for cancer are performed.

CHAPTER 4

Vascular Invasion

CRITICAL ELEMENTS

- En Bloc Resection of Adjacent Blood Vessels Directly Involved by Primary Tumor and/or Tumor Thrombus

1. EN BLOC RESECTION OF ADJACENT BLOOD VESSELS DIRECTLY INVOLVED BY PRIMARY TUMOR AND/OR TUMOR THROMBUS

Recommendation: If direct invasion of the inferior vena cava (IVC), renal vein, or renal artery by adrenal cancer is suspected intraoperatively, the vascular structure(s) should be resected en bloc with the primary adrenal tumor if technically feasible.

Type of Data: Retrospective reports, case series, or case-control studies

Strength of Recommendation: Strong recommendation, low-quality evidence

Rationale

Adrenocortical carcinoma (ACC) may present as a locally advanced tumor that invades adjacent vascular structures with or without associated tumor thrombus.[100–102] Although malignant vascular involvement is more commonly encountered in patients with ACC than in those with pheochromocytoma, the latter may also directly invade vasculature and/or be associated with tumor thrombus.[103] Thus, upon resection of these primary tumors, excision of any involved vasculature and removal of large vessel tumor thrombus should be performed when technically possible.

In general, patients with ACC and large vessel involvement have a worse prognosis than those without involvement of major blood vessels.[23] In patients with tumor thrombus extending into the IVC, venous obstruction may ultimately result in Budd-Chiari syndrome, symptomatic edema, and even death. Embolism of tumor thrombus to the lungs may also occur, so patients with venous thrombus should be anticoagulated.

103

Much of the evidence supporting resection of vascular structures directly invaded by ACC is translated from experience and outcomes associated with other types of malignancies (renal cell cancer, sarcomas). These related experiences may or may not be entirely applicable to ACC; however, in most circumstances in which invasion into the IVC, renal vein, or renal artery is suspected or confirmed in a patient with an otherwise resectable cancer, en bloc resection of the involved vascular structure with the primary tumor is recommended. In those with tumor thrombus and no evidence of external invasion of the vessel wall, thrombectomy may be performed, although tumor thrombus can be adherent to the inside of the vessel, mandating resection of the involved vein. Neoadjuvant chemotherapy may improve the ability to perform an R0 resection in patients with such tumors and should, therefore, be considered prior to surgery.[48] Ultimately, careful selection of patients for surgery with ACC (or malignant pheochromocytoma) involving a major vessel is necessary and should incorporate multidisciplinary input.

Direct invasion into the renal vein or renal artery (without involvement of the vena cava or aorta) in the setting of a left adrenal cancer most often necessitates nephrectomy; however, in rare circumstances, venous or arterial reconstruction may be possible. Preservation of renal function is particularly important if chemotherapy is anticipated because cisplatin, part of first-line chemotherapy, is nephrotoxic. Autotransplantation of the kidney may also be considered if sufficient artery, vein, and renal parenchyma remain following resection.

Adherence to or direct invasion of the IVC wall with or without IVC tumor thrombus should prompt IVC resection en bloc with the tumor. Extension of tumor thrombus into the renal vein or IVC without invasion of the vein wall can occur on either side. On the right, tumor thrombus extension most often occurs through the right adrenal vein. On the left, extension to the IVC occurs through the left renal vein via the left adrenal vein. In most circumstances, invasion of the aorta, celiac axis, superior mesenteric artery, or portal vein should prompt consideration of nonsurgical therapy.

The data specifically supporting resection of vascular structures invaded by ACC are limited. Nearly all existing reports concentrate on tumor involvement of venous structures alone. In a series of 65 patients with locally advanced ACC, those with direct tumor invasion of the IVC or tumor thrombus requiring resection had similar postoperative morbidity, mortality, and 12-month disease-specific survival when compared with patients who underwent resection of tumors without IVC invasion or tumor thrombus. Survival of patients with IVC involvement who underwent R0 resection was significantly shorter beginning three years after surgery.[100] A multicenter survey of physicians caring for 38 patients with ACC that involved the IVC revealed a 13% 30-day mortality rate. At the time of the survey, median time to death of those who had died (25/38) was 5 months (range, 2 to 61 months). Of the 13 surviving patients, 7 had metastatic disease, and 6 had no signs of distant disease with a median follow-up of 16 months (range, 2 to 58 months).[102]

Appropriate management of vascular involvement by ACC or malignant pheochromocytoma requires extensive preoperative planning in a multidisciplinary fashion.[41,100,103–105] Depending on the extent of vascular invasion or intravascular tumor thrombus and other features of the primary tumor, experience of the primary surgeon, and practice patterns and capabilities of the health system, a multidisciplinary surgical team is often beneficial and may include vascular, hepatobiliary, transplant, cardio-thoracic, general, endocrine, urologic, and/or surgical oncology teams.[105]

Technical Aspects

Exposure of the inferior vena cava

If direct invasion or IVC tumor thrombus is suspected, the IVC should be fully exposed prior to resection or thrombectomy. Exposure of the IVC requires full mobilization of the duodenum and head of the pancreas with a Kocher maneuver. Mobilization should extend proximally from the porta hepatis to the ligament of Treitz. The head of the pancreas should be mobilized to the extent that the left renal vein may be identified and controlled. The aorta will also be identified. If necessary, medial visceral rotation of the ascending colon allows for full exposure of the infrarenal vena cava.

Exposure of the retrohepatic and suprahepatic IVC should be performed as needed to achieve vascular control of the IVC cranial to the tumor and thrombus (Fig. 2-5). When vascular control cranial to the hepatic veins is required, this is best accomplished by fully mobilizing both lobes of the liver. The phrenic veins are ligated and divided during this process. The caudate lobe is mobilized from the IVC by ligating and dividing small direct veins draining into the IVC. This can be performed with the caudate lobe rotated cranially and to the right. The hepatocaval ligament should be ligated and divided, which allows the liver to be fully mobilized from the vena cava. The IVC is then fully exposed and can be controlled cranial to the level of the hepatic vein confluence. If more cranial control is necessary, the suprahepatic IVC can be exposed and controlled in the sub- or supradiaphragmatic space by incising the pericardium and clamping as high as the base of the atrium. Incision of the pericardium from within the abdomen allows access to the supradiaphragmatic cava and right atrium, in most cases not requiring cardiopulmonary bypass, but sternal extension of the incision with sternotomy may be required in some.

Vascular control

If direct invasion and/or tumor thrombus of the IVC is known or suspected, venous control should be obtained proximal and distal to the site of disease. The method and extent of vascular control will be defined by the location and extent of invasion and/or tumor thrombus.

Cranial control of the IVC can be obtained above or below the renal veins. The site chosen for caudal control will depend on the location of the caudal extent of the ACC in relation to the right renal vein. If the tumor is small and the site of vascular invasion is near the adrenal vein, the IVC may often be controlled cranial to the renal vein confluence with the IVC. Both right and left renal veins should be in view and exposed in case of need for vascular control. When dissecting the IVC circumferentially, care should be taken to avoid injuring a posterior lumbar vein, as these are found in approximately 40% of patients.[106] In those with significant thrombus in the vena cava or near occlusion, veins feeding the azygous system and others may reconstitute and can be quite large. If venous isolation is necessary for resection of a portion of the IVC,

Left

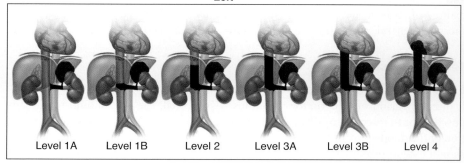

Level 1A Level 1B Level 2 Level 3A Level 3B Level 4

Right

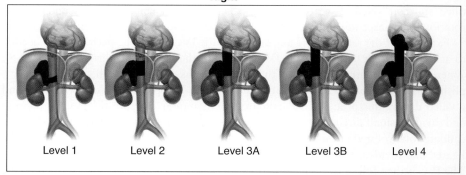

Level 1 Level 2 Level 3A Level 3B Level 4

FIGURE 2-5 Classification of extent of tumor thrombus within the vena cava. *Left*: Level 1A—thrombus contained within the adrenal and/or renal vein; level 1B—minimal extension of thrombus into the vena cava; level 2—extension of thrombus to a level inferior to the hepatic veins; level 3A—thrombus extending cranial to the hepatic veins but caudal to the diaphragm; level 3B—thrombus extending cranial to the diaphragm without intracardiac extension; level 4—extension of thrombus into the atrium and beyond. *Right*: Level 1—minimal extension of thrombus into the vena cava at the level of the right adrenal vein or caudal; level 2—extension of thrombus >2 cm cranial to the adrenal vein remaining caudal to the hepatic veins; level 3A—thrombus extending cranial to the hepatic veins but caudal to the diaphragm; level 3B—thrombus extending cranial to the diaphragm without intracardiac extension; level 4—extension of thrombus into the atrium and beyond.

lumbar and other veins can be ligated and divided, as back bleeding can be brisk after venotomy. If control of the IVC cranial to the renal vein confluence is not possible, control may be obtained more caudally. The site of cranial venous control will depend on the level of vascular invasion and/or extent of IVC tumor thrombus relative to the hepatic veins, diaphragm, and right atrium (Fig. 2-5).

Infrahepatic
If the most cranial extent of disease is caudal to the confluence of the hepatic veins, control of the IVC caudal to the hepatic veins suffices. This will require full mobilization of the right lobe of the liver, including the caudate lobe from the IVC as previously described. A Pringle maneuver is not typically required.

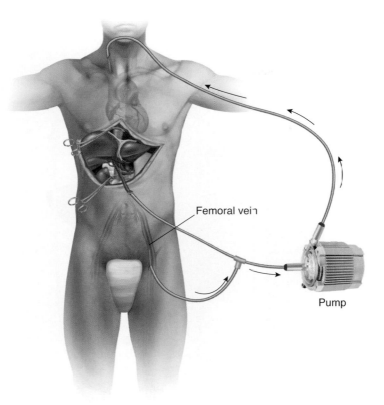

Femoral vein

Pump

FIGURE 2-6   Diagram of a venovenous bypass circuit. Outflow is most commonly achieved through a femoral vein and either the inferior mesenteric vein or portal vein. Vascular access for venous inflow is most commonly provided via the right internal jugular vein, although an axillary vein may also be used.

Retro- and Suprahepatic but below the Diaphragm

If the most cranial extent of disease is at or above the level of the hepatic vein conflu-ence, the IVC can be controlled above the hepatic vein confluence but still below the diaphragm. In this setting, the hepatic veins will also need to be controlled by per-forming a Pringle maneuver. Depending on tolerance of the patient to clamping, ve-novenous bypass (Fig. 2-6) may be required. This is rarely necessary if there has been adequate volume resuscitation prior to clamping. Hypothermic perfusion of the liver may also be considered, especially in cases in which total hepatic vascular exclusion is expected to be prolonged (Fig. 2-7).

Infracardiac Inferior Vena Cava and Intra-atrial

If the cranial extent of disease is at or above the diaphragm and a clamp can be placed above the tumor or area of involvement of the vena cava, this may be able to be treated as if below the diaphragm. If a clamp cannot be placed to allow for

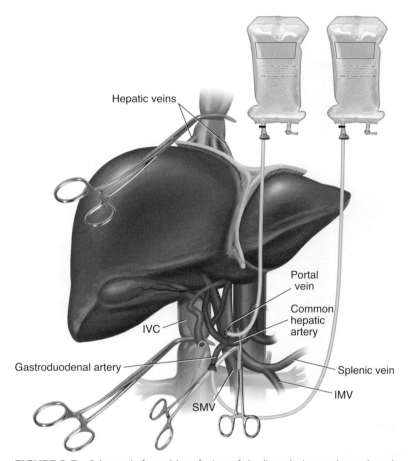

FIGURE 2-7   Schematic for cold perfusion of the liver during prolonged total hepatic vascular exclusion. Cold perfusate is instilled through the portal vein and gastroduodenal artery stump. For simplicity and visualization of the figure, a portion of the bile duct has been removed. IMV: inferior mesenteric vein; IVC: inferior vena cava; SMV: superior mesenteric vein.

reconstruction or the tumor extends into the right atrium, cardiopulmonary bypass with deep hypothermic circulatory arrest is usually required to ensure complete tumor removal.[101]

Extraction of tumor thrombus; resection and reconstruction of the IVC

Once venous vascular control has been safely obtained both proximally and distally as previously described based on extent of disease, resection can commence. If mobile tumor thrombus is encountered with minimal invasion of the IVC wall, thrombus can often be extracted with excision of only a small portion of the IVC wall adjacent to the ostium of the adrenal vein (or other relevant tributary). Even with tumor thrombus extending into the right atrium, invasion may be minimal. In this circumstance, under cardiopulmonary bypass with or without hypothermic circulatory arrest, the cardiac surgeon can open the right atrium and provide retrograde pressure from above while another surgeon opens the IVC and extracts the tumor thrombus. If only a small portion of the IVC wall is involved, the IVC may be closed primarily without clinically relevant narrowing. If, however, there is concern for direct invasion into the IVC, resection should be performed en bloc with a portion of IVC to ensure a negative margin. Reconstruction of the IVC in this circumstance may require patch closure with bovine pericardium or other suitable material to ensure adequate luminal diameter. In situations in which full segmental resection of the IVC is required, the IVC may be replaced with a prosthetic interposition graft (20-mm ringed polytetrafluoroethylene). Intraoperative heparin is usually administered, and systemic anticoagulation is continued postoperatively as soon as hemostasis is ensured.

Adrenal Key Question 2

In patients with stage IV adrenocortical carcinoma (ACC), does surgical resection of the primary tumor, with or without metastasectomy, improve overall survival (OS) relative to nonsurgical therapy?

INTRODUCTION

A complete microscopic (R0) resection of adrenocortical cancer prolongs the survival of patients with local or locoregional ACC.[20,23,41,67,75] Patients diagnosed at presentation with stage IV ACC generally have a poor prognosis and short survival. Although a limited number of patients with stage IV disease may benefit from surgery to reduce the sequelae of hormone excess or to alleviate local symptoms caused by a large, invasive mass, resection of the primary tumor with or without metastasectomy has historically not been pursued. Patients with stage IV ACC are instead most often treated with mitotane and systemic chemotherapy.

Over the past two decades, more has been learned about ACC, its biology, and the disease course. Enthusiasm has begun to grow regarding "potentially curative" resection in the setting of stage IV disease. The purpose of this work was to evaluate the impact of surgical resection of the primary tumor, with or without metastasectomy, in patients with stage IV ACC on OS, compared with nonsurgical therapy.

METHODOLOGY

A systematic search of PubMed was performed from 1990 through 2019 beginning January 2018. A final search was performed on September 1, 2019. Medical Subject Headings (MeSH) terms included "Adrenal Cortex Neoplasm," "Adrenal Cancer," "Adrenocortical Cancer," "Adrenocortical Carcinoma," and "Neoplasm Metastases." Searches were restricted to English language and human subjects. Case reports were excluded. Findings are reported in accordance with the Preferred Reporting Items for Systematic Reviews and Meta-Analyses (PRISMA).[78]

The initial search yielded 529 publications (Fig. 2-8). A total of 462 publications were excluded without review, including 25 reviews, 68 case reports, 17 articles that did not include surgical treatment, 23 ex vivo studies, 326 studies that did not address ACC, and 3 editorials. A total of 67 abstracts were reviewed, with 33 excluded because they did not address the primary topic. Studies that passed the title/abstract review were retrieved for full-text review. Of these 34 studies, 25 were excluded due to small cohort size, poor methodology, heterogeneity in treatment, or inadequate follow-up. The remaining 9 were carefully examined, and 4 studies met all the criteria for inclusion in this systematic review.[2,48,65,107]

Data were extracted from individual studies by the writing group. Each article was reviewed and assigned a quality of evidence based on the Grading of Recommendations,

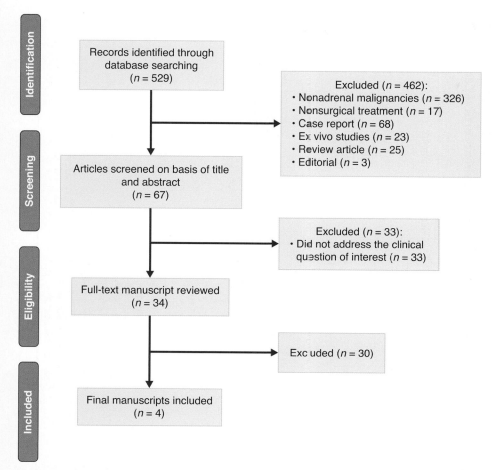

FIGURE 2-8 Preferred Reporting Items for Systematic Reviews and Meta-Analyses diagram for literature regarding surgical resection of the primary tumor, with or without metastasectomy, for patients with stage IV adrenocortical cancer.

Assessment, Development, and Evaluation (GRADE) system.[79] The quality of the data and size of the studies precluded the ability to perform a meta-analysis.

Four studies were included in the qualitative systematic review (Table 2-7). All were retrospective studies. Of these four full-text studies, there was one single-institution study, one dual-institution study, one study using a statewide cancer registry, and one study using a national registry. Overall, the quality of the evidence was very low.

Given the rarity of ACC and the paucity of patients operated on with metastatic disease at presentation, no randomized trials have been performed for this subpopulation of patients with stage IV disease at presentation and none are likely to be performed in the future. All previously reported studies and conclusions are limited by the retrospective design, limited sample size, and inherent selection bias.

TABLE 2-7 Synopsis of Studies Evaluating Outcomes after Surgery in Patients with Stage IV Adrenocortical Carcinoma

Author, Year	Data Source	Study Patients with Stage IV Disease, *n*	Resection Status R0, R1, R2	OS	Grade of Evidence*	Comments
Bednarski et al.,[48] 2014	MD Anderson	53 6 stage IV undergoing surgery	R0—5/6 R2—1/6 Resection of metastatic disease not reported	Survival of stage IV patients treated with mitotane and/or chemotherapy prior to surgery: deaths at 29 and 38 mo in 2/6 Alive mean length of follow-up: 24.6 mo	++	Studied patients with borderline resectable tumors, including stage IV patients. Patients either underwent surgery or neoadjuvant chemotherapy +/– mitotane prior to surgery to study feasibility and outcomes of neoadjuvant therapy.
Dy et al.,[65] 2015	Two-institution study	27	R0—11 R2—15	Median R0, 860 d Median R2, 390 d (P = .02) 1-y OS R0, 69.9% 1-y OS R2, 53% (P = .02)	++	Sex, age, location of metastasis not correlated with OS after surgery 12/14 (86%) had improvement in symptoms of cortisol excess and pain, duration not reported.
Kerkhofs et al.,[2] 2013	Dutch Adrenal Network hospitals	72 34 surgery 38 no surgery	Not reported	Surgery OS, 10 mo No surgery OS, 2 mo (P < .001)	++	—
Livhits et al.,[107] 2014	California Cancer Registry	167 69 surgery	Not reported	Median OS, stage IV—0.3 y Stage IV median survival, 0.4 y for those treated with surgery alone, 0.3 y for those treated with chemotherapy/ radiation therapy, 1.1 y for surgery plus chemotherapy/ radiation therapy, and 0.1 y for no treatment (P < .001)	++	—

OS: overall survival.
*Grade of evidence: ++ low.

FINDINGS

Interpreting available outcomes data relating to the treatment of metastatic ACC is subject to a number of inherent limitations. First, the widely used ACC staging systems of the American Joint Committee on Cancer (AJCC) and European Network for the Study of Adrenal Tumors (ENSAT) defined stage IV variably in the past.[108,109] The most recent versions of each of these sets of guidelines align regarding the definition of stage IV disease as the presence of distant metastasis.[25] However, in previous editions of the *AJCC Cancer Staging Manual*, the presence of a T4 tumor (regardless of tumor size or the presence or absence of nodal metastases) was considered stage IV ACC. Therefore, published series—except those in which tumor node metastasis (TNM) variables are clearly stated—can be difficult to interpret. Second, comparing outcomes of patients managed surgically can also be challenging given that many (but not all) such patients may have received inadequate preoperative evaluations or may have received preoperative or postoperative radiation, ablation, mitotane, and/or chemotherapy. Third, many of the existing datasets include a heterogeneous mix of patients with both synchronous and metachronous metastases.

In a small, retrospective study that evaluated data from two institutions, Dy et al.[65] reported 27 patients who underwent resection of primary ACC with synchronous metastatic disease (ENSAT stage IV). Eleven of the 27 patients underwent an R0 resection. The median OS of patients who underwent R0 resection was longer than that of patients who underwent R2 resection (860 vs. 390 days; $P = .02$); 1- and 2-year OS was 69.9% for R0 versus 46.9% for R2 and 53.0% for R0 versus 22.1% for R2, respectively. Patients in this series did not receive identical therapy: 9 patients received combination chemotherapy plus mitotane or mitotane alone prior to surgery. A nonsignificant trend toward prolonged survival was observed among patients who received neoadjuvant treatment. Notably, all patients in this report were managed surgically; data were not compared with a group of patients who received nonsurgical therapy.

Some population-based data also exist. In a study using data from the Dutch Cancer Registry, patients with ENSAT stage IV ACC who underwent resection had a longer median OS than patients who did not (median OS, 10 vs. 2 months; $P < .001$; 95% confidence interval, 4 to 16 months).[2] However, completeness of resection and specific tumor characteristics were not reported in this study. A similar review of data from the California Cancer Registry demonstrated that patients who underwent resection with or without chemotherapy lived longer than untreated patients (surgery alone, 0.4 years; chemotherapy/radiation alone, 0.3 years; surgery plus chemotherapy/radiation, 1.1 years; no treatment, 0.1 years; $P < .001$).[107] However, in this study, the staging system used was not clearly stated, and evaluation of outcomes was, therefore, confounded by lack of detail regarding extent of disease.

A fourth study to evaluate the impact of neoadjuvant chemotherapy in borderline resectable ACC patients included six stage IV patients.[48] Although these patients were not the sole focus of the study, the OS of this subgroup was more than 2 years. These patients were clearly a carefully selected group chosen for certain features suggesting a better chance for longer survival. R0 resection was achieved in five (83%) patients; one underwent an R1 resection.

Although these studies may suggest a role for surgery in patients with stage IV ACC, the quality of existing evidence is low, and thus, great caution is required before making a recommendation to any specific patient. Patients in these studies undergoing surgery were carefully selected. In practice, multiple variables should be examined when considering surgery for patients with metastatic ACC, given that recurrent metastatic disease will occur in the same organ in as many as approximately 70% to 95% of patients.[58,110] Variables that should be considered include tempo of disease progression, tumor grade, number and site(s) of metastases, ability to resect all disease, and the potential for use of chemotherapy or other adjuncts before or after surgery.[58]

Recommendations regarding surgery in the setting of metastatic disease are best developed in a setting in which providers representing multiple disciplines can weigh the risks and benefits of and alternatives to all available therapies, including surgery. In addition, quality of life and patient preferences should be at the forefront of any decision-making, and extensive counseling should be provided to each patient. The possibility of complications from surgery leading to delayed recovery and diminished quality of life must be strongly considered in any patient anticipated to have a limited lifespan or disease-free interval after resection.

Surgery is most appropriately considered in patients with tumors and synchronous metastases that can be completely resected to negative margins. In some cases, limited and technically resectable metastatic disease may occur in the setting of a locally invasive or "borderline" resectable primary tumor. These patients may benefit from neoadjuvant chemotherapy, which may potentially eliminate or reduce the burden of metastatic disease and/or convert primary tumors that initially appear unresectable or at high risk of R1 or R2 resection to one in which R0 resection is more likely.[48] Again, the decision to proceed with surgery in this setting should be made carefully in a multidisciplinary fashion. Ultimately, surgery should be reserved for carefully selected patients.

Finally, it should be noted that in rare and highly selected circumstances, resection of the primary tumor may be beneficial even when resection of all metastatic disease cannot be anticipated. ACC may grow to become so large that it results in intolerable locoregional symptoms, and hormone production by the dominant local tumor may become difficult to manage. However, rapid control of hormone excess with medication (metyrapone, mifepristone, osilodrostat) is often able to be achieved; high-risk surgery is, therefore, rarely necessary for this purpose, and nonsurgical strategies should be favored in general. If surgery is used in this setting, it should be viewed as palliative, as most patients who undergo R2 resection live no longer than those who receive nonoperative treatment.[58,110] Ultimately, surgery in this context is most appropriate for physiologically robust patients in whom clinical evidence suggests a reasonable likelihood of durable symptom relief and in whom resection can be accomplished with low morbidity and preservation of vital structures.[48,58,65,110]

CONCLUSION

The strength of the data supporting surgery in the setting of metastatic ACC is of extraordinarily low quality, and it is compromised by both selection bias and heterogeneity. Caution should, therefore, be exercised before recommending surgery to any patient with metastatic ACC.

When both the primary tumor and all sites of metastatic disease can be completely resected (or treated with other therapies) with low morbidity, surgery may be reasonable in patients who have an acceptable performance status and when other factors contributing to long-term survival are identified. Conversely, resection of an asymptomatic primary ACC in the setting of an unresectable burden of metastatic disease is rarely justified. Resection of an ACC with synchronous metastases that cannot be completely resected may be considered if locoregional symptoms related to the primary tumor or severe hormone excess cannot be treated by other means. In this setting, the impact of resection on survival is unclear, and surgery should be considered palliative.

CHAPTER 5

Lymphadenectomy

CRITICAL ELEMENTS

● Resection of Regional Lymph Nodes Involved by Metastatic Adrenal Cancer

1. RESECTION OF REGIONAL LYMPH NODES INVOLVED BY METASTATIC ADRENAL CANCER

Recommendation: If regional lymph nodes are clinically suspected to be involved by metastatic adrenal cancer, a complete, en bloc nodal dissection of the affected lymph node basin(s) should be performed. An extended prophylactic lymphadenectomy is not recommended. If en bloc dissection is not possible, any nodal tissue that is removed separately from the primary specimen should be marked and labeled as a distinct specimen for pathologic analysis. The station(s) of origin of any involved lymph nodes should be specifically noted in the operative and pathology reports.

Type of Data: Retrospective reports, case series, or case-control studies

Strength of Recommendation: Strong recommendation, low-quality evidence

Rationale
The goal of adrenalectomy for cancer is to remove all gross and microscopic locoregional disease.[23] In addition to the primary tumor, metastatic disease within the regional nodal basins must also be considered, as it represents a frequent site of locoregional dissemination and postoperative recurrence.[46,111,112]

Data to suggest the true impact of nodal dissection, however, are limited. This is due to a lack of consensus with respect to the anatomic definitions of an optimal nodal dissection, the infrequency with which lymphadenectomy of any type is actually performed for adrenocortical carcinoma (ACC), and the characteristically low yield of nodes in the retroperitoneal space cranial to the renal vessels.[112–114] Furthermore, existing studies are

116

largely retrospective in nature and are limited by bias, reporting error (the station of origin of the lymph nodes dissected may be unknown—in certain instances, nodes identified within the surgical specimen may be extraregional nodes removed as part of multivisceral resections), and incomplete data. Finally, any putative impact of lymphadenectomy on survival may be secondary to an improvement in staging and the identification of patients for whom subsequent treatment with mitotane, chemotherapy, and/or radiation therapy is appropriate and pursued. Similar data to inform staging and the delivery of postoperative therapies may be able to be obtained from microscopic analysis of small intra- or peritumoral lymphatic channels and vessels and may have the same impact on staging, thereby making specific prophylactic removal of lymph nodes unnecessary.[115]

The burden of disease within locoregional lymph nodes can be difficult to assess both prior to surgery and intraoperatively. Close inspection of the basins of concern with comprehensive and current preoperative imaging is imperative, as ACC can progress rapidly.[41] Patterns of disease spread are currently best described by patterns of regional lymph node recurrence and by historical studies that describe lymphatic drainage from the adrenal glands (Fig. 2-9).[111,116] Intraoperatively, the soft tissue removed with the

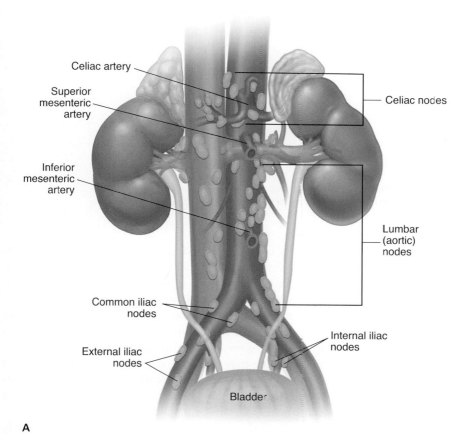

A

FIGURE 2-9 **A:** Distribution pattern of retroperitoneal lymph nodes.

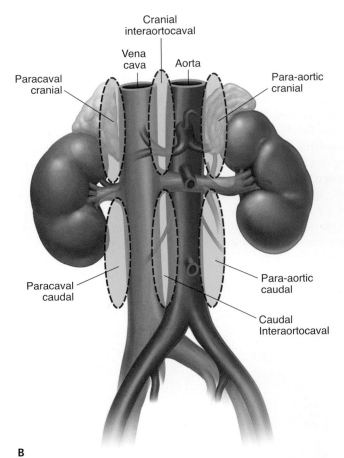

B

FIGURE 2-9 *(continued)* **B:** Nomenclature of nodal basins commonly involved by adrenocortical carcinomas.

primary tumor from the suprarenal, paracaval, and para-aortic (lateral to those vessels) regions rarely yields any lymph nodes. Additional sites of interest include the renal hilum, interaortocaval space, celiac trunk, superior mesenteric artery, infrarenal paracaval and para-aortic areas, and aortic bifurcation. However, further visceral mobilization and dissection are required to gain access to these areas, and existing data do not support prophylactic nodal dissection at the time of initial tumor resection (see Adrenal Key Question 3).[111,116] Consideration of preoperative imaging findings as well as any intraoperative gross evidence of disease may guide the surgeon to expand the field of dissection to include the listed areas. Although helpful for this purpose, ^{18}F-2-deoxy-d-glucose positron emission tomography/computed tomography (FDG-PET/CT) has not yet been formally recommended in any guidelines for the routine preoperative assessment of regional lymph nodes but is likely to be included in the near future. Very rarely does the lymphatic drainage cross the midline of the aorta.[111,116]

Technical Aspects

During resection of a right adrenal cancer, resection margins of the primary tumor can be extended to include the paracaval soft tissue extending posteriorly to the left side of the inferior vena cava. In one study, nodal metastases after right adrenalectomy for ACC in 20 patients were most commonly found cranial to the renal hilum in the perirenal (dorsal 55% and ventral 47%), interaortocaval (35%), renal (10%), and/or paracaval (15%) adipose tissue.[111] This study, however, was limited methodologically given that nodal recurrences were not biopsy proven in most cases and some identified foci could have been local tumor recurrence after seeding from the primary tumor, especially those reported in the suprarenal perirenal fat. Few lymph nodes are retrieved during dissection of this area at the time of initial resection when including all retroperitoneal soft tissue with the primary tumor as described in a previous chapter. (See Chapter 3.) Interaortocaval lymph nodes may be removed separately when indicated by preoperative or intraoperative findings; however, the porta hepatis can make dissection cranial and posterior to the left lobe of the liver and adjacent to the caudate lobe more difficult. Dissection of lymph nodes of the renal hilum, especially on the left, where the tumor more often drains to this nodal basin, requires care so as not to divide small arterial branches to portions of the kidney, cause hemorrhage from posterior venous communications between the renal vein and lumbar veins, or injure the ureter.

Reibetanz et al.[111] reported that most nodal recurrences on the left were located in the left renal hilum (50%) and the infrarenal para-aortic (47%) and interaortocaval (22%) basins. Involvement of the aortic bifurcation was noted very rarely. Left adrenal cancers have additional sites to which they may metastasize. Periadrenal tissue borders the aorta medially, the diaphragm cranially, and the renal vessels caudally. Extending the dissection medially, the surgeon has the option to further dissect out the lymph nodes in the region of the celiac trunk and superior mesenteric artery origin depending on preoperative or intraoperative findings. Close inspection of preoperative imaging can also help the surgeon anticipate any unusual vascular variants.

Therapeutic nodal dissection should be pursued if all disease is technically resectable and no distant metastatic disease exists. In order to visualize the infrarenal nodal basins, a full medial visceral rotation is required to mobilize the colon and, on the right side, the duodenum off the inferior vena cava. When working posterior to the vena cava, great care should be taken to identify (and divide when needed) lumbar venous branches. In addition, while working along the infrarenal paracaval or para-aortic basins, early identification and protection of the ureter and gonadal vessels is necessary.

The site of origin of any involved lymph nodes should be noted in the operative (see Synoptic Operative Report) and pathology reports, and any lymph nodes that are not resected en bloc with the primary specimen and oriented with marking sutures should be clearly labeled prior to submission for pathologic analysis. Not only will this knowledge provide valuable information if radiation therapy is delivered postoperatively in an adjuvant fashion, but it should also aid in better understanding the impact of nodal dissection on recurrence and survival of patients with ACC in future studies.

■ Adrenal Key Question 3

In patients with adrenocortical carcinoma (ACC), does prophylactic lymph-adenectomy concurrent with adrenalectomy have a favorable impact on local recurrence or disease-free survival compared with no lymphadenectomy?

INTRODUCTION

Although several guidelines and studies cite open adrenalectomy with en bloc lymph-adenectomy as the procedure of choice for ACC, the role of prophylactic lymphade-nectomy for ACC remains poorly defined.[23,41,46,113,116–118] Patients in whom metastatic ACC is present in locoregional lymph nodes have shorter overall survival than pa-tients in whom locoregional lymph nodes are not involved by cancer.[112] Locoregional recurrence following potentially curative resection occurs frequently, and recurrence in locoregional lymph nodes is common.[41,111] Autopsy studies have found that two-thirds to three-quarters of patients with ACC had nodal involvement at the time of their death.[112] The purpose of this work was to evaluate whether prophylactic lymph-adenectomy concurrent with resection of the primary tumor in patients with ACC has a favorable effect on the rate of local recurrence and/or length of disease-free survival compared with no lymphadenectomy.

METHODOLOGY

A systematic search of PubMed was performed from 1990 to 2019 beginning January 2018. A final search was performed on June 24, 2019. Medical Subject Headings (MeSH) terms included "Adrenocortical Carcinoma" AND "Lymph Node"; "Adrenocortical Carcinoma" AND "Lymphadenectomy"; "Adrenocortical Carcinoma" AND "Lymph-adenopathy"; "Adrenocortical Carcinoma" AND "Nodal Metastasis"; "Adrenocorti-cal Carcinoma" AND "Lymph Node Metastasis"; "Adrenocortical Carcinoma" AND "Lymph Node Dissection"; "Adrenocortical Carcinoma" AND "Nodal Dissection"; and "Retroperitoneal Lymph Node Dissection" AND "Adrenal." Searches were restricted to English language and human subjects. Findings are reported in accordance with the Pre-ferred Reporting Items for Systematic Reviews and Meta-Analyses (PRISMA).[78]

The initial search yielded 155 publications (Fig. 2-10). After duplicates were re-moved, 115 abstracts were excluded due to being animal studies (2), single-case reports (17), review articles (4), studied malignancies of nonadrenal origin (90), or studied the pediatric population (2). A total of 40 abstracts were reviewed in detail. An additional 12 were excluded as they did not address the clinical question of inter-est, leaving 28 full-text manuscripts to review in detail. Three were removed as they were letters to the editor (1), a reply to a letter (1), and an erratum (1). Final manu-scripts were then fully reviewed. Eight of the 25 full-text reviews were not included in the systematic review due to small cohort size, poor methodology, or inadequate long-term follow-up. Seventeen studies were ultimately included in the qualitative systematic review (Table 2-8).[46,70–72,74,112,114,117,119–128]

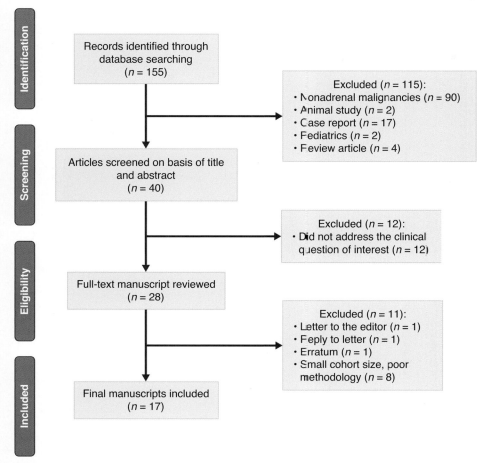

FIGURE 2-10 Preferred Reporting Items for Systematic Reviews and Meta-Analyses diagram for literature regarding prophylactic lymphadenectomy concurrent with adrenalectomy in patients with adrenocortical carcinoma.

Data were extracted from individual studies by the writing group. Each article was reviewed and assigned a quality of evidence based on the Grading of Recommendations, Assessment, Development, and Evaluation (GRADE) system.[93] The quality of the data and size of the studies precluded the ability to perform a meta-analysis.

All studies were performed in retrospective fashion. National registries were used in 13 studies, 1 study used a regional database, and 3 studies reported data from multiple institutions. Quality of evidence was considered very low in all studies.

Given the rarity of ACC, no randomized controlled trials have been performed that compare outcomes related to prophylactic lymphadenectomy. All previously reported studies and conclusions were limited by the retrospective design, relatively limited sample size, and inherent selection bias. These reports had multiple different study designs

TABLE 2-8 Summary of Retrospective Reviews of the Surgical Management of Adrenocortical Carcinoma

Author, Year	Country of Origin, Dataset, Years of Study	No. of Patients	No. with LAD (% of Total)	No. with Positive Nodes (% of Those with LAD)	Survival	Grade of Evidence*	Comments
Alanee et al.,[119] 2015	United States, SEER, 1991–2011	1,037 (treated with surgery)	58 (5.6)	18 (31)	Not reported	+	—
Gerry et al.,[112] 2016	United States, ACC Study Group, 1993–2014	120 (with R0 resection, no metastatic disease)	32 (27)	8 (25)	LAD independently associated with decreased risk of death (HR, 0.17; P = .006)	+	Only included patients with localized (nonmetastatic) disease and who underwent R0 resection; classified LAD based on surgeon documentation on intent to perform LAD; analysis focused on comparison of outcome based on performance of LAD
Gratian et al.,[120] 2014	United States, National Cancer Database, 1998–2011	2,756	538 (19.5)	152 (28)	Positive LN status independently associated with higher risk of death (HR, 1.25 [1.05–1.49])	+	Focus of study was on hospital volume. LAD and positive LN were independently reported results.

Study	Location/Registry/Years	N			Survival finding		Comments
Icard et al.,[70] 2001	France, French Association of Endocrine Surgeons Network, 1978–1997	253	89 (32.5)	Data not provided	Not reported	+	Did not provide data regarding rate of LN involvement; survival data based on MacFarlane classification stage and, for stage IV patients, based on mitotane usage
Lombardi et al.,[121] 2012	Italy, Italian Registry for ACC, 2003–2010	278	45 (16.1)	19 (20)	Not provided based on LN status or LAD	+	Survival data based on where patient was managed (high-volume vs. low-volume center).
Margonis et al.,[71] 2016	United States, ACC Study Group, 1993–2014	165	51 (31)	14 (27)	Positive LN status predictive of worse recurrence-free survival (HR, 2.70; P = .04) but not OS (HR, 2.73; P = .15)	+	Same overall dataset as Gerry et al., but focus of this study was on R0 vs. R1 resection and associated outcomes. This resulted in a larger pool of included patients than with Gerry et al.[112]
Marincola Smith et al.,[74] 2018	United States, ACC Study Group, 1993–2014	167	37 (22)	16 (43)	Performance of LAD predictive of improved OS (HR, 0.29; P = .014), positive LN status not predictive (HR, 1.73; P = .36)	+	Same overall dataset as Gerry et al., but focus of this study was on multivisceral resection at time of adrenalectomy. Additional patients in this manuscript compared with Gerry et al. and Margonis et al.[71]

(continued)

TABLE 2-8 Summary of Retrospective Reviews of the Surgical Management of Adrenocortical Carcinoma (continued)

Author, Year	Country of Origin, Dataset, Years of Study	No. of Patients	No. with LAD (% of Total)	No. with Positive Nodes (% of Those with LAD)	Survival	Grade of Evidence*	Comments
Maurice et al,[117] 2017	United States, National Cancer Database, 2010–2013	481	44 (9.1)	Did not provide this data— LN status designated as "clinical" not "pathologic"	Not reported	+	Focus of study was on minimally invasive vs. open surgical approach.
Nilubol et al,[114] 2016	United States, SEER, 1973–2011	802	67 (8.4)	22 (34)	Performance of LAD did not alter disease-specific survival in months ($P = .3$), but regional LN metastasis did ($P < .01$). Regional LN metastasis was predictive of disease-related mortality (HR, 1.7; $P < .01$).	+	—
Panjwani et al,[122] 2017	United States, National Cancer Database, 2004–2013	827	159 (19) Defined as at least 1 LN examined	35 (22)	Analysis only focused on those who had at least one LN removed. OS better when ≥4 LN were assessed ($P = .02$).	+	Excluded T4 disease, distant metastatic disease, multivisceral resection

Punjani et al.,[123] 2018	Canada, London Regional Cancer Program, 1990–2015	29	8 (33)	4 (50%)	No survival data provided with regard to LAD or LN status	+	—
Reibetanz et al.,[46] 2012	Germany, German ACC Registry, 2003–2009	283	47 (16.6)	12 (25.5%) 13 of 236 (5.5%) did not undergo LAD but had positive LN.	Recurrence-free survival and disease-specific survival better with LAD (P = .042 and P = .049, respectively)	+	—
Saade et al.,[124] 2015	United States, SEER18, 1988–2009	259	16 (6.2)	7 (44) 5 did not undergo formal LAD but had positive LN of 35 with LN in specimen (14%).	LAD not found to affect disease-specific survival on multivariate analysis (P = .69)	+	Stage I–III patients only
Tella et al.,[12] 2018	United States, National Cancer Database, 2004–2015	806 (stages I–III disease and underwent surgery)	149 (18)	11 (7)	For all stages, LAD associated with worse OS (HR, 1.18; P = .02) No difference in OS for stages I–III (P = .15); improved OS for stage IV (P < .01)	+	—
Tran et al.,[125] 2016	United States, SEER, 1988–2009	320	83 (26)	29 (35)	Improved disease-specific survival for stage IV (P = .044)	+	Study only looked at stages III and IV.

(continued)

TABLE 2-8 Summary of Retrospective Reviews of the Surgical Management of Adrenocortical Carcinoma (continued)

Author, Year	Country of Origin, Dataset, Years of Study	No. of Patients	No. with LAD (% of Total)	No. with Positive Nodes (% of Those with LAD)	Survival	Grade of Evidence*	Comments
Wang et al.,[126] 2017	United States, SEER, 1973–2014	118 (patients with surgery at primary site)	39 (33)	No data on positive LNs	Univariate analysis, LAD was not associated with OS (P = .35).	+	Stage IV patients only
Wang et al.,[127] 2017	United States, SEER, 1973–2014	749	145 (21)	94 (65)	LAD was not predictive of OS (HR, .819; P = .103), but having stage N1 was predictive of a worse OS (HR, 1.84; P < .001).	+	All stages

ACC: adrenocortical carcinoma; HR: hazard ratio; LAD: lymphadenectomy; LN: lymph node; OS: overall survival; SEER: Surveillance, Epidemiology, and End Results.
*Grade of evidence: + very low.

and included retrospective multi-institutional studies, retrospective single-institutional studies, meta-analyses, national database series, and consensus statements. None of them specifically addressed the key question as formulated.

FINDINGS

ACC is a rare cancer that often presents as advanced disease. Further, the conduct of lymphadenectomy concurrent with adrenalectomy has been infrequently reported in the surgical literature. In studies when it has been reported, the rate of performance ranges from 5% to 33%; however, it is even less frequently reported if lymphadenectomy was performed with prophylactic or therapeutic intent (Table 2-8). For these reasons, the ability to offer strong, data-driven recommendations with respect to the conduct of prophylactic lymphadenectomy is severely limited.

For those patients who have been reported to have undergone some form of lymphadenectomy, 20% to 65% have had metastatic disease identified within locoregional lymph nodes on final pathologic assessment. However, in such circumstances, lymphadenectomy has often been performed in the setting of multivisceral resection. Lymph node resection in the setting of multivisceral resection is often incidental rather than done in a purposeful manner. Further, the basin of origin of positive nodes often cannot be determined in this circumstance, as it is rarely stated clearly in the pathology report. Therefore, the specific anatomic distribution of nodal metastases is not easily verified in retrospective studies, such as those evaluated herein.

Another confounding issue is that consensus exists neither for the specific technique to be used for lymphadenectomy nor the specific nodal basins that should be dissected. The literature does describe thresholds of nodal counts that might be obtained at lymphadenectomy: four lymph nodes in one study[14] from the National Institutes of Health and five lymph nodes from another study.[46] However, these thresholds were set for the purpose of having a dichotomized variable rather than to suggest a complete lymphadenectomy had been performed or that an adequate number of lymph nodes had been sampled to inform treatment or affect outcome. Indeed, it is unclear that resection of any specific number of nodes directly affects patients' durations of disease-free or overall survival.[70–72,74,112,114,117,119–129] Regardless, the knowledge that lymphadenectomy provides with respect to the presence or absence of lymphatic dissemination is likely ultimately meaningful, as it may be used both for staging and to inform the delivery of subsequent therapies.

Extrapolation from studies of patterns of recurrence following surgery may provide some insight into the true frequency of lymph node involvement over the course of the disease. Reibetanz et al.[111] examined the patterns of lymph node recurrence following primary tumor resection using the European Network for the Study of Adrenal Tumors registry. A total of 56 patients were included in the study; these patients had a median time to lymph node recurrence of 17.5 (range, 4 to 74) months. Intentional lymphadenectomy had been performed at the initial resection in only 6 patients (10.7%). Importantly, nodal recurrence was defined on the basis of radiographic findings; histologic evidence of nodal recurrence was not required. Therefore, some of the "lymphatic recurrence" could have been nonlymphatic deposits of recurrent tumor.

In a separate study of data from 1,592 patients included in the Surveillance, Epidemiology, and End Results registry, the presence of regional nodal metastases increased as primary tumor size increased.[114] Compared with patients with T1 and T2 tumors, the authors reported a higher rate of lymphadenectomy performed in patients with primary tumors greater than 10 cm (12.4% vs. 4.2%; $P < .01$) and in those with T3 and T4 tumors or distant metastasis (12.4% and 12.0% vs. 5.1%, respectively; $P < .01$). Lymph node metastasis was present in 12.8% of patients overall—19.2% in patients with T3 or T4 tumors. Ultimately, lymphadenectomy was not associated with improved disease-specific survival on univariate analysis ($P = .30$), regardless of tumor size or staging. The authors did conclude that lymphadenectomy may be warranted in the setting of large or advanced tumors given the higher incidence of nodal metastases but could not demonstrate an improvement in disease-free or overall survival.

In sum, the high rate of locoregional nodal recurrence following resection of ACC suggests microscopic disease is present at the time of initial surgery in many patients, including those in whom preoperative radiologic studies do not demonstrate visible disease. As extrapolation of these data fuels the debate over the potential benefit of prophylactic lymphadenectomy concurrent with adrenalectomy, higher-level data will need to be generated before consensus regarding a formal recommendation for prophylactic lymphadenectomy can be reached.

CONCLUSION

Currently, data do not support routine performance of prophylactic locoregional lymphadenectomy concurrent with adrenalectomy in patients with ACC because existing data are insufficient to definitively characterize the impact of prophylactic lymphadenectomy on local recurrence and disease-free survival. Prospective studies designed to evaluate the role of prophylactic lymphadenectomy concurrent with adrenalectomy for ACC are necessary, but conduct of such trials would be difficult in practice given the rarity with which ACC is treated at most institutions. If any study is ultimately performed, a standardized anatomic definition of the extent of recommended lymphadenectomy, an optimal surgical technique for dissection of these nodal basins, and a uniform reporting methodology will be critical.

REFERENCES

1. Kebebew E, Reiff E, Duh Q-Y, Clark OH, McMillan A. Extent of disease at presentation and outcome for adrenocortical carcinoma: have we made progress? *World J Surg.* 2006;30(5):872-878. doi:10.1007/s00268-005-0329-x
2. Kerkhofs TM, Verhoeven RH, Bonjer HJ, et al. Surgery for adrenocortical carcinoma in The Netherlands: analysis of the national cancer registry data. *Eur J Endocrinol.* 2013;169(1):83-89. doi:10.1530/EJE-13-0142
3. Almeida MQ, Bezerra-Neto JE, Mendonça BB, Latronico AC, Fragoso M. Primary malignant tumors of the adrenal glands. *Clinics (Sao Paulo).* 2018;73(suppl 1):e756s. doi:10.6061/clinics /2018/e756s
4. Fassnacht M, Libé R, Kroiss M, Allolio B. Adrenocortical carcinoma: a clinician's update. *Nat Rev Endocrinol.* 2011;7(6):323-335. doi:10.1038/nrendo.2010.235
5. Berruti A, Baudin E, Gelderblom H, et al. Adrenal cancer: ESMO Clinical Practice Guidelines for diagnosis, treatment and follow-up. *Ann Oncol.* 2012;23(suppl 7):VII131-VII138. doi:10.1093 /annonc/mds231

6. Petr EJ, Else T. Genetic predisposition to endocrine tumors: diagnosis, surveillance and challenges in care. *Semin Oncol.* 2016;43(5):582-590. doi:10.1053/j.seminoncol.2016.08.007

7. Else T, Kim AC, Sabolch A, et al. Adrenocortical carcinoma. *Endocr Rev.* 2014;35(2):282-326. doi:10.1210/er.2013-1029

8. Ferreira AM, Brondani VB, Helena VP, et al. Clinical spectrum of Li-Fraumeni syndrome/Li-Fraumeni-like syndrome in Brazilian individuals with the TP53 p.R337H mutation. *J Steroid Biochem Mol Biol.* 2019;190:250-255. doi:10.1016/j.jsbmb.2019.04.011

9. Petr EJ, Else T. Adrenocortical carcinoma (ACC): when and why should we consider germline testing? *Presse Med.* 2018;47(7-8, pt 2):e119-e125. doi:10.1016/j.lpm.2018.07.004

10. Lenders JW, Duh Q-Y, Eisenhofer G, et al. Pheochromocytoma and paraganglioma: an Endocrine Society clinical practice guideline. *J Clin Endocrinol Metab.* 2014;99(6):1915-1942. doi:10.1210/jc.2014-1498

11. Adler JT, Meyer-Rochow GY, Chen H, et al. Pheochromocytoma: current approaches and future directions. *Oncologist.* 2008;13(7):779-793. doi:10.1634/theoncologist.2008-0043

12. Ilias I, Pacak K. A clinical overview of pheochromocytomas/paragangliomas and carcinoid tumors. *Nucl Med Biol.* 2008;35(suppl 1):S27-S34. doi:10.1016/j.nucmedbio.2008.04.007

13. Gimenez-Roqueplo AP, Dahia PL, Robledo M. An update on the genetics of paraganglioma, pheochromocytoma, and associated hereditary syndromes. *Horm Metab Res.* 2012;44(5):328-333. doi:10.1055/s-0031-1301302

14. Neumann HP, Bausch B, McWhinney SR, et al. Germ-line mutations in nonsyndromic pheochromocytoma. *N Engl J Med.* 2002;346(19):1459-1466. doi:10.1056/NEJMoa020152

15. Hamidi O, Young WF Jr, Gruber L, et al. Outcomes of patients with metastatic phaeochromocytoma and paraganglioma: a systematic review and meta-analysis. *Clin Endocrinol (Oxf).* 2017;87(5):440-450. doi:10.1111/cen.13434

16. Jimenez P, Tatsui C, Jessop A, Thosani S, Jimenez C. Treatment for malignant pheochromocytomas and paragangliomas: 5 years of progress. *Curr Oncol Rep.* 2017;19(12):83. doi:10.1007/s11912-017-0643-0

17. Lloyd RV, Osamura RY, Klöppel G, et al, eds. *WHO Classification of Tumours of Endocrine Organs.* Vol 10. 4th ed. International Agency for Research on Cancer; 2017.

18. Hescot S, Curras-Freixes M, Deutschbein T, et al. Prognosis of malignant pheochromocytoma and paraganglioma (MAPP-Prono study): a European Network for the Study of Adrenal Tumors retrospective study. *J Clin Endocrinol Metab.* 2019;104(6):2367-2374. doi:10.1210/jc.2018-01968

19. Kerkhofs TM, Ettaieb MH, Hermsen IG, Haak HR. Developing treatment for adrenocortical carcinoma. *Endocr Relat Cancer.* 2015;22(6):R325-R338.

20. Bilimoria KY, Shen WT, Elaraj D, et al. Adrenocortical carcinoma in the United States: treatment utilization and prognostic factors. *Cancer.* 2008;113(11):3130-3136. doi:10.1530/ERC-15-0318

21. Sturgeon C, Shen WT, Clark OH, Duh Q-Y, Kebebew E. Risk assessment in 457 adrenal cortical carcinomas: how much does tumor size predict the likelihood of malignancy? *J Am Coll Surg.* 2006;202(3):423-430. doi:10.1016/j.jamcollsurg.2005.11.005

22. Fassnacht M, Terzolo M, Allolio B, et al. Combination chemotherapy in advanced adrenocortical carcinoma. *N Engl J Med.* 2012;366(23):2189-2197. doi:10.1056/NEJMoa1200966

23. Fassnacht M, Dekkers OM, Else T, et al. European Society of Endocrinology Clinical Practice Guidelines on the management of adrenocortical carcinoma in adults, in collaboration with the European Network for the Study of Adrenal Tumors. *Eur J Endocrinol.* 2018;179(4):G1-G46. doi:10.1530/EJE-18-0608

24. Amin MB, Greene FL, Edge SB, et al. The Eighth Edition *AJCC Cancer Staging Manual*: continuing to build a bridge from a population-based to a more "personalized" approach to cancer staging. *CA Cancer J Clin.* 2017;67(2):93-99. doi:10.3322/caac.21388

25. Amin MB, Edge SB, Greene F, et al, eds. *AJCC Cancer Staging Manual.* 8th ed. Springer; 2017.

26. Gonzalez KD, Noltner KA, Buzin CH, et al. Beyond Li Fraumeni syndrome: clinical characteristics of families with p53 germline mutations. *J Clin Oncol.* 2009;27(8):1250-1256. doi:10.1200/JCO.2008.16.6959

27. Tinat J, Bougeard G, Baert-Desurmont S, et al. 2009 Version of the Chompret criteria for Li Fraumeni syndrome. *J Clin Oncol.* 2009;27(26):e108-e110. doi:10.1200/JCO.2009.22.7967

28. van Hulsteijn LT, Dekkers OM, Hes FJ, Smit JW, Corssmit EP. Risk of malignant paraganglioma in SDHB-mutation and SDHD-mutation carriers: a systematic review and meta-analysis. *J Med Genet.* 2012;49(12):768-776. doi:10.1136/jmedgenet-2012-101192

29. Vanbrabant T, Fassnacht M, Assie G, Dekkers OM. Influence of hormonal functional status on survival in adrenocortical carcinoma: systematic review and meta-analysis. *Eur J Endocrinol.* 2018;179(6):429-436. doi:10.1530/EJE-18-0450

30. Else T, Williams AR, Sabolch A, Jolly S, Miller BS, Hammer GD. Adjuvant therapies and patient and tumor characteristics associated with survival of adult patients with adrenocortical carcinoma. *J Clin Endocrinol Metab.* 2014;99(2):455-461. doi:10.1210/jc.2013-2856

31. Libè R, Fratticci A, Bertherat J. Adrenocortical cancer: pathophysiology and clinical management. *Endocr Relat Cancer.* 2007;14(1):13-28. doi:10.1677/erc.1.01130

32. Fassnacht M, Kenn W, Allolio B. Adrenal tumors: how to establish malignancy? *J Endocrinol Invest.* 2004;27(4):387-399. doi:10.1007/BF03351068

33. Funder JW, Carey RM, Mantero F, et al. The management of primary aldosteronism: case detection, diagnosis, and treatment: an Endocrine Society clinical practice guideline. *J Clin Endocrinol Metab.* 2016;101(5):1889-1916. doi:10.1210/jc.2015-4061

34. Mackie GC, Shulkin BL, Ribeiro RC, et al. Use of [18F]fluorodeoxyglucose positron emission tomography in evaluating locally recurrent and metastatic adrenocortical carcinoma. *J Clin Endocrinol Metab.* 2006;91(7):2665-2671. doi:10.1210/jc.2005-261

35. Groussin L, Bonardel G, Silvéra S, et al. 18F-fluorodeoxyglucose positron emission tomography for the diagnosis of adrenocortical tumors: a prospective study in 77 operated patients. *J Clin Endocrinol Metab.* 2009;94(5):1713-1722. doi:10.1210/jc.2008-2302

36. Deandreis D, Leboulleux S, Caramella C, Schlumberger M, Baudin E. FDG PET in the management of patients with adrenal masses and adrenocortical carcinoma. *Horm Cancer.* 2011;2(6):354-362. doi:10.1007/s12672-011-0091-5

37. Chang CA, Pattison DA, Tothill RW, et al. 68Ga-DOTATATE and 18F-FDG PET/CT in paraganglioma and pheochromocytoma: utility, patterns and heterogeneity. *Cancer Imaging.* 2016;16(1):22. doi:10.1186/s40644-016-0084-2

38. Ctvrtlik F, Koranda P, Schovanek J, Skarda J, Hartmann I, Tudos Z. Current diagnostic imaging of pheochromocytomas and implications for therapeutic strategy. *Exp Ther Med.* 2018;15(4):3151-3160. doi:10.3892/etm.2018.5871

39. Canu L, Van Hemert JAW, Kerstens MN, et al. CT characteristics of pheochromocytoma: relevance for the evaluation of adrenal incidentaloma. *J Clin Endocrinol Metab.* 2019;104(2):312-318. doi:10.1210/jc.2018-01532

40. Fassnacht M, Arlt W, Bancos I, et al. Management of adrenal incidentalomas: European Society of Endocrinology Clinical Practice Guideline in collaboration with the European Network for the Study of Adrenal Tumors. *Eur J Endocrinol.* 2016;175(2):G1-G34. doi:10.1530/EJE-16-0467

41. Gaujoux S, Mihai R; for Joint Working Group of ESES and ENAT. European Society of Endocrine Surgeons (ESES) and European Network for the Study of Adrenal Tumours (ENSAT) recommendations for the surgical management of adrenocortical carcinoma. *Br J Surg.* 2017;104(4):358-376. doi:10.1002/bjs.10414

42. Bancos I, Tamhane S, Shah M, et al. Diagnosis of endocrine disease: the diagnostic performance of adrenal biopsy: a systematic review and meta-analysis. *Eur J Endocrinol.* 2016;175(2):R65-R80. doi:10.1530/EJE-16-0297

43. Williams AR, Hammer GD, Else T. Transcutaneous biopsy of adrenocortical carcinoma is rarely helpful in diagnosis, potentially harmful, but does not affect patient outcome. *Eur J Endocrinol.* 2014;170(6):829-835. doi:10.1530/EJE-13-1033

44. Vanderveen KA, Thompson SM, Callstrom MR, et al. Biopsy of pheochromocytomas and paragangliomas: potential for disaster. *Surgery.* 2009;146(6):1158-1166. doi:10.1016/j.surg.2009.09.013

45. Miller BS, Else T; for the AACE Adrenal Scientific Committee. Personalized care of patients with adrenocortical carcinoma: a comprehensive approach. *Endocr Pract.* 2017;23(6):705-715. doi:10.4158/EP161719.RA

46. Reibetanz J, Jurowich C, Erdogan I, et al. Impact of lymphadenectomy on the oncologic outcome of patients with adrenocortical carcinoma. *Ann Surg.* 2012;255(2):363-369. doi:10.1097/SLA.0b013e3182367ac3

47. Miller BS, Gauger PG, Hammer GD, Doherty GM. Resection of adrenocortical carcinoma is less complete and local recurrence occurs sooner and more often after laparoscopic adrenalectomy than after open adrenalectomy. *Surgery.* 2012;152(6):1150-1157. doi:10.1016/j.surg.2012.08.024

48. Bednarski BK, Habra MA, Phan A, et al. Borderline resectable adrenal cortical carcinoma: a potential role for preoperative chemotherapy. *World J Surg.* 2014;38(6):1318-1327. doi:10.1007/s00268-014-2484-4

49. Palazzo F, Dickinson A, Phillips B, et al. Adrenal surgery in England: better outcomes in high-volume practices. *Clin Endocrinol (Oxf).* 2016;85(1):17-20. doi:10.1111/cen.13021

50. Park HS, Roman SA, Sosa JA. Outcomes from 3144 adrenalectomies in the United States: which matters more, surgeon volume or specialty? *Arch Surg.* 2009;144(11):1060-1067. doi:10.1001/archsurg.2009.191

51. Lindeman B, Hashimoto DA, Bababekov YJ, et al. Fifteen years of adrenalectomies: impact of specialty training and operative volume. *Surgery*. 2018;163(1):150-156. doi:10.1016/j.surg .2017.05.024

52. Hermsen IG, Kerkhofs TM, den Butter G, et al. Surgery in adrenocortical carcinoma: importance of national cooperation and centralized surgery. *Surgery*. 2012;152(1):50-56. doi:10.1016/j.surg .2012.02.005

53. Nieman LK, Biller BM, Findling JW, et al. The diagnosis of Cushing's syndrome: an Endocrine Society Clinical Practice Guideline. *J Clin Endocrinol Metab*. 2008;93(5):1526-1540. doi:10.1210/ jc.2008-0125

54. Eller-Vainicher C, Morelli V, Salcuni AS, et al. Post-surgical hypocortisolism after removal of an adrenal incidentaloma: is it predictable by an accurate endocrinological work-up before surgery? *Eur J Endocrinol*. 2010;162(1):91-99. doi:10.1530/EJE-09-0775

55. Lentschener C, Gaujoux S, Tesniere A, Dousset B. Point of controversy: perioperative care of patients undergoing pheochromocytoma removal—time for a reappraisal? *Eur J Endocrinol*. 2011;165(3):365-373. doi:10.1530/EJE-11-0162

56. Goldstein RE, O'Neill JA Jr, Holcomb GW 3rd, et al. Clinical experience over 48 years with pheochromocytoma. *Ann Surg*. 1999;229(6):755-764. doi:10.1097/00000658-199906000-00001

57. Pacak K. Preoperative management of the pheochromocytoma patient. *J Clin Endocrinol Metab*. 2007;92(11):4069-4079. doi:10.1210/jc.2007-1720

58. Glenn JA, Else T, Hughes DT, et al. Longitudinal patterns of recurrence in patients with adrenocortical carcinoma. *Surgery*. 2019;165(1):186-195. doi:10.1016/j.surg.2018.04.068

59. Strajina V, Dy BM, Farley DR, et al. Surgical treatment of malignant pheochromocytoma and paraganglioma: retrospective case series. *Ann Surg Oncol*. 2017;24(6):1546-1550. doi:10.1245 /s10434-016-5739-5

60. Ellis RJ, Patel D, Prodanov T, et al. Response after surgical resection of metastatic pheochromocytoma and paraganglioma: can postoperative biochemical remission be predicted? *J Am Coll Surg*. 2013;217(3):489-496. doi:10.1016/j.jamcollsurg.2013.04.027

61. Gonias S, Goldsby R, Matthay KK, et al. Phase II study of high-dose [131I]metaiodobenzylguanidine therapy for patients with metastatic pheochromocytoma and paraganglioma. *J Clin Oncol*. 2009;27(25):4162-4168. doi:10.1200/JCO.2008.21.3496

62. Rudisile S, Gosewisch A, Wenter V, et al. Salvage PRRT with 177Lu-DOTA-octreotate in extensively pretreated patients with metastatic neuroendocrine tumor (NET): dosimetry, toxicity, efficacy, and survival. *BMC Cancer*. 2019;19(1):788. doi:10.1186/s12885-019-6000-y

63. Amini N, Margonis GA, Kim Y, et al. Curative resection of adrenocortical carcinoma: rates and patterns of postoperative recurrence. *Ann Surg Oncol*. 2016;23(1):126-133. doi:10.1245 /s10434-015-4810-y

64. Tierney JF, Chivukula SV, Poirier J, et al. National treatment practice for adrenocortical carcinoma: have they changed and have we made any progress? *J Clin Endocrinol Metab*. 2019;104(12):5948-5956. doi:10.1210/jc.2019-00915

65. Dy BM, Strajina V, Cayo AK, et al. Surgical resection of synchronously metastatic adrenocortical cancer. *Ann Surg Oncol*. 2015;22(1):146-151. doi:10.1245/s10434-014-3944-7

66. Gara SK, Lack J, Zhang L, Harris E, Cam M, Kebebew E. Metastatic adrenocortical carcinoma displays higher mutation rate and tumor heterogeneity than primary tumors. *Nat Commun*. 2018;9(1):4172. doi:10.1038/s41467-018-06366-z

67. Paton BL, Novitsky YW, Zerey M, et al. Outcomes of adrenal cortical carcinoma in the United States. *Surgery*. 2006;140(6):914-920. doi:10.1016/j.surg.2006.07.035

68. Kendrick ML, Lloyd R, Erickson L, et al. Adrenocortical carcinoma: surgical progress or status quo? *Arch Surg*. 2001;136(5):543-549. doi:10.1001/archsurg.136.5.543

69. Dackiw AP, Lee JE, Gagel RF, Evans DB. Adrenal cortical carcinoma. *World J Surg*. 2001;25(7): 914-926. doi:10.1007/s00268-001-0030-7

70. Icard P, Goudet P, Charpenay C, et al. Adrenocortical carcinomas: surgical trends and results of a 253-patient series from the French Association of Endocrine Surgeons study group. *World J Surg*. 2001;25(7):891-897. doi:10.1007/s00268-001-0047-y

71. Margonis GA, Kim Y, Prescott JD, et al. Adrenocortical carcinoma: impact of surgical margin status on long-term outcomes. *Ann Surg Oncol*. 2016;23(1):134-141. doi:10.1245/s10434-015-4803-x

72. Tella SH, Kommalapati A, Yaturu S, Kebebew E. Predictors of survival in adrenocortical carcinoma: an analysis from the National Cancer Database. *J Clin Endocrinol Metab*. 2018;103(9):3566-3573. doi:10.1210/jc.2018-00918

73. Ruffolo LI, Nessen MF, Probst CP, et al. Open adrenalectomy through a makuuchi incision: a single institution's experience. *Surgery*. 2018;164(6):1372-1376. doi:10.1016/j.surg.2018.06.045

74. Marincola Smith P, Kiernan CM, Tran TB, et al. Role of additional organ resection in adrenocortical carcinoma: analysis of 167 patients from the U.S. Adrenocortical Carcinoma Database. *Ann Surg Oncol.* 2018;25(8):2308-2315. doi:10.1245/s10434-018-6546-y

75. Zeiger MA, Thompson GB, Duh Q-Y, Kebebew E. American Association of Clinical Endocrinologists and American Association of Endocrine Surgeons medical guidelines for the management of adrenal incidentalomas: executive summary of recommendations. *Endocr Pract.* 2009;15(5):450-453. doi:10.1016/j.jamcollsurg.2005.11.00

76. Varghese J, Habra MA. Update on adrenocortical carcinoma management and future directions. *Curr Opin Endocrinol Diabetes Obes.* 2017;24(3):208-214. doi:10.1097/MED.0000000000000332

77. Grubbs EG, Callender GG, Xing Y, et al. Recurrence of adrenal cortical carcinoma following resection: surgery alone can achieve results equal to surgery plus mitotane. *Ann Surg Oncol.* 2010;17(1):263-270. doi:10.1245/s10434-009-0716-x

78. Moher D, Liberati A, Tetzlaff J, Altman DG; for PRISMA Group. Preferred Reporting Items for Systematic Reviews and Meta-Analyses: the PRISMA statement. *PLoS Med.* 2009;6(7):e1000097. doi:10.1371/journal.pmed.1000097

79. Fosså A, Røsok BI, Kazaryan AM, et al. Laparoscopic versus open surgery in stage I-III adrenocortical carcinoma—a retrospective comparison of 32 patients. *Acta Oncol.* 2013;52(8):1771-1777. doi:10.3109/0284186X.2013.765065

80. Gonzalez RJ, Shapiro S, Sarlis N, et al. Laparoscopic resection of adrenal cortical carcinoma: a cautionary note. *Surgery.* 2005;138(6):1078-1086. doi:10.1016/j.surg.2005.09.012

81. Huynh KT, Lee DY, Lau BJ, Flaherty DC, Lee J, Goldfarb M. Impact of laparoscopic adrenalectomy on overall survival in patients with nonmetastatic adrenocortical carcinoma. *J Am Coll Surg.* 2016;223(3):485-492. doi:10.1016/j.jamcollsurg.2016.05.015

82. Leboulleux S, Deandreis D, Al Ghuzlan A, et al. Adrenocortical carcinoma: is the surgical approach a risk factor of peritoneal carcinomatosis? *Eur J Endocrinol.* 2010;162(6):1147-1153. doi:10.1530/EJE-09-1096

83. Lombardi CP, Raffaelli M, De Crea C, et al. Open versus endoscopic adrenalectomy in the treatment of localized (stage I/II) adrenocortical carcinoma: results of a multiinstitutional Italian survey. *Surgery.* 2012;152(6):1158-1164. doi:10.1016/j.surg.2012.08.014

84. Miller BS, Ammori JB, Gauger PG, Broome JT, Hammer GD, Doherty GM. Laparoscopic resection is inappropriate in patients with known or suspected adrenocortical carcinoma. *World J Surg.* 2010;34(6):1380-1385. doi:10.1007/s00268-010-0532-2

85. Mir MC, Klink JC, Guillotreau J, et al. Comparative outcomes of laparoscopic and open adrenalectomy for adrenocortical carcinoma: single, high-volume center experience. *Ann Surg Oncol.* 2013;20(5):1456-1461. doi:10.1245/s10434-012-2760-1

86. Porpiglia F, Fiori C, Daffara F, et al. Retrospective evaluation of the outcome of open versus laparoscopic adrenalectomy for stage I and II adrenocortical cancer. *Eur Urol.* 2010;57(5):873-878. doi:10.1016/j.eururo.2010.01.036

87. Wu K, Liu Z, Liang J, et al. Laparoscopic versus open adrenalectomy for localized (stage 1/2) adrenocortical carcinoma: experience at a single, high-volume center. *Surgery.* 2018;164(6):1325-1329. doi:10.1016/j.surg.2018.07.026

88. Zheng GY, Li HZ, Deng JH, Zhang XB, Wu XC. Open adrenalectomy versus laparoscopic adrenalectomy for adrenocortical carcinoma: a retrospective comparative study on short-term oncologic prognosis. *Onco Targets Ther.* 2018;11:1625-1632. doi:10.2147/OTT.S157518

89. Suzuki K, Ushiyama T, Ihara H, Kageyama S, Mugiya S, Fujita K. Complications of laparoscopic adrenalectomy in 75 patients treated by the same surgeon. *Eur Urol.* 1999;36(1):40-47. doi:10.1159/000019925

90. Iino K, Oki Y, Sasano H. A case of adrenocortical carcinoma associated with recurrence after laparoscopic surgery. *Clin Endocrinol (Oxf).* 2000;53(2):243-248. doi:10.1046/j.1365-2265.2000.01036.x

91. Sgourakis G, Lanitis S, Kouloura A, et al. Laparoscopic versus open adrenalectomy for stage I/II adrenocortical carcinoma: meta-analysis of outcomes. *J Invest Surg.* 2015;28(3):145-152. doi:10.3109/08941939.2014.987886

92. Autorino R, Bove P, De Sio M, et al. Open versus laparoscopic adrenalectomy for adrenocortical carcinoma: a meta-analysis of surgical and oncological outcomes. *Ann Surg Oncol.* 2016;23(4):1195-1202. doi:10.1245/s10434-015-4900-x

93. Balshem H, Helfand M, Schunemann HJ, et al. GRADE guidelines: 3. Rating the quality of evidence. *J Clin Epidemiol.* 2011;64(4):401-406. doi:10.1016/j.jclinepi.2010.07.015

94. Brix D, Allolio B, Fenske W, et al. Laparoscopic versus open adrenalectomy for adrenocortical carcinoma: surgical and oncologic outcome in 152 patients. *Eur Urol.* 2010;58(4):609-615. doi:10.1016/j.eururo.2010.06.024

95. Cooper AB, Habra MA, Grubbs EG, et al. Does laparoscopic adrenalectomy jeopardize onco-logic outcomes for patients with adrenocortical carcinoma? *Surg Endosc.* 2013;27(11):4026-4032. doi:10.1007/s00464-013-3034-0

96. Donatini G, Caiazzo R, Do Cao C, et al. Long-term survival after adrenalectomy for stage I/II adrenocortical carcinoma (ACC): a retrospective comparative cohort study of laparoscopic versus open approach. *Ann Surg Oncol.* 2014;21(1):284-291. doi:10.1245/s10434-013-3164-6

97. Lee CW, Salem AI, Schneider DF, et al. Minimally invasive resection of adrenocortical carci-noma: a multi-institutional study of 201 patients. *J Gastrointest Surg.* 2017;21(2):352-362. doi:10.1007/s11605-016-3262-4

98. Pommier RF, Brennan MF. An eleven-year experience with adrenocortical carcinoma. *Surgery.* 1992;112(6):963-971.

99. Deckers S, Derdelinckx L, Col V, Hamels J, Maiter D. Peritoneal carcinomatosis following lapa-roscopic resection of an adrenocortical tumor causing primary hyperaldosteronism. *Horm Res.* 1999;52(2):97-100. doi:10.1159/000023442

100. Laan DV, Thiels CA, Glasgow A, et al. Adrenocortical carcinoma with inferior vena cava tumor thrombus. *Surgery.* 2017;161(1):240-248. doi:10.1016/j.surg.2016.07.040

101. Zhu P, Du S, Chen S, et al. The role of deep hypothermic circulatory arrest in surgery for renal or adrenal tumor with vena cava thrombus: a single-institution experience. *J Cardiothorac Surg.* 2018;13(1):85. doi:10.1186/s13019-018-0772-z

102. Mihai R, Iacobone M, Makay O, et al. Outcome of operation in patients with adrenocortical cancer invading the inferior vena cava—a European Society of Endocrine Surgeons (ESES) sur-vey. *Langenbecks Arch Surg.* 2012;397(2):225-231. doi:10.1007/s00423-011-0876-6

103. Gregory SH, Yalamuri SM, McCartney SL, et al. Perioperative management of adrenalectomy and inferior vena cava reconstruction in a patient with a large, malignant pheochromocytoma with vena caval extension. *J Cardiothorac Vasc Anesth.* 2017;31(1):365-377. doi:10.1053/j.jvca.2016.07.019

104. Kato S, Tanaka T, Kitamura H, et al. Resection of the inferior vena cava for urological mal-gnancies: single-center experience. *Int J Clin Oncol.* 2013;18(5):905-909. doi:10.1007/s10147-012-0473-x

105. Spelde A, Steinberg T, Patel PA, et al. Successful team-based management of renal cell carcinoma with caval extension of tumor thrombus above the diaphragm. *J Cardiothorac Vasc Anesth.* 2017;31(5):1883-1893. doi:10.1053/j.jvca.2017.02.036

106. Abbasi A, Johnson TV, Kleris R, et al. Posterior lumbar vein off the retrohepatic inferior vena cava: a novel anatomical variant with surgical implications. *J Urol.* 2012;187(1):296-301. doi:10.1016/j.juro.2011.09.009

107. Livhits M, Li N, Yeh MW, Harari A. Surgery is associated with improved survival for adreno-cortical cancer, even in metastatic disease. *Surgery.* 2014;156(6):1531-1541. doi:10.1016/j.surg.2014.08.047

108. Edge SB, Byrd DR, Compton CC, Fritz A, Greene F, Trotti A, eds. *AJCC Cancer Staging Manual.* 7th ed. Springer; 2010.

109. Lughezzani G, Sun M, Perrotte P, et al. The European Network for the Study of Adrenal Tumors staging system is prognostically superior to the international union against cancer-staging system: a North American validation. *Eur J Cancer.* 2010;46(4):713-719. doi:10.1016/j.ejca.2009.12.007

110. Erdogan I, Deutschbein T, Jurowich C, et al. The role of surgery in the management of recurrent ad-renocortical carcinoma. *J Clin Endocrinol Metab.* 2013;98(1):181-191. doi:10.1210/jc.2012-2559

111. Reibetanz J, Rinn B, Kunz AS, et al. Patterns of lymph node recurrence in adrenocortical carci-noma: possible implications for primary surgical treatment. *Ann Surg Oncol.* 2019;26(2):531-538. doi:10.1245/s10434-018-6999-z

112. Gerry JM, Tran TB, Postlewait LM, et al. Lymphadenectomy for adrenocortical carcinoma: is there a therapeutic benefit? *Ann Surg Oncol.* 2016;23(suppl 5):708-713. doi:10.1245/s10434-016-5535-1

113. Dickson PV, Kim L, Yen TWF, et al. Evaluation, staging, and surgical management for adreno-cortical carcinoma: an update from the SSO Endocrine and Head and Neck Disease Site Working Group. *Ann Surg Oncol.* 2018;25(12):3460-3468. doi:10.1245/s10434-018-6749-2

114. Nilubol N, Patel D, Kebebew E. Does lymphadenectomy improve survival in patients with adrenocortical carcinoma? A population-based study. *World J Surg.* 2016;40(3):697-705. doi:10.1007/s00268-015-3283-2

115. Miller BS, Doherty GM. Regional lymphadenectomy for adrenocortical carcinoma. *Ann Surg.* 2013;257(4):e13-e14. doi:10.1097/SLA.0b013e3182891ee5

116. Gaujoux S, Brennan MF. Recommendation for standardized surgical management of primary adrenocortical carcinoma. *Surgery.* 2012;152(1):123-132. doi:10.1016/j.surg.2011.09.030

117. Maurice MJ, Bream MJ, Kim SP, Abouassaly R. Surgical quality of minimally invasive adrenalectomy for adrenocortical carcinoma: a contemporary analysis using the National Cancer Database. *BJU Int.* 2017;119(3):436-443. doi:10.1111/bju.13618

118. Miller BS. 5th International ACC Symposium: surgical considerations in the treatment of adrenocortical carcinoma: 5th International ACC Symposium session: who, when and what combination? *Horm Cancer.* 2016;7(1):24-28. doi:10.1007/s12672-015-0243-0

119. Alanee S, Dynda D, Holland B. Prevalence and prognostic value of lymph node dissection in treating adrenocortical carcinoma: a national experience. *Anticancer Res.* 2015;35(10):5575-5579.

120. Gratian L, Pura J, Dinan M, et al. Treatment patterns and outcomes for patients with adrenocortical carcinoma associated with hospital case volume in the United States. *Ann Surg Oncol.* 2014;21(11):3509-3514. doi:10.1245/s10434-014-3931-z

121. Lombardi CP, Raffaelli M, Boniardi M, et al. Adrenocortical carcinoma: effect of hospital volume on patient outcome. *Langenbecks Arch Surg.* 2012;397(2):201-207. doi:10.1007/s00423-011-0866-8

122. Panjwani S, Moore MD, Gray KD, et al. The impact of nodal dissection on staging in adrenocortical carcinoma. *Ann Surg Oncol.* 2017;24(12):3617-3623. doi:10.1245/s10434-017-6064-3

123. Punjani N, Clark R, Izawa J, Chin J, Pautler SE, Power N. The impact of patient-, disease-, and treatment-related factors on survival in patients with adrenocortical carcinoma. *Can Urol Assoc J.* 2018;12(4):98-103. doi:10.5489/cuaj.4650

124. Saade N, Sadler C, Goldfarb M. Impact of regional lymph node dissection on disease specific survival in adrenal cortical carcinoma. *Horm Metab Res.* 2015;47(11):820-825. doi:10.1055/s-0035-1549877

125. Tran TB, Postlewait LM, Maithel SK, et al. Actual 10-year survivors following resection of adrenocortical carcinoma. *J Surg Oncol.* 2016;114(8):971-976. doi:10.1002/jso.24439

126. Wang S, Gao W-C, Chen S-S, et al. Primary site surgery for metastatic adrenocortical carcinoma improves survival outcomes: an analysis of a population-based database. *Onco Targets Ther.* 2017;10:5311-5315. doi:10.2147/OTT.S147352

127. Wang S, Chen SS, Gao WC, et al. Prognostic factors of adrenocortical carcinoma: an analysis of the Surveillance Epidemiology and End Results (SEER) database. *Asian Pac J cancer Prev.* 2017;18(10):2817-2823. doi:10.22034/APJCP.2017.18.10.2817

128. Icard P, Louvel A, Chapuis Y. Survival rates and prognostic factors in adrenocortical carcinoma. *World J Surg.* 1992;16(4):753-758. doi:10.1007/BF02067377

129. Langenhuijsen J, Birtle A, Klatte T, Porpiglia F, Timsit MO. Surgical management of adrenocortical carcinoma: impact of laparoscopic approach, lymphadenectomy, and surgical volume on outcomes—a systematic review and meta-analysis of the current literature. *Eur Urol Focus.* 2016;1(3):241-250. doi:10.1016/j.euf.2015.12.001

Synoptic Operative Report: Adrenal

Date of procedure _____   Surgeon(s) _____

_____

Clinical Information

Side
- ☐ Right
- ☐ Left
- ☐ Bilateral

Clinical stage by preoperative and intraoperative assessment
- ☐ I
- ☐ II
- ☐ III
- ☐ IV

Radiologic necrosis
- ☐ Yes
- ☐ No

Hormone excess
- ☐ Yes
  - ☐ Hormone(s) _____
  - ☐ Complete biochemical evaluation
  - ☐ Incomplete biochemical evaluation
- ☐ No

Preoperative treatment
- ☐ None
- ☐ Mitotane
- ☐ Chemotherapy
- ☐ Radiation
- ☐ Other _____

Synoptic Operative Report: Adrenal

Date of procedure _____   Surgeon(s) _____

_____

Intraoperative Findings

Peritoneal disease
☐ Yes
☐ No

Clinical adenopathy
☐ Yes

Location
☐ Renal
☐ Paracaval
☐ Suprarenal
☐ Infrarenal
☐ Para-aortic
☐ Suprarenal
☐ Infrarenal
☐ Interaortocaval
☐ Celiac
☐ Superior mesenteric artery
☐ Other _____

☐ No

Distant metastatic disease
☐ Yes

Location _____
☐ No

Gross or suspected extra-adrenal
extension into periadrenal
fat/tissues
☐ Yes

Location _____
☐ No

Gross or suspected invasion
of adjacent organs
☐ Yes

Organ(s) invaded

_____

☐ No

Synoptic Operative Report: Adrenal

Date of procedure _____   Surgeon(s) _____

_____

Vascular invasion of vessel wall   ☐   Yes
  (with or without thrombus)   Location _____
         ☐   No

Venous tumor thrombus   ☐   Yes
                       Location
                       ☐   Vena cava
                       ☐   Right renal vein
                       ☐   Left renal vein
                       Extent
                       ☐   Adrenal vein
                       ☐   Renal vein
                       ☐   Infrahepatic
                       ☐   Retrohepatic caudal to or
                             at hepatic veins
                       ☐   Retrohepatic cranial to
                             hepatic veins
                       ☐   Suprahepatic at or below
                             diaphragm
                       ☐   Suprahepatic above
                             diaphragm
                       ☐   Intracardiac
                       ☐   Or use figure to describe
                             extent—levels 1–4:
         ☐   No

Frozen section   ☐   Performed
                       Location _____
                       Result _____
         ☐   Not performed

Synoptic Operative Report: Adrenal

Date of procedure _____   Surgeon(s) _____

_____

Operative Details

Approach

- ☐ Open
- ☐ Laparoscopic
  - ☐ With hand assist
  - ☐ Without hand assist
- ☐ Robot-assisted
- ☐ Laparoscopic converted to open (reason)

_____

Complete exploration of peritoneal cavity

- ☐ Yes
- ☐ No

Inclusion of periadrenal fat with specimen

- ☐ Yes
- ☐ No

Adjacent organs resected if suspected of invasion

- ☐ Yes
  - Organ(s) removed
    - ☐ Total
    - ☐ Partial
    - ☐ En bloc
      - ☐ Yes
      - ☐ No
- ☐ No

Synoptic Operative Report: Adrenal

Date of procedure _____ Surgeon(s) _____

_____

Lymph nodes removed ☐ Yes
      ☐ Formal dissection
      ☐ Sampling/"berry picking"
      Location(s) of nodes removed
        ☐ Renal
        ☐ Paracaval
          ☐ Suprarenal
          ☐ Infrarenal
        ☐ Para-aortic
          ☐ Suprarenal
          ☐ Infrarenal
        ☐ Interaortocaval
        ☐ Celiac
        ☐ Superior mesenteric artery
        ☐ Other _____
☐ No

Venous thrombectomy ☐ Yes
☐ No

Venous reconstruction ☐ Yes
      ☐ Primary repair
      ☐ Patch
      ☐ Graft
☐ No

Need for bypass ☐ Yes
      ☐ Venovenous
      ☐ Cardio-pulmonary bypass
      with hypothermic circulatory
      arrest in situ liver perfusion
☐ No

Synoptic Operative Report: Adrenal

Date of procedure _____ Surgeon(s) _____

_____

Resection of metastatic disease   ☐ Yes

Location _____

☐ No

Capsular disruption   ☐ Yes

Tumor spillage
☐ Yes
☐ No

☐ No

Clinical resection status   ☐ R0
☐ R1
☐ R2

COMMENTARY: ADRENAL SECTION

Nancy D. Perrier, MD, FACS
Ruth and Walter Sterling Tenured Professor of Surgery
Chief of Surgical Endocrinology
Department of Surgical Oncology
MD Anderson Cancer Center
Houston, Texas

The authors of the primary adrenal malignancy section of the *Operative Standards for Cancer Surgery*, Volume 3, had an arduous task and are to be congratulated for a detailed review of the cortical and medullary aspects of this organ. Central to the section for adrenocortical carcinoma (ACC) is that surgery is the only cure. Removal without shed of cells outside the capsule is the most important determinant of outcome. This responsibility is totally surgeon dependent. The data comparing laparoscopic to the open technique is problematic because the most controversial group—those who required conversion from laparoscopic to open—were excluded from analysis. As such, adrenal malignancy management should not be left to the surgical ego in deciding what is best. If malignancy is in the differential, the resection should be performed in the safest possible fashion to prevent any cell spillage.

In this section, the technical aspects are strong and appropriately emphasize that the sequence of ACC treatment requires recognition of the fact that there is an ideal window to operate amidst hormonal management and oncologic therapy. This is especially true when there are gross metabolic deviations or consideration for nephrotoxic systemic therapy is anticipated.

Understanding that the complexity of perioperative management is fundamental to excellent surgical care is as important as the technical aspects. Highlights include distinguishing incomplete fluid resuscitation from bleeding or hypoperfusion in the perioperative period. This requires unique mastery beyond technical or laboratory interpretation. Knowledge of the effects of metyrapone and ketoconazole is necessary due to the resulting reaction and fibrosis that can significantly complicate the technical aspects of resection. Familiarity of all aspects of incisions (traditional subcostal midclavicular to midaxillary versus Makuuchi) is vital to strategic planning because debilitating pain may delay recovery and oncologic treatment. Dissection principles, from areas of known to unknown and releasing tension without accepting as true the misconception that early adrenal vein ligation, are absolutely necessary. Technically, prevention of thrombus dislodgment is also vital; preparation of instruments such as a Satinsky side clamp and sponge on a stick are indispensable for dissection around and behind the vena cava. Sequencing of staged procedures for oligometastatic disease after primary tumor resection may drastically improve metabolic derangement.

With regard to the medulla-based carcinoma, the most recent American Joint Committee on Cancer (AJCC) staging system includes elements and definitions to take into account the unique characteristics of these tumors. Simply stated, on any tumor >5 cm is categorized to stage II, any peritumor invasion or nodal involvement is upgraded to stage III, and any metastases stage IV. Standardized use of staging will improve communication among physicians and provide data to better understand prognostic indicators of survival.

It is worthy to highlight that clinical germline testing is recommended for the presurgical workup of patients with concerning features for metastatic disease. If metastatic disease is suspected, somatostatin receptor (SSTR) positron emission tomography/computed tomography (PET/CT) should be a first-line functional imaging modality, given its high sensitivity. Functional scanning can determine if the patient is likely to benefit from potential peptide receptor radionuclide therapy (PRRT). ^{18}F-fluoro-2-deoxy-d-glucose ([18]FDG)-PET/CT may be useful in patients with *SDHB*-associated metastatic pheochromocytoma and paraganglioma or rapidly progressive disease, and ^{123}I-metaiodobenzylguanidine (MIBG) imaging is required to select patients for ^{131}I-MIBG therapy. Neoadjuvant approaches remain individualized within multidisciplinary teams with careful patient selection criteria. Radioguided surgery may have utility in patients to localize occult nodal metastases, determining adequacy of surgical margins, and to detect small tumors that might not be visible. Different isotopes are available, but the timing of exploration after injection, radiation exposure, and scatter differ. Embolization and chemoembolization either prior to adrenalectomy for large or ruptured pheochromocytoma or to control symptoms from unresectable primary and metastatic lesions are highly selective options. The decision to perform aortic sidewall resection may be considered to enable an R0 resection but has no objective data to prove benefit. The most recent North American Neuroendocrine Tumor Society Consensus Guidelines recommendation encourages primary tumor resection if it will improve medical management of hormone excess and allow for targeted nuclear medicine ablation of metastases.

The section highlights that the location of distant metastases is important. Bone metastases are most common, and patients who have only skeletal metastasis have a longer survival compared with patients with or without skeletal metastasis but with metastasis in other organs such as the liver and lungs. Percutaneous image-guided thermal ablation performed under alpha-blockade and monitored anesthesia is effective for symptom control and prevention of skeletal-related events from oligometastatic disease. The rate of disease progression of 6 to 12 months is a good marker for overall prognosis.

As William Mayo, a founding adrenal surgical giant, stated, "The best interest of the patient is the only interest to be considered, and in order that the sick may have the benefit of advancing knowledge, union of forces is necessary."[1] The section reiterates that malignancy of the adrenal gland requires union of advanced multidisciplinary resources.

REFERENCES

1. Mayo WJ. The necessity of cooperation in medicine. *Mayo Clin Proc*. 2000;75(6):553-556.

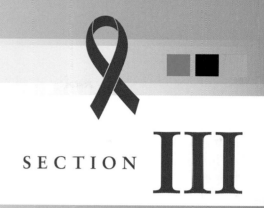

SECTION **III**

NEUROENDOCRINE

INTRODUCTION

Neuroendocrine neoplasms (NENs) are now, per World Health Organization (WHO) guidelines published in 2019, regarded as two entirely separate and independent entities: neuroendocrine *tumors* (NETs) and neuroendocrine *carcinomas* (NECs).[1-4] These require entirely different staging and management algorithms. A summary of the WHO 2019 classification of NENs is shown in Table 3-1.

This section focuses primarily on operations used for NENs that are not described elsewhere in the *Operative Standards for Cancer Surgery* manuals. These include small bowel (including duodenal) resections and parenchyma-preserving pancreas resections.

Neuroendocrine Tumors

NETs are by definition well-differentiated neoplasms encompassing the entities that were previously called carcinoids and islet cell tumors/carcinomas. These are low-grade malignancies and may be cured by resection if early stage. NETs are graded 1 to 3 on the basis of Ki-67 index and mitotic count.[4] Although mitotic count is used to grade tumors, it has been shown to have poorer reproducibility and seldom, if ever, trumps Ki-67 grade.[5] Grade 3 NETs (Ki-67 >20%) are rare and behave significantly more aggressively than lower-grade lesions. However, they are associated with significantly better survival than the poorly differentiated NECs.[6,7] In contrast, the survival difference between Grade 1 and Grade 2 cases is not appreciable, and the management of patients with these tumors is generally similar.

In earlier classifications including WHO 2004, an attempt was made to recognize a "benign" subset of NETs; however, careful studies with extended follow-ups have

TABLE 3-1 World Health Organization 2019 Classification of Gastrointestinal Neuroendocrine Neoplasms

WHO 2019 Classification	Grade	Differentiation	Ki-67 Index	Mitotic Rate (mitoses/2 mm²)
Neuroendocrine Tumor				
G1	Low	Well	<3%	<2
G2	Intermediate	Well	3-20%	2–20
G3	High	Well	>20%	>20
Neuroendocrine Carcinoma				
Small cell type	High	Poor	>20%	>20
Large cell type	High	Poor	>20%	>20
Mixed neuroendocrine-non-neuroendocrine neoplasms	Variable	Well or poor	Variable	Variable

established that even small, incidentally found lesions have a real risk of progression over the long term. Hence, these tumors are now uniformly regarded as malignancies.[8] The exception to this is minute tumorlets, which are dysplastic-type lesions that can develop in syndromic conditions or certain medical diseases; they are graded, staged, and managed as such.

For some rare conditions, the underlying setting that leads to the development of a NET can be the crucial determinant of behavior and management. For example, a conservative watchful-waiting approach is appropriate for type A (type 1, enterochromaffin cell) gastric "carcinoids" arising in the context of autoimmune gastritis.[9] These tumors arise in the setting of compensatory hypergastrinemia reacting to hypochlorhydria, which leads to multifocal proliferation of enterochromaffin cells. In contrast, for the sporadic (type C, or type 3) gastric NETs, which are typically solitary, resection is recommended, as these tumors often behave in an aggressive manner.[9]

Tumor location is also associated with behavior. In the earlier literature, NETs arising anywhere within the gastrointestinal (GI) tract were typically analyzed as a group. However, it has become clear that GI NETs have vastly different phenotypes and natural histories. For example, although type 3 gastric or transverse-colonic tumors are fairly aggressive, those in the appendix and rectum appear to have significantly more indolent behavior.[10] This difference may reflect biologic properties of the site-dependent neuroendocrine cell types (e.g., L cell versus G cell) from which they presumably arise.[11] Similarly, in the pancreas, most insulin-producing NETs behave in an indolent fashion, but glucagon-secreting examples seem to be more aggressive. This may be attributable, at least in part, to the biology of different cell types.[12-14] Regardless, these factors naturally affect the management approach to NETs and should be taken into consideration in the design of surgical and other therapies.

NETs are most common in the GI tract, pancreas, lungs, and adrenal glands. The age-adjusted incidence rate of NETs increased 6.4-fold from 1973 (1.09 per 100,000) to 2012 (6.98 per 100,000) across all sites, stages, and grades. In the Surveillance, Epidemiology, and End Results (SEER) 18 registry grouping (2000 to 2012), the highest incidence rate was 3.56 per 100,000 people for gastroenteropancreatic sites, which is the focus of this discussion.[15]

Approximately 25% of NETs have a corresponding hereditary predisposition.[16] These are summarized in Table 3-2.[4,17,18] Among the manifestations of NETs that are the most challenging and devastating to quality of life are their functional capacity to secrete vasoactive substances (e.g., serotonin and 5-hydroxytryptamine, among others) or hormones (e.g., insulin, glucagon, gastrin). The classic carcinoid syndrome (CS) is characterized by diarrhea, flushing, and bronchospasm, and long-term sequelae may be evident as fibrotic changes to the mesentery and cardiac valves.[19] The syndrome is seen in association with midgut NETs but can occur in patients with tumors of other sites.[20] The liver is a site of vasoactive peptide inactivation to the inactive 5-hydroxyindoleacetic acid. Thus, CS is generally seen in patients with liver metastases.[21] Zollinger-Ellison syndrome is characterized by abdominal pain, nausea, vomiting, diarrhea, and severe peptic ulcer disease due to a gastrin-producing NET, or gastrinoma. These tumors are most often located in the pancreas, duodenum, or both.[22]

TABLE 3-2   Hereditary Syndromes Associated with Neuroendocrine Neoplasms

Syndrome	Gene Mutation	Associated NENs
MEN 1	Menin	Pancreatic NET, gastric NET
MEN 2/3	RET	Pheochromocytoma
MEN 4	CDKN1B	Pancreatic, lung, and gastric NET
Von Hippel-Lindau	VHL	Pheochromocytoma, pancreatic NET
Tuberous sclerosis complex	TSC 1/2	Pheochromocytoma, pancreatic NET
Neurofibromatosis type 1	NF1	Paraganglioma, pheochromocytoma, pancreatic NET, gastrointestinal NET

MEN: multiple endocrine neoplasia; NEN: neuroendocrine neoplasm; NET: neuroendocrine tumor.

Neuroendocrine Carcinomas

NECs are regarded entirely separately from NETs. They are poorly differentiated, high-grade cancers. Differentiating them from other cancers such as high-grade lymphomas, undifferentiated carcinomas not otherwise specified, medullary carcinomas, and melanomas can be challenging. An analysis from the SEER database reported that only 9% of NECs were extrapulmonary.[23]

There does not seem to be a continuum between NETs and NECs; transformation into a (poorly differentiated) NEC from an NET is extremely rare. It is likewise uncommon to find a well-differentiated NET and poorly differentiated NEC within the same tumor. In contrast, NECs commonly occur concurrent with adenocarcinoma. NECs also show molecular genetic findings that are more typical of adenocarcinoma lineage (such as p53 and, in the pancreas, SMAD4 loss), which indicates that their cell of origin and mechanism are in fact closer to the glandular epithelial cells.[3,6] NETs seldom occur in conjunction with adenocarcinomas, and those reported NETs occurring at the base of "adenomas" of the GI tract may in fact be reactive hyperplastic changes rather than frank NETs. The molecular profile of NETs are also vastly different than both adenocarcinomas and NECs (such as neurofibromatosis type 1 [NF1] alterations or loss of ATRX/DAXX).[3] Whereas NETs are typically highlighted by DOTATATE scan (because they express the somatostatin receptor), NECs are typically not.[24]

NECs are characterized by aggressive behavior. They have a very high proliferation rate, with the Ki-67 labeling index typically greater than 50%. Unlike NETs, which are slow growing but typically intractable to chemotherapy, NECs often show striking, albeit transient, response to platinum-based therapies and, in some studies, to radiotherapy as well.[3,17,24] Therefore, when devising treatment strategies for patients with NEC, the aggressive behavior and early metastatic nature of these tumors should be carefully considered. Thorough staging is critical because NECs are often associated with distant metastases in various locations that may be difficult to detect. Although resection thus may be considered for some highly selected patients, most experience cancer recurrence and progression following surgery—usually rapidly.[6]

Mixed Tumors

Tumors with mixed neuroendocrine differentiation also occur. These have been termed variably as "mixed adeno-neuroendocrine carcinoma" and are now regarded under the conceptual category of "mixed neuroendocrine non-neuroendocrine neoplasms" per WHO 2019.[25] Typically, the neuroendocrine component is high grade and seems to be the main driver in such cases, even when it is small. It should be noted here that the tumor type that used to be called goblet cell carcinoid, which was previously thought to be a NEN (a peculiar form of mixed or amphicrine type of neoplasm), has now been proven to be a form of adenocarcinoma and reclassified as goblet cell adenocarcinoma or crypt cell adenocarcinoma.[4]

CLINICAL STAGING

Staging of gastroenteropancreatic NENs is usually achieved with cross-sectional, multiphase contrast imaging, typically with computed tomography (CT) or magnetic resonance imaging (MRI). CT and MRI provide high-quality anatomic images to assess for regional and distant metastases. Endoscopic ultrasound is also useful for locoregional assessment of disease in gastroduodenal, pancreatic, and rectal NENs and allows for biopsy. Another important and relatively novel imaging technique for NETs is based on their expression of high-affinity somatostatin receptors. Positron emission tomography (PET) using the radiolabeled somatostatin analogue (SSA) gallium-68 DOTATATE was approved by the US Food and Drug Administration in 2016. This imaging modality has been shown to be extremely sensitive and allows for identification of the primary tumor site and extent of metastatic disease and is predictive of response to somatostatin receptor-based therapies.

The *American Joint Commission on Cancer (AJCC) Cancer Staging Manual*, Eighth Edition,[26] includes nine separate TNM staging systems for NETs of the stomach, duodenum/ampulla of Vater, jejunum/ileum, colon/rectum, appendix, pancreas, adrenal (pheochromocytoma and paraganglioma), lung, and thymus.[17] NETs are staged slightly differently from the adenocarcinomas of the corresponding organs. In some sites, the size of the lesion is incorporated into the T stage for NETs. Stage is a fairly reliable prognosticator for these tumors. Selected TNM staging systems of NETs of the duodenum/ampulla of Vater, jejunum/ileum, and pancreas are shown in Tables 3-3, 3-4, and 3-5. NECs are defined and staged by the criteria used in the lungs for small cell carcinoma or large cell NEC.[17]

MULTIDISCIPLINARY CARE

A multidisciplinary team is important for optimal management of patients with NENs. The myriad disciplines potentially involved include medical oncology, surgical oncology, interventional radiology, nuclear medicine, gastroenterology, cardiology,

TABLE 3-3 American Joint Committee on Cancer Staging Criteria for Neuroendocrine Tumors of the Duodenum and Ampulla of Vater, Eighth Edition

TABLE 3-3A Definition of Primary Tumor (T)

T Stage	Criteria
Tx	Not able to assess
T1	Duodenum: ≤1 cm size and invades mucosa or submucosa Ampulla: ≤1 cm size and confined to sphincter of Oddi
T2	Duodenal: >1 cm size OR invades muscularis propria Ampulla: tumor >1 cm OR invades duodenal submucosa or muscularis propria
T3	Invades pancreas or peripancreatic adipose tissue
T4	Invades serosa or other organs/structures

TABLE 3-3B Definition of Regional Lymph Node (N)

N Stage	Criteria
Nx	Not able to assess
N0	No regional lymph node metastases
N1	Any regional node metastases

TABLE 3-3C Definition of Distant Metastasis (M)

M Stage	Criteria
M0	No distant metastases
M1	Distant metastases present
M1a	Liver-only metastases
M1b	Distant extrahepatic metastases only
M1c	Hepatic and extrahepatic metastases

TABLE 3-3D American Joint Committee on Cancer Prognostic Stage Groups

T Stage	N Stage	M Stage	Group Stage
T1	N0	M0	I
T2	N0	M0	II
T3	N0	M0	II
T4	N0	M0	III
Any T stage	N1	M0	III
Any T stage	Any N stage	M1	IV

Note: American Joint Committee on Cancer staging and TNM classification for neuroendocrine tumors of the duodenum and ampulla of Vater.[26] Used with permission of the American Joint Committee on Cancer (AJCC), Chicago, Illinois. The original and primary source for this information is the *AJCC Cancer Staging Manual*, Eighth Edition (2017) published by Springer International Publishing.

TABLE 3-4 American Joint Committee on Cancer Staging Criteria for Neuroendocrine Tumors of the Jejunum and Ileum, Eighth Edition

TABLE 3-4A Definition of Primary Tumor (T)

T Stage	Criteria
Tx	Not able to assess
T0	No evidence of primary tumor
T1	<1 cm size AND invades lamina propria or submucosa
T2	>1 cm size OR invades muscularis propria
T3	Invades through muscularis propria without penetration of serosa
T4	Invades serosa or other organs/structures

TABLE 3-4B Definition of Regional Lymph Node (N)

N Stage	Criteria
Nx	Not able to assess
N0	No regional lymph node metastases
N1	<12 regional node metastases
N2	≥12 nodal metastases AND/OR mesenteric masses >2 cm OR encasement of superior mesenteric vessels

TABLE 3-4C Definition of Distant Metastasis (M)

M Stage	Criteria
M0	No distant metastases
M1	Distant metastases present
M1a	Liver-only metastases
M1b	Distant extrahepatic metastases only
M1c	Hepatic and extrahepatic metastases

TABLE 3-4D American Joint Committee on Cancer Prognostic Stage Groups

T Stage	N Stage	M Stage	Group Stage
Tx or T0	Any	M1	IV
T1	N0	M0	I
T1	N1–N2	M0	III
T1	Any	M1	IV
T2	N0	M0	II
T2	N1–N2	M0	III
T2	Any	M1	IV
T3	N0	M0	II
T3	N1–N2	M0	III
T3	Any	M1	IV
T4	N0	M0	III
T4	N1–N2	M0	III
T4	Any	M1	IV

Note: American Joint Committee on Cancer staging and TNM classification for neuroendocrine tumors of the jejunum and ileum.[26] Used with permission of the American Joint Committee on Cancer (AJCC), Chicago, Illinois. The original and primary source for this information is the *AJCC Cancer Staging Manual*, Eighth Edition (2017) published by Springer International Publishing.

TABLE 3-5   American Joint Committee on Cancer Staging Criteria for Pancreatic Neuroendocrine Tumors, Eighth Edition

TABLE 3-5A   Definition of Primary Tumor (T)

T Stage	Criteria
Tx	Not able to assess
T1	<2 cm size AND limited to pancreas
T2	2–4 cm size AND limited to pancreas
T3	>4 cm size AND limited to pancreas OR invades duodenum or common bile duct
T4	Invades adjacent organs OR the wall of large blood vessels

TABLE 3-5B   Definition of Regional Lymph Node (N)

N Stage	Criteria
Nx	Not able to assess
N0	No regional lymph node metastases
N1	Any regional node metastases

TABLE 3-5C   Definition of Distant Metastasis (M)

M Stage	Criteria
M0	No distant metastases
M1	Distant metastases present
M1a	Liver-only metastases
M1b	Distant extrahepatic metastases only
M1c	Hepatic and extrahepatic metastases

TABLE 3-5D   American Joint Committee on Cancer Prognostic Stage Groups

T Stage	N Stage	M Stage	Group Stage
T1	N0	M0	I
T2	N0	M0	II
T3	N0	M0	II
T4	N0	M0	III
Any T stage	N1	M0	III
Any T stage	Any N stage	M1	IV

Note: American Joint Committee on Cancer staging and TNM classification for pancreatic neuroendocrine tumors.[26] Used with permission of the American Joint Committee on Cancer (AJCC), Chicago, Illinois. The original and primary source for this information is the *AJCC Cancer Staging Manual*, Eighth Edition (2017) published by Springer International Publishing.

endocrinology, transplant surgery, and genetics. Treatment decisions are driven by consideration of anatomy, tumor category definition, tumor type definition, degree of differentiation, grade (mitotic activity, Ki-67 labeling index, presence of necrosis), and presence of hormonal hypersecretion (vasoactive substances).[2] Despite the relative rarity of these tumors, there remains intense clinical interest in identifying novel agents and combinatorial therapy for NENs, both for symptom control and for disease control.

Surgical resection is the mainstay of therapy for patients with locoregional gastroenteropancreatic NETs.[17,27-29] A selective role for surgery may also exist in the metastatic setting. Systemic therapy options for functional and nonfunctional NENs are also abundant and are increasing in number. Impressive long-term oncologic outcomes have been achieved with aggressive surgical treatment, including cytoreductive surgery and liver transplantation for liver-only disease.[30,31] Owing to the prolonged natural history of low-grade and intermediate NETs, extended surveillance is advisable.

Carcinoid Syndrome

For patients with CS, octreotide and lanreotide (with dose escalation and use of supplemental octreotide), which target somatostatin receptor subtype 2, are recommended as first-line therapy.[28,32] Second-line options include interferon, locoregional therapy, everolimus, or peptide receptor radionuclide therapy (PRRT), in no particular order of preference. Despite the lack of randomized data, locoregional options include hepatic segment resection, radiofrequency ablation, cryosurgery, bland embolization, chemoembolization, or radioembolization. Serotonin pathway inhibitors cyproheptadine and ondansetron may be added in refractory cases.[33,34] A novel serotonin synthesis inhibitor named telotristat ethyl was tested in phase III trials, and a favorable effect of telotristat ethyl on diarrhea was shown in 40% to 44% of patients, compared with 0% to 20% of patients treated with placebo.[35]

Patients with CS should be evaluated for valvular heart disease. Most patients present with symptoms of right heart failure secondary to severe dysfunction of the tricuspid and pulmonary valves.[36] Transthoracic echocardiography is indicated at baseline. Cardiology and cardiothoracic surgery evaluation should be considered for potential valvular repair.[30,31]

Locally Advanced and Metastatic Disease

Numerous trials have shown efficacy of various drugs to control disease proliferation and prolong patients' progression-free and overall survival in the metastatic setting. The use of the SSA octreotide was evaluated in the PROMID study, in which 85 treatment-naïve patients were randomly assigned to monthly octreotide LAR 30 mg or placebo until tumor progression or death.[37] The median overall survival of all 85 patients was 84.7 months, with 107.6 months in the low tumor load ($n = 64$) and 57.5 months in the high tumor load ($n = 21$) subgroups (hazard ratio [HR], 2.49; 95% confidence interval [CI], 1.36 to 4.55; $P = .002$). There was a trend toward improved overall survival in patients with a low hepatic tumor load receiving octreotide compared with placebo ("median not reached" and 87.2 months; HR, 0.59; 95% CI, 0.29 to 1.2; $P = .142$). Crossover may have confounded the overall survival data.

A randomized, double-blind, placebo-controlled study of patients with advanced, well-differentiated or moderately differentiated, nonfunctioning, somatostatin receptor–positive NETs of grade 1 or 2 and documented disease-progression status showed that lanreotide was associated with significantly prolonged progression-free survival (median not reached vs. median of 18.0 months, $P < .001$) relative to observation.[38] Everolimus, an inhibitor of mechanistic target of rapamycin (mTOR), was evaluated in pancreatic NETs, displaying a progression-free survival of 11.0 months with everolimus as compared with 4.6 months with placebo, representing a 65% reduction in the estimated risk of progression or death.[39] The multi-tyrosine kinase inhibitor sunitinib is currently only approved for pancreatic NET. A phase III trial, including a total of 171 patients with progressive disease who were continuously treated with either sunitinib 37.5 mg daily or placebo, displayed a median progression-free survival of 11.4 versus 5.5 months (HR, 0.42; 95% CI, 0.26 to 0.66).[40] The oral alkylating agent temozolomide, evaluated in 144 patients with pancreatic NETs treated with temozolomide alone or with capecitabine, was generally active and more effective than monotherapy (progression-free survival, 22.7 vs. 14.4 months; HR, 0.58), with a response rate of about 30%.[41] Immunotherapy is a valid treatment option for patients with high-grade, poorly differentiated NECs, but results in patients with low- and intermediate-grade, well-differentiated tumors have not been robust.[42]

The advent of extremely sensitive diagnostic imaging like the ^{68}Ga-DOTATATE PET, a single-day procedure with higher spatial resolution, improved dosimetry, and the ability to semiquantify the activity in a given region as the standard uptake value,[43] allows for identification of the primary tumor site, extent of metastatic disease, predictive response to SSA therapy, and PRRT.[43] A randomized phase 3 study assigned 229 patients who had well-differentiated metastatic midgut NETs to receive either ^{177}Lu-DOTATATE (116 patients) or octreotide LAR alone (113 patients). Treatment with ^{177}Lu-DOTATATE resulted in markedly longer progression-free survival and a significantly higher response rate (18%) when compared with octreotide.[27,30,31,35,36,44]

Finally, appropriate molecular profiling may delineate agents to be used in this relatively rare tumor type, irrespective of the histology, and may enable personalized combination therapy.[45] Predictive studies are not without precedent, as seen with pancreatic NETs being treated with temozolomide. Four of five patients with O6-methylguanine-DNA methyltransferase (MGMT)-deficient tumors (all pancreatic NETs) and 0 of 16 patients with tumors showing intact MGMT expression responded to treatment ($P = .001$).[46] Regardless of different cancer types, mTOR pathway–activating mutations confer sensitivity to everolimus. Genomic alterations with activating effect on mTOR signaling were identified in 10 of 22 (45%) patients with clinical benefit, and these include mTOR, TSC1, TSC2, NF1, PIK3CA, and PIK3CG mutations.[47] Selective therapies could be chosen based on genomic profiling rather than unselected clinical trials.[37–39,48]

PERIOPERATIVE CARE

Patients with localized gastroenteropancreatic NETs who are symptomatic due to hormone secretion should be treated with SSAs such as octreotide or lanreotide for symptom control in the perioperative setting.[27] Patients with CS are at risk of developing a carcinoid crisis during minor or major surgery, arterial embolization, radiofrequency ablation, endoscopic procedures, diagnostic procedures, or treatment with PRRT. Awareness of this possible event is critical. The presence of carcinoid heart disease and high 5-hydroxyindoleacetic acid (5-HIAA) levels represent predictors of an emerging carcinoid crisis.[44] Patients with high-grade or type III gastric NETs may develop atypical CS. Antihistamine receptor therapy with loratadine or ranitidine may also be considered for these patients.[27] For patients with gastrinoma, high-dose proton pump inhibitor therapy is recommended in addition to SSAs and should be continued for as long as 3 months postoperatively. Additional considerations in perioperative therapy include nutritional optimization for patients with diarrhea, for example, in the setting of VIPoma. As previously mentioned, telotristat ethyl has been shown to be effective for management of diarrhea perioperatively. Patients with insulinoma require close glucose monitoring in the perioperative period, and surgery should be expedited for these patients once a diagnosis is made. Diazoxide can be considered for perioperative glucose control, but expeditious surgery is optimal.[27] Close communication with the anesthesia team in the peri- and intraoperative setting is critically important for patients with functional tumors so that appropriate intravenous access, monitoring, and immediate availability of medications, particularly pressors and antihypertensive agents, is in place. The European Neuroendocrine Tumor Society published consensus guidelines for pre- and perioperative therapy for patients with NETs in 2009; these were updated in 2017.[27,49]

QUALITY MEASURES

Historically, there have been no widely accepted quality performance measures for NENs. This is in part because of the rarity of these tumors and also because of their heterogeneity. However, CommNET, a collaboration between NET experts in Canada, Australia, and New Zealand, used rigorous methodology to establish ten consensus quality performance measures for NENs: documentation of the primary site, proliferative index, differentiation, tumor board review, use of a structured pathology report, documentation of the presence of distant metastasis, and 5- and 10-year disease-free and overall survival.[29]

Guidelines from the National Comprehensive Cancer Network, European Neuroendocrine Tumor Society, and North American Neuroendocrine Tumor Society describe general surgical approaches to NENs. These guidelines do not, however, provide detailed recommendations on the individual steps of operations that likely contribute to oncologic outcome, as is the aim of this publication.

CHAPTER 6

Small Bowel Resection

CRITICAL ELEMENTS

- Intraoperative Evaluation and Identification of Primary Tumor(s)
- Regional Lymphadenectomy along Segmental Vessels
- Resection of the Primary Tumor

1. INTRAOPERATIVE EVALUATION AND IDENTIFICATION OF PRIMARY TUMOR(S)

Recommendation: In patients with a small bowel neuroendocrine tumor (NET), intraoperative exploration should include assessment of the entirety of the small bowel at laparotomy. In patients with Zollinger-Ellison syndrome in whom a gastrinoma cannot be localized radiographically, the entire gastrinoma triangle should be inspected at laparotomy, and intraoperative ultrasound (IOUS) of the pancreas should be performed. If no gastrinoma can be identified using these techniques, the duodenal mucosa should be completely visualized and inspected through a lateral duodenotomy.

Type of Data: Retrospective reports, case series, or case-control studies

Strength of Recommendation: Strong recommendation, low-quality evidence

Rationale

The incidence of NETs is rising; their incidence was 6.98 cases per 100,000 population in 2012. Small bowel (jejunal and ileal) NETs account for 25% of gastroenteropancreatic NETs.[15] Resection of the primary tumor and associated lymphadenectomy can be curative for patients with gastroenteropancreatic NETs and a limited extent of disease. Surgery may even benefit select patients with metastatic tumors, in whom resection may prevent the development of future symptoms and prolong survival.

Gastrinomas, a rare functional subtype of NET that typically arise in the duodenum or pancreas, should also be considered for surgical resection.

Small bowel NETs, including gastrinomas, may be difficult to identify preoperatively and may also be multifocal. For this reason, a thorough surgical exploration with manual palpation of the bowel is critical.

Intraoperative exploration for duodenal neuroendocrine tumors/ gastrinoma

More than 80% of gastrinomas are located in the gastrinoma triangle, which is defined as the area within a triangle drawn from the cystic duct/common bile duct junction cranially, the junction of the second and third portions of the duodenum inferolaterally, and the junction of the neck and body of the pancreas inferomedially (Fig. 3-1).[50,51] If preoperative imaging studies do not definitively localize a primary tumor in a patient with clinical evidence of gastrinoma, surgical exploration is necessary to localize the tumor. An estimated 30% of patients with sporadic Zollinger-Ellison syndrome have primary tumors that cannot be successfully localized prior to surgery; the rate is closer to 60% among patients with tumors smaller than 1 cm.[50,52] An inability to locate the primary tumor radiographically may unnecessarily delay surgical treatment. A prospective study by Norton et al.[53] reported a mean delay of 8.9 years in this subset of patients. As is true for other small bowel NETs,

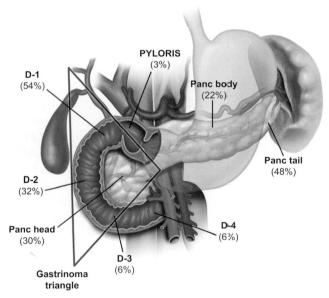

FIGURE 3-1 Illustration of gastrinoma triangle, the location of more than 80% of gastrinomas. The *triangle* is defined by the cystic duct/common bile duct junction cranially, the junction of the second and third portions of the duodenum inferolaterally, and the junction of the neck and body of the pancreas inferomedially.

open exploration is the recommended approach for gastrinoma when the operation is intended to be curative.[50]

IOUS has been known to identify pancreatic tumors as small as 5 mm. However, IOUS has limited sensitivity for identification of duodenal primaries.[54,55] Therefore, although IOUS should be performed routinely for patients with gastrinoma, it should not be considered definitive if no gastrinoma is found. Instead, the duodenum should be examined via duodenotomy with transillumination and direct palpation. Duodenotomy is particularly critical to the identification of small tumors, allowing for localization of up to 90% of gastrinomas measuring less than 1 cm.[55,56]

Intraoperative exploration for jejunal/ileal neuroendocrine tumors

Peritoneal metastases and liver metastases are found in 20% to 61% of patients with small bowel NETs. Further, primary small bowel NETs are typically small and are multifocal in 15% to 54% of patients.[57–59] In addition to a complete examination of the liver and peritoneal surfaces, careful examination and manual palpation of the entire small bowel is required to identify intramural, subcentimeter tumors.

The role of minimally invasive surgery in the evaluation and treatment of small bowel NET has yet to be defined because minimally invasive techniques do not typically allow complete manual palpation of the bowel. Further, a minimally invasive approach may increase the risk of inadequate nodal dissection and may not allow thorough peritoneal debulking, when indicated. There may be a role for limited palliative resection/cytoreduction procedures performed via a minimally invasive approach. Irrespective of the surgical approach taken, the goals of safety and quality of life must be considered in the context of patient physiology and comorbidities. Both the North American Neuroendocrine Tumor Society and the European Neuroendocrine Tumor Society endorse laparotomy for patients with small bowel NET.[58,60]

Hybrid approaches may allow for laparoscopic or minimally invasive assisted surgery with manual palpation of the bowel. Current literature evaluating the use of these approaches still favors manual palpation to identify primary and multifocal disease.[61–63] Options for evaluation of the small bowel in this manner include the use of a hand-assisted laparoscopic device (i.e., Gelport; Applied Medical Resources, Rancho Santa Margarita, CA) or the creation of a small incision through which the jejunum and ileum can be exteriorized and palpated.[61] Massimino et al.[62] evaluated a total of 63 patients with occult small bowel NETs with biopsy-proven nodal or hepatic metastases. Laparoscopic surgery was performed in 46 of these patients with successful primary tumor localization in 61%, suggesting that laparoscopic exploration may be superior to preoperative imaging and endoscopy for this subset of patients. In their study, 14 patients had conversion to open surgery, and only 2 of these were converted for palpation of the bowel.[62]

Owing to limited data supporting the use of laparoscopic techniques, open surgery remains the preferred approach for patients with small bowel NET. Laparoscopic-assisted approaches are reasonable if manual palpation of the entire small bowel can be performed (Fig. 3-2).

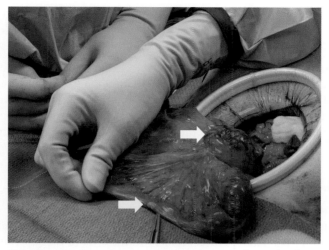

FIGURE 3-2   Gross intraoperative photograph shows the classic scenario of large, bulky mesenteric nodal disease (*white arrow*) with a small primary tumor (*yellow arrow*) that was not able to be localized on preoperative imaging studies. This highlights the importance of thorough intraoperative exploration for the primary tumor with careful manual palpation of the entire small bowel, which is not possible with a strictly laparoscopic approach.

Technical Aspects

Gastrinoma

The gastrinoma triangle (triangle drawn from the cystic duct/common bile duct junction cranially, the junction of the second and third portions of the duodenum inferolaterally, and the junction of the neck and body of the pancreas inferomedially) should be explored at the time of surgery. The duodenum should be fully mobilized by kocherization. It should then be manually palpated between the thumb and forefinger. Any suspicious lesions should be noted. If visual inspection and manual palpation do not identify any lesions, intraoperative upper endoscopy should be performed for transillumination of the duodenal wall. Areas of tumor will be represented by areas of light defect.

To examine the duodenal mucosa, a longitudinal duodenotomy should be created along the antimesenteric porion, and the mucosa should be visualized and subsequently palpated. Small gastrinomas may resemble areas of dimpling in the mucosa and be associated with palpation of small nodules. Attention should be paid to avoid injury to the ampulla of Vater, which can be mistaken for a gastrinoma.

The pancreatic head and body should also be inspected. The lesser sac along the avascular plane of the transverse colon should be opened. The caudal border of the pancreas should be dissected free so that the body and tail can be palpated between two fingers. An IOUS can then be used to identify lesions and may be helpful in identifying lesions as small as 5 mm.[64]

Lymph nodes should also be evaluated. Any grossly positive lymph nodes in the paraduodenal, peripancreatic, and periportal regions should be resected, and lymph node biopsies should be taken in patients who have no evidence of gross disease.

Jejunal/ileal neuroendocrine tumors

The pelvis, paracolic gutters, mesentery, ovaries, and bilateral diaphragms should be evaluated, and the liver should be carefully palpated. The entire small intestine from the ligament of Treitz to the ileocecal valve should be visually inspected and palpated by running the bowel gently between the thumb and forefinger. The entire mesentery should also be palpated for firm or enlarged lymph nodes.

2. REGIONAL LYMPHADENECTOMY ALONG SEGMENTAL VESSELS

Recommendation: Regional lymphadenectomy for jejunal and ileal small bowel NETs should include removal of all lymph nodes along the segmental vessels associated with the tumor-containing bowel segment to the level of the superior mesenteric artery and vein. For duodenal tumors treated with segmental resection or local excision, periportal and hepatic artery nodes should be sampled for lesions in D1 or D2, and proximal jejunal and adjacent retroperitoneal nodes posterior to the duodenum should be sampled for lesions in D3/D4. A minimum of eight lymph nodes should be examined for accurate pathologic staging.

Type of Data: Retrospective reports, case series, or case-control studies

Strength of Recommendation: Strong recommendation, low-quality evidence

Rationale

The aim of a curative operation for small bowel NET(s) should be a complete resection of all primary tumor(s), regional lymph nodes, and mesenteric fibrosis whenever feasible. Nodal metastases have been reported in 46% to 98% of patients when complete nodal dissection is conducted.[65–69] Lymph node metastases can be present in up to 67% of patients with gastrinoma, and routine removal of peripancreatic, periduodenal, and/or periportal lymph nodes has been advocated by many.[70–72]

Regional lymphadenectomy should include a thorough lymphatic dissection to the superior mesenteric artery and superior mesenteric vein.[58,60] A study by Wang et al.[68] investigated the use of lymphatic mapping with a subserosal injection of isosulfan blue to better define the lymphatic drainage of small bowel NETs.[68,73] This approach resulted in a selective nodal basin resection, altered the extent of resection in 98% of cases, and allowed for sparing of the ileocecal valve in 44% of terminal ileal tumors. There were no recurrences in a 1- to 5-year follow-up of 112 patients.[68] Although this mapping technique is not considered standard practice, it does nicely illustrate the extent of lymphatic spread associated with small bowel NETs (Fig. 3-3).

Among patients with duodenal gastrinoma, rates of nodal metastasis are also high. In a series of patients with sporadic duodenal gastrinoma, most of whom had primary tumors under 1 cm in size, the rate of nodal metastasis was 60%.[22] In this study of

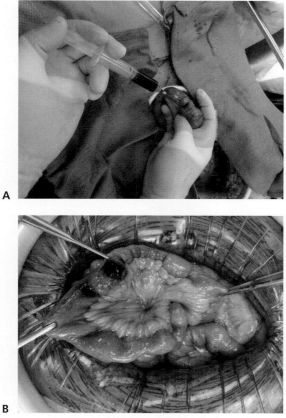

FIGURE 3-3 Photographs demonstrating lymphatic mapping achieved by injection of a small bowel primary neuroendocrine tumor with isosulfan blue dye. **A:** Intramural injection of isosulfan blue at the site of the primary tumor. **B:** Distribution of isosulfan blue through peritumoral lymphatics showing the potential path of lymphatic spread.

63 patients who underwent surgical resection for sporadic duodenal gastrinoma, the authors clearly illustrated the location of nodal metastases relative to the primary tumor location in the duodenum (Fig. 3-4). Lymph node sampling is recommended for small duodenal and pancreatic NETs treatable by local excision, but formal resection with pancreatoduodenectomy is not mandated. This is because of the potential morbidity of the procedure and because lymph node resection has not been definitively shown to affect survival for these lesions.[71,74,75] Formal resection with regional lymphadenectomy is recommended for patients with jejunoileal NETs, however, as the clinical significance of regional nodal disease and improved survival with radical resection have been established.[58,60,76]

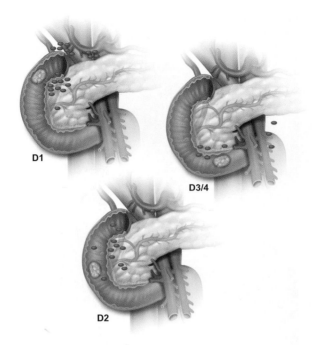

FIGURE 3-4 Location of lymph node metastases relative to primary tumor location for duodenal gastrinoma. The pertinent lymph nodes are similar for tumors in D1 and D2 and include those around the porta hepatis, along the hepatic artery, and around the proximal duodenum. For tumors in D3 or D4, the nodes are along the distal duodenum and proximal jejunum.

The minimum number of lymph nodes that should be removed at surgery for small bowel NET has not been informed by any randomized controlled studies. Data from the Surveillance, Epidemiology, and End Results (SEER) database have shown that a lymph node ratio of less than 0.29 is associated with favorable survival when more than seven nodes have been examined.[58] It is therefore recommended that at least eight lymph nodes are examined in the lymphadenectomy specimen. However, a conglomeration of matted nodes in the mesentery may often preclude an accurate count.

Inadequate resection of the lymph nodal basin may lead to proximal nodal recurrence. The consequences of mesenteric encasement with bulky adenopathy and fibrosis are variable but can and often do include intractable abdominal pain, intestinal ischemia, recurrent obstruction, malnutrition, and intestinal gangrene.[58,77] When the nodal metastases encase the mesenteric root, an extensive dissection may be required to prevent or treat these complications. Extensive nodal metastases can be safely resected at experienced centers (Fig. 3-5). In many cases, because the tumors are slow growing, patients can develop sufficient collateral circulation and will avoid symptomatic intestinal ischemia. However, mesenteric foreshortening and intestinal obstruction can still occur.

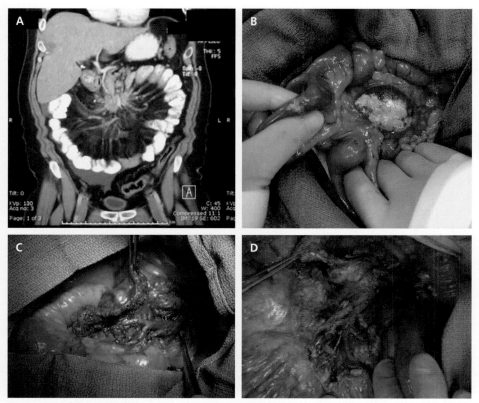

FIGURE 3-5 Computed tomographic image (**A**) and gross photograph (**B**) of bulky nodal disease encasing the mesenteric root. This was able to be safely resected by first unroofing the mesenteric vessels at the base of the mesentery (**C**). This image shows the root of the mesentery being elevated with the aorta and aortic bifurcation posteriorly. The mesenteric vasculature is then carefully skeletonized (**D**).

Technical Aspects

Duodenum

After a Kocher maneuver has been performed and intraoperative localization of primary tumors has been completed as described earlier, periduodenal, peripancreatic, periportal, and adjacent retroperitoneal nodes posterior to the duodenum near the vena cava and aorta, and celiac lymph nodes should be inspected. The peritoneum along the cranial aspect of the pancreas and overlying the porta hepatis should be opened with cautery, and lymph nodes should be carefully manually palpated. The hepatic artery lymph node should be dissected off of the underlying common hepatic artery and small lymphatics and vessels entering it. Once the duodenum is able to be rotated off of the retroperitoneum, retroperitoneal nodes sitting behind the duodenum along the vena cava and aorta should be inspected. Nodes extending along the posterior aspect of the porta hepatis can also be inspected at this time. Any grossly abnormal or suspicious nodes should be made note of and resected. If nodes appear grossly normal, focused sampling should be performed. For primary tumors in D1/D2, this should include nodes along the hepatic artery, porta hepatis, and celiac axis. For those in D3/D4, this should include adjacent retroperitoneal nodes and proximal jejunal nodes.

Jejunum and ileum

An overly aggressive dissection at the mesenteric root can result in a vascular catastrophe if critical collateral vessels and the main superior mesenteric arterial and/or venous trunks are sacrificed. The first jejunal branch of the mesenteric vein must be preserved. Careful dissection of this area may be successfully accomplished, but it can be a tedious and time-consuming process. An asymptomatic calcified fibrotic mass encasing the mesenteric root should be left in place in inexperienced hands.[58] Some specialized neuroendocrine centers have developed methods to surgically remove these nodal metastases at the root. They have reported a lower incidence of obstruction and intestinal angina, and they have avoided mesenteric ischemia and intestinal gangrene.[58,65,68,77–79]

The mesenteric root dissection proceeds from the root of the mesentery outward, in a counterclockwise fashion, preferably incising the mesenteric peritoneum in an uninvolved area. Every effort should be expended to preserve collateral vessels as they are encountered while the main tumor mass is approached proximal to distal. Often, a plane can be developed between the vessels and the fibrotic reaction surrounding the tumor, as frequently, the tumors encase the vessels without invasion. IOUS may be a useful adjunct to locate patent vessels. Temporary occlusion of the vessels to be ligated and divided with vascular clamps is recommended in cases in which bowel length may be of concern. This allows for accurate assessment of the length of viable bowel that will remain before any irreversible steps are taken. Clamps need to be placed on the central vessels to be divided as well as on the marginal arteries near the bowel wall at the planned sites of bowel division. All involved nodes should be resected when feasible. The bowel is resected after the dissection is complete in order to minimize loss of bowel length and maximize sparing of vascularized intestine. The lengths of residual and resected bowel should be measured and recorded in the operative note. Generally, patients with less than 200 cm of combined jejunum-ileum are at risk of short gut syndrome.[80]

3. RESECTION OF THE PRIMARY TUMOR

Recommendation: Full-thickness local excision is appropriate for low-grade NETs of the duodenum, including gastrinomas, that do not involve the ampulla of Vater. Lesions should be excised with a grossly negative margin of normal duodenal mucosa. For lesions of the jejunum and ileum, segmental resection is recommended, with the length of bowel to be resected dictated by the degree of lymphadenectomy.

Type of Data: Retrospective reports, case series, or case-control studies

Strength of Recommendation: Strong recommendation, low-quality evidence

Rationale

Full-thickness local excision is appropriate for selected duodenal NETs as a means of preserving normal anatomy and optimizing long-term digestive function and quality of life for patients. Local excision is not appropriate for jejunal/ileal tumors, however, because segmental resection with lymphadenectomy is generally low risk and well tolerated with minimal long-term effects on digestive function.

Technical Aspects

Duodenum

Proximal duodenal NETs, including gastrinomas, that do not invade into surrounding structures can be removed with local excision. For lesions of the second and proximal third portions of the duodenum, a lateral duodenotomy should be created on the second portion. Lesions on the lateral wall of the duodenum should be excised using a full-thickness, elliptical incision. Lesions on the pancreatic aspect of the duodenum may be excised in the submucosal plane by incising the normal mucosa immediately adjacent to the lesion through the duodenotomy. In either case, a margin of grossly normal tissue should be sought to ensure a negative margin. Tumors that involve the ampulla of Vater may require pancreatoduodenectomy, although ampullectomy may be considered in selected cases.

If the location of the ampulla of Vater in relation to a duodenal lesion is not clear, a cholecystectomy should be performed. A ballooned catheter can then be passed into the duodenum via the cystic duct to localize the ampulla. The duodenotomy should be closed in a transverse fashion to prevent narrowing of the duodenum.

For lesions of the distal third or fourth portion of the duodenum, segmental resection with duodenojejunostomy may be performed.

Jejunum/ileum

Local excision is not appropriate for jejunal/ileal NETs, regardless of size. Segmental resection is recommended due to the propensity for regional lymphatic dissemination. The length of the bowel to be resected is usually dictated by the extent of lymphadenectomy performed, as described above. Once the extent of lymphadenectomy is defined, the bowel is divided at the closest possible sites proximal and distal to the lesion where it remains well perfused. Perfusion can be assessed grossly by appearance of the tissue, with Doppler ultrasound and/or with an intravenously administered visual agent such as fluorescein or indocyanine green. None of these individual techniques has been shown to be superior.

Neuroendocrine Key Question 1

In patients with small bowel neuroendocrine tumors (NETs) with regional nodal disease undergoing surgical resection, is prophylactic cholecystectomy indicated to reduce the incidence of subsequent cholestasis-related pathology?

INTRODUCTION

The somatostatin analogues octreotide or lanreotide are mainstays of medical therapy for metastatic NETs. Somatostatin is an inhibitory hormone in the digestive system. Similar effects are exerted by its synthetic analogues.[81–83] These analogues exhibit their effects via binding to somatostatin receptor subtypes 1 to 5, and they have variable affinity for these receptors.[81] They have shown to be efficacious in controlling many of the secretory symptoms in patients with hormonally active NETs. They also demonstrate antiproliferative properties in this setting.[81]

The antisecretory effects of somatostatin analogues are thought to increase the rate of gallstone formation. In addition, many patients with NETs develop hepatic metastasis, for which liver-directed therapies (resection, ablation, chemoembolization, or radioembolization) are indicated. The presence of a gallbladder may affect the ability to provide these therapies or raise the complication potential associated with them.

The purpose of this work was to evaluate whether a prophylactic cholecystectomy is beneficial at the time of primary tumor resection to prevent future cholestasis-related pathology in patients with small bowel NETs.

METHODOLOGY

A systematic search of PubMed, EMBASE, and Cochrane review was performed from January 1990 to September 2019. The Medical Subject Headings (MeSH) terms included "Neuroendocrine Tumor," "Prophylactic Cholecystectomy," "Octreotide," "Incidence," and "Symptomatic Gallstones." Findings are reported in accordance with the Preferred Reporting Items for Systematic Reviews and Meta-Analyses (PRISMA).[84]

The initial search yielded 85 publications (Fig. 3-6). Five were excluded because they were not written in English or were published before 1990. The remaining articles were screened on the basis of their titles and abstract content. Of these 80 studies, 64 were excluded because they were duplicates, not specific to gallbladder disease, literature review only, and case reports. Sixteen met all the criteria for inclusion in this systematic review (Table 3-6).

Data were extracted from individual studies and evaluated by a single author. Each article was reviewed and assigned a quality of evidence based on the Grading of Recommendations, Assessment, Development, and Evaluation (GRADE) system.[101]

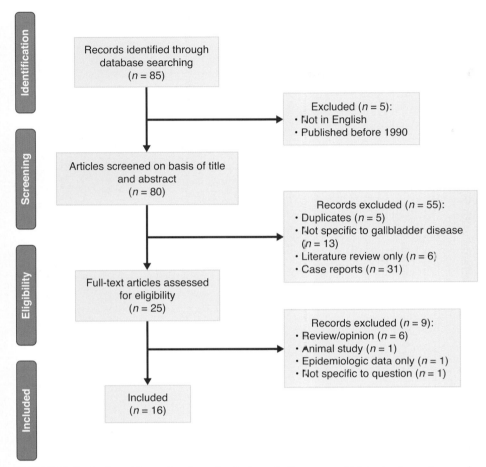

FIGURE 3-6 Preferred Reporting Items for Systematic Reviews and Meta-Analyses diagram for prophylactic cholecystectomy in patients with small bowel neuroendocrine tumors with regional nodal disease undergoing surgical resection.

FINDINGS

Gallstone formation is a common problem. More than 700,000 cholecystectomies are performed annually for symptoms in the United States. The prevalence of gallstones varies by ethnicity; formation rates range from 10% to 70% in developed countries.[102] The formation of gallstones is thought to be related to three factors: supersaturation of bile in the gallbladder, an imbalance between stone promoters and inhibitors, and bile stasis with decreased gallbladder emptying.[88]

Somatostatin analogues are frequently used to treat patients with NETs and those with acromegaly. An increase in the frequency of gallstone formation and symptoms has been noted in these patients.[83,85,87,89,95,98,100] The increased rate of gallstone formation in these patients is thought to be multifactorial.

TABLE 3-6 Review of Literature for Prophylactic Cholecystectomy in Patients with Small Bowel NET with Regional Nodal Disease Undergoing Surgical Resection

Authors, Year	Number of Patients	Main Objective	Study Design	Comments	Grade of Evidence*
Attanasio et al.,[85] 2008	459	Review the prevalence and clinical and biochemical correlates of gallstones in acromegalic patients	Retrospective	Retrospective study of acromegalic patients on octreotide. Gallstones occur frequently but not commonly symptomatic and do not commonly require surgery.	++
Bigg-Wither et al.,[86] 1992	25	Follow 15 acromegalic patients with 10 control patients on octreotide with ultrasound to assess stone formation and gallbladder volumes	Quasi-experimental	Patients with acromegaly or nonacromegalic volunteers receiving octreotide showing increased incidence of gallstone formation and impaired gallbladder motility. This was reversible with medication withdrawal.	+++
Catnach et al.,[87] 1993	77	Compare the effects of octreotide on acromegalic patients between groups with and without octreotide treatment	Cohort	Cohort study of acromegalic patients showing gallstone formation in patients treated with octreotide compared with controls (34% vs. 16%, $P < .005$) and increased postprandial gallbladder volume ($P < .001$) in treated patients	++
Dowling et al.,[88] 1997	32	Compare small bowel transit time between acromegalic patients on octreotide treatment with controls	Quasi-experimental	Quasi-experimental design study demonstrating octreotide-induced prolonged GI transit time in the bowel which may contribute to etiology of gallstone formation	+++
Eastman et al.,[89] 1992	17	Determine the effects of octreotide on gallbladder function during treatment of acromegaly	Observational	Prospective, observational study showing biliary particulate matter forming in the first 6 mo of octreotide therapy in 12 of 17 patients with acromegaly	++

Reference	N	Objective	Design	Results	
Ewins et al.,[90] 1992	9	Determine the effects of octreotide on cholecystokinin release and gallbladder emptying in acromegalic patients	Observational	Observational study showing diminished gallbladder ejection fraction and impaired release of postprandial cholecystokinin levels ($P < .01$) following the initiation of octreotide therapy in acromegalic patients	++
Hussaini et al.,[91] 1994	25	Assess the effects of octreotide treatment on bile composition via gallbladder aspiration	Observational	Observational study with gallbladder aspiration showing greater saturation indices and bile alterations promoting stone formation in patients treated with octreotide similar to control patients who have gallstones	++
Hussaini et al.,[92] 1995	14	Evaluate the composition and dissolvability of gallstones in patients treated with octreotide	Observational	Observational study showing gallstones in patients receiving octreotide are small, multiple, and cholesterol rich. Only 22% dissolve with UDCA treatment.	++
Hussaini et al.,[93] 1996	32	Study the roles of gallbladder emptying and intestinal transit on gallstone formation in subjects treated with octreotide	Observational	Observational study showing impaired gallbladder emptying and prolonged intestinal transit time in patients treated with octreotide	++
Moschetta et al.,[94] 2001	7	Assess the effects of long-acting octreotide formulation on gastric and gallbladder emptying	Observational	Observational study showing significantly impaired gastric and gallbladder emptying with long-acting octreotide treatment similar to short-acting formulations	++
Norlén et al.,[95] 2010	187	Retrospective review of patients with midgut carcinoids to evaluate the incidence of gallstone-related disease between those treated or not treated with octreotide	Retrospective	Patients with midgut carcinoids treated with octreotide have increased incidence of gallstones (63% octreotide vs. 55% untreated) and required subsequent cholecystectomy within 5 y (2.3% vs. 19%) that was not significant. The authors recommended consideration of prophylactic cholecystectomy during laparotomy for primary tumor, especially if liver metastases are present.	++

(continued)

TABLE 3-6 Review of Literature for Prophylactic Cholecystectomy in Patients with Small Bowel NET with Regional Nodal Disease Undergoing Surgical Resection (continued)

Authors, Year	Number of Patients	Main Objective	Study Design	Comments	Grade of Evidence*
Shi et al.,[96] 1993	20	Examine changes in gallbladder function in acromegaly patients treated with octreotide	Observational	Acromegalic patients treated with octreotide showing diminished gallbladder emptying and new gallstone formation	++
Sinnamon et al.,[97] 2018	1,300	Review of the NSQIP database for patients with small bowel NETs who underwent surgery for the NET	Retrospective database	Concurrent cholecystectomy at time of small bowel NET resection is associated with longer operating time but no significant change in morbidity or mortality	+++
Trendle et al.,[98] 1997	45	Retrospective chart review of patients with NETs on investigational protocols for octreotide treatment	Observational	Subgroup analysis of patients on octreotide treatment protocols for NETs showing that more than 50% developed cholelithiasis but only 6.8% of those required emergent cholecystectomy. The authors recommended monitoring for symptoms when treated with octreotide.	++
Turner et al.,[99] 1999	11	Prospective trial to assess and compare the effects of two long-acting somatostatin analogues on gallbladder motility in patients with acromegaly	Observational	Long-acting octreotide analogues led to larger fasting gallbladder volumes, residual volumes, and decreased ejection fractions compared with pretreatment.	++
Wymenga et al.,[100] 1999	55	Evaluate the long-acting lanreotide formulation effects on symptoms and quality of life for patients with gastrointestinal NETs	Observational	Prospective study demonstrating efficacy and safety of lanreotide treatment in gastrointestinal NETs. 8/30 patients developed gallstones.	+++

GI: gastrointestinal; NET: neuroendocrine tumor; NSQIP: National Surgical Quality Improvement Program; UDCA: ursodeoxycholic acid.
*Grade: ++ low; +++ moderate.

Pathogenesis of Gallstones Secondary to Somatostatin Analogues

The composition of bile in patients who have gallstones is different from that of people who do not have gallstones. An early study of prairie dogs found that administration of octreotide alters the composition of bile to favor gallstone formation while increasing bile stasis.[82] Human patients treated with octreotide have been shown to have bile supersaturation that is similar to patients with gallstones. The bile of patients with gallstones and of patients treated with octreotide both have elevated levels of biliary deoxycholic acid compared with bile of patients who do not have stones. Biliary deoxycholic acid leads to biliary cholesterol hypersecretion, increased saturation, and subsequent stone formation. The deoxycholic acid levels have been shown to double following initiation of treatment with octreotide.[88] These increased deoxycholic acid levels may be related to a decrease in intestinal transit.[88,93] A study by Hussaini et al.[91] evaluated bile aspirates of patients with acromegaly who were treated with octreotide. All patients under treatment, whether they had stones or not, developed greater bile saturation indices after initiating treatment than did patients with acromegaly who were not treated with octreotide. These bile saturation changes have a profile similar to previous reports on patients in the general population with gallstones.[91]

Hussaini et al.[92] performed a follow-up study to assess the composition of gallstones and the efficacy of dissolution therapy with ursodeoxycholic acid. Eight out of 12 patients with gallstones on octreotide therapy were found to have stones consistent with cholesterol-rich composition on computed tomography (CT) analysis. Ten of these 12 patients were treated with ursodeoxycholic acid; 2 had complete dissolution at 4 months, and 3 others had partial dissolution within 1 year. The authors concluded that concurrent octreotide treatment does not necessarily impede the efficacy of ursodeoxycholic acid dissolution therapy.[92]

Somatostatin analogues have also been shown to inhibit gallbladder emptying, leading to cholestasis.[89,90,94,96] In 25 patients with acromegaly who were treated with long-acting octreotide, the rate of gallstone formation was 32%, and they had an increase in the volumes of their gallbladders, suggesting impaired emptying and increased stasis.[86] Ewins et al.[90] demonstrated a decrease in gallbladder ejection fraction within 24 hours as well as a decrease in postprandial serum in cholecystokinin following initiation of octreotide therapy. Some patients had recovery of gallbladder emptying after 6 months of therapy, but 75% of those with continued impairment developed stones.[90] Moschetta et al.[94] confirmed impaired gallbladder emptying with impaired postprandial cholecystokinin release with gallstone formation in 6 out of 7 patients on long-acting octreotide within 8 months of initiating treatment.[94]

In a study by Eastman et al.,[89] 17 patients underwent gallbladder ultrasound before and after initiation of octreotide treatment. There was a significant increase in echogenic particles in the gallbladder in 70% of patients within 6 months of starting treatment.[89] A single study of 11 patients evaluated the effects of gallbladder motility when comparing octreotide and lanreotide in acromegaly; impaired motility was noted with both agents, but less impairment was associated with lanreotide.[99] In a study evaluating the efficacy of lanreotide in patients with gastrointestinal NETs, lanreotide was noted to significantly improve hypersecretory symptoms in 38% to 67% of patients, depending on which hormone was secreted. However, new gallstone formation was noted in 8 of 30 (27%) evaluable patients.[100]

Frequency of Gallstone Formation in Patients Treated with Somatostatin Analogues

The largest published study was a retrospective multicenter chart review of patients with acromegaly from Italy. The authors reviewed 459 patients and found a prevalence of gallstones of 8.3% at the time of their diagnosis. Somatostatin analogues were used in 357 patients, with a mean follow-up of 7.1 years. Gallstones developed in an additional 34.2% of males and 35.5% of females after a median 3 years of follow-up on therapy. Symptoms related to gallstone disease were reported in 17.6% of the patients with stones; the others were diagnosed using surveillance ultrasound. Among the patients who developed stones during treatment with somatostatin analogues, 16.8% required cholecystectomy, and one-half of their operations were emergent. On multivariate analysis of all patients, independent predictors of gallstone occurrence were obesity, dyslipidemia, and somatostatin analogue treatment.[85]

In the setting of NETs, fewer studies exist, and those that do exist report data generated from smaller patient populations. One of the earliest studies, by Trendle et al.,[98] was a retrospective chart review of patients who were treated with octreotide as part of a clinical trial. This study included 44 patients who had not undergone prior cholecystectomy who were evaluated for the development of stones. However, the finding of presence or absence of stones was based on ultrasound or CT scans, which can underreport the frequency of stones. In this study, 52.3% of the patients developed sludge or stones in the gallbladder, which occurred after a median of 28 months of treatment. Patients were divided into three groups based on their octreotide dose. Gallstones or sludge were found to develop in a dose-dependent fashion relative to their octreotide dose. Stones were of differing composition. Overall, eight (18%) of the patients in this study required cholecystectomy. The authors proposed using the lowest efficacious dose so as to avoid this adverse effect.[98]

Multiple reports indicate that new gallstones arise in up to 50% of treated patients.[98] The abundance of the evidence that suggests an increase in stone incidence is taken from studies of patients treated for acromegaly, who may have a slightly increased rate of gallstone formation compared with the general population. This was confirmed in a prospective study comparing gallstone formation in acromegaly patients treated with octreotide and without somatostatin analogues at 20 months (34% vs. 16%; $P < .005$).[87] An increased duration of treatment of 3 months or greater may be associated with an increased risk of gallstone formation but not in a strictly time-dependent fashion. Data provided courtesy of Sandoz Pharmaceuticals showed a plateau in stone formation within 1 year of initiating treatment. Notably, most of the gallstones remained asymptomatic in these varied patient populations.[83] The authors of this study recommended timing the octreotide regimen around meals, but this requires use of a short-acting formulation with multiple daily injections rather than the monthly long-acting formulation. Return to normal cholecystokinin response can take 4 to 8 hours after administration of a short-acting somatostatin agonist. Another consideration was periodic cessation of treatment to prevent gallstone formation.[83] This would be particularly problematic for patients with symptomatic secretory NETs.

A retrospective chart review of an institutional database in Sweden studied patients with midgut NETs. Of 187 patients in the study who had not previously undergone cholecystectomy, 43 did not receive somatostatin analogues and did not develop any complications of cholelithiasis. The prevalence of gallstones in this group of patients, who were followed for almost 7 years on average, was 55%. The remaining 144 patients were administered somatostatin analogues and were observed for a comparable period. Gallstones were found on radiologic images of 63% of the patients with available information. In this group, 22% required cholecystectomy after their original operation for the NET owing to gallstone complications such as acute cholecystitis, cholangitis, or pancreatitis. The 5-year cumulative risk of requiring a cholecystectomy was 2.3% in untreated patients and 19% in patients treated with somatostatin analogues. Subsequently, 23 patients underwent liver-directed embolic therapy for metastasis, with 3 patients developing gallbladder complications related to this.[95]

Prophylactic Cholecystectomy in Patients Treated for Metastatic Neuroendocrine Tumors

Although routine cholecystectomy for the presence of gallstones is not recommended,[103] several papers have recommended prophylactic cholecystectomy at the time of surgery for metastatic NETs.[58,95,104–106] This recommendation has been controversial because most of these patients might never require cholecystectomy. However, risks of gallbladder-associated complications in patients undergoing treatment for NETs have been described. Biliary complications may arise related to the gallstones themselves or secondary to liver-directed therapies used to treat metastatic tumors.

A review of the American College of Surgeons National Surgical Quality Improvement Program database was undertaken by Sinnamon et al.[97] Of 1,300 patients who underwent resection of a small bowel NET, 11% overall underwent a concurrent cholecystectomy. Of those with documented disseminated disease, 36% underwent concurrent cholecystectomy. In the patients who did undergo prophylactic cholecystectomy, operative time was significantly longer (median 172 vs. 123 minutes; $P < .001$), but this was not stratified by extent of disease. Of note, there was no significant difference in operative morbidity, mortality, or 30-day readmission rates in patients who underwent cholecystectomy.[97]

CONCLUSION

Long-term data regarding the prevalence of gallstone formation and complications in patients treated with somatostatin analogues are limited, but there does appear to be an increased risk of stone development in patients treated with these agents. These patients are not likely to require a cholecystectomy related to gallstone disease. However, there is some evidence that patients may develop complications from their gallbladder related to percutaneous treatment of hepatic metastases. Patients undergoing operations in the setting of hepatic metastatic NETs, who are likely to be treated with somatostatin analogues in the future, may be safely observed in most cases. When patients who are not undergoing operations for other indications are treated initially with somatostatin analogues, they can be safely followed routinely, and an intensive monitoring program or prophylactic cholecystectomy does not appear warranted.

Neuroendocrine Key Question 2

In patients with metastatic neuroendocrine tumors to the liver, does incomplete resection and/or ablation of liver metastases lead to improved survival compared with alternative therapies? If so, what degree of hepatic debulking is necessary?

INTRODUCTION

Gastrointestinal neuroendocrine tumors (GI-NETs) derive from peptide-producing cells that originate from throughout the gastrointestinal tract and pancreas. The incidence of GI-NETs has been rising worldwide, with an estimated incidence of 7 per 100,000 individuals per year in the United States.[15,107]

Approximately 50% of these tumors have metastasized by the time of presentation, with the liver being the most common site of metastasis in more than 80% of cases. The presence of liver metastases, in addition to tumor grade, is the most important predictor of survival in patients with GI-NETs.[108,109] Among those patients who die of their disease, approximately 80% succumb to liver failure due to progressive liver involvement.[57] In a recent analysis of the National Cancer Database, no difference in median overall survival was identified between 5,569 patients with GI-NET and isolated hepatic metastases and 995 patients with both hepatic and extrahepatic metastases.[110] What is unclear, however, is how to accurately predict the biologic behavior of these tumors, as some patients with low- or intermediate-grade tumors and liver metastases seem to experience very little or no tumor progression for years and others progress rapidly despite treatments. Because of this variation in biologic behavior and the lack of randomized controlled studies comparing treatment effects on GI-NET liver metastases, there currently are no definitive clinical guidelines available that dictate which treatment option should be used first, alone, or in combination with others, after a patient is diagnosed.

Although most surgeons believe surgical removal of metastatic liver disease is beneficial for symptom control and may be associated with longer survival if 70% to 90% of the tumor burden can be removed, no prospective study data exist to support this approach.[58] Additionally, medical oncologists, who most commonly treat patients with stage IV GI-NETs, may underestimate the resectability of diffuse liver metastases. In one study of colorectal cancer patients with liver metastases, there was a substantial discrepancy between the perception of resectability among medical oncologists and liver surgeons.[111] Surgical resection or debulking of liver metastases in a patient with an NET may be overlooked by clinicians treating patients with GI-NETs that have metastasized to the liver.

Besides surgery, other interventional treatment options in patients with stage IV GI-NETs with liver metastasis include transarterial chemoembolization, selective intra-arterial radiation therapy, or percutaneous ablation. The effect of such therapy on overall survival of patients with GI-NETs and liver metastases is unknown. Clinicians treating patients with GI-NETs also have a multiplicity of systemic treatment options that include somatostatin analogues, mechanistic target of rapamycin–inhibitors, vascular endothelial growth factor inhibitors, oral chemotherapy with capecitabine and temozolomide, as well as peptide receptor radionuclide therapy. These treatment options are commonly used in patients with GI-NETs and metastatic liver disease, sometimes after surgical consultation has deemed the patient to have "unresectable" disease or without consideration of surgical options or liver-directed therapy. The purpose of this work was to evaluate whether incomplete resection and/or ablation of liver metastases lead to improved survival in patients with metastatic neuroendocrine tumors to the liver, compared with alternative therapies, and if so, what degree of hepatic debulking is necessary.

It should be noted that palliative cytoreduction, or debulking, for patients with symptoms related to hormonal hypersecretion is a different topic entirely and is not the focus of this key question.

METHODOLOGY

A systematic search of PubMed, Embase, and Cochrane review was performed from January 1990 to September 2019. The Medical Subject Headings (MeSH) terms included "Neuroendocrine Tumor," "Debulking," "Asymptomatic," "Liver Metastases," "Peritoneal Metastases," "Nodal Metastases," and "Resection." Findings are reported in accordance with the Preferred Reporting Items for Systematic Reviews and Meta-Analyses (PRISMA).[84]

The initial search yielded 419 publications (Fig. 3-7). Sixty-two manuscripts of the original 419 were excluded because they were not written in English, included pediatric populations, or were published before 1990. The remaining articles were screened on the basis of their titles and abstract content. Of these 357 abstracts, 254 were excluded because they were duplicates, focused on the wrong subtype of neuroendocrine tumor (pulmonary), literature reviews with no unique content, focused on nonmetastatic primary NETs, or case reports. A total of 103 manuscripts were included in the full manuscript review and application of inclusion criteria. A total of 51 articles were further excluded because they were on topics that did not focus on direct surgical or medical treatment of metastatic disease (i.e., imaging, surveillance, histology review, etc.) or included extra-abdominal metastases. A final total of 51 manuscripts met all criteria for inclusion in this systematic review.[15,35,37–39,57,58,65–67,69,78,107–145]

Data were extracted from individual studies and evaluated by a single author. Each article was reviewed and assigned a quality of evidence based on the Grades of Recommendation, Assessment, Development, and Evaluation (GRADE) system.[101]

FINDINGS

The more recent studies are summarized in Table 3-7. Early reports suggested that a cytoreductive threshold of 90% liver clearance be used, whereas more recent reports have lowered that threshold to 70%.

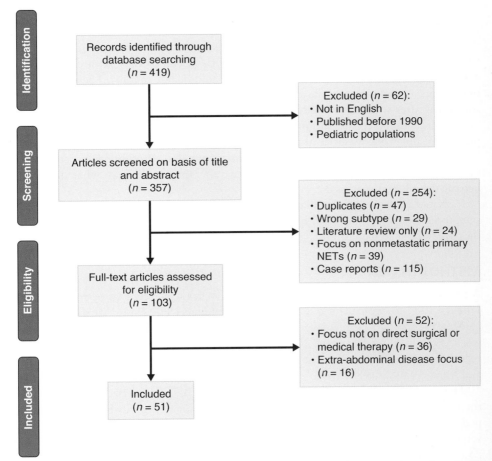

FIGURE 3-7   Preferred Reporting Items for Systematic Reviews and Meta-Analyses diagram for incomplete resection and/or ablation of liver metastases in patients with metastatic neuroendocrine tumors (NETs) to the liver.

The reports are all retrospective series that include patients with a variety of GI-NETs who have undergone disparate therapies in addition to liver resection. Updating earlier work by Maxwell et al.,[131] Scott et al.[141] looked specifically at outcomes based on cytoreduction of less than 70% versus 70% to 90% and greater than 90% cytoreduction and found that patients with a less than 70% cytoreduction had a shorter median overall survival duration as compared with patients with greater than 70% cytoreduction (134 vs. 38 months).[141] There were no overall survival differences between the 70%-to-90% and greater-than-90% groups (median not reached vs. 134 months), but there was a difference in progression-free survival (20.6 vs. 56.1 months). There were several factors that were significantly different between the less-than-70%, 70%-to-90%, and greater-than-90% cytoreduction groups. These included number

TABLE 3-7   Review of Literature for Hepatic Cytoreduction in GI-NETs

Authors, Year	Cytoreduction	Survival	Number of Patients	Grade of Evidence*
Chakedis et al.,[119] 2019	Unspecified	89 mo overall	51	++
Graff-Baker et al.,[128] 2014	>70% vs. >90% vs. 100%	Nonsignificant	52	−+
Maxwell et al.,[131] 2016†	>70% vs. <70%	Improved progression-free survival	108	++
Morgan et al.,[134] 2018	>70% vs. >90% vs. 100%	Nonsignificant	42	++
Scott et al.,[141] 2019	>70% vs. <70%	134 vs. 38 mo overall	188	++

GI-NET: gastrointestinal neuroendocrine tumor.
*Grade: ++ low.
†These patients are a subset of those reported in Scott et al.[141]

of metastatic lesions (median of 22, 11, and 2 lesions in the <70%, 70% to 90%, and >90% groups, respectively), the number of lesions treated (seven, nine, and three), and percentage of liver replacement (30%, 12%, and 2%). Other reports showed no difference in outcomes for those who underwent greater than 70% versus greater than 90% cytoreduction. Surgical techniques used in these series include major resections, wedge resections, enucleation, and liver ablations, with a trend toward parenchymal-sparing approaches in more recent series.[128,131,134,141] It should be noted that in studies in which the causes of mortality are reported, approximately 80% of patients succumb to liver failure secondary to liver replacement by tumor.

Cytoreduction of NET liver metastases may be beneficial even for some patients with disease metastatic to sites other than the liver. Small bowel NETs often grow through the serosa of the bowel and gain access to the peritoneal cavity, which results in peritoneal carcinomatosis in up to 20% of patients. Limited areas of disease can be managed with peritoneal stripping; however, it must be realized that this procedure is not curative. Cytoreductive surgery coupled with hyperthermic intraperitoneal chemotherapy has been used anecdotally with some success, although no prospective trials are available for review.[58]

The overall conclusion rendered is that a lower cytoreductive target of greater than 70% increases the number of patients that *may* benefit in terms of survival from being offered liver cytoreduction. However, there are no studies that offer a prospective assessment of the extent of cytoreduction or its relative role as compared with other therapies. Additionally, the use of local ablative techniques in concert with resectional surgery, although recommended by most surgeons to increase cytoreduction but preserve liver parenchyma, has not been subject to the scrutiny of prospective trials.

Patients may also be considered for cytoreduction for palliation of symptoms as the primary goal. It should be made clear in these cases that palliation is the primary goal of surgery, and patients may not have a survival benefit if greater than 70% cytoreduction cannot be achieved. Therefore, those with higher tumor burdens (>25%) and lesion number (>10 to 20) are less likely to benefit. Similarly, patients with significant medical comorbidities, carcinoid heart disease, or grade 3 tumors are also less likely to benefit from an aggressive surgical approach at cytoreduction.

CONCLUSION

Cytoreduction of liver disease may confer a survival advantage in some patients with metastatic GI-NETs. Although the evidence to support this recommendation is relatively low, patients with tumors metastatic to the liver should be considered for cytoreduction of their liver metastases if 70% or more of the metastatic burden can be safely resected.

CHAPTER 7

Parenchyma-Preserving Pancreatectomy

CRITICAL ELEMENTS

- Intraoperative Ultrasound Prior to Enucleation
- Resection of the Primary Tumor
- Regional Lymph Node Sampling of the Peripancreatic and Celiac Lymph Nodes

1. INTRAOPERATIVE ULTRASOUND PRIOR TO ENUCLEATION

Recommendation: Intraoperative ultrasound (IOUS) should be performed routinely prior to enucleation of a pancreatic neuroendocrine tumor (pNET) both to localize the tumor(s) and to evaluate the anatomic relationship between the tumor(s) and the pancreatic duct.

Type of Data: Retrospective reports, case series, or case-control studies

Strength of Recommendation: Strong recommendation, low-quality evidence

Rationale

Enucleation is generally accepted for small, benign or low-grade, peripherally located pNETs as long as complete excision can be achieved. Because the malignant potential of pNETs correlates with tumor size, enucleation should generally be reserved for lesions 2 cm or smaller, except in the case of insulinoma.[146] Additionally, lesions should have a distance from the main pancreatic duct of at least 2 to 3 mm, along with benign histology.[147]

IOUS has been used only selectively as described in published series of enucleation for pNET. However, the technique should be used routinely to localize tumor(s), assess for multifocality, evaluate for evidence of invasion, and measure tumor proximity to the pancreatic duct. Hackert et al.[148] performed IOUS in 45 of 53 cases of pancreatic enucleation for pNET and identified additional lesions that had not been identified on

179

preoperative imaging in nine cases (17%).[148] Several larger studies of parenchyma-preserving techniques of pancreatic resection for pNET used IOUS to decide between enucleation and central pancreatectomy or more extended resection.[147,149,150]

Technical Aspects

IOUS should be performed to scan the pancreatic parenchyma for possible additional lesions and to evaluate the features of the known lesion. The pancreas should be fully mobilized. A Kocher maneuver should be performed by first mobilizing the hepatic flexure of the colon and then opening the peritoneum overlying the lateral aspect of the duodenum. Retroperitoneal attachments to the duodenum and posterior aspect of the pancreatic head should then be divided. The lesser sac should be opened by dividing the gastrocolic ligament as well as any attachments between the pancreatic capsule and the posterior wall of the stomach. The ultrasound probe should be placed directly against the pancreatic parenchyma and the entire gland scanned.

The size of all tumors should be noted, as should the distance between the tumor and the main pancreatic duct. Any evidence of invasion into the surrounding parenchyma or lack of a clear peritumoral capsule or plane should prompt more definitive resection with a margin of normal parenchyma, such as central pancreatectomy (see below), distal pancreatectomy, or pancreatoduodenectomy. IOUS can also be used to assess for abnormal or enlarged-appearing peripancreatic lymph nodes. Frozen section should be considered for assessment for malignancy if ultrasonographic features suggestive of invasion are identified.

2. RESECTION OF THE PRIMARY TUMOR

Recommendation: Pancreatic neuroendocrine tumors selected for enucleation should be completely separated from adjacent normal parenchyma by careful blunt dissection. Intraoperative histopathologic analysis should be used if there is any concern for tissue invasion. For well-differentiated tumors in the body of the pancreas not amenable to enucleation, a central pancreatectomy or spleen-preserving distal pancreatectomy may be performed in order to preserve normal pancreatic parenchyma and the spleen.

Type of Data: Retrospective reports, case series, or case-control studies

Strength of Recommendation: Weak recommendation, low-quality evidence

Rationale

Enucleation

Pancreatic enucleation is appropriate for low-grade, well-differentiated pNETs 2 cm or less in size. In addition to these criteria, tumors should also be peripherally located on the gland and more than 3 mm from the main pancreatic duct (Fig. 3-8). If concern exists for tissue invasion, intraoperative histopathologic analysis should be performed, as a more formal pancreatectomy is more appropriate in this circumstance.

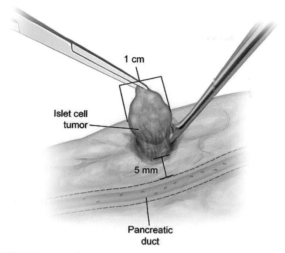

FIGURE 3-8 Illustration showing a pancreatic neuroendocrine tumor with optimal characteristics for enucleation, specifically location of greater than 2 mm from the main pancreatic duct and less than 2 cm in size.

Enucleation involves bluntly dissecting a lesion away from the surrounding pancreatic parenchyma without resection of any adjacent normal parenchyma. Proposed benefits of enucleation include avoidance of pancreatic insufficiency postoperatively and improved intestinal function long term due to avoidance of complex gastrointestinal reconstruction and preservation of normal anatomy. Although enucleation carries a lower risk of postoperative mortality than major pancreatic resection, it is not associated with a lower rate of short-term morbidity. Reported rates of postoperative morbidity in recent series range from 20% to 57%.[146–152] The incidence of clinically significant pancreatic fistula following enucleation has been highly variable in recent series, ranging from 0% to 43%.[151] No randomized prospective trials have been conducted to evaluate various techniques for enucleation, and, unfortunately, most published series do not provide detailed information on the surgical technique used.

Dissection of the pancreatic parenchyma should employ clips, ties, and energy sealing devices. In one of the few studies that described the methods used, Hackert et al.[148] described clip closure of vascular and ductal structures or use of nonabsorbable sutures, with avoidance of coagulation in the parenchyma. These authors also described reapproximation of the pancreatic capsule after the enucleation was complete with simple reabsorbable sutures. In this study, the incidence of clinically significant postoperative pancreatic fistula was 20.8%.[143] Series of minimally invasive enucleation tend to be more descriptive on the technique of parenchymal transection, and most use energy sealing devices such as ultrasonic shears.[150,152,153] Although there are no prospective studies comparing minimally invasive versus open techniques for enucleation, the minimally invasive approach has been associated with lower rates of clinically significant postoperative pancreatic fistula and similar long-term oncologic outcomes.[152,153] There is likely selection bias, however, as patients felt to be candidates for minimally invasive enucleation are likely to have more superficial lesions on the anterior surface of the gland.

Central and spleen-preserving distal pancreatectomy

Central pancreatectomy or spleen-preserving distal pancreatectomy may be used for well-differentiated tumors located in the neck, body, or tail of the pancreas when enucleation is not possible due to proximity to the pancreatic duct. Central pancreatectomy offers the benefit of preservation of normal pancreatic parenchyma for proximal lesions that do not require wide margins of resection.[147] Spleen-preserving distal pancreatectomy is more appropriate for distal lesions. No prospective studies have compared different operative techniques for these procedures.

An enteropancreatic anastomosis should be created to the pancreatic body when the distal pancreas is preserved. There are no clinical trials studying the utility of pancreatojejunostomy versus pancreaticogastrostomy in this setting. However, several clinical trials have established similar outcomes for these two reconstructive techniques for pancreatoduodenectomy.[154–156] If desired, a pancreatojejunostomy (using a Roux-en-Y approach) can be constructed in the manner described for a Beger procedure. More recently, direct end-to-end pancreatic anastomosis has been reported using the robotic surgery platform. Wang et al.[157] performed this procedure in 11 patients and found a rate of clinically significant postoperative pancreatic fistula of 64%.[157] Given the extremely limited data on this technique, the current recommendation is for enteric anastomosis.

Technical Aspects

Enucleation

Once the pancreas is adequately mobilized and the lesion is exposed, enucleation should be initiated by bluntly separating the lesion from the adjacent parenchyma. In open surgery, microsurgical loupes should be used to assist in identifying small vascular and ductal structures. These should be carefully ligated with clips or monofilament sutures and divided. Using a laparoscopic or robotic approach, the lesion should similarly be bluntly separated from the surrounding parenchyma, and the small bridging structures should be controlled with a fine-tipped energy sealing device. Methods to reapproximate the capsule or fill the space with omentum or other tissue have not been definitely associated with lower leak rates. Excess sutures and trauma to what is typically soft, normal pancreatic parenchyma should be avoided.

Central and spleen-preserving distal pancreatectomy

The lesser sac is opened by dissecting the omentum off of the transverse colon, including ligating and dividing the short gastric vessels as needed to facilitate exposure of the pancreatic body. The celiac axis should be dissected to isolate the splenic artery should control be needed. If the splenic artery is not separable from the pancreas in the region of the lesion, the operation may be converted to a distal pancreatectomy.

The peritoneum should be incised on the caudal border of the pancreas. The pancreas is typically soft, and great care should be exercised while mobilizing the gland.

A tunnel behind the neck of the pancreas should be created bluntly to separate the gland from the portomesenteric venous confluence or splenic vessels. The pancreas should then be dissected off of the splenic vessels from a right to left approach. Individual retropancreatic splenic vein tributaries must be identified, ligated, and divided. A generous portion of the pancreas should be mobilized to the left of the tumor.

The pancreas should be divided proximal to the tumor. The proximal pancreas can be divided sharply and the pancreas oversewn, or, alternatively, a linear stapler can be used. Recommendations on the technique in dividing the pancreas is extrapolated from data on distal pancreatectomy. No one technique has been shown to be definitively superior to another.[158–160] There is no convincing evidence that bioabsorbable staple line reinforcement improves closure. The distal pancreas should be divided, if appropriate, either sharply or using electrocautery. If necessary, additional pancreatic body should be mobilized free from the splenic vein and artery. The splenic artery can usually be separated from the body while identifying small arteries feeding the pancreas. If mobilization requires ligation of the pancreatica magna, the remaining distal pancreas should be removed to avoid ischemia to the remnant. For reconstruction at central pancreatectomy, either pancreaticogastrostomy or pancreaticojejunostomy are acceptable.

3. REGIONAL LYMPH NODE SAMPLING OF THE PERIPANCREATIC AND CELIAC LYMPH NODES

Recommendation: Regional lymph node sampling of the peripancreatic and celiac lymph nodes should be considered for pNETs greater than 1.5 to 2.0 cm in size at the time of parenchyma-preserving resection.

Type of Data: Retrospective reports, case series, or case-control studies

Grade of Recommendation: Weak recommendation, low-quality evidence

Rationale

Multiple recent studies from the US Neuroendocrine Tumor Study Group have evaluated the incidence and prognostic implication of lymph node metastases in nonfunctional pNETs.[161–163] Factors consistently shown to predict lymph node metastasis are tumor size greater than 2 cm, location in the head of the pancreas, Ki-67 index greater than 3%, and moderate differentiation. Even for patients without any of these risk factors, nodal metastases are still present in approximately 9% to 23% of cases and are associated with poorer long-term survival.

Regional lymphadenectomy is inherent in pancreaticoduodenectomy and distal pancreatectomy with splenectomy. Because of the significant risk of nodal involvement in lesions greater than 1.5 cm, regional nodal sampling is similarly recommended if it can be performed safely in parenchyma-preserving resection for staging and prognostication. This is because tumors of this size have been shown to have a greater than 40% risk of nodal metastasis.[75,152] Although there is no set number of nodes deemed adequate for staging in this setting, it has been reported that seven or more lymph nodes were required to detect a difference in 5-year recurrence-free survival in node-negative versus node-positive patients with pNET treated with distal pancreatectomy.[163]

Technical Aspects

For tumors in the head of the pancreas being managed with enucleation, gross inspection should be performed to identify any abnormal or suspicious-appearing nodes anterior or posterior to the head of the gland. Retroperitoneal nodes posterior to the uncinate process as well as periportal nodes in the posterior aspect of the porta hepatis should be sampled. For tumors in the neck, body, or tail region, lymph nodes along the celiac axis, particularly the hepatic and splenic artery nodes, are pertinent (Fig. 3-9). The peritoneum along the cranial border of the pancreas should be carefully opened with cautery, and lymph nodes along the hepatic, splenic, and celiac vessels should be carefully excised with the same technique. The gross appearance of nodes and the location of any suspicious-appearing nodes should be carefully documented in the operative report.

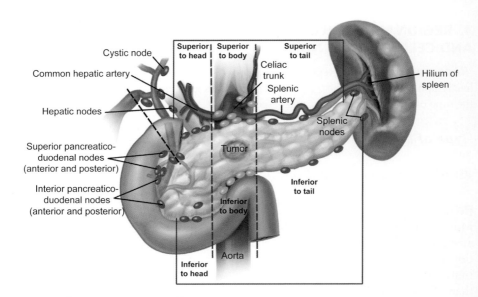

FIGURE 3-9   Illustration depicting peripancreatic lymph nodes that should be sampled at the time of parenchyma-preserving resection of pancreatic neuroendocrine tumors.

Neuroendocrine Key Question 3

In patients with low-grade nonfunctional pancreatic neuroendocrine tumors (NF-pNETs), does regional lymphadenectomy result in improved survival compared with margin-negative resection without lymphadenectomy?

INTRODUCTION

The incidence of pancreatic neuroendocrine tumors (pNETs) is increasing, prompting renewed interest in pathophysiology and disease treatment. pNETs are rare tumors that account for less than 3% of pancreatic tumors and are biologically distinct from pancreatic ductal adenocarcinoma. The natural history of pNETs is highly variable, but most patients experience an indolent disease course.[164] This favorable overall prognosis as well as relative rarity of the disease has presented significant challenges in the prospective study and identification of prognostic and predictive factors. Current evidence for management of this disease is therefore largely based on retrospective studies. In functional pNETs other than insulinoma, for example, glucagonoma and VIPoma, the rate of lymph node metastasis (LNM) is relatively high, and regional lymphadenectomy is often necessary to eliminate the hormonally mediated metabolic derangements.[165,166] However, the role of regional lymphadenectomy in NF-pNET is more controversial.

Small (<2 cm), low-grade NF-pNETs are generally thought to be clinically indolent with low risk of nodal metastasis, supporting the recommendation of observation versus limited resection without lymph node sampling at many high-volume centers.[167,168] However, several studies suggest that even small pNETs can exhibit more aggressive biology.[169,170] In either case, the impact of LNM on survival is unclear in low-grade pNET. Although some studies report better survival outcomes in patients without LNM,[162,171] others have shown presence of distant metastasis and tumor grade to be the major drivers of prognosis, with LNM conveying no significant prognostic relevance.[164,172] Current National Comprehensive Cancer Network (NCCN) guidelines recommend resection with lymphadenectomy for pNETs greater than 2 cm and consideration of lymphadenectomy for tumors 1 to 2 cm, acknowledging the limited data to support this recommendation.[173]

Based on these studies, the prognostic and/or therapeutic role of routine regional lymphadenectomy for pNET remains unclear, and debate continues around maximizing treatment benefit while mitigating surgical morbidity. The purpose of this work was to evaluate whether the presence of LNM has prognostic relevance in low-grade NF-pNET, and if so, whether regional lymphadenectomy results in improved survival in patients with low-grade NF-pNETs, compared with margin-negative resection without lymphadenectomy.

METHODOLOGY

A systematic search of PubMed, Embase, and Cochrane review was performed from January 1990 to September 2019. Medical Subject Headings (MeSH) terms included "Pancreatic Neuroendocrine Tumor," "Islet Cell Carcinoma," "Pancreas Neuroendocrine Neoplasm," "Lymph Node," "Metastasis," and "Surgery." Findings are reported in accordance with the Preferred Reporting Items for Systematic Reviews and Meta-Analyses (PRISMA).[84]

The initial search yielded 420 publications (Fig. 3-10). Sixty-two manuscripts of the original 420 were excluded because they were not written in English ($n = 36$), did not involve human adults ($n = 15$), or were published before 1990 ($n = 11$). The 358 articles included were screened on the basis of title and abstract content. A total of 266 articles were excluded because they were inapplicable to the question; focused

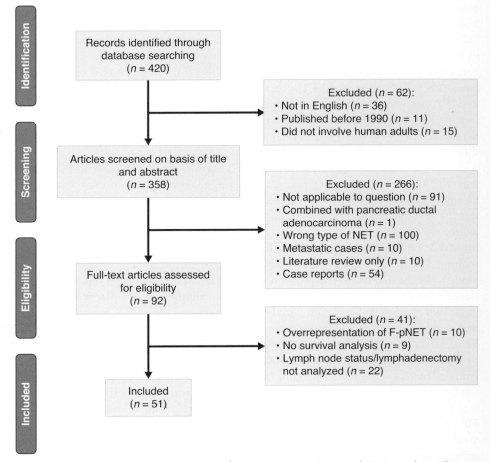

FIGURE 3-10 Preferred Reporting Items for Systematic Reviews and Meta-Analyses diagram for regional lymphadenectomy in patients with low-grade nonfunctional pancreatic neuroendocrine tumors. F-pNET: functional pancreatic neuroendocrine tumor. NET: neuroendocrine tumor.

on the wrong subtype of neuroendocrine tumor (duodenal, small bowel, or functional pNET only) or metastatic NF-pNET; were literature reviews with no unique content; or were case reports. A total of 92 manuscripts were included in the full manuscript review and application of inclusion criteria. Forty-one articles were further excluded because of overrepresentation of functional pNET in the study cohorts or exclusion of lymph node status or lymphadenectomy from survival analysis. A final total of 51 manuscripts were identified and used in the systematic review (Tables 3-8 and 3-9).

Data were extracted from individual studies by a single author. Each study was reviewed and assigned a quality of evidence according to the Grading of Recommendations, Assessment, Development, and Evaluation (GRADE) system.[101]

FINDINGS

Impact of Lymph Node Status on Recurrence-Free Survival

Twenty-eight studies retrospectively analyzed the impact of LNM or lymphadenectomy on recurrence-free survival (RFS) (Table 3-8). Eighteen (64%) studies found that the presence of LNM was associated with worse RFS after curative resection of pNET. Partelli et al.[187] were among the first to report their experience with 181 resected NF-pNETs, demonstrating that node-positive disease was associated with increased risk of tumor recurrence. Hashim et al.[162] noted the same finding that LNM was associated with decreased median RFS and concluded that routine regional lymphadenectomy was critically indicated in the surgical management of pNET to optimize outcomes.[162] Zaidi et al.[198] presented the largest cohort from a multi-institutional, international database of patients who underwent pancreatectomy for NF-pNET to identify risk factors for disease recurrence. Symptomatic tumors, tumor size greater than 2 cm, Ki-67 greater than 3%, and LNM were associated with increased tumor recurrence on multivariable analysis.[198] Multiple analyses from the US Neuroendocrine Tumor Study Group demonstrated similar findings.

In terms of the therapeutic value of lymphadenectomy, Wu et al.[196] and the US Neuroendocrine Tumor Study Group investigated the therapeutic index of regional lymphadenectomy in 647 patients after curative resection of pNET. LNM was associated with decreased 5-year RFS, 56.0% versus 83.3% ($P < .001$) when compared with node-negative patients.[196] Lymphadenectomy was associated with a therapeutic index of 13.8 for the entire cohort, with increasing benefit observed in patients with tumors 2 cm or larger, moderately or poorly differentiated tumors, Ki-67 3% and greater, and tumors in the head of the pancreas.[196] Other analyses from the group demonstrated similar decreased RFS with LNM even in small, less-than-2 cm NF-pNETs and a two-fold increased risk of LNM in tumors less than 1.5 cm.[161,163,185] Other cohorts from both Western and Eastern countries have found LNM to be a poor prognostic factor for RFS.[175–177,179–182,186,188,191,194]

Ten studies reported that lymph node metastases and/or lymphadenectomy has no effect on RFS. Lee et al.[183] reviewed their experience with small NF-pNETs less than 4 cm in size and compared survival outcomes between 77 patients who underwent nonoperative management and 56 patients who underwent resection. They reported no progression in the nonoperative group after a median follow-up of 45 months

TABLE 3-8 Review of Literature Reporting Impact of Lymph Node Metastasis on Recurrence-Free Survival in pNET

Authors, Year	Study Duration	Study Location	Cohort	N	Median Follow-up, mo	LNM, %	LNM Prognostic of RFS?	Grade of Evidence*
Dong et al.,[161] 2019†	1997–2016	United States	NF-pNET ≤2 cm	328	34	12.8	Yes HR, 3.06; $P = .026$ Tumor <1.5 cm 2-fold increase risk of LNM (OR, 2.59; $P = .022$)	++
Furukori et al.,[174] 2014	1996–2012	Japan	NF-pNET	9	NS	11.1	No	+
Ge et al.,[175] 2017	2007–2013	China	NF-pNET	48	46	25.0	Yes OR, 44.53; $P = .003$	+
Genç et al.,[176] 2018	1992–2016	Netherlands	NF-pNET	280	62	23.2	Yes HR, 3.36; $P = .004$	++
Genç et al.,[177] 2018	1992–2015	Netherlands, Italy	NF-pNET	211	51	24.2	Yes HR, 2.44; $P = .017$	++
Harimoto et al.,[178] 2019‡	2008–2017	Japan	NF-pNET (65%) F-pNET (35%)	55	47	18.2	No	+
Harimoto et al.,[179] 2019‡	2008–2017	Japan	NF-pNET (77%) F-pNET (23%)	84	25	14.3	Yes HR, 3.30; $P = .03$	+
Hashim et al.,[162] 2014	1994–2012	United States	NF-pNET (94%) F-pNET (6%)	136	59	37.5	Yes LNM associated with decreased median RFS, 4.5 y vs. 14.6 y; $P < .001$	++

Jiang et al.,[180] 2015	2004–2014	China	NF-pNET	100	NS	20.0	Yes HR, 3.995; $P = .003$	++
Kaltenborn et al.,[181] 2016	1990–2009	Germany	pNET	41	42	NS	Yes OR, 1.172; $P = .026$	+
Kim et al.,[182] 2019	1990–2017	South Korea	NF-pNET (80%) F-pNET (20%)	542	60	12.4	Yes HR, 2.46; $P = .009$	++
Lee et al.,[183] 2012	2000–2011	United States	NF-pNET <4 cm	133 Nonoperative = 77 Operative = 56	45 52	NA 9.6	No	++
Lopez-Aguiar et al.,[184] 2018	2000–2013	United States	NF-pNET Ki-67 <3%	72	39	18.1	No	++
Lopez-Aguiar et al.,[163] 2019†	2000–2016	United States	NF-pNET	695	36	22.7	Yes HR, 3.7; $P < .001$ 5-y RFS, 60% vs. 86% (LNM vs. no LNM); $P < .001$	++
Lopez-Aguiar et al.,[185] 2019†	2000–2016	United States	NF-pNET <2 cm	309	35	7.1	Yes HR, 5.9; $P = .016$ 5-y RFS, 80% vs. 96% (LNM vs. no LNM); $P = .007$	++
Masui et al.,[186] 2019	2000–2018	Japan	NF-pNET ≤2 cm	69	NS	27.5	Yes 5-y RFS, 89.7% vs. 95.7% (LNM vs. no LNM); $P = .006$ 10-y RFS, 53.2% vs. 71.4% (LNM vs. no LNM); $P = .006$	++
Partelli et al.,[187] 2013	1993–2009	France, Italy	NF-pNET	181	55	30.3	Yes HR, 5.21; $P = .001$	++

(continued)

TABLE 3-8 Review of Literature Reporting Impact of Lymph Node Metastasis on Recurrence-Free Survival in pNET *(continued)*

Authors, Year	Study Duration	Study Location	Cohort	N	Median Follow-up, mo	LNM, %	LNM Prognostic of RFS?	Grade of Evidence*
Postlewait et al.,[188] 2016	2000–2014	United States	NF-pNET (79%) F-pNET (21%)	164	18	24.4	Yes HR, 3.04; P = .04 LNM associated with decreased median RFS, 42.6 mo vs. median not reached; P < .001	++
Sallinen et al.,[189] 2018	1999–2014	Europe	NF-pNET ≤2 cm	210	36	10.6	No	++
Sarmiento et al.,[190] 2002	1980–1995	United States	NF-pNET (69%) F-pNET (31%)	29	105	55.2	No	+
Sho et al.,[191] 2019	1989–2015	United States	NF-pNET (86%) F-pNET (14%)	140	56	22.1	Yes HR, 4.28; P = .006	++
Taki et al.,[192] 2017	2001–2014	Japan	NF-pNET (75%) F-pNET (25%)	83	NS	20.5	No	+
Tsutsumi et al.,[193] 2014	1987–2011	Japan	NF-pNET (90%) F-pNET (10%)	70	46	11.4	No	++
Wang et al.,[194] 2011	1974–2008	Taiwan	NF-pNET (58%) F-pNET (42%)	93	40	22	Yes 5-y RFS, 31.0% vs. 96.2% (LNM vs. no LNM); P < .001	+

Study	Years	Country	Type	N					Grade
Wong et al.,[195] 2014	1999–2012	United States	NF-pNET (93%) F-pNET (7%)	150	52	28.3	No		++
Wu et al.,[196] 2019†	1997–2016	United States	NF-pNET (88%) F-pNET (12%)	647	34	24.6	Yes	5-y RFS, 56.0% vs. 83.3% (LNM vs. no LNM); P < .001 Lymphadenectomy carried a therapeutic index value of 13.8.	++
Yoo et al.,[197] 2015	2005–2014	South Korea	NF-pNET Left sided	35	38	NS	No		+
Zaidi et al.,[198] 2019‡	2000–2016	United States, Italy	NF-pNET	1,006	41	23.1	Yes	LNM associated with a 1.9 OR of recurrence; P = .039	++

F-pNET: functional pancreatic neuroendocrine tumors; HR: hazard ratio; LNM: lymph node metastasis; NA: not applicable; NF-pNET: nonfunctional pancreatic neuroendocrine tumors; NS: not stated; OR: odds ratio; pNET: pancreatic neuroendocrine tumors; RFS: recurrence-free survival.
*Grade: + very low; ++ low.
†Studies with overlapping cohorts from the US Neuroendocrine Tumor Study Group.
‡Studies with overlapping patient cohort from the Gunma University Hospital System.

TABLE 3-9 Studies Reporting Impact of Lymph Node Metastasis on Overall Survival in pNET

Authors, Year	Study Duration	Study Location/Data	Cohort	N	Median Follow-up, mo	LNM, %	LNM Prognostic of OS?	Grade of Evidence*
Bilimoria et al.,[164] 2008	1985–2004	NCDB	NF-pNET (84%) F-pNET (16%)	3,851	51	52.8	Yes 5-y OS, 53.6% vs. 60.2% (LNM vs. no LNM). *P* < .001 Not significant on multivariate analysis	++
Cherenfant et al.,[170] 2013	1998–2011	United States	NF-pNET	128	33	24.2	No	++
Chung et al.,[199] 2007	1995–2004	South Korea	NF-pNET (89%) F-pNET (11%)	28	25	31.8	No	+
Conrad et al.,[200] 2016	1998–2012	SEER	pNET	981	NS	32.3	Yes LNM was associated with decreased OS in T1–T2 tumors (*P* < .001) but not T3–T4 (*P* = .789).	++
Curran et al.,[201] 2015	1988–2010	SEER	NF-pNET (71%) F-pNET (29%)	1,915	40	38.0	Yes 5-y DSS, 69% vs. 81% (LNM vs. no LNM); *P* < .001 LNM independently associated with an increase in risk of mortality (HR, 1.57; 95% CI, 1.23–1.95).	++
Demir et al.,[202] 2011	1964–2006	Germany	NF-pNET (68%) F-pNET (32%)	82	72	42.7	No	+

Study	Years	Country	Type	N			LNM	Comments	
Dima et al.,[203] 2018	2000–2014	Romania	NF-pNET (59%) F-pNET (41%)	120	NS	15.8	No		+
Fitzgerald et al.,[204] 2016	1988–2012	SEER	pNET	561	NS	30.1	Yes	5-y OS, 72.4% vs. 82.9% (LNM vs. no LNM); $P = .003$; HR, 2.02	++
Ge et al.,[175] 2017	2007–2013	China	NF-pNET	48	46	25.0	No		++
Genç et al.,[177] 2018	1992–2015	Netherlands, Italy	NF-pNET	211	51	24.2	No		++
Han et al.,[205] 2014	1999–2011	China	NF-pNET (74%) F-PNET (26%)	104	51.6	42.9	Yes	LNM decreased OS (HR, 4.9; 95% CI, 1.9–21.8; $P = .033$) on univariate analysis.	+
Harimoto et al.,[179] 2019†	2008–2017	Japan	NF-pNET (77%) F-pNET (23%)	84	25	14.3	No		+
Hashim et al.,[162] 2014	1994–2012	United States	NF-pNET (94%) F-pNET (6%)	136	59	37.5	No		++
Haynes et al.,[169] 2011	1977–2009	United States	NF-pNET	139	34	20.1	Yes	5-y OS, 55.1% vs. 94.1% (LNM vs. no LNM); $P < .001$	++
Jin et al.,[206] 2017	2003–2015	China	NF-pNET (87%) F-pNET (13%)	162	NS	24.7	Yes	LNM decreased OS (HR, 4.802; 95% CI, 1.824-12.645; $P - .001$) on univariate analysis.	++
Jutric,[207] 2017	1998–2011	NCDB	NF pNET	2,735	60	51%	Yes	LNM decreased OS (HR, 1.5, 95% CI, 1.14–2.05; $P = .017$).	++

(continued)

TABLE 3-9 Studies Reporting Impact of Lymph Node Metastasis on Overall Survival in pNET *(continued)*

Authors, Year	Study Duration	Study Location/Data	Cohort	N	Median Follow-up, mo	LNM, %	LNM Prognostic of OS?	Grade of Evidence*
Kaltenborn et al.,[181] 2016	1990–2009	Germany	pNET	41	42	NS	Yes LNM decreased OS (HR, 1.18; 95% CI, 1.04–1.352; P = .031) on univariate analysis.	+
Kazanjian et al.,[208] 2006	1990–2005	United States	NF-pNET (71%) F-pNET (29%)	70	50	30.0	No	+
Li et al.,[209] 2019	2004–2014	SEER	pNET	4,608	NS	21.33	No	++
Liu et al.,[210] 2017	2004–2014	SEER	pNET	1,273	NS	41.7	Yes LNM decreased OS (HR, 1.914; 95% CI, 1.467–2.497; P < .001) on univariate analysis.	++
Madeira et al.,[211] 1998	1991–1997	France	NF-pNET (54%) F-pNET (46%)	82	32	63.5	No	+
Masui et al.,[186] 2019	2000–2018	Japan	NF-pNET ≤2 cm	69	NS	27.5	No	++
Matthews et al.,[212] 2000	1984–1999	United States	NF-pNET (74%) F-pNET (26%)	38	42	NS	Yes Median survival for node-negative patients, 124 mo; for node-positive patients, 75 mo (P = .003)	+
Sarmiento et al.,[190] 2002	1980–1995	United States	NF-pNET (69%) F-pNET (31%)	29	105	55.2	Yes 5-y OS, 67% vs. 100% (LNM vs. no LNM); P = .04	+

Study	Years	Country	Tumor type	n			LNM prognostic	Findings	Rating
Schurr et al.,[213] 2007	1987–2004	Germany	NF-pNET (74%) F-pNET (26%)	62	31	NS	No		+
Sharpe et al.,[214] 2015	1998–2006	NCDB	pNET ≤2 cm	380	60	29.0	Yes	5-y DSS, 84.1% vs. 93.8% (LNM vs. no LNM); $P < .001$ LNM independently associated with an increase in risk of mortality (HR, 2.01; 95% CI, 1.199–3.369; $P = .008$).	++
Song et al.,[215] 2016	1995–2010	South Korea	NF-pNET	225	70	NS	Yes	LNM independently associated with an increase in risk of mortality (HR, 7.85; 95% CI, 2.35–26.19; $P = .001$).	++
Taki et al.,[192] 2017	2001–2014	Japan	NF-pNET (75%) F-pNET (25%)	83	NS	20.5	Yes	LNM decreased OS (HR, 6.89; 95% CI, 1.8–32.8; $P = .005$) on univariate analysis.	+
Tomassetti et al.,[171] 2005	1978–2003	United States	NF-pNET (63%) F-pNET (19%)	83	30	59.5	Yes	LNM decreased OS (HR, 4.97; 95% CI, 1.91–12.90; $P = .001$).	+
Toste et al.,[216] 2013	1989–2012	United States	NF-pNET	116	47	27.6	Yes	LNM independently associated with an increase in risk of mortality (HR, 4.4; 95% CI, 1.6–12.2; $P = .005$).	++

(continued)

TABLE 3-9 Studies Reporting Impact of Lymph Node Metastasis on Overall Survival in pNET (continued)

Authors, Year	Study Duration	Study Location/Data	Cohort	N	Median Follow-up, mo	LNM, %	LNM Prognostic of OS?	Grade of Evidence*
Tsutsumi et al.,[166] 2012	1987–2010	Japan	NF-pNET (52%) F-pNET (48%)	66	NS	18.2	Yes 5-y OS, 46.9% vs. 100% (LNM vs. no LNM); P < .001	+
Wang et al.,[194] 2011	1974–2008	Taiwan	NF-pNET (58%) F-pNET (42%)	93	40	22	Yes 5-y OS, 60.3% vs. 96.1% (LNM vs. no LNM); P < .001	+
Watzka et al.,[217] 2020	1990–2018	Germany	NF-pNET	155	NS	39.4	Yes 10-y OS, 65.7% vs. 81.3% (LNM vs. no LNM); P = .032	++
Wong et al.,[195] 2014	1999–2012	United States	NF-pNET (93%) F-pNET (7%)	150	52	28.3	No	++
Wu et al.,[196] 2019‡	1997–2016	United States	NF-pNET (88%) F-pNET (12%)	647	34	24.6	Yes 5-y OS, 84.1% vs. 93.8% (LNM vs. no LNM); P < .001	++

CI: confidence interval; DSS: disease-specific survival; F-pNET: functional pancreatic neuroendocrine tumors; HR: hazard ratio; LNM: lymph node metastasis; NCDB: National Cancer Database; NF-pNET: nonfunctional pancreatic neuroendocrine tumors; NS: not stated; OS: overall survival; pNET: pancreatic neuroendocrine tumor; SEER: Surveillance, Epidemiology, and End Results.

*Grade: + very low; ++ low.

†Studies with overlapping patient cohort from the Gunma University Hospital System.

‡Studies with overlapping cohorts from the US Neuroendocrine Tumor Study Group.

and no recurrences in the operative group at 52-month follow-up.[183] Sallinen et al.[189] similarly evaluated their cohort of resected 2 cm or smaller NF-pNETs and found no difference in RFS between those undergoing formal resection with lymphadenectomy and those who had parenchymal-sparing surgery without lymph node sampling, suggesting that routine lymphadenectomy conferred no therapeutic benefit.[189] In a single institutional cohort of 72 patients with localized low-grade (Ki-67 <3%) NF-pNETs who underwent curative resection, LNM was found to be associated with shorter RFS on univariate analysis; however, in the multivariate model, only R1 resection and Ki-67 remained significant.[184] Other cohorts of mixed functional and NF-pNET also failed to demonstrate prognostic relevance of LNM on RFS.[174,178,190,192,193,195,197]

In summary, the preponderance of data suggests LNM is predictive of shorter RFS. Resection with regional lymphadenectomy is, therefore, recommended for tumors greater than 2 cm and with high Ki-67 proliferative indices. It is unclear if regional lymphadenectomy in and of itself affects RFS, but it may. In addition, it does provide staging information to inform prognosis and surveillance.

Impact of Lymph Node Status on Overall Survival

Thirty-five studies retrospectively analyzed the impact of LNM and/or lymphadenectomy on overall survival (OS) (Table 3-9). Twenty-one (58%) studies found that the presence of LNM was associated with worse OS after curative resection of pNET. Bilimoria et al.[164] reported their analysis of 3,851 patients diagnosed with both functional and NF-pNET in the National Cancer Database (NCDB) from 1985 to 2004. On univariate analysis, LNM was associated with worse 5-year OS, 53.6% versus 60.2% (LNM vs. no LNM; $P < .001$); however, on multivariate analysis, LNM was not independently prognostic.[164] In an NCDB cohort of 2,735 patients with NF-pNET only, LNM was independently associated with decreased OS (hazard ratio [HR], 1.5; 95% confidence interval [CI], 1.14 to 2.05; $P = .017$).[207] The same database was interrogated to assess the prognostic impact on LNM and other clinicopathologic factors in 2 cm or smaller, localized pNETs. Sharpe et al.[214] found positive lymph nodes were an independent predictor of worse OS in resected small pNETs, with a 5-year disease-specific survival of 84.1% versus 93.8% (LNM vs. no LNM; $P < .001$) and an increased risk of disease-related mortality (HR, 2.01; 95% CI, 1.199 to 3.369; $P = .008$). The Surveillance, Epidemiology, and End Results (SEER) database has also been queried to investigate the impact of LNM on OS in resected pNET. Curran et al.[201] reported their analysis of 1,915 patients undergoing pNET resection with curative intent and found a decreased 5-year disease-specific survival of 69% in patients with LNM when compared with 81% in node-negative patients ($P < .001$). LNM was independently associated with an increase in risk of mortality (HR, 1.57; 95% CI, 1.23 to 1.95).[201] Others have found similar associations of LNM with worse survival outcomes in SEER database analyses,[200,204,210] although another more recent SEER analysis showed no such correlation.[209] In the previously mentioned study by Wu et al.[196] and the US Neuroendocrine Tumor Study Group, LNM was associated with decreased 5-year OS, 84% versus 94% ($P < .001$), when compared with node-negative patients. There was a benefit in patients undergoing lymphadenectomy.[196] In patients with incidental NF-pNET, Haynes et al.[169]

also reported worse 5-year OS rate with LNM of 55% versus 94% ($P < .001$). Other multi-institutional and single-institutional studies from both Western and Eastern countries have found LNM to be a poor prognostic factor for OS on either univariate or multivariate analysis.[166,171,181,190,192,194,205,206,212,215–217]

Fifteen studies reported that lymph node metastases and/or lymphadenectomy have no effect on OS after curative-intent pancreatectomy for pNET. Except for the previously discussed SEER data analysis by Li et al.,[209] most of these studies were smaller cohort studies.[162,170,175,177,179,186,195,199,202,203,208,211,213]

In summary, most analyses from large databases, multi-institutional collaborations, and large single-center series report an association of LNM with worse OS, suggesting that resection with regional lymphadenectomy may improve outcomes when compared with margin-negative resection without lymphadenectomy.

CONCLUSION

Patients with low-grade NF-pNETs 2 cm or larger should undergo resection with regional lymphadenectomy. In tumors smaller than 2 cm, special attention should be paid to preoperative imaging, patient symptoms, and Ki-67.

REFERENCES

1. Nagtegaal ID, Odze RD, Klimstra D, et al. The 2019 WHO classification of tumours of the digestive system. *Histopathology*. 2020;76(2):182-188. doi:10.1111/his.13975
2. Rindi G, Klimstra DS, Abedi-Ardekani B, et al. A common classification framework for neuroendocrine neoplasms: an International Agency for Research on Cancer (IARC) and World Health Organization (WHO) expert consensus proposal. *Mod Pathol*. 2018;31(12):1770-1786. doi:10.1038/s41379-018-0110-y
3. Sorbye H, Baudin E, Perren A. The problem of high-grade gastroenteropancreatic neuroendocrine neoplasms: well-differentiated neuroendocrine tumors, neuroendocrine carcinomas, and beyond. *Endocrinol Metab Clin North Am*. 2018;47(3):683-698. doi:10.1016/j.ecl.2018.05.001
4. WHO Classification of Tumours Editorial Board, eds. *Digestive System Tumours*. World Health Organization; 2019. *WHO Classification of Tumours*. 5th ed; vol 1.
5. Adsay V. Ki67 labeling index in neuroendocrine tumors of the gastrointestinal and pancreatobiliary tract: to count or not to count is not the question, but rather how to count. *Am J Surg Pathol*. 2012;36(12):1743-1746. doi:10.1097/PAS.0b013e318272ff77
6. Sorbye H, Welin S, Langer SW, et al. Predictive and prognostic factors for treatment and survival in 305 patients with advanced gastrointestinal neuroendocrine carcinoma (WHO G3): the NORDIC NEC study. *Ann Oncol*. 2013;24(1):152-160. doi:10.1093/annonc/mds276
7. Yachida S, Vakiani E, White CM, et al. Small cell and large cell neuroendocrine carcinomas of the pancreas are genetically similar and distinct from well-differentiated pancreatic neuroendocrine tumors. *Am J Surg Pathol*. 2012;36(2):173-184. doi:10.1097/PAS.0b013e3182417d36
8. Hochwald SN, Zee S, Conlon KC, et al. Prognostic factors in pancreatic endocrine neoplasms: an analysis of 136 cases with a proposal for low-grade and intermediate-grade groups. *J Clin Oncol*. 2002;20(11):2633-2642. doi:10.1200/JCO.2002.10.030
9. Norton JA, Kim T, Kim J, et al. SSAT state-of-the-art conference: current surgical management of gastric tumors. *J Gastrointest Surg*. 2018;22(1):32-42. doi:10.1007/s11605-017-3533-8
10. Shebani KO, Souba WW, Finkelstein DM, et al. Prognosis and survival in patients with gastrointestinal tract carcinoid tumors. *Ann Surg*. 1999;229(6):815-823. doi:10.1097/00000658-199906000-00008
11. Gastrointestinal Pathology Study Group of Korean Society of Pathologists, Sohn JH, Cho M-Y, et al. Prognostic significance of defining L-cell type on the biologic behavior of rectal neuroendocrine tumors in relation with pathological parameters. *Cancer Res Treat*. 2015;47(4):813-822. doi:10.4143/crt.2014.238

12. Chan CS, Laddha SV, Lewis PW, et al. ATRX, DAXX or MEN1 mutant pancreatic neuroendocrine tumors are a distinct alpha-cell signature subgroup. *Nat Commun.* 2018;9(1):4158. doi:10.1038/s41467-018-06498-2
13. Scarpa A, Chang DK, Nones K, et al. Whole-genome landscape of pancreatic neuroendocrine tumours. *Nature.* 2017;543(7643):65-71. doi:10.1038/nature21063
14. Tang LH. Pancreatic neuroendocrine neoplasms: landscape and horizon. *Arch Pathol Lab Med.* 2020;144(7):816:828. doi:10.5858/arpa.2019-0654-RA
15. Dasari A, Shen C, Halperin D, et al. Trends in the incidence, prevalence, and survival outcomes in patients with neuroendocrine tumors in the united states. *JAMA Oncol.* 2017;3(10): 1335-1342. doi:10.1001/jamaoncol.2017.0589
16. Schernthaner-Reiter MH, Trivellin G, Stratakis CA. MEN1, MEN4, and Carney complex: pathology and molecular genetics. *Neuroendocrinology.* 2016;103(1):18-31. doi:10.1159/000371819
17. Neuroendocrine and adrenal tumors. National Comprehensive Cancer Network. Accessed July 16, 2020. https://www.nccn.org/professionals/physician_gls/pdf/neuroendocrine.pdf
18. Gut P, Komarowska H, Czarnywojtek A, et al. Familial syndromes associated with neuroendocrine tumours. *Contemp Oncol (Pozn).* 2015;19(3):176-183 doi:10.5114/wo.2015.52710
19. van der Lely AJ, de Herder WW. Carcinoid syndrome: diagnosis and medical management. *Arq Bras Endocrinol Metabol.* 2005;49(5):850-860. doi:10.1590/s0004-27302005000500028
20. Halperin DM, Shen C, Dasari A, et al. Frequency of carcinoid syndrome at neuroendocrine tumour diagnosis: a population-based study. *Lancet Oncol.* 2017;18(4):525-534. doi:10.1016/S1470-2045(17)30110-9
21. Grahame-Smith DG. Progress report: the carcinoid syndrome. *Gut.* 1970;11(2):189-192. doi:10.1136/gut.11.2.189
22. Zogakis TG, Gibril F, Libutti SK, et al. Management and outcome of patients with sporadic gastrinoma arising in the duodenum. *Ann Surg.* 2003;238(1):42-48. doi:10.1097/01.SLA.0000074963.87688.31
23. Dasari A, Mehta K, Byers LA, Sorbye H, Yao JC. Comparative study of lung and extrapulmonary poorly differentiated neuroendocrine carcinomas: a SEER database analysis of 162,983 cases. *Cancer.* 2018;124(4):807-815. doi:10.1002/cncr.31124
24. Sanli Y, Garg I, Kandathil A, et al. Neuroendocrine tumor diagnosis and management: ^{68}Ga-DOTATATE PET/CT. *AJR Am J Roentgenol.* 2018;211(2):267-277. doi:10.2214/AJR.18.19881
25. Tang LH, Untch BR, Reidy DL, et al. Well-differentiated neuroendocrine tumors with a morphologically apparent high-grade component: a pathway distinct from poorly differentiated neuroendocrine carcinomas. *Clin Cancer Res.* 2016;22(4):1011-1017. doi:10.1158/1078-0432.CCR-15-0548
26. Amin MB, Edge SB, Greene F, et al, eds. *AJCC Cancer Staging Manual.* 8th ed. Springer; 2017.
27. Kaltsas G, Caplin M, Davies P, et al. ENETS consensus guidelines for the standards of care in neuroendocrine tumors: pre- and perioperative therapy in patients with neuroendocrine tumors. *Neuroendocrinology.* 2017;105(3):245-254. doi:10.1159/000461583
28. Strosberg JR, Halfdanarson TR, Bellizzi AM, et al. The North American Neuroendocrine Tumor Society consensus guidelines for surveillance and medical management of midgut neuroendocrine tumors. *Pancreas.* 2017;46(6):707-714. doi:10.1097/MPA.0000000000000850
29. Woodhouse B, Pattison S, Segelov E, et al. Consensus-derived quality performance indicators for neuroendocrine tumour care. *J Clin Med.* 2019;8(9):1455. doi:10.3390/jcm8091455
30. Blonski WC, Reddy KR, Shaked A, Siegelman E, Metz DC. Liver transplantation for metastatic neuroendocrine tumor: a case report and review of the literature. *World J Gastroenterol.* 2005;11(48):7676-7683. doi:10.3748/wjg.v11.i48.7676
31. Woltering EA, Voros BA, Beyer DT, et al. Aggressive surgical approach to the management of neuroendocrine tumors: a report of 1,000 surgical cytoreductions by a single institution. *J Am Coll Surg.* 2017;224(4):434-447. doi:10.1016/j.jamcollsurg.2016.12.032
32. Jaïs P, Terris B, Ruszniewski P, et al. Somatostatin receptor subtype gene expression in human endocrine gastroentero-pancreatic tumours. *Eur J Clin Invest.* 1997;27(8):639-644. doi:10.1046/j.1365-2362.1997.1740719.x
33. Kiesewetter B, Duan H, Lamm W, et al. Oral ondansetron offers effective antidiarrheal activity for carcinoid syndrome refractory to somatostatin analogs. *Oncologist.* 2019;24(2):255-258. doi:10.1634/theoncologist.2018-0191
34. Moertel CG, Kvols LK, Rubin J. A study of cyproheptadine in the treatment of metastatic carcinoid tumor and the malignant carcinoid syndrome. *Cancer.* 1991;67(1):33-36. doi:10.1002/1097-0142(19910101)67:1<33::aid-cncr2820670107>3.0.co;2-e

35. Strosberg J, El-Haddad G, Wolin E, et al. Phase 3 trial of ^{177}Lu-Dotatate for midgut neuroendocrine tumors. *N Engl J Med.* 2017;376(2):125-135. doi:10.1056/NEJMoa1607427

36. Johnston SD, Johnston PW, O'Rourke D. Carcinoid constrictive pericarditis. *Heart.* 1999; 82(5):641-643. doi:10.1056/NEJMoa1607427

37. Rinke A, Müller H-H, Schade-Brittinger C, et al. Placebo-controlled, double-blind, prospective, randomized study on the effect of octreotide LAR in the control of tumor growth in patients with metastatic neuroendocrine midgut tumors: a report from the PROMID Study Group. *J Clin Oncol.* 2009;27(28):4656-4663. doi:10.1200/JCO.2009.22.8510

38. Caplin ME, Pavel M, wikła JB, et al. Lanreotide in metastatic enteropancreatic neuroendocrine tumors. *N Engl J Med.* 2014;371(3):224-233. doi:10.1056/NEJMoa1316158

39. Yao JC, Fazio N, Singh S, et al. Everolimus for the treatment of advanced, non-functional neuroendocrine tumours of the lung or gastrointestinal tract (RADIANT-4): a randomised, placebo-controlled, phase 3 study. *Lancet.* 2016;387(10022):968-977. doi:10.1016/S0140-6736(15)00817-X

40. Raymond E, Dahan L, Raoul J-L, et al. Sunitinib malate for the treatment of pancreatic neuroendocrine tumors. *N Engl J Med.* 2011;364(6):501-513. doi:10.1056/NEJMoa1003825

41. Kunz PL, Catalano PJ, Nimeiri H, et al. A randomized study of temozolomide or temozolomide and capecitabine in patients with advanced pancreatic neuroendocrine tumors: a trial of the ECOG-ACRIN Cancer Research Group (E2211). *J Clin Oncol.* 2018;36(15):4004. doi:10.1200/JCO.2018.36.15_suppl.4004

42. Maggio I, Manuzzi L, Lamberti G, Ricci AD, Tober N, Campana D. Landscape and future perspectives of immunotherapy in neuroendocrine neoplasia. *Cancers (Basel).* 2020;12(4):832. doi:10.3390/cancers12040832

43. Bodei L, Sundin A, Kidd M, Prasad V, Modlin IM. The status of neuroendocrine tumor imaging: from darkness to light? *Neuroendocrinology.* 2015;101(1):1-17. doi:10.1159/000367850

44. Kinney MA, Warner ME, Nagorney DM, et al. Perianaesthetic risks and outcomes of abdominal surgery for metastatic carcinoid tumours. *Br J Anaesth.* 2001;87(3):447-452. doi:10.1093/bja/87.3.447

45. Sicklick JK, Kato S, Okamura R, et al. Molecular profiling of cancer patients enables personalized combination therapy: the I-PREDICT study. *Nat Med.* 2019;25(5):744-750. doi:10.1038/s41591-019-0407-5

46. Kulke MH, Hornick JL, Frauenhoffer C, et al. O[6]-methylguanine DNA methyltransferase deficiency and response to temozolomide-based therapy in patients with neuroendocrine tumors. *Clin Cancer Res.* 2009;15(1):338-345. doi:10.1158/1078-0432.CCR-08-1476

47. Lim SM, Park HS, Kim S, et al. Next-generation sequencing reveals somatic mutations that confer exceptional response to everolimus. *Oncotarget.* 2016;7(9):10547-10556. doi:10.18632/oncotarget.7234

48. Chan DL, Segelov E, Singh S. Everolimus in the management of metastatic neuroendocrine tumours. *Therap Adv Gastroenterol.* 2017;10(1):132-141. doi:10.1177/1756283X16674660

49. Akerström G, Falconi M, Kianmanesh R, et al. ENETS consensus guidelines for the standards of care in neuroendocrine tumors: pre- and perioperative therapy in patients with neuroendocrine tumors. *Neuroendocrinology.* 2009;90(2):203-208. doi:10.1159/000225949

50. Shao Q-Q, Zhao B-B, Dong L-B, Cao H-T, Wang W-B. Surgical management of Zollinger-Ellison syndrome: classical considerations and current controversies. *World J Gastroenterol.* 2019;25(32):4673-4681. doi:10.3748/wjg.v25.i32.4673

51. Stabile BE, Morrow DJ, Passaro E Jr. The gastrinoma triangle: operative implications. *Am J Surg.* 1984;147(1):25-31. doi:10.1016/0002-9610(84)90029-1

52. Alexander HR, Fraker DL, Norton JA, et al. Prospective study of somatostatin receptor scintigraphy and its effect on operative outcome in patients with Zollinger-Ellison syndrome. *Ann Surg.* 1998;228(2):228-238. doi:10.1097/00000658-199808000-00013

53. Norton JA, Fraker DL, Alexander HR, Jensen RT. Value of surgery in patients with negative imaging and sporadic Zollinger–Ellison syndrome. *Ann Surg.* 2012;256(3):509-517. doi:10.1097/SLA.0b013e318265f08d

54. Krampitz GW, Norton JA. Current management of the Zollinger-Ellison syndrome. *Adv Surg.* 2013;47:59-79. doi:10.1016/j.yasu.2013.02.004

55. Norton JA. Intra-operative procedures to localize endocrine tumours of the pancreas and duodenum. *Ital J Gastroenterol Hepatol.* 1999;31(suppl 2):S195-S197.

56. Cho MS, Kasi A. *Zollinger Ellison Syndrome.* StatPearls; 2020.

57. Farley HA, Pommier RF. Surgical treatment of small bowel neuroendocrine tumors. *Hematol Oncol Clin North Am.* 2016;30(1):49-61. doi:10.1016/j.hoc.2015.09.001

58. Howe JR, Cardona K, Fraker DL, et al. The surgical management of small bowel neuroendocrine tumors: consensus guidelines of the North American Neuroendocrine Tumor Society. *Pancreas.* 2017;46(6):715-731. doi:10.1097/MPA.000000000000084€

59. Pasquer A, Walter T, Hervieu V, et al. Surgical management of small bowel neuroendocrine tumors: specific requirements and their impact on staging and prognosis. *Ann Surg Oncol.* 2015;22(suppl 3):S742-S749. doi:10.1245/s10434-015-4620-2

60. Niederle B, Pape U-F, Costa F, et al. ENETS consensus guidelines update for neuroendocrine neoplasms of the jejunum and ileum. *Neuroendocrinology.* 2016;103(2):125-138. doi:10.1159/000443170

61. Figueiredo MN, Maggiori L, Gaujoux S, et al. Surgery for small-bowel neuroendocrine tumors: is there any benefit of the laparoscopic approach? *Surg Endosc.* 2014;28(5):1720-1726. doi:10.1007/s00464-013-3381-x

62. Massimino KP, Han E, Pommier SJ, Pommier RF. Laparoscopic surgical exploration is an effective strategy for locating occult primary neuroendocrine tumors. *Am J Surg.* 2012;203(5): 628-631. doi:10.1016/j.amjsurg.2011.12.010

63. Wang SC, Parekh JR, Zuraek MB, et al. Identification of unknown primary tumors in patients with neuroendocrine liver metastases. *Arch Surg.* 2010;145(3):276-280. doi:10.1001/archsurg.2010.10

64. Chambers AJ, Pasieka JL. Gastrinoma. *Cancer Treat Res.* 2010;153:213-233. doi:10.1007/978 -1-4419-0857-5_12

65. Boudreaux JP, Klimstra DS, Hassan MM, et al. The NANETS consensus guideline for the diagnosis and management of neuroendocrine tumors: well-differentiated neuroendocrine tumors of the jejunum, ileum, appendix, and cecum. *Pancreas.* 2010;39(6):753-766. doi:10.1097 /MPA.0b013e3181ebb2a5

66. Landerholm K, Zar N, Andersson RE, Falkmer SE, Järhult J. Survival and prognostic factors in patients with small bowel carcinoid tumour. *Br J Surg.* 2011;98(11):1617-1624. doi:10.1002 /bjs.7649

67. Landry CS, Lin HY, Phan A, et al. Resection of at-risk mesenteric lymph nodes is associated with improved survival in patients with small bowel neuroendocrine tumors. *World J Surg.* 2013;37(7):1695-1700. doi:10.1007/s00268-013-1918-8

68. Wang Y-Z, Carrasquillo JP, McCord E, et al. Reappraisal of lymphatic mapping for midgut neuroendocrine patients undergoing cytoreductive surgery. *Surgery.* 2014;156(6):1498-1503. doi:10.1016/j.surg.2014.05.028

69. Watzka FM, Fottner C, Miederer M, et al. Surgical treatment of NEN of small bowel: a retrospective analysis. *World J Surg.* 2016;40(3):749-758. doi:10.1007/s00268-016-3432-2

70. Jensen RT, Cadiot G, Brandi ML, et al. ENETS consensus guidelines for the management of patients with digestive neuroendocrine neoplasms: functional pancreatic endocrine tumor syndromes. *Neuroendocrinology.* 2012;95(2):98-119. doi:10.1159/000335591

71. Bartsch DK, Waldmann J, Fendrich V, et al. Impact of lymphadenectomy on survival after surgery for sporadic gastrinoma. *Br J Surg.* 2012;99(9):1234-1240. doi:10.1002/bjs.8843

72. Krampitz GW, Norton JA, Poultsides GA, Visser BC, Sun L, Jensen RT. Lymph nodes and survival in pancreatic neuroendocrine tumors. *Arch Surg.* 2012;147(9):820-827. doi:10.1001 /archsurg.2012.1261

73. Wang Y-Z, Diebold A, Woltering E, et al. Radioguided exploration facilitates surgical cytoreduction of neuroendocrine tumors. *J Gastrointest Surg.* 2012;16(3):635-640. doi:10.1007/s11605 -011-1767-4

74. Gamboa AC, Liu Y, Lee RM, et al. Duodenal neuroendocrine tumors: somewhere between the pancreas and small bowel? *J Surg Oncol.* 2019;120(8):1293-1301. doi:10.1002/jso.25731

75. Howe JR, Merchant NB, Conrad C, et al. The North American Neuroendocrine Tumor Society consensus paper on the surgical management of pancreatic neuroendocrine tumors. *Pancreas.* 2020;49(1):1-33. doi:10.1097/MPA.0000000000001454

76. Jann H, Roll S, Couvelard A, et al. Neuroendocrine tumors of midgut and hindgut origin: tumor-node-metastasis classification determines clinical outcome. *Cancer.* 2011;117(15):3332-3341. doi:10.1002/cncr.25855

77. Ohrvall U, Eriksson B, Juhlin C, et al. Method for dissection of mesenteric metastases in mid-gut carcinoid tumors. *World J Surg.* 2000;24(11):1402-1408. doi:10.1007/s002680010232

78. Hellman P, Lundström T, Öhrvall U, et al. Effect of surgery on the outcome of midgut carcinoid disease with lymph node and liver metastases. *World J Surg.* 2002;26(8):991-997. doi:10.1007 /s00268-002-6630-z

79. Kerström G, Hellman P, Hessman O. Midgut carcinoid tumours: surgical treatment and prognosis. *Best Pract Res Clin Gastroenterol.* 2005;19(5):717-728. doi:10.1016/j.bpg.2005.05.005

80. Robinson MK, Wilmore DW. Short bowel syndrome. In: Holzheimer RG, Mannick JA, eds. *Surgical Treatment: Evidence-Based and Problem-Oriented.* Zuckschwerdt; 2001. Accessed March 9, 2022. https://www.ncbi.nlm.nih.gov/books/NBK6974/

81. Delaunoit T, Rubin J, Neczyporenko F, Erlichman C, Hobday TJ. Somatostatin analogues in the treatment of gastroenteropancreatic neuroendocrine tumors. *Mayo Clin Proc.* 2005;80(4): 502-506. doi:10.4065/80.4.502

82. Ahrendt SA, McGuire GE, Pitt HA, Lillemoe KD. Why does somatostatin cause gallstones? *Am J Surg.* 1991;161(1):177-183. doi:10.1016/0002-9610(91)90381-m

83. Redfern JS, Fortuner WJ II. Octreotide-associated biliary tract dysfunction and gallstone formation: pathophysiology and management. *Am J Gastroenterol.* 1995;90(7):1042-1052.

84. Moher D, Liberati A, Tetzlaff J, Altman DG, Prisma Group. Preferred reporting items for systematic reviews and meta-analyses: the PRISMA statement. *PLoS Med.* 2009;6(7):e1000097. doi:10.1371/journal.pmed.1000097

85. Attanasio R, Mainolfi A, Grimaldi F, et al. Somatostatin analogs and gallstones: a retrospective survey on a large series of acromegalic patients. *J Endocrinol Invest.* 2008;31(8):704-710. doi:10.1007/BF03346419

86. Bigg-Wither GW, Ho KK, Grunstein RR, Sullivan CE, Doust BD. Effects of long term octreotide on gall stone formation and gall bladder function. *BMJ.* 1992;304(6842):1611-1612. doi:10.1136/bmj.304.6842.1611

87. Catnach SM, Anderson JV, Fairclough PD, et al. Effect of octreotide on gall stone prevalence and gall bladder motility in acromegaly. *Gut.* 1993;34(2):270-273. doi:10.1136/gut.34.2.270

88. Dowling RH, Veysey MJ, Pereira SP, et al. Role of intestinal transit in the pathogenesis of gallbladder stones. *Can J Gastroenterol.* 1997;11(1):57-64. doi:10.1155/1997/532036

89. Eastman RC, Arakaki RF, Shawker T, et al. A prospective examination of octreotide-induced gall-bladder changes in acromegaly. *Clin Endocrinol (Oxf).* 1992;36(3):265-269. doi:10.1111/j.1365-2265.1992.tb01442.x

90. Ewins DL, Javaid A, Coskeran PB, et al. Assessment of gall bladder dynamics, cholecystokinin release and the development of gallstones during octreotide therapy for acromegaly. *Q J Med.* 1992;83(300):295-306.

91. Hussaini SH, Murphy GM, Kennedy C, Besser GM, Wass JA, Dowling RH. The role of bile composition and physical chemistry in the pathogenesis of octreotide-associated gallbladder stones. *Gastroenterology.* 1994;107(5):1503-1513. doi:10.1016/0016-5085(94)90556-8

92. Hussaini SH, Pereira SP, Murphy GM, et al. Composition of gall bladder stones associated with octreotide: response to oral ursodeoxycholic acid. *Gut.* 1995;36(1):126-132. doi:10.1136/gut.36.1.126

93. Hussaini SH, Pereira SP, Veysey MJ, et al. Roles of gall bladder emptying and intestinal transit in the pathogenesis of octreotide induced gall bladder stones. *Gut.* 1996;38(5):775-783. doi:10.1136/gut.38.5.775

94. Moschetta A, Stolk MF, Rehfeld JF, et al. Severe impairment of postprandial cholecystokinin release and gall-bladder emptying and high risk of gallstone formation in acromegalic patients during Sandostatin LAR. *Aliment Pharmacol Ther.* 2001;15(2):181-185. doi:10.1046/j.1365-2036.2001.00924.x

95. Norlén O, Hessman O, Stålberg P, Akerström G, Hellman P. Prophylactic cholecystectomy in midgut carcinoid patients. *World J Surg.* 2010;34(6):1361-1367. doi:10.1007/s00268-010-0428-1

96. Shi YF, Zhu XF, Harris AG, Zhang JX, Dai Q. Prospective study of the long-term effects of somatostatin analog (octreotide) on gallbladder function and gallstone formation in Chinese acromegalic patients. *J Clin Endocrinol Metab.* 1993;76(1):32-37. doi:10.1210/jcem.76.1.8421099

97. Sinnamon AJ, Neuwirth MG, Vining CC, et al. Prophylactic cholecystectomy at time of surgery for small bowel neuroendocrine tumor does not increase postoperative morbidity. *Ann Surg Oncol.* 2018;25(1):239-245. doi:10.1245/s10434-017-6093-y

98. Trendle MC, Moertel CG, Kvols LK. Incidence and morbidity of cholelithiasis in patients receiving chronic octreotide for metastatic carcinoid and malignant islet cell tumors. *Cancer.* 1997;79(4):830-834. doi:10.1002/(sici)1097-0142(19970215)79:4<830::aid-cncr20>3.0.co;2-#

99. Turner HE, Lindsell DR, Vadivale A, Thillainayagam AV, Wass JA. Differing effects on gallbladder motility of lanreotide SR and octreotide LAR for treatment of acromegaly. *Eur J Endocrinol.* 1999;141(6):590-594. doi:10.1530/eje.0.1410590

100. Wymenga AN, Eriksson B, Salmela PI, et al. Efficacy and safety of prolonged-release lanreotide in patients with gastrointestinal neuroendocrine tumors and hormone-related symptoms. *J Clin Oncol.* 1999;17(4):1111. doi:10.1200/JCO.1999.17.4.1111

101. Balshem H, Helfand M, Schünemann HJ, et al. GRADE guidelines: 3. Rating the quality of evidence. *J Clin Epidemiol.* 2011;64(4):401-406. doi:10.1016/j.jclinepi.2010.07.015
102. Shaffer EA. Gallstone disease: epidemiology of gallbladder stone disease. *Best Pract Res Clin Gastroenterol.* 2006;20(6):981-996. doi:10.1016/j.bpg.2005.05.004
103. Sakorafas GH, Milingos D, Peros G. Asymptomatic cholelithiasis: is cholecystectomy really needed? A critical reappraisal 15 years after the introduction of laparoscopic cholecystectomy. *Dig Dis Sci.* 2007;52(5):1313-1325. doi:10.1007/s10620-006-9107-3
104. Jayakrishnan TT, Groeschl RT, George B, Thomas JP, Clark Gamblin T, Turaga KK. Review of the impact of antineoplastic therapies on the risk for cholelithiasis and acute cholecystitis. *Ann Surg Oncol.* 2014;21(1):240-247. doi:10.1245/s10434-013-3300-3
105. Doherty G. Surgical treatment of neuroendocrine tumors (including carcinoid). *Curr Opin Endocrinol Diabetes Obes.* 2013;20(1):32-36. doi:10.1097/MED.0b013e32835b7efa
106. Falconi M, Bettini R, Boninsegna L, Crippa S, Butturini G, Pederzoli P. Surgical strategy in the treatment of pancreatic neuroendocrine tumors. *JOP.* 2006;7(1):150-156.
107. Hallet J, Law CH, Cukier M, Saskin R, Liu N, Singh S. Exploring the rising incidence of neuroendocrine tumors: a population-based analysis of epidemiology, metastatic presentation, and outcomes. *Cancer.* 2015;121(4):589-597. doi:10.1002/cncr.29099
108. Frilling A, Modlin IM, Kidd M, et al. Recommendations for management of patients with neuroendocrine liver metastases. *Lancet Oncol.* 2014;15(1):e8-e21. doi:10.1016/S1470-2045(13)70362-0
109. Pape U-F, Berndt U, Müller-Nordhorn J, et al. Prognostic factors of long-term outcome in gastroenteropancreatic neuroendocrine tumours. *Endocr Relat Cancer.* 2008;15(4):1083-1097. doi:10.1677/ERC-08-0017
110. Keutgen XM, Schadde E, Pommier RF, Halfdanarson TR, Howe JR, Kebebew E. Metastatic neuroendocrine tumors of the gastrointestinal tract and pancreas: a surgeon's plea to centering attention on the liver. *Semin Oncol.* 2018;45(4):232-235. doi:10.1053/j.seminoncol.2018.07.002
111. Choti MA, Thomas M, Wong SL, et al. Surgical resection preferences and perceptions among medical oncologists treating liver metastases from colorectal cancer. *Ann Surg Oncol.* 2016;23(2):375-381. doi:10.1245/s10434-015-4925-1
112. Ahmed A, Turner G, King B, et al. Midgut neuroendocrine tumours with liver metastases: results of the UKINETS study. *Endocr Relat Cancer.* 2009;16(3):885-894. doi:10.1677/ERC-09-0042
113. Åkerström G, Hellman P, Hessman O, Osmak L. Management of midgut carcinoids. *J Surg Oncol.* 2005;89(3):161-169. doi:10.1002/jso.20188
114. Bertani E, Falconi M, Grana C, et al. Small intestinal neuroendocrine tumors with liver metastases and resection of the primary: prognostic factors for decision making. *Int J Surg.* 2015;20:58-64. doi:10.1016/j.ijsu.2015.06.019
115. Bertani E, Fazio N, Radice D, et al. Resection of the primary tumor followed by peptide receptor radionuclide therapy as upfront strategy for the treatment of G1–G2 pancreatic neuroendocrine tumors with unresectable liver metastases. *Ann Surg Oncol.* 2016;23(suppl 5):981-989. doi:10.1245/s10434-016-5550-3
116. Boudreaux JP, Putty B, Frey DJ, et al. Surgical treatment of advanced-stage carcinoid tumors. *Ann Surg.* 2005;241(6):839-846. doi:10.1097/01.sla.0000164073.08093.5d
117. Boudreaux JP, Wang Y-Z, Diebold AE, et al. A single institution's experience with surgical cytoreduction of stage IV, well-differentiated, small bowel neuroendocrine tumors. *J Am Coll Surg.* 2014;218(4):837-844. doi:10.1016/j.jamcollsurg.2013.12.035
118. Capurso G, Rinzivillo M, Bettini R, Boninsegna L, Fave GD, Falconi M. Systematic review of resection of primary midgut carcinoid tumour in patients with unresectable liver metastases. *Br J Surg.* 2012;99(11):1480-1486. doi:10.1002/bjs.8842
119. Chakedis J, Beal EW, Lopez-Aguiar AG, et al. Surgery provides long-term survival in patients with metastatic neuroendocrine tumors undergoing resection for non-hormonal symptoms. *J Gastrointest Surg.* 2019;23(1):122-134. doi:10.1007/s11605-018-3986-4
120. Chambers AJ, Pasieka JL, Dixon E, Rorstad O. The palliative benefit of aggressive surgical intervention for both hepatic and mesenteric metastases from neuroendocrine tumors. *Surgery.* 2008;144(4):645-653. doi:10.1016/j.surg.2008.06.008
121. Citterio D, Pusceddu S, Facciorusso A, et al. Primary tumour resection may improve survival in functional well-differentiated neuroendocrine tumours metastatic to the liver. *Eur J Surg Oncol.* 2017;43(2):380-387. doi:10.1016/j.ejso.2016.10.031
122. Croome KP, Burns JM, Que FG, Nagorney DM. Hepatic resection for metastatic neuroendocrine cancer in patients with bone metastases. *Ann Surg Oncol.* 2016;23(11):3693-3698. doi:10.1245/s10434-016-5274-4

123. Cusati D, Zhang L, Harmsen WS, et al. Metastatic nonfunctioning pancreatic neuroendocrine carcinoma to liver: surgical treatment and outcomes. *J Am Coll Surg.* 2012;215(1):117-125. doi:10.1016/j.jamcollsurg.2012.05.002

124. Ejaz A, Reames BN, Maithel S, et al. Cytoreductive debulking surgery among patients with neuroendocrine liver metastasis: a multi-institutional analysis. *HPB (Oxford).* 2018;20(3):277-284. doi:10.1016/j.hpb.2017.08.039

125. Elias D, David A, Sourrouille I, et al. Neuroendocrine carcinomas: optimal surgery of peritoneal metastases (and associated intra-abdominal metastases). *Surgery.* 2014;155(1):5-12. doi:10.1016/j.surg.2013.05.030

126. Givi B, Pommier SJ, Thompson AK, Diggs BS, Pommier RF. Operative resection of primary carcinoid neoplasms in patients with liver metastases yields significantly better survival. *Surgery.* 2006;140(6):891-898. doi:10.1016/j.surg.2006.07.033

127. Glazer ES, Tseng JF, Al-Refaie W, et al. Long-term survival after surgical management of neuroendocrine hepatic metastases. *HPB (Oxford).* 2010;12(6):427-433. doi:10.1111/j.1477-2574.2010.00198.x

128. Graff-Baker AN, Sauer DA, Pommier SJ, Pommier RF. Expanded criteria for carcinoid liver debulking: maintaining survival and increasing the number of eligible patients. *Surgery.* 2014;156(6):1369-1377. doi:10.1016/j.surg.2014.08.009

129. Kimbrough CW, Beal EW, Dillhoff ME, et al. Influence of carcinoid syndrome on the clinical characteristics and outcomes of patients with gastroenteropancreatic neuroendocrine tumors undergoing operative resection. *Surgery.* 2019;165(3):657-663. doi:10.1016/j.surg.2018.09.008

130. Lesurtel M, Nagorney DM, Mazzaferro V, Jensen RT, Poston GJ. When should a liver resection be performed in patients with liver metastases from neuroendocrine tumours? A systematic review with practice recommendations. *HPB (Oxford).* 2015;17(1):17-22. doi:10.1111/hpb.12225

131. Maxwell JE, Sherman SK, O'Dorisio TM, Bellizzi AM, Howe JR. Liver-directed surgery of neuroendocrine metastases: what is the optimal strategy? *Surgery.* 2016;159(1):320-333. doi:10.1016/j.surg.2015.05.040

132. Mayo SC, de Jong MC, Pulitano C, et al. Surgical management of hepatic neuroendocrine tumor metastasis: results from an international multi-institutional analysis. *Ann Surg Oncol.* 2010;17(12):3129-3136. doi:10.1245/s10434-010-1154-5

133. McEntee GP, Nagorney DM, Kvols LK, Moertel CG, Grant CS. Cytoreductive hepatic surgery for neuroendocrine tumors. *Surgery.* 1990;108(6):1091-1096.

134. Morgan RE, Pommier SJ, Pommier RF. Expanded criteria for debulking of liver metastasis also apply to pancreatic neuroendocrine tumors. *Surgery.* 2018;163(1):218-225. doi:10.1016/j.surg.2017.05.030

135. Norlén O, Stålberg P, Öberg K, et al. Long-term results of surgery for small intestinal neuroendocrine tumors at a tertiary referral center. *World J Surg.* 2012;36(6):1419-1431. doi:10.1007/s00268-011-1296-z

136. Que FG, Nagorney DM, Batts KP, Linz LJ, Kvols LK. Hepatic resection for metastatic neuroendocrine carcinomas. *Am J Surg.* 1995;169(1):36-43. doi:10.1016/s0002-9610(99)80107-x

137. Rozenblum L, Mokrane F-Z, Yeh R, et al. The role of multimodal imaging in guiding resectability and cytoreduction in pancreatic neuroendocrine tumors: focus on PET and MRI. *Abdom Radiol (NY).* 2019;44(7):2474-2493. doi:10.1007/s00261-019-01994-5

138. Sarmiento JM, Heywood G, Rubin J, Ilstrup DM, Nagorney DM, Que FG. Surgical treatment of neuroendocrine metastases to the liver. *J Am Coll Surg.* 2003;197(1):29-37. doi:10.1016/S1072-7515(03)00230-8

139. Saxena A, Chua TC, Chu F, Al-Zahrani A, Morris DL. Optimizing the surgical effort in patients with advanced neuroendocrine neoplasm hepatic metastases: a critical analysis of 40 patients treated by hepatic resection and cryoablation. *Am J Clin Oncol.* 2012;35(5):439-445. doi:10.1097/COC.0b013e31821bc8dd

140. Schindl M, Kaczirek K, Passler C, et al. Treatment of small intestinal neuroendocrine tumors: is an extended multimodal approach justified? *World J Surg.* 2002;26(8):976-984. doi:10.1007/s00268-002-6628-6

141. Scott AT, Breheny PJ, Keck KJ, et al. Effective cytoreduction can be achieved in patients with numerous neuroendocrine tumor liver metastases (NETLMs). *Surgery.* 2019;165(1):166-175. doi:10.1016/j.surg.2018.04.070

142. Sham JG, Ejaz A, Gage MM, et al. The impact of extent of liver resection among patients with neuroendocrine liver metastasis: an international multi-institutional study. *J Gastrointest Surg.* 2018;23(3):484-491. doi:10.1007/s11605-018-3862-2

143. Tsilimigras DI, Ntanasis-Stathopoulos I, Kostakis ID, et al. Is resection of primary midgut neuroendocrine tumors in patients with unresectable metastatic liver disease justified? A systematic review and meta-analysis. *J Gastrointest Surg.* 2019;23(5):1044-1054. doi:10.1007/s11605-018-04094-9

144. Wang Y-Z, Chauhan A, Rau J, et al. Neuroendocrine tumors (NETs) of unknown primary: is early surgical exploration and aggressive debulking justifiable? *Chin Clin Oncol.* 2016;5(1):4. doi:10.3978/j.issn.2304-3865.2016.02.03

145. Veerendaal LM, Borel Rinkes IH, Lips CJ, van Hillegersberg R. Liver metastases of neuroendocrine tumours; early reduction of tumour load to improve life expectancy. *World J Surg Oncol.* 2006;4:35. doi:10.1186/1477-7819-4-35

146. Ramage JK, Ahmed A, Ardill J, et al. Guidelines for the management of gastroenteropancreatic neuroendocrine (including carcinoid) tumours (NETs). *Gut.* 2012;61(1):6-32. doi:10.1136/gutjnl-2011-300831

147. Falconi M, Zerbi A, Crippa S, et al. Parenchyma-preserving resections for small nonfunctioning pancreatic endocrine tumors. *Ann Surg Oncol.* 2010;17(6):1621-1627. doi:10.1245/s10434-010-0949-8

148. Hackert T, Hinz U, Fritz S, et al. Enucleation in pancreatic surgery: indications, technique, and outcome compared to standard pancreatic resections. *Langenbecks Arch Surg.* 2011;396(8):1197-1203. doi:10.1007/s00423-011-0801-z

149. Crippa S, Zerbi A, Boninsegna L, et al. Surgical management of insulinomas: short- and long-term outcomes after enucleations and pancreatic resections. *Arch Surg.* 2012;147(3):261-266. doi:10.1001/archsurg.2011.1843

150. Hu M, Zhao G, Luo Y, Liu R. Laparoscopic versus open treatment for benign pancreatic insulinomas: an analysis of 89 cases. *Surg Endosc.* 2011;25(12):3831-3837. doi:10.1007/s00464-011-1800-4

151. Dalla Valle R, Cremaschi E, Lamecchi L, Guerini F, Rosso E, Iaria M. Open and minimally invasive pancreatic neoplasms enucleation: a systematic review. *Surg Endosc.* 2019;33(10):3192-3199. doi:10.1007/s00464-019-06967-9

152. Tian F, Hong X-F, Wu W-M, et al. Propensity score-matched analysis of robotic versus open surgical enucleation for small pancreatic neuroendocrine tumours. *Br J Surg.* 2016;103(10):1358-1364. doi:10.1002/bjs.10220

153. Strobel O, Cherrez A, Hinz U, et al. Risk of pancreatic fistula after enucleation of pancreatic tumours. *Br J Surg.* 2015;102(10):1258-1266. doi:10.1002/bjs.9843

154. Figueras J, Sabater L, Planellas P, et al. Randomized clinical trial of pancreaticogastrostomy versus pancreaticojejunostomy on the rate and severity of pancreatic fistula after pancreaticoduodenectomy. *Br J Surg.* 2013;100(12):1597-1605. doi:10.1002/bjs.9252

155. Penninck D, d'Anjou M-A, eds. *Atlas of Small Animal Ultrasonography.* 2nd ed. Wiley; 2015.

156. Yeo CJ, Cameron JL, Maher MM, et al. A prospective randomized trial of pancreaticogastrostomy versus pancreaticojejunostomy after pancreaticoduodenectomy. *Ann Surg.* 1995;222(4):580-592. doi:10.1097/00000658-199510000-00014

157. Wang Z-Z, Zhao G-D, Zhao Z-M, et al. An end-to-end pancreatic anastomosis in robotic central pancreatectomy. *World J Surg Oncol.* 2019;17(1):67. doi:10.1186/s12957-019-1609-5

158. Ce ka F, Jon B, Subrt Z, Ferko A. Surgical technique in distal pancreatectomy: a systematic review of randomized trials. *Biomed Res Int.* 2014;2014:432906. doi:10.1155/2014/482906

159. Ratnayake CBB, Wells C, Hammond J, French JJ, Windsor JA, Pandanaboyana S. Network meta-analysis comparing techniques and outcomes of stump closure after distal pancreatectomy. *Br J Surg.* 2019;106(12):1580-1589. doi:10.1002/bjs.11291

160. Zhang H, Zhu F, Shen M, et al. Systematic review and meta-analysis comparing three techniques for pancreatic remnant closure following distal pancreatectomy. *Br J Surg.* 2015;102(1):4-15. doi:10.1002/bjs.9653

161. Dong D-H, Zhang X-F, Poultsides G, et al. Impact of tumor size and nodal status on recurrence of nonfunctional pancreatic neuroendocrine tumors </=2 cm after curative resection: a multi-institutional study of 392 cases. *J Surg Oncol.* 2019;120(7):1071-1079. doi:10.1002/jso.25716

162. Hashim YM, Trinkaus KM, Linehan DC, et al. Regional lymphadenectomy is indicated in the surgical treatment of pancreatic neuroendocrine tumors (PNETs). *Ann Surg.* 2014;259(2):197-203. doi:10.1097/SLA.0000000000000348

163. Lopez-Aguiar AG, Zaidi MY, Beal EW, et al. Defining the role of lymphadenectomy for pancreatic neuroendocrine tumors: an eight-institution study of 695 patients from the US Neuroendocrine Tumor Study Group. *Ann Surg Oncol.* 2019;26(8):2517-2524. doi:10.1245/s10434-019-07367-y

164. Bilimoria KY, Talamonti MS, Tomlinson JS, et al. Prognostic score predicting survival after resection of pancreatic neuroendocrine tumors: analysis of 3851 patients. *Ann Surg.* 2008;247(3): 490-500. doi:10.1097/SLA.0b013e31815b9cae

165. Grant CS. Surgical management of malignant islet cell tumors. *World J Surg.* 1993;17(4): 498-503. doi:10.1007/BF01655109

166. Tsutsumi K, Ohtsuka T, Mori Y, et al. Analysis of lymph node metastasis in pancreatic neuroendocrine tumors (PNETs) based on the tumor size and hormonal production. *J Gastroenterol.* 2012;47(6):678-685. doi:10.1007/s00535-012-0540-0

167. Chua TC, Yang TX, Gill AJ, Samra JS. Systematic review and meta-analysis of enucleation versus standardized resection for small pancreatic lesions. *Ann Surg Oncol.* 2016;23(2):592-599. doi:10.1245/s10434-015-4826-3

168. Partelli S, Mazza M, Andreasi V, et al. Management of small asymptomatic nonfunctioning pancreatic neuroendocrine tumors: limitations to apply guidelines into real life. *Surgery.* 2019;166(2):157-163. doi:10.1016/j.surg.2019.04.003

169. Haynes AB, Deshpande V, Ingkakul T, et al. Implications of incidentally discovered, nonfunctioning pancreatic endocrine tumors: short-term and long-term patient outcomes. *Arch Surg.* 2011;146(5):534-538. doi:10.1001/archsurg.2011.102

170. Cherenfant J, Stocker SJ, Gage MK, et al. Predicting aggressive behavior in nonfunctioning pancreatic neuroendocrine tumors. *Surgery.* 2013;154(4):785-793.

171. Tomassetti P, Campana D, Piscitelli L, et al. Endocrine pancreatic tumors: factors correlated with survival. *Ann Oncol.* 2005;16(11):1806-1810. doi:10.1016/j.surg.2013.07.004

172. Ellison TA, Wolfgang CL, Shi C, et al. A single institution's 26-year experience with nonfunctional pancreatic neuroendocrine tumors: a validation of current staging systems and a new prognostic nomogram. *Ann Surg.* 2014;259(2):204-212. doi:10.1097/SLA.0b013e31828f3174

173. National Comprehensive Cancer Network. Neuroendocrine and adrenal tumors (version 1.2019). National Comprehensive Cancer Network. Accessed April 10, 2020. https://www.nccn.org/professionals/physician_gls/pdf/neuroendocrine_blocks.pdf

174. Furukori M, Imai K, Karasaki H, et al. Clinicopathological features of small nonfunctioning pancreatic neuroendocrine tumors. *World J Gastroenterol.* 2014;20(47):17949-17954. doi:10.3748/wjg.v20.i47.17949

175. Ge W, Zhou D, Xu S, Wang W, Zheng S. Surveillance and comparison of surgical prognosis for asymptomatic and symptomatic non-functioning pancreatic neuroendocrine tumors. *Int J Surg.* 2017;39:127-134. doi:10.1016/j.ijsu.2017.01.088

176. Genç CG, Falconi M, Partelli S, et al. Recurrence of pancreatic neuroendocrine tumors and survival predicted by Ki67. *Ann Surg Oncol.* 2018;25(8):2467-2474. doi:10.1245/s10434-018-6518-2

177. Genç CG, Jilesen AP, Partelli S, et al. A new scoring system to predict recurrent disease in grade 1 and 2 nonfunctional pancreatic neuroendocrine tumors. *Ann Surg.* 2018;267(6):1148-1154. doi:10.1097/SLA.0000000000002123

178. Harimoto N, Hoshino K, Muranushi R, et al. Prognostic significance of neutrophil-lymphocyte ratio in resectable pancreatic neuroendocrine tumors with special reference to tumor-associated macrophages. *Pancreatologys.* 2019;19(6):897-902. doi:10.1016/j.pan.2019.08.003

179. Harimoto N, Hoshino K, Muranushi R, et al. Significance of lymph node metastasis in resectable well-differentiated pancreatic neuroendocrine tumor. *Pancreas.* 2019;48(7):943-947. doi:10.1097/MPA.0000000000001355

180. Jiang Y, Jin J-B, Zhan Q, Deng X-X, Shen BY. Impact and clinical predictors of lymph node metastases in nonfunctional pancreatic neuroendocrine tumors. *Chin Med J (Engl).* 2015;128(24):3335-3344.

181. Kaltenborn A, Matzke S, Kleine M, et al. Prediction of survival and tumor recurrence in patients undergoing surgery for pancreatic neuroendocrine neoplasms. *J Surg Oncol.* 2016;113(2): 194-202. doi:10.1002/jso.24116

182. Kim H, Song KB, Hwang DW, Lee JH, Alshammary S, Kim SC. Time-trend and recurrence analysis of pancreatic neuroendocrine tumors. *Endocr Connect.* 2019;8(7):1052-1060. doi:10.1530/EC-19-0282

183. Lee LC, Grant CS, Salomao DR, et al. Small, nonfunctioning, asymptomatic pancreatic neuroendocrine tumors (PNETs): role for nonoperative management. *Surgery.* 2012;152(6):965-974. doi:10.1016/j.surg.2012.08.038

184. Lopez-Aguiar AG, Ethun CG, Postlewait LM, et al. Redefining the Ki-67 index stratification for low-grade pancreatic neuroendocrine tumors: improving its prognostic value for recurrence of disease. *Ann Surg Oncol.* 2018;25(1):290-298. doi:10.1245/s10434-017-6140-8

185. Lopez-Aguiar AG, Ethun CG, Zaidi MY, et al. The conundrum of < 2-cm pancreatic neuroendocrine tumors: a preoperative risk score to predict lymph node metastases and guide surgical management. *Surgery.* 2019;166(1):15-21. doi:10.1016/j.surg.2019.03.008
186. Masui T, Sato A, Nakano K, et al. Predictive value of the Ki67 index for lymph node metastasis of small non-functioning pancreatic neuroendocrine neoplasms. *Surg Today.* 2019;49(7): 593-600. doi:10.1007/s00595-019-01779-9
187. Partelli S, Gaujoux S, Boninsegna L, et al. Pattern and clinical predictors of lymph node involvement in nonfunctioning pancreatic neuroendocrine tumors (NF-PanNETs). *JAMA Surg.* 2013;148(10):932-939. doi:10.1001/jamasurg.2013.3376
188. Postlewait LM, Ethun CG, Baptiste GG, et al. Pancreatic neuroendocrine tumors: preoperative factors that predict lymph node metastases to guide operative strategy. *J Surg Oncol.* 2016;114(4):440-445. doi:10.1002/jso.24338
189. Sallinen VJ, Le Large TYS, Tieftrunk E, et al. Prognosis of sporadic resected small (≤2 cm) nonfunctional pancreatic neuroendocrine tumors—a multi-institutional study. *HPB (Oxford).* 2018;20(3):251-259. doi:10.1016/j.hpb.2017.08.034
190. Sarmiento JM, Farnell MB, Que FG, Nagorney DM. Pancreaticoduodenectomy for islet cell tumors of the head of the pancreas: long-term survival analysis. *World J Surg.* 2002;26(10): 1267-1271. doi:10.1007/s00268-002-6714-9
191. Sho S, Court CM, Winograd P, et al. A prognostic scoring system for the prediction of metastatic recurrence following curative resection of pancreatic neuroendocrine tumors. *J Gastrointest Surg.* 2019;23(7):1392-1400. doi:10.1007/s11605-018-4011-7
192. Taki K, Hashimoto D, Nakagawa S, et al. Significance of lymph node metastasis in pancreatic neuroendocrine tumor. *Surg Today.* 2017;47(9):1104-1110. doi:10.1007/s00595-017 -1485-y
193. Tsutsumi K, Ohtsuka T, Fujino M, et al. Analysis of risk factors for recurrence after curative resection of well-differentiated pancreatic neuroendocrine tumors based on the new grading classification. *J Hepatobiliary Pancreat Sci.* 2014;21(6):418-425. doi:10.1002/jhbp.47
194. Wang S-E, Su C-H, Kuo Y-J, et al. Comparison of functional and nonfunctional neuroendocrine tumors in the pancreas and peripancreatic region. *Pancreas.* 2011;40(2):253-259. doi:10.1097 /MPA.0b013e3181f94cc4
195. Wong J, Fulp WJ, Strosberg JR, Kvols LK, Centeno BA, Hodul PJ. Predictors of lymph node metastases and impact on survival in resected pancreatic neuroendocrine tumors: a single-center experience. *Am J Surg.* 2014;208(5):775-780. doi:10.1016/j.amjsurg.2014.04.003
196. Wu L, Sahara K, Tsilimigras DI, et al. Therapeutic index of lymphadenectomy among patients with pancreatic neuroendocrine tumors: a multi-institutional analysis. *J Surg Oncol.* 2019;120(7):1080-1086. doi:10.1002/jso.25689
197. Yoo YJ, Yang SJ, Hwang HK, Kang CM, Kim H, Lee WJ. Overestimated oncologic significance of lymph node metastasis in G1 nonfunctioning neuroendocrine tumor in the left side of the pancreas. *Medicine (Baltimore).* 2015;94(36):e1404. doi:10.1097/MD.0000000000001404
198. Zaidi MY, Lopez-Aguiar AG, Switchenko JM, et al. A novel validated recurrence risk score to guide a pragmatic surveillance strategy after resection of pancreatic neuroendocrine tumors: an international study of 1006 patients. *Ann Surg.* 2019;270(3):422-433. doi:10.1097 /SLA.0000000000003461
199. Chung JC, Choi DW, Jo SH, Heo JS, Choi SH, Kim YI. Malignant nonfunctioning endocrine tumors of the pancreas: predictive factors for survival after surgical treatment. *World J Surg.* 2007;31(3):579-585. doi:10.1007/s00268-006-0585-4
200. Conrad C, Kutlu OC, Dasari A, et al. Prognostic value of lymph node status and extent of lymphadenectomy in pancreatic neuroendocrine tumors confined to and extending beyond the pancreas. *J Gastrointest Surg.* 2016;20(12):1966-1974.
201. Curran T, Pockaj BA, Gray RJ, Halfdanarson TR, Wasif N. Importance of lymph node involvement in pancreatic neuroendocrine tumors: impact on survival and implications for surgical resection. *J Gastrointest Surg.* 2015;19(1):152-160. doi:10.1007/s11605-014-2624-z
202. Demir R, Pohl J, Agaimy A, et al. Necrosis and angioinvasion predict adverse outcome in pancreatic neuroendocrine tumors after curative surgical resection: results of a single-center series. *World J Surg.* 2011;35(12):2764-2772. doi:10.1007/s00268-011-1262-9
203. Dima SO, Dumitrascu T, Pechianu C, et al. Prognostic factors in patients with surgical resection of pancreatic neuroendocrine tumours. *Acta Endocrinol (Buchar).* 2018;14(3):389-393. doi:10.4183/aeb.2018.389
204. Fitzgerald TL, Mosquera C, Vora HS, Vohra NA, Zervos EE. Indications for surgical resection in low-grade pancreatic neuroendocrine tumors. *Am Surg.* 2016;82(8):737-742.

205. Han X, Xu X, Jin D, Wang D, Ji Y, Lou W. Clinicopathological characteristics and prognosis-related factors of resectable pancreatic neuroendocrine tumors: a retrospective study of 104 cases in a single Chinese center. *Pancreas*. 2014;43(4):526-531. doi:10.1097/MPA.0000000000000065

206. Jin K, Luo G, Xu J, et al. Clinical outcomes and prognostic factors of resected pancreatic neuro-endocrine neoplasms: a single-center experience in China. *Oncol Lett*. 2017;13(5):3163-3168. doi:10.3892/ol.2017.5834

207. Jutric Z, Grendar J, Hoen HM, et al. Regional metastatic behavior of nonfunctional pancre-atic neuroendocrine tumors: impact of lymph node positivity on survival. *Pancreas*. 2017;46(7): 898-903. doi:10.1097/MPA.0000000000000861

208. Kazanjian KK, Reber HA, Hines OJ. Resection of pancreatic neuroendocrine tumors: results of 70 cases. *Arch Surg*. 2006;141(8):765-770. doi:10.1001/archsurg.141.8.765

209. Li G, Tian M-L, Bing Y-T, et al. Clinicopathological features and prognosis factors for survival in elderly patients with pancreatic neuroendocrine tumor: a STROBE-compliant article. *Medicine (Baltimore)*. 2019;98(11):e14576. doi:10.1097/MD.0000000000014576

210. Liu P, Zhang X, Shang Y, et al. Lymph node ratio, but not the total number of examined lymph nodes or lymph node metastasis, is a predictor of overall survival for pancreatic neuroendo-crine neoplasms after surgical resection. *Oncotarget*. 2017;8(51):89245-89255. doi:10.18632/oncotarget.19184

211. Madeira I, Terris B, Voss M, et al. Prognostic factors in patients with endocrine tumours of the duodenopancreatic area. *Gut*. 1998;43(3):422-427. doi:10.1136/gut.43.3.422

212. Matthews BD, Heniford BT, Reardon PR, Brunicardi FC, Greene FL. Surgical experience with nonfunctioning neuroendocrine tumors of the pancreas. *Am Surg*. 2000;66(12):1116-1123.

213. Schurr PG, Strate T, Rese K, et al. Aggressive surgery improves long-term survival in neuro-endocrine pancreatic tumors: an institutional experience. *Ann Surg*. 2007;245(2):273-281. doi:10.1097/01.sla.0000232556.24258.68

214. Sharpe SM, In H, Winchester DJ, Talamonti MS, Baker MS. Surgical resection provides an overall survival benefit for patients with small pancreatic neuroendocrine tumors. *J Gastrointest Surg*. 2015;19(1):117-123.

215. Song KB, Kim SC, Kim JH, et al. Prognostic factors in 151 patients with surgically resected non-functioning pancreatic neuroendocrine tumours. *ANZ J Surg*. 2016;86(7-8):563-567. doi:10.1111/ans.12738

216. Toste PA, Kadera BE, Tatishchev SF, et al. Nonfunctional pancreatic neuroendocrine tumors <2 cm on preoperative imaging are associated with a low incidence of nodal metastasis and an excellent overall survival. *J Gastrointest Surg*. 2013;17(12):2105-2113. doi:10.1007/s11605-013-2360-9

217. Watzka FM, Meyer F, Staubitz JI, et al. Prognostic assessment of non-functioning neuroen-docrine pancreatic neoplasms as a basis for risk-adapted resection strategies. *World J Surg*. 2020;44(2):594-603. doi:10.1007/s00268-019-05220-7

Synoptic Operative Report: Pancreatic Neuroendocrine Tumor

Date of procedure _____   Surgeon(s) _____

_____

Operative Staging

Operative intent
☐ Curative
☐ Palliative

Intraoperative biopsies
☐ Extrapancreatic biopsy specimens and results of immediate histopathologic analysis:

_____

Final operative stage
☐ Resectable
☐ Metastatic

Procedure Summary

Pancreatectomy type
☐ Enucleation
☐ Pancreaticoduodenectomy
☐ Central
☐ Distal with splenectomy
☐ Distal spleen-sparing

Plane of dissection retroperitoneal
☐ Superficial to posterior fascia
☐ Alternate plane

Extent of lymphadenectomy
☐ Description of basins resected:

_____

Synoptic Operative Report: Small Bowel Neuroendocrine Tumor

Date of procedure _____ Surgeon(s) _____

_____

Operative Staging

Operative intent
- ☐ Curative
- ☐ Palliative

Intraoperative biopsies
- ☐ Biopsy specimens and results of immediate histopathologic analysis: _____

Final operative stage
- ☐ Resectable
- ☐ Metastatic

Extent of lymphadenectomy
- ☐ Description of basins resected:

_____

Residual nodal disease present
- ☐ Yes
- ☐ No

Multifocality
- ☐ No other small bowel masses palpated
- ☐ Other sites of palpable masses: _____

COMMENTARY: NEUROENDOCRINE SECTION

James R. Howe, MD, FACS, FSSO
Professor of Surgery
Chief, Division of Surgical Oncology and Endocrine Surgery
University of Iowa Carver College of Medicine

Neuroendocrine tumors (NETs) were once considered rare, but they have been diagnosed with increasing frequency over the past several decades. The prevalence of NETs has also increased because these patients tend to live a long time after diagnosis, even with advanced disease. Therefore, these tumors are being encountered more often by general surgeons and surgical subspecialists. Surgeons need to be aware of the many nuances relating to these tumors, and the neuroendocrine section of *Operative Standards for Cancer Surgery*, Volume 3, accomplishes this important objective. The first chapter provides a strong framework of how to manage patients with NETs of the small bowel (SBNETs), which have surpassed adenocarcinoma as the leading histologic type of cancer of the small intestine. The second chapter, on parenchyma-preserving pancreatectomy, covers the appropriate selection of patients with pancreatic NETs (PNETs) for these procedures and the operative techniques. Within them, several key questions are carefully examined with thorough literature reviews to shine a light on current areas of confusion and controversy.

For management of patients with SBNETs, it is important to understand that these tumors are often small and within the bowel wall (typically <1–2 cm); yet, they can give rise to large nodal and liver metastases. This explains why the primary tumors are often not found in routine imaging studies but can be readily identified between the fingertips of the surgeon. They occur most frequently in the ileum and are commonly multifocal; therefore, it is important to palpate the entire small bowel. If the surgeon only identifies the most obvious tumor causing obstruction or other symptoms, the patient may be left with additional tumor(s) that could lead to future problems. If the surgeon uses a minimally invasive approach, it is important to deliver and palpate the bowel through the incision to be used for extracorporeal anastomosis. Even when exploration is performed open, the associated mesenteric nodal disease may also present significant challenges, as it often extends beyond the segmental branches and may encase the main superior mesenteric vein or superior mesenteric artery. These nodal resections can be quite difficult, and it is important not to jeopardize the blood supply to the remaining intestine. Patients may also have metastases to aortocaval, left pararenal, posterior pancreatic, and other retroperitoneal nodes, and even to more distant sites, such as left supraclavicular, cardiophrenic, and mediastinal nodes. These nodes may be difficult to locate and remove, rarely cause symptoms, and the survival benefits of resecting them is not clear, as patients can still live a long time with this involvement. When present, the ovaries should be carefully examined for metastases, as these are frequent when there is advanced disease.

Peritoneal carcinomatosis occurs when small bowel tumors grow through the serosa and may manifest as numerous peritoneal lesions, or implants throughout the mesentery, diaphragmatic surfaces, and pelvic structures. These implants can cause future small bowel and sigmoid colon obstructions and should be cyto-reduced as much as possible, with removal of larger lesions (if this can be done safely) and thermal ablation (cautery or argon beam) of smaller lesions. The decision of how much peritoneal cytoreduction and nodal resection to perform is often difficult, and one must carefully balance minimizing harm with trying to improve survival.

The important question of whether prophylactic cholecystectomy should be performed in patients with nodal disease or metastases is addressed through an extensive review of the available literature. Patients with advanced disease may be placed on long-term somatostatin analogues, and the risk of developing gallstones is 50% to 60% in this population. Those having embolization of liver metastases are also at risk of gallbladder necrosis. About a quarter of patients with surgically resected SBNETs, left with an intact gallbladder, and receiving somatostatin analogues will require a later cholecystectomy. This review suggests that patients can generally be safely observed with the gallbladder left in place. On the other hand, it can generally be removed quite safely and with a low complication rate while performing surgery for the primary tumor and/or metastases, and this is an important option to discuss with patients preoperatively.

Many patients with SBNETs (and PNETs) present with liver metastases or will develop them in follow-up. These may be accompanied by high levels of hormones that bypass metabolism in the liver, giving rise to carcinoid syndrome. Cytoreduction of liver metastases can help control symptoms and may also extend survival, as liver failure is the leading cause of death in these patients. Because these metastases are often many and involving both lobes of the liver, parenchymal-preserving approaches to cytoreduction, including wedge resections, enucleations, and ablations, are being used with increasing frequency in place of large resections. Recurrence within the liver is nearly universal within 5 years, so it is important to use a rational approach to achieve the objective of reducing tumor volume to improve symptoms and/or survival. This chapter examines the key question of whether less than total cytoreduction of liver tumors benefits patients and what a reasonable target would be for the degree of cytoreduction to derive benefit. The literature on this subject contains only retrospective studies likely influenced by selection bias but suggest that cytoreduction helps to alleviate symptoms and improve survival relative to historical controls with stage IV NETs. Older series opined that to be effective for improving either symptoms or survival, 90% of metastatic disease needed to be removed. A few recent series have shown that improvement in progression-free and overall survival may be achieved even in patients who achieve a lower threshold of 70% cytoreduction. Removing or ablating as much liver disease as possible, preferably using parenchymal-preserving methods to reach a 70% or 90% threshold, allows patients to start over with a lower tumor burden and thereby lengthen the time until the liver is replaced by metastases. There is also evidence that peptide receptor radionuclide therapy has greater efficacy in smaller tumors, which is one of the most effective adjuvant treatments for patients with advanced SBNETs.

The decision of when to use parenchymal-preserving approaches for PNETs depends on several factors, which include whether there is familial disease (where there will be multifocal and metachronous lesions), the size and location of a lesion, and its likelihood of demonstrating malignant behavior. A subset of functional tumors, such as insulinomas, are ideally suited for this, although most other secreting PNETs behave more aggressively. Smaller (1–2 cm), nonfunctional lesions may be candidates for enucleation, but completely removing these tumors and sampling regional nodes is important. For enucleation, tumors should be 3 mm away from the pancreatic or bile duct to avoid the potential for a difficult to manage fistula. The technique and indications for splenic preservation and central pancreatectomy are also discussed, where the benefit of preserving endocrine and exocrine function must be weighed against the higher risk of pancreatic leak. This chapter also nicely outlines the locations of important regional nodes and reviews in depth the key question of whether regional lymphadenectomy improves survival for patients with non-functional PNETs. Taken together, these chapters covering basic principles of managing SBNETs and PNETs will be a valuable guide to practicing surgeons encountering these increasingly common tumors.

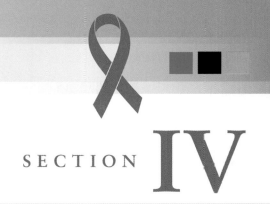

SECTION IV

PERITONEAL MALIGNANCIES

INTRODUCTION

Peritoneal surface malignancies encompass a wide range of disease processes ranging from the rare malignant peritoneal mesothelioma to the more common disseminated colon and ovarian carcinomas. Successful management of peritoneal metastasis requires multidisciplinary management, with the crux of treatment resting on cytoreductive surgery (CRS) and the intraperitoneal delivery of hyperthermic intraperitoneal chemotherapy (HIPEC). Peritoneal metastasis from appendiceal neoplasms, colorectal carcinoma, peritoneal mesothelioma, gastric adenocarcinoma, and ovarian carcinoma have all been shown to derive a benefit from CRS/HIPEC (Table 4-1).

CLINICAL STAGING

The most widely used and accepted classification scheme to quantify peritoneal disease burden is the peritoneal cancer index (PCI).[1] In this anatomic system, the abdomen is divided into nine regions by two transverse planes and two sagittal planes, and the small bowel is divided into four regions (upper and lower jejunum and upper and lower ileum). Each region is assigned a lesion size (LS) score based on the amount of macroscopic disease present. If no tumor is present, the region is assigned LS 0. If the maximum diameter of the lesions is less than or equal to 5 mm, the region is assigned LS 1. Tumor with a maximum diameter greater than 5 mm and up to 5 cm is assigned LS 2, and any tumor greater than 5 cm or a confluence of disease is assigned LS 3. The cumulative total score for all 13 regions is recorded as the PCI, which carries a minimum score of 0 and a maximum of 39. The PCI provides prognostic information for peritoneal metastases, and the score is used to estimate the potential curative value of CRS/HIPEC in several disease processes.[2–4]

Most peritoneal malignancies do not easily lend themselves to the typical tumor node metastasis (TNM) staging system. For appendiceal neoplasms in particular, there has been a persistent lack of uniform diagnostic terminology, resulting in an absence of an appendix-specific staging system until only recently. In an effort to provide standardized classifications and definitions to be used for more accurate staging,

---

TABLE 4-1 Peritoneal Malignancies Treated with Cytoreduction and Hyperthermic Intraperitoneal Chemotherapy

CRS and HIPEC: Indications
Appendiceal neoplasms
Colorectal carcinoma
Peritoneal mesothelioma
Gastric adenocarcinoma
Ovarian carcinoma

CRS: cytoreductive surgery; HIPEC: hyperthermic intraperitoneal chemotherapy.

in 2016, an international modified Delphi consensus process was instigated by the Peritoneal Surface Oncology Group International.[5] Consensus was achieved on pathologic classification of primary appendiceal neoplasms, enabling standardized reporting and meaningful comparison of results. Following this consensus on terminology, the *American Joint Committee on Cancer (AJCC) Cancer Staging Manual*, Eighth Edition, now includes cancers of the appendix (Table 4-2).[6] Two staging systems for appendiceal neoplasms exist: one for all carcinomas of the appendix and a separate system for well-differentiated neuroendocrine appendiceal tumors. For carcinomas, the primary tumor designation is based on depth of invasion, with T1 and T2 designations not used for low-grade mucinous neoplasms, Tis, T3, and T4. Nodal disease is

TABLE 4-2 American Joint Committee on Cancer Staging Criteria for Appendiceal Carcinoma Cancer, Eighth Edition

TABLE 4-2A Definition of Primary Tumor (T)

T Category	T Criteria
TX	Primary tumor cannot be assessed
T0	No evidence of primary tumor
Tis	Carcinoma in situ (intramucosal carcinoma; invasion of the lamina propria or extension into but not through the muscularis mucosae)
Tis (LAMN)	Low-grade appendiceal mucinous neoplasm confined by the muscularis propria. Acellular mucin or mucinous epithelium may invade into the muscularis propria
	T1 and T2 are not applicable to LAMN. Acellular mucin or mucinous epithelium that extends into the subserosa or serosa should be classified as T3 or T4a, respectively
T1	Tumor invades the submucosa (through the muscularis mucosa but not into the muscularis propria)
T2	Tumor invades the muscularis propria
T3	Tumor invades through the muscularis propria into the subserosa or the mesoappendix
T4	Tumor invades the visceral peritoneum, including the acellular mucin or mucinous epithelium involving the serosa of the appendix or mesoappendix, and/or directly invades adjacent organs or structures
T4a	Tumor invades through the visceral peritoneum, including the acellular mucin or mucinous epithelium involving the serosa of the appendix or serosa of the mesoappendix
T4b	Tumor directly invades or adheres to adjacent organs or structures

LAMN: low-grade appendiceal mucinous neoplasm.

TABLE 4-2B Definition of Regional Lymph Node (N)

N Category	N Criteria
NX	Regional lymph nodes cannot be assessed
N0	No regional lymph node metastasis
N1	One to three regional lymph nodes are positive (tumor in lymph node measuring $\geq$0.2 mm) or any number of tumor deposits is present, and all identifiable lymph nodes are negative
N1a	One regional lymph node is positive
N1b	Two or three regional lymph nodes are positive
N1c	No regional lymph nodes are positive, but there are tumor deposits in the subserosa or mesentery
N2	Four or more regional lymph nodes are positive

TABLE 4-2C Definition of Distant Metastasis (M)

M Category	M Criteria
M0	No distant metastasis
M1	Distant metastasis
M1a	Intraperitoneal acellular mucin, without identifiable tumor cells in the disseminated peritoneal mucinous deposits
M1b	Intraperitoneal metastasis only, including peritoneal mucinous deposits containing tumor cells
M1c	Metastasis to sites other than peritoneum

Note: American Joint Committee on Cancer staging and TNM classification for appendiceal carcinoma.[6] Used with permission of the American Joint Committee on Cancer (AJCC), Chicago, Illinois. The original and primary source for this information is the *AJCC Cancer Staging Manual*, Eighth Edition (2017) published by Springer International Publishing.

graded on the number of positive regional lymph nodes. Metastatic disease includes presence of intraperitoneal acellular mucin (M1a), intraperitoneal mucinous deposits with tumor cells (M1b), and extraperitoneal metastases (M1c). When a tumor has cellular intraperitoneal metastases, tumor grade (well, moderately, or poorly differentiated) is used in addition to pTNM status to assign overall combined tumor stage. Well-differentiated neuroendocrine tumors of the appendix are staged using a separate system. The primary tumor designation depends on size and perforation, and nodal disease is either present (N1) or absent (N0). Peritoneal disease is considered distant metastasis (M1), with divisions for hepatic metastases (M1a), metastases in extrahepatic sites (M1b), and both hepatic and extrahepatic metastases (M1c).[6]

Peritoneal metastases secondary to colon and gastric cancer are staged with the primary tumor by the AJCC. For colon cancer, M1a and M1b disease denotes metastases to distant organ sites without peritoneal metastases; M1c denotes peritoneal metastases. For gastric malignancies, the presence of peritoneal metastasis is considered M1 disease.[6] In clinical practice, the extent of peritoneal metastases is further quantified using the PCI.

For malignant peritoneal mesothelioma, diffuse spread throughout the abdomen and rare nodal or extra-abdominal metastatic spread makes staging with a traditional TNM approach even more challenging. The *AJCC Cancer Staging Manual* has a staging system for pleural mesothelioma but does not have a staging system for malignant peritoneal mesothelioma. To address this issue, a novel TNM staging system was proposed by Yan et al.[7] In this system, T was assigned based on extent of disease burden quantified by intraoperative PCI and divided into four subgroups: T1 (PCI 1 to 10), T2 (PCI 11 to 20), T3 (PCI 21 to 30), and T4 (PCI 31 to 39). Node status was assigned based on presence (N1) or absence (N0) of positive lymph nodes on histopathology of surgical specimens. Any extra-abdominal metastasis discovered on preoperative imaging was assigned M1. Stage I disease included T1N0M0, stage II included T2-3N0M0, and stage III included T4N0M0 and N1 or M1 disease [7]

MULTIDISCIPLINARY CARE

As with other malignancies, multidisciplinary care is critical to the optimal treatment of all patients with peritoneal surface malignancy. Prior to the introduction of CRS/HIPEC, systemic chemotherapy was the only option for patients with peritoneal malignancies. Outcomes were dismal, with most patients progressing to death owing to bowel obstruction in less than a year.[8] However, with the addition of aggressive CRS/HIPEC, median overall survival (OS) has risen to more than 29 months in combined tumor types,[9] and OS associated with systemic chemotherapy alone has nearly doubled in prospective trials.[10]

Multidisciplinary discussion is imperative to ensure that all patients with peritoneal malignancies receive the optimal treatment for the rare diseases for which CRS/HIPEC is typically performed. For example, because appendiceal carcinoma is rarely encountered and clinical practice guidelines do not exist, it is tempting to provide systemic chemotherapeutic treatment using recommendations for similar and more frequently encountered colon adenocarcinoma. However, for peritoneal metastases of low-grade appendiceal origin, there is no difference in OS or progression-free survival between patients who receive systemic chemotherapy and CRS/HIPEC and those who receive CRS/HIPEC alone.[11] Recent studies have even questioned the utility of HIPEC in peritoneal disease from a colorectal primary. PRODIGE 7, a randomized multicenter phase 3 trial from France, demonstrated no improvement in OS in patients who underwent CRS/HIPEC with oxaliplatin compared with patients who underwent CRS alone.[12] However, the study has received significant criticism for its short HIPEC perfusion time and perfusate itself, and the final trial results remain unpublished. High-volume peritoneal malignancy centers still perform CRS/HIPEC for colorectal peritoneal disease, and thus, both surgeons and medical oncologists need to understand their continued role in treatment.

PERIOPERATIVE CARE

Patient History and Physical

The presentation of peritoneal metastases is variable, nonspecific, and dependent on the primary histopathologic diagnosis. Complaints of abdominal pain, distension, and fatigue are common. The most common presentation of appendiceal neoplasms is suspected acute appendicitis, followed by increasing abdominal distention, and in women, suspected ovarian mass.[13] Malignant peritoneal mesothelioma, however, slowly spreads along peritoneal surfaces and thus may only present with vague, nonspecific symptoms dependent on the extent of spread. Patients most commonly complain of increasing diffuse abdominal pain and distention, usually secondary to ascites.[14,15] Gastric adenocarcinoma is often first diagnosed when symptoms of dyspepsia, weight loss, hematemesis, melena, or anemia prompt further investigation with esophagogastroduodenoscopy.[16] Peritoneal metastasis is often occult on imaging and found only on laparoscopy for staging.[17] Presentation of colon adenocarcinoma with peritoneal metastases can also be quite variable and nonspecific, with common complaints including fatigue, abdominal pain, distension, melena, and anemia.[18] In all patients with peritoneal metastases, potential physical examination findings may include a protuberant abdomen with a fluid wave or palpable mass.

Tumor Markers

Baseline preoperative tumor markers including carcinoembryonic antigen, cancer antigen 19-9, and cancer antigen 125 should be routinely obtained. Elevated levels may allow for continued surveillance following CRS/HIPEC or potentially guide response to systemic chemotherapy.[19] If preoperative tumor markers are not elevated, they need not be obtained at future follow-up visits.

Imaging

Preoperative contrast-enhanced computed tomography (CT) scan of the chest, abdomen, and pelvis is a necessity for treatment planning to evaluate for both distant and unresectable disease. The presence of extra-abdominal metastasis is an absolute contraindication for CRS and HIPEC in most disease processes, unless the disease is low volume and potentially resectable. Unresectable disease includes extensive infiltration of small bowel loops and mesentery and involvement of the ligament of Treitz, porta hepatis, lesser sac, or suprahepatic veins that would not allow for adequate cytoreduction.[20]

In patients with potentially resectable disease, preoperative CT is useful for localizing and quantifying the degree of peritoneal metastases. Nodular or plaque lesions show various levels of enhancement with intravenous contrast, and identification often depends on anatomic location.[21] Small lesions less than 5 mm are more easily distinguished on the surfaces of the liver or spleen. Lesions on curved surfaces, such as the diaphragm and paracolic gutters, often require image visualization on different planes.[21] Peritoneal metastases from nonmucinous gastrointestinal malignancies is unfortunately not well visualized on CT, as lesions often conform to the normal contours of the abdominopelvic structures rather than distorting local structures, especially on the surface of the small bowel or colon and its mesentery.[22]

Involvement of the greater omentum, or omental caking, can appear as a thick layer of heterogenous density between the bowel and abdominal wall.[21] Bowel loops can be warped or tethered to each other, indicating bowel or mesentery involvement even when disease is not readily apparent. If the disease infiltrates the small bowel mesentery, the mesentery may have a pleated appearance, whereas the mesenteric vessels have an uncharacteristically straight course.[23] Free or entrapped ascites is found in more than 70% of cases.[21]

Diagnosis

To definitively diagnose peritoneal metastases, pathologic evaluation is required, with the method of diagnosis dependent on the primary. In appendiceal malignancies, for example, most patients have already undergone appendectomy and present to a peritoneal malignancy referral center with a diagnosis. Outside pathology reports and slides are typically re-reviewed by dedicated pathologists to confirm diagnosis. Meticulous review of operative reports for location and extent of peritoneal disease should also be undertaken, as small metastases are often not well visualized on cross-sectional imaging.[22]

If a histologic diagnosis has not been obtained but imaging is suggestive of peritoneal metastases, the preferred diagnostic modality is direct tissue sampling via diagnostic laparoscopy. Diagnostic laparoscopy also offers the advantage of direct visualization of the abdominal cavity with improved assessment of tumor burden. Many studies have demonstrated the failure of CT scans to detect all peritoneal metastases, with a sensitivity in determining disease of only 70% to 88%, depending on the region of the abdomen.[22] If diagnostic laparoscopy is performed, it is incumbent on the surgeon to define the extent of disease as well as to obtain tissue sufficient for accurate pathologic analysis.

Surgical Management

The surgical techniques of CRS/HIPEC are discussed in depth in the following chapters, with the overall goal of a complete resection of all macroscopic tumor followed by hyperthermic perfusion with intra-abdominal chemotherapy.

Postoperative Care

Although little data exist to inform a routine postoperative surveillance strategy, clinical follow-up should occur 1 month after surgery and then at least every 6 months for 3 to 5 years. After 5 years, follow-up should occur on a yearly basis. Abdominal and pelvic CT scan with intravenous contrast as well as tumor markers, if they were initially elevated, should be drawn at each visit.[9]

QUALITY MEASURES

Although CRS/HIPEC for peritoneal metastases was developed over 30 years ago, the true incidence of patients in the United States undergoing CRS/HIPEC and their surgical outcomes remains difficult to estimate. A diverse range of histologies may benefit from CRS/HIPEC, resulting in varied ICD-10 codes, and there is no current procedural terminology code that includes CRS/HIPEC.[24] Cancer registries such as the National Cancer Database or Surveillance, Epidemiology, and End Results Program do not capture these patients separately, nor do they include pertinent perioperative information such as PCI. Additionally, even among high-volume peritoneal metastasis centers, significant differences exist with respect to surgical technique, perfusate, and perfusion time.[18,25,26] This high clinical variability and lack of consistent reporting make developing quality reporting challenging.

Despite early reports of poor morbidity and mortality associated with CRS/HIPEC, most contemporary studies have demonstrated acceptable rates, with morbidities ranging from 10% to 30% and mortality from 1% to 5%.[9,27,28] According to data from the National Surgical Quality Improvement Program, mortality for CRS/HIPEC was actually lower than other well-accepted, high-risk surgical oncology procedures such as esophagectomy and pancreaticoduodenectomy.[28]

The association between hospital volume and surgical outcomes has been well established, with significantly lower mortality rates for complex surgical procedures completed at high-volume hospitals versus low-volume hospitals.[29] This volume-outcome relationship has never been studied in CRS/HIPEC, however, likely owing to the challenges associated with obtaining appropriate patients from large databases. Furthermore, based on studies examining the learning curve for technical expertise, 140 to 220 CRS/HIPEC cases per hospital or 33 to 70 cases per individual surgeon would need to be performed to attain such expertise.[24] Because of the rarity of many peritoneal metastases, such volumes are currently only encountered at a few major regional centers. Thus, the argument for increased surgical mentorship, established training programs at high-volume centers, and standardized systems of perioperative care seems more rational than volumetric cutoffs alone.

CHAPTER 8

Cytoreduction

CRITICAL ELEMENTS

- Supracolic Greater Omentectomy
- Resection of Mesenteric Disease
- Cytoreduction of the Diaphragm
- Cytoreduction within the Pelvis
- Abdominal Visceral Resections

1. SUPRACOLIC GREATER OMENTECTOMY

Recommendation: A supracolic greater omentectomy should be performed as part of all complete cytoreductive operations conducted for any peritoneal surface malignancy. In contrast, the lesser omentum should be resected only when gross tumor is identified on the structure.

Type of Data: Retrospective reports, case series, or case-control studies

Strength of Recommendation: Strong recommendation, low-quality evidence

Rationale

The greater omentum has long been referred as the "policeman of the abdomen" given its predilection to contain intra-abdominal pathologic processes and immunologic functions. Although the omentum predominantly comprises adipose tissue, it also contains lymphoid aggregates (milky spots) that contribute to peritoneal immunity. Milky spots collect pathogens, antigens, and even metastatic cancer cells.[30] Evidence also suggests that tumor cells preferentially hone to the greater omentum and that the omentum promotes tumor growth.[31] For these reasons, the greater omentum is the most common site of peritoneal metastasis from intrabdominal malignancies (Fig. 4-1). In a prospective

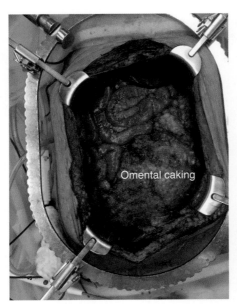

FIGURE 4-1 Image of extensive omental involvement in a patient with peritoneal carcinomatosis. Supracolic omentectomy with or without en bloc resection of adjacent organs is necessary to achieve complete cytoreduction.

study that examined the distribution of peritoneal disease in 129 patients with a variety of intra-abdominal malignancies including colon, appendix, and ovarian cancer, tumor involvement of the greater omentum was seen in more than 80% of the patients.[32]

The importance of complete cytoreduction in achieving long-term survival benefit in patients with peritoneal carcinomatosis undergoing cytoreductive surgery (CRS) was unequivocally demonstrated by two prospective randomized controlled trials.[10,33] A phase III trial by Verwaal et al.[10] that compared systemic therapy plus cytoreduction and hyperthermic intraperitoneal chemotherapy (HIPEC) with systemic therapy alone in patients with appendix or colon peritoneal carcinomatosis reported a median survival duration of 48 months and a 5-year survival rate of 45% in patients in whom complete cytoreduction was achieved. Several retrospective studies have also confirmed the importance of resection of all gross disease.[9,34,35] Although it would be impossible to study the impact of an individual component such as greater omentectomy on the long-term survival outcome of a multicomponent cytoreduction, extrapolation based on the biological predisposition and the frequency of greater omental involvement in carcinomatosis implies that resection of the greater omentum is necessary in all patients to achieve complete cytoreduction. Greater omentectomy is therefore indicated in all cytoreductive operations performed with curative intent, whether or not omental tumor deposits are grossly visible.

However, the lesser omentum does not share the same immunologic functions as the greater omentum, and it is often free of cancer even when tumors are identified elsewhere in the abdomen. Lesser omentectomy need be performed only when macroscopic disease on the structure is identified.

Technical Aspects

Greater omentectomy

A supracolic omentectomy is standard for greater omentectomy. The greater omentum should be elevated and separated from the transverse colon along its avascular attachment from the hepatic to the splenic flexure.[36–38] The peritoneum overlying the transverse mesocolon should be dissected with the omentum to the caudal border of the pancreas. This allows for resection of a portion of the omental bursa. Extreme care should be taken to avoid injury to the middle colic vessels during this step. In the absence of macroscopic involvement of the stomach or the gastroepiploic arcade, the branches of the gastroepiploic arcade to the omentum should be divided and the arcade preserved.[37,38] If the extent of disease warrants, the gastroepiploic branches to the greater curvature of the stomach should be dissected and divided to separate the omentum from the stomach. The short gastric vessels should be preserved. The technique of greater omentectomy can be changed based on the extent of disease, exposure, and the need for en bloc resection of the colon, spleen, or stomach due to bulky disease (Fig. 4-2).

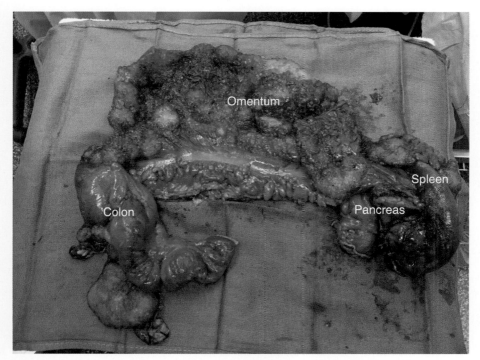

FIGURE 4-2 Specimen photograph depicting greater omentectomy with en bloc resection of terminal ileum, appendix, colon, distal pancreas, and spleen in a patient with appendiceal mucinous adenocarcinoma. Multivisceral resections are often required to perform a complete greater omentectomy in patients with extensive disease.

Lesser omentectomy

The left triangular ligament should be divided to retract the left lateral segment of the liver and to thereby expose the entire hepatogastric ligament. The lesser omentum should be separated from the gastrohepatic fissure that separates segments 2, 3, and 4 of the liver from the caudate lobe.[36–40] Care should be taken to identify and preserve an aberrant left hepatic artery, which may arise from the left gastric artery. If present, tumor nodules from the anterior surface of the caudate lobe should be dissected using electrocautery. The left gastric artery should be skeletonized and preserved. The lesser omentum should be separated from the lesser curvature of the stomach, with every effort made to preserve the vascular arcade, particularly the major branches of the left gastric artery and the anterior vagus nerve. This is especially important if the short gastric vessels and gastroepiploic arcade were resected, as the blood supply of the stomach will be solely dependent on the left gastric branches. The lesser omentum should be separated from the gastric antrum by dividing the antral branches (Fig. 4-3). In the setting of bulky disease in the subpyloric space, the lesser omentum should be left in continuity with the antrum, and a distal gastrectomy should be performed to achieve complete clearance. It is important to examine the cranial portion of the omental bursa by elevating the caudate lobe, as tumor nodules in this area could be

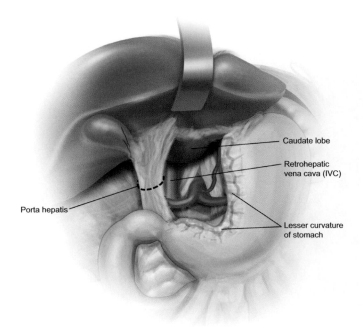

FIGURE 4-3 The illustration depicts resection of the lesser omentum and exposure of the cranial recess of the omental bursa with anterior retraction of the caudate lobe. Examination of the cranial recess of the omental bursa should be routinely performed during cytoreduction to avoid missing disease in this location.

easily missed. If tumor is present, this portion of omental bursa should be removed by stripping the peritoneum that overlies the retrohepatic vena cava and the right crus of the diaphragm.

2. RESECTION OF MESENTERIC DISEASE

Recommendation: The entire small intestine and mesentery should be systematically evaluated from the ligament of Treitz to the cecum. All visible mesenteric disease should be resected either by mesenteric peritonectomy or by resection of mesentery with the associated segment of bowel. Thermal ablation with high-voltage electrocautery, electrovaporization, or ultrasonic dissection may also be used to destroy mesenteric tumor nodules when complete cytoreduction cannot otherwise be safely performed.

Type of Data: Retrospective reports, case series, or case-control studies

Strength of Recommendation: Strong recommendation, low-quality evidence

Rationale

The small bowel serosa and mesentery are frequently involved by peritoneal surface malignancies, and the extent of disease on the small bowel often determines whether optimal CRS can be performed.[41] A review of 350 patients referred for CRS and HIPEC determined that 23% of patients underwent incomplete cytoreduction owing to widespread disease with extensive small bowel and mesenteric involvement.[42]

Assessment of small bowel and mesenteric disease prior to CRS and HIPEC remains a challenge, as small tumors may not be detected radiographically.[43,44] A review of 102 patients who underwent diagnostic laparoscopy with the goal of detecting occult disease demonstrated that 37% of patients were found to have significant small bowel and mesenteric tumors that were not identified radiographically.[45]

The extent of small bowel resection and mesenteric peritonectomy necessary to perform complete cytoreduction varies with the extent of disease involvement. In the setting of extensive small bowel and/or mesenteric disease, the benefit of a potentially incomplete resection and peritonectomy must be balanced with the risks for short intestinal length, fistula formation, and malnutrition. The number of anastomoses required to resect all disease, as well as the potential need for diversion, should also be considered. Ultimately, the decision to perform small bowel resection must be made in the context of the mesenteric peritonectomy necessary to achieve complete cytoreduction.

In rare circumstances, tumor deposits may be limited to either the small bowel serosa or the mesentery, and each may be addressed separately. More commonly, disease is present on both the small bowel serosa and the mesentery; in this circumstance, the resection and peritonectomy procedures necessary to safely remove all disease require thoughtful consideration. The optimal technique for mesenteric peritonectomy has not been defined: although a variety of mesenteric peritonectomy techniques using cautery, vaporization, ultrasonic dissection, and ablation are available, the specific method used should be based on surgeon preference and institutional resources, as no data exist to support the superiority of any specific modality.

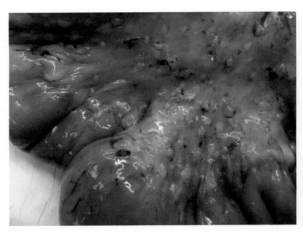

FIGURE 4-4 Small bowel mesenteric disease in a patient with poorly differentiated adenocarcinoma of the colon. Extensive mesenteric peritonectomy with or without small bowel resection is required to achieve complete cytoreduction.

Technical Aspects

Small bowel mesenteric peritonectomy

At the time of exploration, the entire small intestine and mesentery should be systematically evaluated from the ligament of Treitz to the cecum. Both sides of the mesentery must be evaluated. The ligament of Treitz is a particularly common location for tumor nodules.

Small-volume mesenteric disease may be excised with scissors or a scalpel or vaporized with cautery. In the setting of moderate- or high-volume mesenteric disease, parietal peritonectomy of both sides of the mesentery may be required (Fig. 4-4).[46] If removal of all gross disease is not possible, tissue ablation with high-voltage electrocautery, electrovaporization, and/or ultrasonic dissection may also be used to perform mesenteric peritonectomy. Irrespective of the technique chosen, it is important to avoid vascular trauma to the underlying mesenteric vessels, which may result in inadequate blood supply and need for additional intestinal resection. In the absence of gross mesenteric disease, mesenteric peritonectomy should not be performed.

3. CYTOREDUCTION OF THE DIAPHRAGM

Recommendation: Cytoreduction of disease on the peritoneal surface of the diaphragm should typically be accomplished via subdiaphragmatic peritonectomy, but full-thickness resection of the diaphragm may occasionally be required to resect cancer that invades deep into this structure.

Type of Data: Retrospective reports, case series, or case-control studies

Strength of Recommendation: Strong recommendation, low-quality evidence

Rationale

Regardless of the source and type of peritoneal disease (e.g., colon adenocarcinoma or low-grade appendiceal mucinous neoplasm), a "redistribution phenomenon" exists in which the diaphragm becomes seeded from distant sites, particularly on the right side.[47,48] The process of distribution is related to several factors including peritoneal fluid circulation/absorption, bowel peristalsis, and gravity.[49] The circulation of peritoneal fluid is continuous toward the diaphragms, allowing for peritoneal fluid to be absorbed into subperitoneal lymphatic capillaries. The main driver of this cranial to caudal to cranial pattern of circulation is from the negative pressure generated in the thorax by the diaphragms during respiration. Although bowel peristalsis also contributes to peritoneal circulation directed at the diaphragms, gravity in the recumbent position appears to influence deposition of tumor between the liver and the right diaphragm recesses.[48] Therefore, the diaphragmatic surfaces represent a common area for implantation of tumor and a frequent site of parietal peritonectomy or full-thickness resection during cytoreduction surgery (Figs. 4-5 and 4-6).[50]

A complete cytoreduction of all peritoneal disease has repeatedly been shown to be a major determinant of postoperative survival.[51] Following complete cytoreduction, patients with diaphragmatic implants who undergo diaphragmatic stripping/resection have similar oncological outcomes to patients who do not have tumor on the diaphragm. The median survival of patients following complete cytoreduction with or without full-thickness diaphragmatic resection was similar for those with low-grade appendiceal or colorectal cancer (Fig. 4-7).[52] Morbidity is potentially higher when diaphragmatic resection, rather than peritonectomy, is performed, but mortality and overall survival appear unaffected.[53] The issue of seeding the pleural space and how to

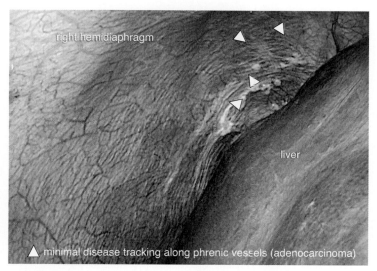

FIGURE 4-5 Relatively minor involvement of diaphragm peritoneum with metastases from adenocarcinoma of colon. This will require a fairly minor diaphragmatic stripping. *Arrowheads* indicate minimal disease tracking along phrenic vessels (adenocarcinoma).

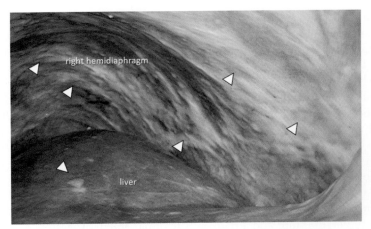

FIGURE 4-6 Confluent involvement of diaphragm peritoneum with metastases from adenocarcinoma of colon. This will entail a more challenging diaphragmatic stripping and possibly even a full-thickness diaphragm resection. *Arrowheads* indicate coalesced disease on right hemidiaphragm and liver surface (adenocarcinoma).

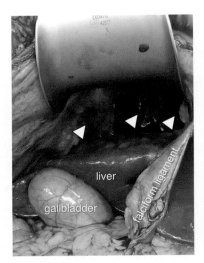

FIGURE 4-7 Extensive involvement of right diaphragm peritoneum and liver capsule with disseminated peritoneal adenomucinosis. Despite extensive subphrenic involvement, complete cytoreduction is possible with complex diaphragmatic peritonectomy alone and stripping of the Glisson's capsule of the liver.

deal with it during cytoreduction/HIPEC is an open question. In a case series, patients who had a full-thickness defect of the diaphragm and underwent chemoperfusion to include the pleural space exhibited less subsequent pleural disease than those who had the defect closed prior to HIPEC.[54] In a more recent and much larger report examining ipsilateral pleural recurrence after no diaphragmatic stripping, parietal stripping only, or full-thickness resection, no differences were noted between the groups and no differences were detected, whether the pleura was perfused or not during HIPEC.[55] Although consensus is lacking from the literature, it does appear that perfusion of the pleural space is tolerated during HIPEC and does not affect respiratory-related morbidity.[54] Additionally, despite the large number of HIPEC cases with diaphragmatic stripping or resection, the rate of respiratory complications and diaphragmatic hernias appears extremely low.[53,56]

Technical Aspects

Subdiaphragmatic peritonectomy

Extraperitoneal parietal peritonectomy should be carried to the upper abdomen into the subdiaphragmatic plane for performance of the diaphragm stripping. Performance of this maneuver early allows placement of a self-retaining multiquadrant retractor, retraction of the abdominal wall, and elevation of the subcostal margin for optimal exposure.

Subphrenic peritonectomy should be performed with a combination of blunt and electrosurgical dissection. The method of dissection is usually dictated by the extent and invasiveness of the disease. The right diaphragmatic peritoneum is involved much more commonly than the left, but cytoreduction of the diaphragmatic component must be complete regardless of laterality.

The falciform ligament and ligamentum teres should be dissected from the abdominal wall. This dissection should be continued in a cranial and posterior direction, stripping the peritoneum with tumor from the underlying diaphragmatic muscle. Elevating the costal margin and exerting downward pressure on the liver facilitate display of the operative field. During dissection of the ligamentum teres, caution should be used during its proximal ligation as injury to the left branch of the portal vein could ensue. Dissection of the falciform ligament should be continued posteriorly onto the anterior and posterior leaflets of the coronary and triangular ligaments of the liver, taking great care to avoid injury to the hepatic veins and the suprahepatic inferior vena cava (IVC) and the right phrenic vein.

The peritoneum overlying the right Gerota's fascia and the adrenal gland should be resected, and the dissection should be extended to the lateral right triangular ligament attachments to the liver. Dividing the right triangular ligament allows the liver to be rotated anteriorly and medially to further expose the deep subphrenic recess for completion of the right subdiaphragmatic peritoneal stripping. The entire diaphragmatic peritoneum can thus be stripped onto the bare area of the liver and carried onto the Glisson's capsule should the disease distribution dictate this. The degree of difficulty in clearing the peritoneum of the right hemidiaphragm is dependent on the invasiveness and extent of the disease, with the central tendon often representing a challenge if involved. A blunt technique may allow for these areas to be cleared in

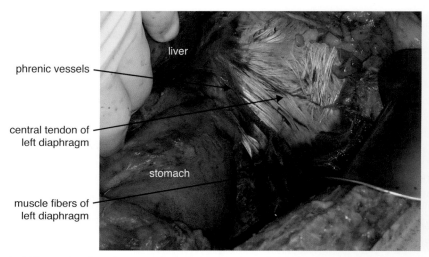

FIGURE 4-8 The photograph depicts stripping of the left diaphragmatic peritoneum. A complete diaphragmatic peritonectomy, including both muscle and central tendon, is performed without formal diaphragmatic resection.

continuity without disrupting the central tendon or phrenic vessels, but a directed force is required to separate the peritoneum and underlying musculature. Alternatively, techniques using the "cut" setting on electrocautery, an argon beam coagulator, or a Cavitron Ultrasonic Surgical Aspirator device have been described.

The retroperitoneal dissection on the left side is usually less extensive, but this depends on the individual patient and on the distribution of disease around the spleen. The left lobe of the liver is readily mobilized and can facilitate exposure of the entire left hemidiaphragm. Sometimes, the left subphrenic peritonectomy is extended in an extraperitoneal fashion onto the splenic suspensory ligaments, rotating the spleen anteromedially for performance of an en bloc splenectomy, if needed. Regardless, this maneuver is facilitated by upward and outward retraction on the subcostal margin by the fixed retractor as well as strong traction on the tumor specimen inferomedially. Posterior lateral dissection of the peritoneum off the left hemidiaphragm may extend to expose the left adrenal gland and the cranial aspect of the perirenal fat, at which point the specimen can be detached (Fig. 4-8).

Full-thickness resection of the diaphragm

Diaphragmatic peritoneal stripping will address most patients with diaphragmatic involvement. Less than 30% of patients will require full-thickness resection.[55] It is often not possible to identify which patient will require full diaphragmatic resection without initiation of a blunt technique diaphragmatic stripping at the plane between the diaphragmatic muscle and the peritoneal lining. On exposure of the diaphragmatic muscle, tumor invasion becomes apparent; it is usually limited in extent. By approaching this area via circumferential stripping of the peritoneum, a stapler may be fired in the plicated involved area, avoiding altogether the need for thoracic perfusion.

In cases of large full-thickness diaphragmatic defects, the synchronous instillation of both thoracic and intraperitoneal chemotherapy may be considered as an option. In order to minimize intrathoracic recurrence, the diaphragmatic defect may be left open, or even extended, so that HIPEC can be allowed to bathe the thoracic cavity.

On completion of HIPEC, the diaphragmatic defect should be repaired primarily. In the unusual event of the defect being too broad to close primarily with suture, a patch or mesh may be used to bridge any defect. If there has been violation of the bowel and there is concern regarding infection, a bioprosthetic mesh can be used. Most commonly, the diaphragm should be repaired primarily. As the right hemidiaphragm is usually protected by the liver, herniation of abdominal contents is rare. The left hemidiaphragm, however, is at risk of herniation, and this complication should be a consideration for the type and extent of repair. The thoracic cavity should be evacuated of air and fluid prior to tying down the final suture with a catheter in the thoracic cavity through the defect and sustained positive pressure ventilation by the anesthesiologist. An ipsilateral tube thoracostomy should be performed at the conclusion of the operation, which not only serves to eliminate any pneumothorax in the short term but also drains the eventual pleural effusion associated with an extensive dissection.[57]

4. CYTOREDUCTION WITHIN THE PELVIS

Recommendation: If cancer is visible on the pelvic peritoneal surface, a pelvic peritonectomy should be undertaken to achieve optimal cytoreduction. Visceral and parietal peritoneum that is not grossly involved by tumor need not be excised. Resection of the rectosigmoid colon, bladder wall, ureters, ovaries, and/or uterus should be performed en bloc with the pelvic peritonectomy if these organs appear directly invaded by tumor. A bilateral oophorectomy should be performed routinely for postmenopausal patients with pelvic disease. The role of oophorectomy should be discussed preoperatively with each premenopausal patient in whom direct ovarian involvement is not identified.

Type of Data: Retrospective reports, case series, or case-control studies

Strength of Recommendation: Strong recommendation, low-quality evidence

Rationale

The peritoneum serves as the first line of defense against cancer progression in peritoneal surface malignancy. A knowledge of its pelvic anatomy is thus critical to the optimal conduct of pelvic surgery for these neoplasms (Fig. 4-9).[58] The peritoneum should be reflected off the anterior surface of the rectum to the posterior surface of the bladder or vagina—3 cm or more cranial to the level of the muscular floor of the pelvis. This reflection of the peritoneum forms the floor of the most caudal portion of the peritoneal cavity: the rectovesical pouch in the male or the rectouterine pouch (rectovaginal pouch, or cul-de-sac of Douglas) in the female. These locations are frequently seeded with tumor in patients with peritoneal surface malignancy of any origin.[59] In a study of 129 patients that specifically evaluated the distribution and volume of peritoneal surface malignancy with five different types of tumors, tumor involvement

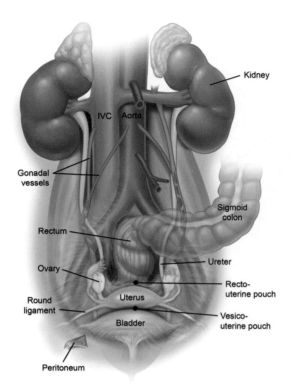

FIGURE 4-9   Pelvic anatomy in a female patient demonstrating the peritoneal reflections. This reflection of the peritoneum forms the floor of the most caudal portion of the peritoneal cavity: the rectovesical pouch in the male or the rectouterine pouch (rectovaginal pouch or cul-de-sac of Douglas) in the female. IVC: inferior vena cava.

of the visceral peritoneum was greatest at three anatomic sites: ileocecal valve region, where the bowel is tethered to the retroperitoneum resulting in slowing of peristaltic motion of the visceral peritoneal surface and pooling of fluid; rectosigmoid colon, which is located in a dependent site within the pelvis and which, within the pelvis, is fixed and secondarily retroperitoneal; and cul-de-sac of Douglas.[32]

In the pelvis, tumor may invade into the bladder or vagina anteriorly or the rectosigmoid colon posteriorly. The ovaries are likewise fertile ground for metastasis. To achieve an optimal cytoreduction within the pelvis, resection of the rectosigmoid colon and ovaries and/or hysterectomy may therefore be required en bloc with pelvic peritonectomy. The tumor distribution within the pelvis and its degree of invasion of pelvic structures dictate the extent of the visceral resections and parietal peritonectomy procedures that are required. In general, visceral and parietal peritoneum and structures that are not grossly involved by tumor need not be excised; only surfaces or structures that are directly implanted by tumor should be resected. However, more extensive peritonectomies may be considered in patients with certain tumor types, such as serous epithelial ovarian cancer, peritoneal mesothelioma, and mucinous appendiceal tumors.[60,61]

When extensive pelvic disease exists, complete pelvic peritonectomy will require stripping of the sidewalls of the pelvis, the peritoneal lining overlying the bladder, and the cul-de-sac and en bloc resection of the rectosigmoid colon. A study of 100 patients concluded that en bloc rectosigmoid resection was justified in this circumstance because deperitonealization with preservation of the rectosigmoid would have left tumor in situ in 73% of patients who had suspected cul-de-sac involvement.[62]

Metastases to the ovary have been shown to be independent predictors of a poor survival outcome.[63,64] Patients with gross tumor involving the ovary should undergo a therapeutic salpingo-oophorectomy. In a female patient who is postmenopausal, a bilateral oophorectomy should be performed routinely, irrespective of obvious tumor involvement, as the ovaries are at high risk of implantation by tumors of a variety of origins.[65] In a study of 194 women who underwent CRS and HIPEC for colorectal cancer carcinomatosis and appendix cancer carcinomatosis, synchronous ovarian metastases were confirmed in at least 52% of patients.[66] Two of every five patients who had undergone an operation for colorectal cancer carcinomatosis in whom ovarian involvement was not obvious at the time of surgery had microscopic disease confirmed at final pathology. Also, 14 (78%) of 18 patients aged younger than 40 years had ovarian metastases. These data notwithstanding, at present no consensus exists regarding the performance of prophylactic oophorectomy for premenopausal patients. Expert opinions range from routine bilateral oophorectomy regardless of age and reproductive status to a more selective approach, depending on the histologic origin of the carcinomatosis, the reproductive age of the woman, and whether there is evidence of macroscopic involvement of the ovaries.[25,46] Based on the existing literature, fertility should be addressed with all young female patients preoperatively, the ovaries need to be carefully evaluated radiographically and at the time of surgery, and the potential role of oophorectomy should be strongly considered in every patient.

Hysterectomy should be performed if invasion of tumor into the organ is identified. This invasion will usually be noted in the cul-de-sac of Douglas, where deep invasion of the anterior wall of the cervix and vagina will necessitate a total abdominal hysterectomy en bloc with pelvic peritonectomy. For women with disease not involving the cervix, a supracervical hysterectomy can be considered.

In patients in whom the bladder or ureters are invaded, resection of the involved portion of the bladder or ureter has been documented to be safe and feasible to achieve a complete cytoreduction.[67,68] Placement of ureteral stents preoperatively can be helpful for patients undergoing CRS and HIPEC if a complex operative pelvis is anticipated. If the patient is noted to have hydronephrosis on preoperative imaging, this concerning radiologic feature should alert the surgeon of the potential need for synchronous urologic procedures. The ureter is noted to be most often involved with peritoneal surface malignancies as it courses over the iliac vessels toward the trigone of the bladder. Prophylactic ureteral stenting can facilitate quick ureteral identification and reduce inadvertent ureteral complications without incurring an increase in urinary tract–related complications.[69,70] Bladder defects, particularly if they are away from the trigone, can typically be closed primarily, whereas ureteral reconstructions with direct implantations into the bladder with a psoas hitch or Boari flap is preferred over ureteroureterostomy owing to the lower risk or urinary fistulas.[71] Cystectomy is rarely if ever indicated given the morbidity and quality-of-life implications and likely poor oncological outcomes from such an extensive and invasive malignancy.

In patients who present with tumor of a low aggressive potential or in those who present with a low peritoneal cancer index, a visceral-sparing pelvic peritonectomy is a viable option.[26] The peritoneum overlying the anterior midrectum is superficial to a layer of fat that allows for peritoneal stripping without damage to the underlying bowel. In contrast, the visceral peritoneum lining the other parts of the rectosigmoid is so tightly adherent to the colon that peritonectomy with an adequate margin and avoidance of an iatrogenic bowel injury is usually impossible. If the extent of pelvic disease is limited, a visceral-sparing pelvic peritonectomy with the rectum stripped of peritoneum may also be possible. In the female patient, hysterectomy may be avoided if the uterus is free of disease.

Technical Aspects

Pelvic peritonectomy

Pelvic peritonectomy usually commences with a centripetal dissection of the peritoneum underlying the posterior aspect of the lower abdominal incision. This dissection should proceed toward the bladder and avoid iatrogenic injury to the muscular layer of the bladder. This phase of the dissection may be facilitated by dissecting out the urachus to use as a lead point. The urachus should be defined and then transected at the cranial aspect of the bladder and used for traction, which is essential to avoid injury to the bladder. Firm traction on the bladder helps to define the proper plane of dissection; likewise, countertraction on the peritoneal lining being stripped allows the surgeon to remain in the correct plane (Fig. 4-10). A low pelvic peritoneal cancer index may suggest that resection of peritoneal metastases without an extensive peritonectomy is appropriate.

Hysterectomy

Invasion of the uterus will usually be noted in the cul-de-sac of Douglas, where deep invasion of the anterior wall of the cervix and vagina denotes need for en bloc total abdominal hysterectomy with the pelvic peritonectomy. In the female patient in whom the uterus is still in place, the round ligaments can be identified as they exit the pelvis via the deep inguinal ring. The round ligaments should be transected at the level of the internal inguinal ring. The peritoneal stripping should be continued within the false and true pelvis, and care should be taken to isolate the gonadal vessels and protect the ureters. The gonadal vessels that run anterior to the ureters should be traced upward to the lower pole of the kidney, where they should be ligated and transected. Next, the uterine arteries and veins that run along the lateral wall of the vagina should be defined; upward traction on the uterus facilitates isolation of these vessels from the ureter, thus allowing them to be safely secured. Transection of the obliterated umbilical artery at the level of the ureter will also aid in separating these tissues.

With upward traction being maintained on the uterus, the end of the cervix should be palpated through the intact vagina wall, thus allowing the distal margin of transection to be defined prior to dividing the anterior aspect of the vagina. Alternatively, a sponge stick can be placed in the anterior fornix and the vagina transected above the

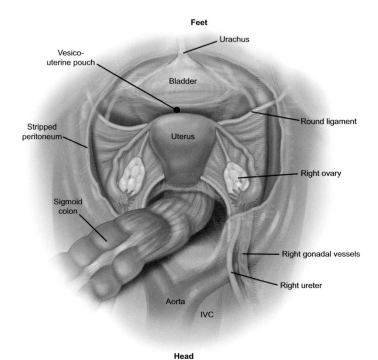

Feet

Urachus

Vesico-
uterine pouch

Bladder

Round ligament

Stripped
peritoneum

Uterus

Right ovary

Sigmoid
colon

Right gonadal vessels

Right ureter

Aorta

IVC

Head

FIGURE 4-10 Pelvic peritonectomy including stripping of the visceral peritoneum from the undersurface of the bladder and its reflection onto the vesicouterine pouch and the rectouterine pouch. IVC: inferior vena cava.

end of the cervix if there is no tumor involvement. Laterally, the vaginal branches of the uterine vessels may be secured to elevate the corners of the vagina as the vessels are ligated. The posterior aspect of the vagina should then be transected below the cul-de-sac of Douglas. To ensure that all tumor deposits within the cul-de-sac are removed en bloc with the specimen following transection of the vaginal cuff anterior and posterior to the cervix, the perirectal fat caudal to the posterior vaginal wall should be encountered and divided beneath the peritoneal reflection. The vaginal cuff should then be closed (Fig. 4-11). A supracervical hysterectomy may be considered if the invasive disease is limited to the uterine fundus. Bilateral salpingo-oophorectomy should be performed routinely for postmenopausal patients with pelvic disease as part of the effort to achieve a complete cytoreduction within the pelvis. The role of oophorectomy should be discussed preoperatively with each premenopausal patient in whom direct ovarian involvement is not identified.

Rectosigmoid resection

Rectosigmoid dissection begins by mobilizing the left colon mesentery off the retroperitoneum. The bowel should typically be divided at the junction of the sigmoid colon and descending colon. A lymphadenectomy is not required. The branches of

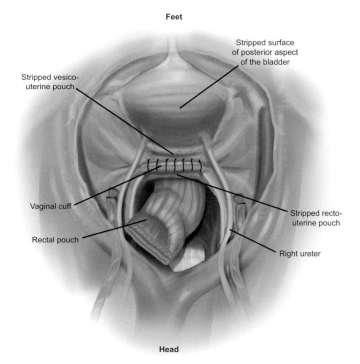

FIGURE 4-11 Completed pelvic peritonectomy in a female patient, including a total abdominal hysterectomy with a bilateral salpingo-oophorectomy, pelvic stripping, and rectosigmoid resection.

the sigmoid vessels on the left colic vessel should be divided. A centripetal dissection should then be begun in the plane of the mesorectal envelope. Branches of the middle hemorrhoidal vessels should be secured, and a strong upward traction on the rectosigmoid stump allows the rectal wall to be cleared of perirectal fat. The rectum should be divided caudal to the peritoneal reflection at approximately the junction of the middle and upper one-third of the rectum (Fig. 4-11). A diverting ostomy (ileostomy/colostomy) should be considered for patients who undergo a low colorectal or coloanal anastomosis as a means of protecting these low anastomoses. A lack of tension on the low colorectal or coloanal anastomosis is a key tenet to help avoid an anastomotic leak. If the need for further proximal mobilization of the left colon to achieve a tension-free anastomosis is seen, the following steps should be followed to accomplish this: The peritoneal fold that constitutes the ligament of Treitz should be mobilized. This maneuver then clearly exposes the inferior mesenteric vein, which should be ligated in continuity and then divided. Next, the inferior mesenteric artery should be identified as it arises from the aorta and ligated in continuity and divided. This will allow for adequate stretching of the left colonic mesentery with preservation of its blood supply, ensuring that the descending colon reaches to the low rectum for an anastomosis that is free of tension. However, rectal resection is not routinely needed to conduct an adequate cytoreduction.

Operating in the setting of prior hysterectomy

Prior hysterectomy may simplify complete pelvic peritonectomy. Scar tissue along the ureter induced by prior dissection is simple to release, and in almost all patients, the uterine arteries and veins have atrophied, which simplifies acquisition of hemostasis along the complete course of the ureter. The round ligaments should be electrosurgically divided as they exit the internal inguinal ring. The obliterated umbilical arteries should be transected just lateral to the ureter, and the ovarian vessels should be ligated at the lower pole of the kidney.

One caution with respect to the conduct of complete pelvic peritonectomy after prior hysterectomy involves dissection of the bladder. As the prior hysterectomy involved the separation of the bladder from the lower uterus and cervix, tumor may have been seeded on the exposed bladder muscle and may have focally invaded the bladder around the old bladder flap. Achieving a clear margin will require careful dissection through bladder muscle deep to the progressive tumor. Normally, the bladder mucosa can be preserved.

The caudal limit of dissection is the cervix.

5. ABDOMINAL VISCERAL RESECTIONS

Recommendation: Fulguration of the hepatic or splenic visceral peritoneum and focal serosal resection of the stomach, small bowel, or colon with primary repair is an option for low-grade appendiceal primaries with limited serosal involvement. In cases of extensive visceral peritoneal involvement not amenable to stripping, visceral resection en bloc with involved surrounding parietal peritoneum is indicated. Parenchymal-preserving partial resections are preferred, as long as complete gross resection of all peritoneal metastasis can be achieved. Lymphadenectomy is generally unnecessary, but in the setting of a synchronous primary malignancy such as high-grade appendix, colon, or gastric cancer, standard oncological lymphadenectomy with high ligation of the blood vessels feeding the primary tumor remains standard.

Type of Data: Retrospective reports, case series, or case-control studies

Strength of Recommendation: Strong recommendation, low-quality evidence

Rationale

Peritoneal surface malignancies often involve the visceral peritoneum overlying the abdominal organs. Complete resection of all gross disease is necessary for optimal surgical outcomes. In general, surgical resection to wide tissue margins is unnecessary. Parenchymal-preserving partial resections are therefore preferred, when possible, if complete resection of all visible peritoneal disease can otherwise be achieved.

Enteric resection

Often, peritoneal metastasis can involve the serosa and/or mesentery of the small and/or large bowel. There is no evidence to suggest that wide radical margin resections are necessary in the context of operations performed for peritoneal surface malignancy, and extensive bowel resections can lead to poor quality of life with malabsorption and diarrhea. Therefore, bowel-preserving approaches to resection are preferred.

The anatomy of the bowel mesentery lends itself to both peritoneal implant excision and/or ablation accomplished with electrocautery, carbon dioxide laser, sharp dissection, argon beam coagulator, and Cavitron Ultrasonic Surgical Aspirator. Serosal tumors, however, must be excised with primary bowel repair. If tumors are more extensive, full-thickness resection of the bowel and anastomosis may be required.

When bowel resection is performed in order to clear serosal disease, no lymphadenectomy is generally necessary, as peritoneal metastases rarely if ever metastasize to the regional lymph nodes. However, in the setting of a synchronous primary malignancy such as high-grade appendix, colon, or gastric cancer, standard oncological lymphadenectomy with high ligation of the blood vessels feeding the primary tumor remains standard. Multiple retrospective series have reported high correlation between lymph node metastasis and peritoneal metastasis in colon and appendiceal cancer.[72–74] The presence and number of lymph node metastases remain prognostic even in the context of peritoneal metastasis and represent an indicator of aggressive biological behavior and risk of extraperitoneal recurrence.[75] As a result, the status of the regional lymph nodes are included in the peritoneal disease severity score, a validated prognostic scoring system for colon and appendiceal cancers.[76,77] Two multiinstitutional retrospective series independently reported improved survival outcomes associated with high ligation and adequate lymphadenectomy during cytoreduction for peritoneal metastasis from colon cancer.[78,79] Furthermore, both the PERISCOPE I trial and the CYTO-CHIP study for gastric cancer included D2 lymphadenectomy as a major component of the potentially curative R0 resection of gastric cancer with limited peritoneal metastasis.[80,81]

An expert panel previously recommended that intestinal anastomosis should be performed following perfusion with HIPEC to avoid the potential adverse effects of heat and chemotherapy on the suture line.[82] However, there is a lack of data to support this recommendation. Furthermore, after HIPEC the bowel may become edematous during perfusion, potentially increasing the risk of anastomotic leak. Further, reevaluation after perfusion is another advantage of anastomosis prior to perfusion. Therefore, in the absence of strong data, the anastomosis can be performed either before or after the perfusion depending on surgeon preference. A multi-institutional study of more than 1,000 patients demonstrated that patient- and tumor-related factors (albumin and anastomotic location), but not technical factors (hand-sewn vs. stapled), were associated with anastomotic failure.[83] Therefore, anastomotic technique may be individualized based on patient considerations and surgeon preference.

Hepatic resection

Long-term outcomes for patients with colon cancer with metastasis to the liver and peritoneum treated with cytoreduction and HIPEC are similar to slightly worse compared with those of patients with peritoneal-only metastasis.[84–86] The best outcomes appear to be for those who have a low peritoneal cancer index and less that three liver metastases.[87] However, formal hepatectomy with cytoreduction and HIPEC has been

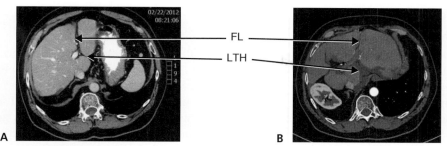

FIGURE 4-12 Possible sequelae of not resecting falciform ligament (FL) and ligamentum teres hepatis (LTH) in patients with carcinomatosis. **A:** CT scan of a patient with pseudomyxoma peritonea post cytoreductive surgery and hyperthermic intraperitoneal chemotherapy in which the FL and LTH were not resected. **B:** CT scan in the same patient showing tumor recurrence in the region of the FL and LTH.

demonstrated to increase operative time, length of stay, risk of reoperation, and postoperative morbidity compared with cytoreduction and HIPEC alone.[88,89] This may be owing to differences in perioperative fluid strategies, increased risk of infection when hepatectomy and bowel resection are performed concomitantly, and/or the hepatic absorption of intraperitoneal chemotherapy across a raw liver surface. Parenchymal-preserving liver wedge resection and/or ablation is therefore preferred if feasible; the selective use of a staged approach for lesions requiring formal hepatectomy may also be considered.[88,90,91] Hepatic lobectomy is only reasonable if complete resection of all hepatic *and* peritoneal disease is achieved.

The omentum, falciform ligament, and ligamentum teres hepatis (LTH) are frequent sites of occult tumor deposits, especially in mucinous tumors and ovarian cancer. Failure to remove tumor nodules from beneath the pons hepatique (bridge of liver parenchyma covering the umbilical fissure) can result in recurrent disease (Fig. 4-12), which is typically difficult to resect. Routine resection is not associated with increased complications and can minimize the likelihood of persistent disease.

Pancreatectomy and/or splenectomy

Pancreatectomy and splenectomy are safe and may be used to achieve complete cytoreduction if there is involvement with peritoneal surface malignancies. Preservation of the spleen and pancreas is feasible when there is only a minor or superficial involvement of the splenic capsule or bursa of the lesser sac; however, more extensive involvement of the left hemidiaphragm may require splenectomy and/or distal pancreatectomy to allow for complete left diaphragmatic peritonectomy.

Although these procedures are associated with increased postoperative complications (e.g., left upper quadrant abscess, pancreatic fistulas, and pleural effusions),[92,93] the increased morbidity is reasonable given the oncological benefits of complete cytoreduction. In case of distal pancreatectomy, routine drain placement is advisable especially in cases of synchronous bowel resection. Interestingly, postsplenectomy leukocytosis appears to protect from the hematologic toxicities of intraperitoneal chemotherapy.[94]

Technical Aspects

Enteric resection

During abdominal cytoreduction, the entire small and large intestine should be evaluated prior to determining the extent of resection. The extent of resection will depend on the invasiveness, size, and extent of disease. Sugarbaker[40] described five types of small bowel involvement by peritoneal surface malignancies (Fig. 4-13). Type 1 are noninvasive nodules often seen in low-grade mucinous appendiceal neoplasms and peritoneal mesothelioma. These nodules have not invaded past the visceral peritoneum and can be elevated with scissors. Often, the serosa is left intact, and seromuscular repair is not necessary. Type 2 are small invasive nodules on the antimesenteric portion of the small bowel that have invaded into the seromuscular layer. These nodules can still be elevated with scissors in a partial-thickness resection. The resulting seromuscular defect is then repaired. Type 3 are moderately sized invasive nodules on the antimesenteric portion of the bowel. The larger size requires a full-thickness resection of the nodule with the bowel wall. The resulting enterotomy is closed in the standard two-layered technique. Type 4 are small invasive nodules at the junction of the bowel and mesentery. These are dealt with in a similar fashion as type 2 or 3 nodules; however, the vascular supply should be evaluated either visually, with a Doppler, or by palpation. If there is concern for vascular compromise of the corresponding vascular arcade, then segmental resection is recommended. Lastly, type 5 are large invasive nodules that require segmental bowel resection with grossly negative proximal and distal margins.

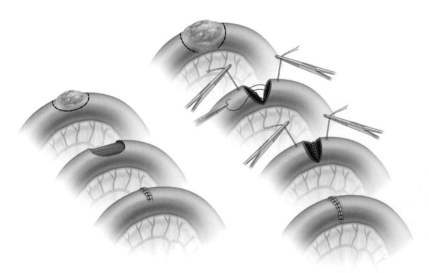

A

FIGURE 4-13 Illustrations of various techniques for complete resection of small bowel serosal implants. Type of resection technique best used depends on the depth of visceral involvement and the size and extent of the tumor. **A:** Noninvasive (type 1) and small invasive (type 2) nodules being locally resected and the resulting serosal defect being repaired.

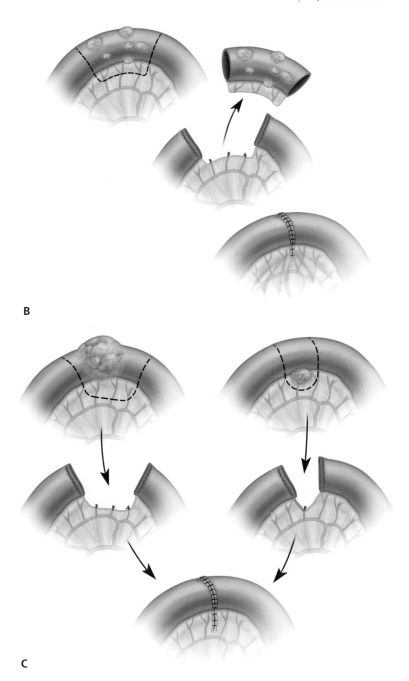

B

C

FIGURE 4-13 *(continued)* **B:** Moderately sized invasive nodules (type 3) undergoing full-thickness resection and anastomosis. **C:** Numerous nodules confined to a local segment of bowel being resected (type 4).

Tumor involving the small bowel serosa should be left intact until the entire stomach and small and large intestines are evaluated. Following complete evaluation, the decision must be made to proceed with resection(s) that preserve(s) as much bowel length as possible, so as to maintain normal nutritional function and minimize the number of intestinal anastomoses. It is particularly important to consider the extent of involvement of the entire gastrointestinal tract because numerous full-thickness resections of the intestines to remove serosal tumor deposits should be avoided. It is preferable to resect multiple smaller lesions within a segment of intestine with a single larger segmental resection. This approach will significantly decrease the risk of intestinal leak and fistulization. Furthermore, the decision on extent of intestinal resection also needs to consider the remaining bowel length, whether or not there is an intact ileocecal valve, remaining colon length, and the presence of a gastrectomy or gastrojejunostomy, as these factors will have significant implications on the nutritional function and enteric output of the patient postoperatively. It is generally recommended to leave at least 120 cm of small bowel beyond the ligament of Treitz after all requisite resections, but more (approximately 200 cm) may be necessary if the patient has an ileostomy or gastrojejunostomy.[95] Extensive small bowel serosal involvement is generally considered a contraindication to cytoreduction and HIPEC, and a thorough assessment of the length of small bowel to be spared should be performed early in the operative procedure. Several large prospective multi-institutional databases demonstrate that the number of intestinal anastomosis and gastrectomy are independent predictors of increased perioperative morbidity.[96–98] Complications not only have impact on patient quality of life but also long-term cancer-specific survival. Therefore, careful patient selection is necessary, as well as the use of organ-sparing techniques when possible.[99,100] In the setting of extensive disease, small nodules on the serosa may need to be left in situ if complete cytoreduction cannot be performed. Small bowel anastomoses may be constructed after HIPEC is completed, or they may be completed at the time of resection. Hand-sewn and stapled anastomotic techniques are both appropriate.[90] Only the mesentery that is involved with peritoneal surface malignancies should be incorporated in the bowel resection if performed. No formal lymphadenectomy is necessary for peritoneal metastasis except in the case of the primary tumor. If the primary tumor is in the appendix, colon, or small intestine, then resection should include oncological high ligation of the feeding vessels (ileocolic and right colic vessels in right-sided colon and appendiceal primaries; the inferior mesenteric artery in left-sided colon cancers; ligation of jejunal or ileal arcade at the takeoff from the superior mesenteric artery in small bowel primaries). If the primary is a gastric adenocarcinoma, then resection would include a D2 lymphadenectomy with lymphadenectomy of stations 1 through 12a for proximal or diffuse gastric primaries. Stations 2, 4sa, 10, and 11d can be omitted in distal gastric primary resections. The viability of the bowel and the anastomoses should be reassessed after the perfusion by visualization, palpation, Doppler, or indocyanine green. Mesenteric defects should be closed to prevent internal herniation and strangulation.

Liver resection

Peritoneal carcinomatosis involving the Glisson's capsule can be stripped by incising sharply and entering the sub-Glissonian space and then bluntly dissecting or using electrocautery to elevate the tumor off the underlying liver parenchyma (Fig. 4-14). Smaller isolated tumor deposits can also be fulgurated.[95] In the setting of no disease and minimal disease, use of an energy device for resection of the falciform ligament-LTH (often required for exposure and when diaphragmatic peritonectomy is required) is safe and feasible. In patients with extensive disease burden, complete eradication of the disease requires resection of the falciform ligament-LTH, opening and division of the pont hepatique (hepatic bridge variably present in patients) if present (Figs. 4-15 and 4-16), along with cholecystectomy and stripping of the hepatoduodenal ligament based on tumor involvement. The pont hepatique can be easily divided using an energy device or by ball-tipped electrosurgery at high voltage with minimal bleeding, as no major vascular or ductal structures are present within this structure. Once divided, the umbilical ligament should be exposed, inspected, and divided. Residual tumor implants can be electroevaporated.[96–98] Care must be taken not to injure the left portal vein at the base of the ligamentum teres. However, some patients, particularly those with colorectal or high-grade appendiceal cancers, will present with synchronous parenchymal liver metastasis that will require resection.

When a liver resection is necessary, a nonanatomic liver wedge resection and/or ablation is preferred if feasible because the greater parenchymal-sparing surgery afforded by a nonanatomic resection results in less morbidity and equivalent oncological outcomes and may be beneficial especially in the setting of intrahepatic recurrent disease, which occurs in up to 50% of colon cancer cases.[99] For larger liver resections,

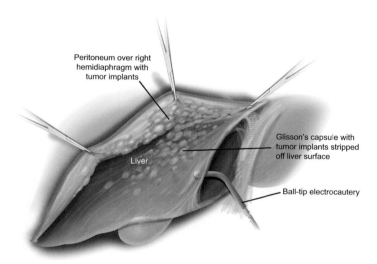

FIGURE 4-14 Depiction of a technique of using ball-tip electrocautery to strip the Glisson's capsule involved with tumor deposits.

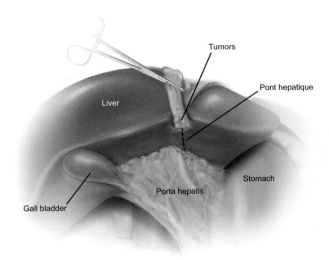

FIGURE 4-15 Illustration showing the presence of occult tumor deposits on the falciform ligament-ligamentum teres hepatis and possible extension under the pont hepatique.

selective use of a staged approach may also be considered depending on the health of the liver and the functional liver remnant. The approach to complex liver resection should start with complete mobilization of the liver to expose the portal veins. Visual inspection, bimanual palpation, and intraoperative ultrasound are recommended to identify the target metastatic lesions as well as evaluate for occult metastasis not visualized on preoperative imaging.[100] Depending on the type of resection necessary,

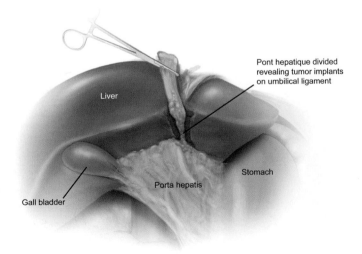

FIGURE 4-16 Illustration showing the presence of tumor deposits on umbilical ligament identified after division of pont hepatique.

vascular occlusion may be achieved through Pringle maneuver and extrahepatic or intrahepatic pedicle ligation. Parenchymal transection can be achieved via crush-clamp method, saline-linked radiofrequency sealer (TissueLink), Cavitron Ultrasonic Surgical Aspirator (CUSA), water-jet dissection (ERBEJET), and vascular staplers. Although the Cochrane database shows that no parenchymal technique is superior to the crush-clamp and vessel ligation technique in regard to bile leaks, bleeding, and liver failure, it does not specifically address the complications in relation to cytoreduction and HIPEC.[101] Regardless of technique, the oncological goal should be to achieve microscopic negative surgical margins and minimize blood loss and morbidity.

For cholecystectomy, the fundus-down approach is preferred. The fundus of the gall bladder should be mobilized off the liver bed, and the mesentery of the gall bladder should be taken down to the level of the porta hepatis, where the peritoneum over the hepatoduodenal ligament should be stripped with dissection of the visceral peritoneum over the entire portal structures, including the left hepatic artery and left portal vein. The cystic artery and cystic ducts should be identified, dissected, and divided. This is an opportune time to open the pars flaccida and palpate the portal structures and the caudate lobe through the foramen of Winslow to evaluate for any peritoneal disease in these spaces.

Visceral peritonectomy of the right upper quadrant

Electrosurgery should also be used to strip visceral peritoneum from beneath the right hemidiaphragm, from the right subhepatic space, and from the surface of the liver. The dissection is greatly facilitated if the tumor specimen is maintained intact and dissection starts by taking down the attachment of the ligamentum teres and falciform ligament from abdominal wall. The dissection continues laterally on the right to encounter, but need not include, the perirenal fat covering the right kidney. Also, the right adrenal gland should be visualized and carefully avoided as tumor is stripped from the right subhepatic space. As the peritoneal reflection at the posterior aspect of the liver is divided, care should be taken not to traumatize the vena cava or to disrupt the caudate lobe veins that pass between the vena cava and segment 1 of the liver.

An alternative technique for stripping visceral peritoneum in the right upper quadrant, especially when complete subphrenic peritonectomy is not required, is to first perform complete mobilization of the right lobe of the liver. The medial to lateral dissection approach for complete mobilization of the cranial attachment of the right lobe is preferred. The attachments of the ligamentum teres and falciform ligament from the abdominal wall should be taken down and dissection continued posteriorly with division of the coronary ligament to the level of the right and middle hepatic veins insertion into the IVC. The right lobe should then be slightly rotated to the left with gentle downward traction while dividing the right triangular ligament to allow identification and mobilization of the bare area of the liver for complete exposure of the right hepatic vein and suprahepatic IVC. Next, the right lobe of the liver should be gently lifted upward and liver mobilization continued from the hilar area toward the diaphragm (caudal to cranial approach), exposing the right side of the IVC. Care should be taken to avoid injury to the right adrenal gland and the hepatic veins to the caudate lobe. Once the right lobe of the liver is completely mobilized, stripping of the Glisson's capsule can be easily completed as previously described.

Pancreatectomy and/or splenectomy

These procedures can be performed en bloc with the omentum to achieve complete visceral and parietal peritonectomy of the left upper quadrant by mobilizing the omentum off the transverse colon and then dissecting the omentum off the greater curvature of the stomach. It has been found that preserving the right gastroepiploic vessels, if possible, may be associated with less delayed gastric emptying. However, this vessel should be divided and resected if involved with disease. The short gastric arteries should be taken down, and the left upper quadrant peritoneum should be elevated off the left hemidiaphragm using a combination of blunt and electrocautery dissection. The peritoneum should then be dissected back to its splenic attachments. The left adrenal gland should be visualized and carefully avoided as tumor is stripped from the left retroperitoneal space. The pancreatic tail can either be transected with a stapler or mobilized away from the splenic hilum if it is going to be preserved.

Splenic capsulectomy is rarely feasible owing to attendant bleeding. If the spleen is to be removed, the splenic artery and vein should then be divided proximal to the left gastroepiploic vessels to facilitate a complete en bloc resection of the omentum, spleen, and distal pancreas if necessary to achieve a complete cytoreduction. If there is significant disease in the hilum of the spleen, the spleen can be mobilized laterally to medially and the vessels taken posteriorly to avoid bleeding and injury to the pancreas.

Drug Delivery and Safety

CRITICAL ELEMENTS

- Hyperthermic Intraperitoneal Chemotherapy following Cytoreduction

1. HYPERTHERMIC INTRAPERITONEAL CHEMOTHERAPY FOLLOWING CYTOREDUCTION

Recommendation: The decision to administer hyperthermic intraperitoneal chemotherapy (HIPEC) should be made on the basis of tumor type, patient physiology, and extent of cytoreduction. When administered, chemotherapy should be perfused following complete cytoreduction, using open or closed techniques, with close monitoring of intraperitoneal/core body temperatures, hemodynamics, and end organ function.

Type of Data: Retrospective reports, case series, or case-control studies

Strength of Recommendation: Strong recommendation, low-quality evidence

Rationale

HIPEC involves perfusion of the peritoneal cavity with heated cytotoxic chemotherapy to potentially eradicate residual microscopic peritoneal disease after cytoreduction. It has been used since the 1980s in patients undergoing complete cytoreduction of peritoneal metastases who have a high risk of peritoneal recurrence.[102] Administration of chemotherapy directly into the peritoneal cavity takes advantage of the peritoneal-plasma barrier and allows for delivery of high local drug concentration and provides lower systemic toxicity than intravenous chemotherapy. Hyperthermia is selectively toxic to malignant cells and has synergistic cytotoxic effects with chemotherapy.[103,104] Retrospective cohort studies and a single randomized controlled trial have found improved survival in patients undergoing combined cytoreduction and HIPEC versus intravenous chemotherapy alone for peritoneal metastases secondary to ovarian and colorectal cancer.[105–107] However, there have been relatively few studies comparing cytoreduction alone versus cytoreduction with HIPEC, including randomized controlled trials, which have shown a significant survival benefit with HIPEC in ovarian cancer, a modest survival benefit in gastric cancer, and only subset survival benefit in colorectal cancer when oxaliplatin was used.[12,33,108] Thus, its utility continues to be debated. An analysis of this debate is the focus of the second key question in this section.

Currently, HIPEC is used most often in peritoneal mesothelioma or in appendiceal, colorectal, and ovarian cancer with peritoneal metastases that are amenable to complete cytoreduction (with resection of all gross peritoneal nodules or residual nodules less than 2.5 mm).[109] Toxicity specifically attributed to HIPEC beyond that associated with cytoreduction itself is somewhat difficult to ascertain; however, it includes leukopenia, thrombocytopenia, hemorrhage, and nephrotoxicity, depending on the drug and dosing used.[12,110,111] In any case, HIPEC should be used only after careful consideration of the known benefits and risks and institutional and surgeon experience. Cytoreduction alone without HIPEC might be reasonable in patients with peritoneal metastases at high operative risk (i.e., in frail patients or those with impaired bone marrow or renal function) or those with little likelihood of seeing any benefit from HIPEC (e.g., in patients with early recurrence after prior HIPEC or, possibly, those with colorectal cancer). The decision to proceed with HIPEC must be made prior to the procedure itself when there is known peritoneal metastasis and conducted only after a complete cytoreduction has been performed.

Open versus closed technique

In vitro studies have shown target hyperthermia of 40°C to 42°C provides optimal cytotoxic effects on neoplastic cells without causing onerous thermal damage on non-neoplastic tissue.[103] HIPEC may be perfused using either an open or a closed technique. Preclinical data using a murine model of HIPEC have shown that peritoneal tissue concentration of the intraperitoneal chemotherapeutic agent is no different between the open or closed technique. However, systemic drug concentrations were higher using the open technique.[112] Most US centers use a closed technique given the potential risks of chemotherapy spillage or vaporization with the open technique as well as the increased ability to maintain hyperthermia and possibly lower complications associated with the closed technique.[113,114] Also, the use of the open technique is not allowed in most US states owing to Occupational Safety and Health Administration rules concerning chemotherapy fumes. If an open approach is considered, applicable rules should be checked with the particular state's occupational safety and health agency. However, there is no outcome data suggesting better outcome with either an open or closed technique.

Technical Aspects

Administration of HIPEC requires adequate equipment (cannulas, tubing, temperature probes and wires, and a perfusion system), medications (intraperitoneal chemotherapeutic agent), personnel (perfusionist and standard operating room nurses and anesthesia personnel), and experience. A discussion of the operative plans with the anesthesia team is mandatory.

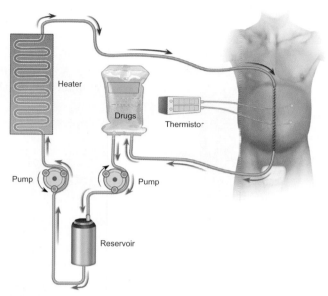

FIGURE 4-17 Critical elements of the hyperthermic intraperitoneal chemotherapy perfusion system. These elements include an extracorporeal pump, heater, reservoir, and thermistors to monitor intraperitoneal temperature. The chemotherapy to be perfused into the peritoneum should be administered into the circuit extracorporeally.

Once a complete cytoreduction has been achieved with comprehensive evaluation of all peritoneal surfaces, all abdominal quadrants and raw surfaces should be carefully examined, and any bleeding and/or residual peritoneal tumors should be addressed, prior to proceeding with HIPEC. All adhesions should be lysed to allow for chemotherapy to reach all peritoneal surfaces. The patient's hemodynamic status and urine output should also be normalized (with a target urine output of 1 mL/kg/h) and the patient allowed to passively cool to approximately 35°C.

Intraoperative peritoneal chemoperfusion should be administered using a perfusion system with an infusion pump, a reservoir with a filter, and a heat exchanger (Fig. 4-17). A trained perfusionist can prepare the perfusion system in the operating room. Inflow and outflow cannulas should then be placed in the peritoneal cavity. Thermistors should be placed in the cannulas and/or directly in the tissue in the peritoneal cavity. The skin must be tightly closed around inflow and outflow cannulas and temperature probe wires (closed technique) or with the abdominal wall open and suspended and sealed around the cannulas and temperature probe wires (open technique) to prevent leakage of perfusate (Fig. 4-18).[115] The circuit should be primed with perfusate until adequate abdominal distension has been achieved—generally 3 to 4 L—and then the perfusate should be circulated until adequate intraperitoneal hyperthermia is reached (40°C to 42°C).

Chemotherapy ordering, preparation, and delivery to the operating room should be performed with strict adherence to the American Society of Clinical Oncology and

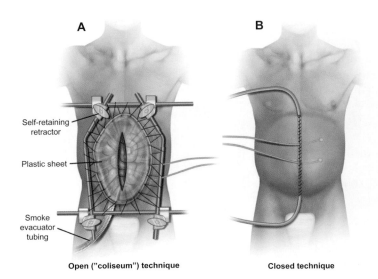

Self-retaining retractor

Plastic sheet

Smoke evacuator tubing

Open ("coliseum") technique   Closed technique

FIGURE 4-18 Open and closed methods of hyperthermic intraperitoneal chemotherapy administration. **A:** Illustration shows the open ("coliseum") technique with a plastic sheet and smoke evacuator to sequester liquid and aerosolized chemotherapy. Thermistors should be placed into the peritoneal cavity to monitor temperature during perfusion. **B:** Illustration shows the closed technique with the skin temporarily closed around the inflow and outflow cannulas and thermistors wires to monitor intraperitoneal temperature.

Oncology Nursing Society chemotherapy administration standards, as adapted to the intraoperative setting.[116] Chemotherapy used for HIPEC should be ordered using a standardized order set, which includes the drug dose (per square meter body surface area or flat dose), base fluid and volume, and date of administration, with prior communication regarding drug availability, timing, concentration, and volume to be delivered. Chemotherapy should then be administered through the perfusion circuit and may be given in a single dose at the time hyperthermia is achieved or in two doses during the chemoperfusion to maintain adequate drug concentration. Standard intraperitoneal chemotherapeutic agents include oxaliplatin, cisplatin, and doxorubicin, although mitomycin C is the most commonly used agent.[117] Chemoperfusion should then be maintained at a minimum of 1 L/min for 60 to 120 minutes, with intermittent or continuous mechanical abdominal agitation during the perfusion.[118]

Precautions should be taken to minimize chemotherapy exposure to staff, as it is considered a hazardous material.[119] These precautions include use of a class II biological safety cabinet during pharmacy drug preparation and personal protective equipment for individuals handling chemotherapy. Leakage of perfusate from the incision or around the cannulas should be stopped typically by placing additional sutures to seal the leak. Patient excreta should be treated as potentially contaminated for 48 hours, handled using universal precautions and generally placed in chemotherapy-designated bins.

Intraperitoneal temperature should be maintained at 40°C to 43°C using a heat exchanger. Core body temperature should be monitored throughout the case, but particular attention should be focused on temperatures during chemoperfusion, using an esophageal, bladder, blood, or rectal temperature sensor. Caution must be used with bladder temperatures, as it may be more representative of perfusate temperature than true core body temperature. The core body temperature should be kept below 40°C using various cooling techniques such as lowered ambient room temperature, removal of forced-air warming blankets, and cooling packs in the axilla and around the neck, if necessary. If persistent overheating of core body temperature occurs (which is rare), the perfusate temperature can be lowered. Ice slurries should not be used against patient skin owing to the risk of frostbite injury. There are retrospective data showing an association between elevation in core body temperature above 40°C and increased postoperative complications.[120]

Patients should be adequately monitored and managed during HIPEC to maintain normal hemodynamics and brisk urine output (ideally, 1 mL/kg/h), using intraoperative measures including intravenous fluid administration, vasopressor therapy, and diuresis depending on the overall fluid status. Sodium thiosulfate should be administered as a bolus and subsequent infusion for prevention of nephrotoxicity when chemoperfusion with high-dose cisplatin is used.[121,122] It is recommended that the chemotherapy used for HIPEC should be suspended in minimal volume (ideally, 50 to 100 mL) when used as the perfusate. Oxaliplatin is not entirely stable when suspended in chloride solutions, and 5% dextrose can be used.[123] However, a 5% dextrose solution should not be used to prime or flush the perfusion circuit, as this can lead to serious electrolyte abnormalities. The chemotherapeutic agent should be prepared as close to the time of use as feasible, as some agents are not entirely stable in solution.

Once chemoperfusion is complete, the circuit should be drained and rinsed with additional perfusate. The abdomen should then be reopened, and all visceral surfaces should be examined for cannula or thermal-related injuries, hemostasis, status of anastomoses if any, position of nasogastric tube, etc. Completion of anastomoses, if necessary and not previously constructed, and creation of any necessary stomas or drain placements should then be performed, followed by definitive closure.

In adult patients with metastatic cancers of colon, appendiceal, or gastric origin who undergo cytoreductive surgery (CRS) and hyperthermic intraperitoneal chemotherapy (HIPEC) with curative intent, is there an optimal peritoneal cancer index (PCI) limit beyond which surgery does not improve outcomes?

INTRODUCTION

CRS and HIPEC have been recently adopted as a treatment option for select patients with colon, appendiceal, and disseminated peritoneal surface disease (PSD). Although several patient- and tumor-related factors are associated with long-term outcome, the disease burden as quantified at the time of CRS/HIPEC and the ability to achieve a complete cytoreduction have been demonstrated to be the strongest independent predictors of survival in patients who undergo CRS/HIPEC with curative intent.[3,124–126] Among the multiple scoring systems that have been devised for quantifying disease burden, the PCI score has been shown to be the most reliable and reproducible.[1,127–132] The PCI score measures the distribution of tumor within 13 abdominopelvic regions, with each region being assigned a score between 0 and 3, for a total score between 0 and 39 (Table 4-3).[133] The PCI forms an essential component of several validated, prognostic scoring systems such as the Peritoneal Disease Severity Score and Colorectal Peritoneal Metastases Prognostic Surgical Score.[76,134,135]

The PCI score has also been associated with perioperative morbidity and mortality.[2,125] Early studies of CRS/HIPEC demonstrated high rates of surgical morbidity and mortality associated with these procedures. Although more recent studies, especially those from high-volume centers, have noted significantly lower complication rates,[2,9,34,136–138] the adverse effect of major surgical morbidity on long-term survival rates remains notable.[139,140] The outcome of patients with PSD treated with CRS/HIPC therefore depends on both the risks (perioperative morbidity) and anticipated benefits (long-term survival) associated with surgery—both of which are associated with the PCI score. Thus, it stands to reason that an optimal PCI score threshold may exist, above which the risks of surgery potentially outweigh any survival benefit. Importantly, because the survival of patients who undergo incomplete cytoreduction is often suboptimal irrespective of the PCI, such a threshold should be defined for patients in whom complete cytoreduction is deemed feasible.[2,34] The completeness of cytoreduction (CC) score is a well-established index that is used to quantify the residual tumor after maximal cytoreduction, with a CC score of 0 or 1 often being used to define a complete cytoreduction (CC0—no visible tumor; CC1—tumor nodules <2.5 mm; CC2—tumor nodules between 2.5 mm and 2.5 cm; CC3—tumor nodules >2.5 cm).[141]

Given the significant variation in the histopathologic subtypes of disease for which CRS/HIPEC is performed, as well as the significant heterogeneity that has historically existed between studies, consensus has not been achieved regarding an acceptable

TABLE 4-3 Peritoneal Cancer Index

Region	Description	Lesion Size Score	Description
0 Central	Midline abdominal incision; entire greater omentum, transverse colon	LS 0	No tumor seen
1 Right upper	Superior surface of right lobe of liver; undersurface of the right hemidia-phragm; right retrohepatic space	LS 1	Tumor up to 0.5 cm
2 Epigastrium	Epigastric fat pad; left lobe of the liver; lesser omentum; falciform ligament	LS 2	Tumor up to 5.0 cm
3 Left upper	Undersurface of the left hemi-diaphragm; spleen; tail of the pancreas; anterior and posterior surfaces of the stomach	LS 3	Tumor >5.0 cm or confluence
4 Left flank	Descending colon; left abdominal gutter		
5 Left lower	Pelvic sidewall lateral to the sigmoid colon; sigmoid colon;		
6 Pelvis	Female internal genitalia with tubes, ovaries and uterus; bladder; pouch of Douglas; rectosigmoid		
7 Right lower	Right pelvic sidewall; cecum; appendix		
8 Right flank	Ascending colon; right abdominal gutter		
10 Upper jejunum			
11 Lower jejunum			
12 Upper ileum			
13 Lower ileum			

Two transverse planes and two sagittal planes divide the abdomen into nine regions. The upper transverse plane is located at the lowest aspect of the costal margin, and the lower transverse plane is located at the anterior superior iliac spine. The sagittal planes divide the abdomen into three equal sectors. Lesion size score (LS) is determined after complete lysis of all adhesions and the complete inspection of all parietal and visceral peritoneal surfaces. It refers to the greatest diameter of the tumor implants that are distributed on the peritoneal surfaces. Primary tumors or localized recurrences at the primary site that can be removed definitively are excluded from the lesion size assessment. If there is confluence of disease matting abdominal or pelvic structures together, this is automatically scored as LS 3 even if it is a thin confluence of cancerous implants.

PCI threshold beyond which a complete CRS/HIPEC is no longer considered beneficial.[124-126,142,143] The purpose of this work was to evaluate whether there is an optimal PCI limit beyond which surgery does not improve outcomes for adult patients with metastatic cancers of colon, appendiceal, or gastric origin who undergo CRS and HIPEC with curative intent.

METHODOLOGY

A systematic search of PubMed (US National Library of Medicine, National Institutes of Health) was conducted for full-text articles between 1990 and 2019 that addressed optimal PCI threshold in patients undergoing CRS/HIPEC. Combinations of the following Medical Subject Headings (MeSH) terms or keywords were used: [(Prognostic Value OR Optimal OR Maximum OR Limit OR Threshold) AND (PCI OR Peritoneal Cancer Index OR PCI Score OR Peritoneal Cancer Index Score) AND (Cytoreductive Surgery OR Cytoreduction OR HIPEC OR Hyperthermic Intraperitoneal Chemotherapy OR Surgery) AND (Curative OR Therapeutic OR Curative Intent OR Complete)]. Findings are reported in accordance with the Preferred Reporting Items for Systematic Reviews and Meta-Analyses (PRISMA).[144]

The initial search yielded 339 publications (Fig. 4-19). Abstracts that were not in English, included nonhuman studies, or did not have full-text availability were excluded. The remaining 177 abstracts were reviewed. Of those, 130 abstracts were excluded because they were duplicates, did not address PCI limits and thresholds, did not include survival and perioperative morbidity, had fewer than 10 patients. Forty-seven articles passed the title and abstract review and were retrieved for full-text review. Of those, 13 were excluded because they didn't address the question. One additional article was included based on reference list review. Thirty-five full-text articles met all criteria for inclusion in this systematic review (Tables 4-4, 4-5, and 4-6). Each article was reviewed by and assigned a quality of evidence based on the Grading of Recommendations, Assessment, Development, and Evaluation (GRADE) system.[145]

Most of these studies were conducted in patients with PSD associated with colorectal cancer, and most were retrospective analyses of data from single, high-volume centers at which CRS/HIPEC is routinely performed. Some studies used pooled data from multiple centers. Although HIPEC was the predominant intraperitoneal chemotherapy (IPC) modality used, many centers used early postoperative IPC, especially early in their institutional experience. Overall, the quality of the evidence was low.

FINDINGS

PCI Limit in PSD Associated with Colorectal Cancer

CC has been regarded as the most important factor associated with survival of patients who undergo CRS/IPC for colorectal cancer–associated PSD. The survival of patients with colorectal cancer who undergo incomplete resection is similar to that of patients who undergo palliative operations.[10,143] Many early studies reported PCI limits above which the likelihood of patients undergoing complete cytoreduction was low.[146] The poor survival outcomes also reported in these studies was primarily due to the inclusion of patients who did not undergo complete cytoreduction, as suggested

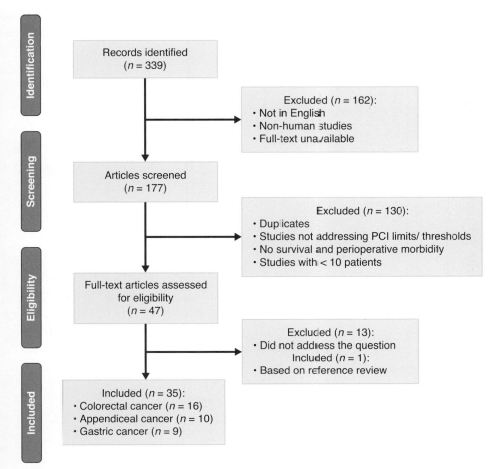

FIGURE 4-19 Preferred Reporting Items for Systematic Reviews and Meta-Analyses diagram for optimal peritoneal cancer index (PCI) limit beyond which surgery does not improve outcomes in adult patients with metastatic cancers of colon, appendiceal, or gastric origin who undergo cytoreductive surgery and hyperthermic intraperitoneal chemotherapy with curative intent.

by the fact that PCI no longer remained a prognostic factor after adjusting for CC score.[146,147] Over time, surgeons have, therefore, become increasingly selective, with CRS/HIPEC being offered only to patients in whom a complete cytoreduction can be anticipated.[148] Table 4-4 summarizes studies to date that have described a PCI limit for colorectal PSD. PCI limits described in these studies should be interpreted in the context of the ability to achieve complete cytoreduction and perioperative morbidity/mortality.[2,125,150]

The earliest attempt to define a PCI threshold was by Elias et al.[150] In a study of 70 patients who underwent complete CRS for metastatic colorectal cancer and PSD, the 3-year survival rate of patients with PCI above 15 was significantly poorer than that of patients with PCI below 15 (32.5% vs. 60.3%; $P = .01$). Although all patients

TABLE 4-4   Studies Assessing PCI Threshold in Metastatic Colorectal Cancer with Peritoneal Dissemination

Author, Year	Study Design	Study Period	Primary Tumor	Number of Patients (Procedures)	Perfusion Technique	Operative Morbidity, %	Operative Mortality, %	Median/ Mean PCI	CCR Score	OS	PCI Threshold	Grade of Evidence*
Barrati et al.,[139] 2014	Multicenter, retrospective observational	2004–2007	CRC	101	HIPEC	23.0	3.0	10	CC0, 87%	Median OS, 32 mo 5-y OS, 43.2%	19 (based on prior study cutoffs and significant decrease in survival for PCI >19, after adjusting for CC score)	+
Brandl et al.,[149] 2018	Single center, retrospective	2008–2015	CRC	51	HIPEC	NR	NR	Mucinous, 20.5 Nonmucinous, 8.9	CC0/1	5-y survival: Mucinous, 56.1% Nonmucinous, 42.2%	16 (only for nonmucinous tumors, based on worse 2-y survival in this subgroup)	+
Cashin et al.,[146] 2014	Single-center, retrospective	2004–2010	CRC	67 (CC0, 56)	HIPEC	39.0	4.0	17.6	CC0, 83.5%	Median OS, 30 mo for CC0	20 (based on predetermined value and decreased survival for PCI >20, not adjusted for CC score)	+
da Silva and Sugarbaker,[124] 2006	Single center, retrospective	1981–2004	CRC	70	EPIC HIPEC	NR	NR	13	CC0	PCI <20, 41 mo PCI ≥20, 16 mo	20 (based on prior studies by the authors and significantly decreased survival in PCI >20)	+

Study	Design	Years / Cancer	N	Regimen				CC status	Outcomes	PCI cutoff	
Elias et al.,[150] 2001	Single center, prospective	1993–1999 CRC	64	EPIC HIPEC	65.6	9.3	15.3	CC0	Median OS, 35.9 mo 3-y OS: PCI ≤ 15, 60.3% PCI > 15, 32.5%	15 (arbitrary cutoff based on significant difference in OS between two PCI groups)	+
Elias et al.,[125] 2010	Multicenter, retrospective	1990–2007 CRC	523 (CC0, 439)	HIPEC EPIC	31.0	3.3	14% with PCI ≥20	CC0, 85%	Median OS, 30.1 mo Median OS in CC0, 33 mo	20 (based on statistically significant poor median OS in patients with PCI ≥20)	+
Elias et al.,[151] 2014	Single center, retrospective	2000–2009 CRC	139	HIPEC	22.0	6.0	13 if SB involved 6 if SB uninvolved	CC0	Median OS, 39 mo 5-y OS, 39%	15 (based on universal involvement of the SB and decreased 5-y survival for PCI >15)	+
Glehen et al.,[34] 2004	Multicenter, retrospective	1987–2002 CRC	506 (533) (CC0, 271)	HIPEC EPIC HIPEC + EPIC	23.0	3.7	<13, 34% ≥13, 66%	CC0 in 270 (19.8%)	PCI <13, 34.8 mo PCI >13, 14 mo CC0 patients: Median OS, 32.4 mo 1 y, 87%; 3 y, 47%; 5 y, 31%	13 (to consolidate groups within Gilly and PCI classification systems and based on statistically significant survival difference; after adjusting for CC score)	+

(continued)

TABLE 4-4 Studies Assessing PCI Threshold in Metastatic Colorectal Cancer with Peritoneal Dissemination (continued)

Author, Year	Study Design	Study Period	Primary Tumor	Number of Patients (Procedures)	Perfusion Technique	Operative Morbidity, %	Operative Mortality, %	Median/Mean PCI	CCR Score	OS	PCI Threshold	Grade of Evidence*
Goéré et al,[152] 2013	Single center, retrospective	1995–2005	CRC	107	HIPEC EPIC	53.0	3.7	11	CC0/1	Median OS: 5 y, 35% 10 y, 15% Median DFS: 5 y, 16% 10 y, 13%	10 (based on ability to achieve cure defined as no recurrence after 5 y)	+
Goéré et al,[143] 2015	Single center, retrospective	2000–2010	CRC	180 (CC0, 139)	HIPEC EPIC	21.7 (intra-abdominal)	5.6	11 in curative group (23 in palliative group)	CC0/1, 77.2% CC2/3, 22.8%	Median OS, 19 mo 3-y OS: 52% for curative 7% for palliative	17 (based on no significant difference in OS between curative and palliative groups)	+
Hompes et al,[153] 2012	Multicenter, prospective observational	2004–2008	CRC	48	HIPEC	52.1	0.0	11	CC0	1 y, 97.9% 2 y, 88.7%	15 (based on statistically significant survival difference in OS and DFS)	+
Huang et al,[147] 2014	Single center, prospective	2005–2013	CRC	60 (CC0, 17)	HIPEC + EPIC	30.2	0.0	PCI >20, 53%	CC0/1, 53%	Median OS, 16 mo 1 y, 70.5% 3 y, 22% 5 y, 22%	20 (based on predetermined value and decreased survival for PCI >20, not adjusted for CC score)	+

Study	Type	Years	Cancer	N	Treatment							Grade
Robella et al.,[148] 2013	Single center, retrospective	1999–2012	CRC	50	HIPEC	34.0	2.0	21 (32% with PCI <16) for group A 11 (100% with PCI <16) for group B	Group A, 65% CC0/1 Group B, 100% CC0	PCI <16, 48 mo	16 (based on higher CC0 rate and OS)	+
Tabrizian et al.,[154] 2014	Single center, retrospective	2007–2012	CRC, HGA	170; 101 (59%) with CRC + HGA	HIPEC	52.4	2.4	14.3	CC0/1, 77.1%	Median OS, 22.8 mo 1 y, 81.6% 3 y, 30.6%	16 (based on significant difference in survival for PCI ≥16, adjusted for CC score)	+
Yan and Morris,[155] 2008	Single center, retrospective	1997–2007	CRC	50	HIPEC HIPEC + EPIC	30.0	0.0	12	CC0, 82%	Median OS, 29 mo 3-y survival, 39%	10 (based on statistically significant decreased survival in PCI ≥10)	+
Yonemura et al.,[142] 2013	Single center, retrospective	2004–2012	CRC	142 (CC0, 108	HIPEC	42.9	0.7	≤10 in 53% of patients	CC0 76%, CC1 24%	Median OS, 25.9 mo 5-y survival, 20% for CC0 patients	10 (based on significant difference in OS after adjusting for CC score)	+

CC: completeness of cytoreduction; CRC: colorectal cancer; DFS: disease-free survival; EPIC: early postoperative intraperitoneal chemotherapy; HGA: high-grade appendiceal; HIPEC: hyperthermic intraperitoneal chemotherapy; NR: not recorded; OS: overall survival; PCI: peritoneal cancer index; SB: small bowel.
*Grade: + very low.

TABLE 4-5 Studies Assessing PCI Threshold in Metastatic Appendiceal Cancer with Peritoneal Dissemination/Pseudomyxoma Peritonei

Author, Year	Study Design	Study Period	Primary Tumor	Number of Patients (Procedures)	Perfusion Technique	Operative Morbidity, %	Operative Mortality, %	Median/Mean PCI	CCR Score	OS	PCI Threshold	Grade of Evidence*
Aziz et al.,[172] 2018	Single center, retrospective	2005–2015	HGA (78% high-grade)	65; CC0, 45	HIPEC	NR	NR	6	CC0, 69%	Median 5-y OS, 55% CC0 5-y OS, 70%	7 (based on significantly decreased 5-y OS for PCI ≥7, not adjusted for CC status)	+
Benhaim et al.,[165] 2019	Single center, retrospective	1992–2014	LGA + HGA	313; CC0, 245 (78%)	HIPEC	PCI <28, 23.0 PCI ≥28, 46.0	PCI <28, 3.0 PCI ≥28, 8.0	PCI <28, 16 PCI ≥28, 37	CC0/1 PCI <28, 95% PCI ≥28, 51%	5-y OS PCI <28, 90% PCI ≥28, 70%	28 (predefined as extensive disease)	+
Chua et al.,[162] 2009	Single center, retrospective	1997–2008	LGA + HGA	106; CC0/1, 93	HIPEC EPIC HIPEC + EPIC	49.0	3.0	21	CC0/1 90.5%	Median OS, 104 mo 5 y, 5% 10 y, 36%	≥20 (based on difference in progression-free survival)	+
Chua et al.,[136] 2012	Multicenter, retrospective	1993–2011	LGA + HGA	2,298; CC0/1, 1,904	HIPEC ± EPIC	2.0	24.0	20	CC0, 1165	Median OS, 16.3 y 10 y OS, 63%	20 (based on significant difference in OS but recommended against using this as threshold)	+
El Halabi et al.,[160] 2012	Single center, retrospective	1999–2010	HGA	77; CC0/1, 58 (75%)	HIPEC	27.1	0.0	PCI ≥20, 68%	CC0/1 rate PCI <20, 96% PCI ≥20, 65%	Median OS, 3.4 y 5-y survival: CC0/1, 52% CC0/1 PCI ≥20, 66% CC0/1 PCI <20, 45% CC 2/3, 0%	≥20 (arbitrary threshold; PCI <20, 96% CC0/1: PCI ≥20, 65% CC0/1)	+

Study	Design	Years	Histology	N; CC	Treatment				CC rate	OS	Threshold (PCI)	Grade*
Elias et al.,[170] 2010	Multicenter, retrospective	1993–2007	LGA + HGA	301; CCO, 206	HIPEC ± EPIC	40.0	4.4	18.5	CCO, 73%	5-y OS, 72.6% 10-y OS, 54.8% PCI <20 5-y OS, >80% PCI ≥20 5-y OS, 57%	20 (based on ability to achieve CCO; and significantly lower OS)	+
Glehen et al.,[2] 2010	Multicenter, retrospective	1989–2007	Nonovarian	1,290 (1,344)	HIPEC EPIC	33.6	4.1	13.1	CCO, 74.7% CC1, 17.1%	Median OS, 34 mo 1 y, 77%; 3 y, 49%; 5 y, 37%	No defined threshold. Each additional point in PCI increased the risk ratio of death by 4.3% (after adjusting for CC score).	+
Jimenez et al.,[163] 2014	Single center, retrospective	1998–2013	LGA + HGA	202; CCO/1, 170	HIPEC	16.0	0.0	PCI <20, 28% PCI ≥20, 72%	CCO/1 rate, 85% PCI <20, 100% PCI ≥20, 78%	5-y OS: PCI <20, 67% PCI ≥20, 54%	20 (based on significant difference in OS)	+
Kitai et al.,[169] 2019	Single institution, retrospective	1999–2017	LGA (39%) + HGA (61%)	49; CCO/1, 40 (81.6%)	HIPEC	PCI <28, 10.0 PCI ≥20, 45.0	PCI <28, 0 PCI ≥28, 5.0	PCI <28, 41% PCI ≥28, 59%	CCO/1 PCI <28, 90% PCI ≥28, 50%	NR; OS comparable between PCI <28 and ≥28 if CCO/1	28 (arbitrarily selected as high tumor burden)	+
Votanopoulos et al.,[171] 2018	Multicenter, retrospective	1993–2015	HGA	521; CCO, 260	HIPEC	NR	NR	18.9	CCO/RO/R1, 50.1%	For CCO: Median, 6.1 y 5 y, 51.7% 10 y, 36.1%	21 (based on ability to achieve a complete cytoreduction; no defined PCI for CCO patients)	++

CC: completeness of cytoreduction; EPIC: early postoperative intraperitoneal chemotherapy; HGA: high-grade appendiceal; HIPEC: hyperthermic intraperitoneal chemotherapy; LGA: low-grade appendiceal; NR: not recorded; OS: overall survival; PCI: peritoneal cancer index.
*Grade: + very low; ++ low.

TABLE 4-6 Studies Assessing PCI Threshold in Metastatic Gastric Cancer with Peritoneal Dissemination

Author, Year	Study Design	Study Period	Primary Tumor	Number of Patients (Procedures)	Perfusion Technique	Operative Morbidity, %	Operative Mortality, %	Median/Mean PCI	CCR Score	OS	PCI Threshold	Grade of Evidence*
Canbay et al.,[181] 2014	Single center, prospective	2005–2012	Gastric	152; CC0/1, 103	BIPSC + HIPEC	23.6	3.9	NR	CC0/1, 68%	15.8 mo; 1 y, 66%; 2 y, 32%; 5 y, 10.7%; CC0/1, 18 mo	6 (based on significantly decreased 5-y OS for PCI ≥7, not adjusted for CC status)	+
Chia et al.,[179] 2016	Multicenter, retrospective	1989–2009	Gastric	81; CC0, 59	HIPEC	44.0	2.5	6 (for CC0 patients)	CC0, 73%; CC1, 27%	Median OS, 17.3 mo; 5-y OS, 18%; 5-y DFS, 11%; PCI <7, 26.4 mo; PCI ≥7, 10.9 mo; CC0, 22.1 mo; CC1, 8.4 mo	7 (based on ability to obtain cure defined as DFS at 5 y)	+
Glehen et al.,[176] 2010	Multicenter, retrospective	1989–2007	Gastric	159; CC0, 89	HIPEC ± EPIC	27.8	6.5	9.4	CC0, 56%; CC1, 25.8%; CC2, 18.2%	Median OS, 9.2 mo; CC0, 15 mo	12 (based on no survival beyond 3 y)	+
Hotopp,[182] 2019	Single center, retrospective	2008–2013	Gastric	26	HIPEC	NR	0.0	10; PCI <12, 53.8%; PCI ≥12, 46.2%	CC0/1	17 mo	12 (based on decrease in OS)	+
Kimbrough et al.,[184] 2019	Multicenter, retrospective	2010–2017	Gastric	28; CC0, 24	HIPEC	18.0	7.0 (90 d)	Median PCI, 12	CC0/1, 86%	10 mo; PCI ≤9, 26 mo; PCI >9, 8 mo	9 (based on survival)	+

Study	Design	Years	Cancer	N; CC	Treatment				CC	Survival		Grade
Manzanedo et al.,[183] 2019	Multicenter, retrospective	2006–2017	Gastric	88; CC0, 80	HIPEC EPIC	31.0	3.1 (90 d)	6	CC0, 91%	Median OS, 21.2 mo; 1 y, 79.9%; 3 y, 30.9%; 5 y, 27.5%; PCI ≤6: Median OS, 26.1 mo; 5-y OS, 46.8%; PCI >6: Median OS, 19.9 mo; 5-y OS, 0%	7 (based on poor survival with PCI ≥7)	+
Rau et al.,[178] 2020	Multicenter institution, retrospective	2011–2016	Gastric	235; CC0, 121	HIPEC	17.0	5.5 (2.6% in high-volume center)	8; 46% with PCI ≤7	CC0, 71.6%	13 mo; 5-y OS, 6%; Median OS: PCI ≤6, 18 mo; PCI ≥16, 5 mo	16 (based on inability to achieve CC and poor OS)	+
Yang et al.,[180] 2010	Single center, retrospective	2005–2009	Gastric	28; CC0/1, 17	HIPEC	14.3	0	NR	CC0/1, 61%	6 mo, 75%; 1 y, 50%; 2 y, 43%; CC0, 43.4 mo; CC1, 9.4 mo; CC2/3, 8.3 mo	≥20 (based on difference in OS; <20, 27.7 mo; ≥20, 6.4 mo; not adjusted for CC status)	+
Yonemura et al.,[177] 2010	Single center, retrospective	NR	Gastric	96; CC0/1, 58 (75%)	NIPC + HIPEC	32.0	2.0	PCI ≤7, 63%	CC0/1 rate: PCI ≤6, 86%; PCI ≥7, 29%	CC0/1; 1-y OS, 65%; 2-y OS, 34%; 5-y OS, 15%	6 (based on ability to obtain CC0/1 and survival difference)	+

BIPSC: bidirectional intraperitoneal and systemic induction chemotherapy; CC: completeness of cytoreduction; DFS: disease-free survival; EPIC: early postoperative intraperitoneal chemotherapy; HIPEC: hyperthermic intraperitoneal chemotherapy; NIPC: neoadjuvant intraperitoneal-systemic chemotherapy; NR: not recorded; OS: overall survival; PCI: peritoneal cancer index.
*Grade: + very low.

underwent a CC0 resection, the PCI threshold was set at 15. Da Silva and Sugarbaker[124] used a PCI threshold of 20 based on prior studies and a significant survival difference noted in patients with PCI below 20 versus 20 or above. In one of the largest multi-institutional, international series performed to date, Glehen et al.[34] grouped 506 patients undergoing CRS and IPC for metastatic colorectal cancer into cohorts with limited or extensive disease based on a PCI cutoff of 13. This arbitrary threshold was selected to allow for consolidation of disease burden between two widely used scoring systems—the Gilly and Sugarbaker PCI scores.[133] After adjusting for CC status, the median overall survival (OS) of patients who had limited disease (PCI < 13) was significantly longer than that of patients with extensive disease (34.8 vs. 14.4 months; $P < .0001$). Given the higher surgical morbidity rate observed among patients with extensive disease, the authors advised caution when recommending CRS to such patients, especially when other negative prognostic factors are present.

Elias et al.[151] conducted a large study of 523 patients with metastatic colorectal cancer and PSD who underwent CRS/IPC at multiple institutions in France. Eighty-five percent of patients underwent a CC0 resection, and only 14% had a PCI of 20 or above. Multivariable analysis demonstrated an association between PCI and poor survival (hazard ratio [HR], 1.054; $P = .0001$). Patients with PCI of 20 or above had a significantly shorter median OS (18 months) and 5-year survival rate (7%) than patients with PCI below 20, leading the authors to recommend against CRS/HIPEC in these patients, especially in the presence of other poor prognostic factors like lymph node involvement or progression during systemic therapy. Additional retrospective analyses have established a similar PCI threshold of 20 or above.[146,147] However, other studies have established a lower PCI threshold of 10 based on the ability to obtain a cure, defined as a 5-year disease-free interval following surgery.[152]

In a study by Goéré et al.,[143] patients were classified as whether or not they had undergone a curative operation, defined as the ability to obtain a CC0/1 resection. For each PCI score, survival was compared between those patients undergoing CC0/1 (curative) and CC2/3 (noncurative or palliative) surgery. No significant difference in OS was noted between the curative and palliative cohorts when the PCI was 17 or above; survival of patients with PCI 17 or above was poor. Based on this, the authors defined a PCI threshold of 17 as a relative contraindication to CRS/HIPEC even when an optimal cytoreduction can be anticipated.

Most recently, the results of the PRODIGE 7 study, a French multicenter randomized controlled trial of CRS alone compared with CRS/HIPEC were published. The trial demonstrated prolonged long-term survival in both arms (>41 months). Only patients with PCI below 25 were included in the trial, and survival of patients with PCI 11 or below was longer than that of patients with PCI 11 to 15 (HR, 1.95; 95% confidence interval [CI], 1.3 to 2.9; $P = .001$) and greater than 15 (HR, 3.28; 95% CI, 2.3 to 4.7; $P < .001$).[156] Although the trial was not designed to establish a PCI cutoff and has been criticized for several reasons, it has demonstrated the negative impact of a higher PCI score (>11) in patients with colorectal PSD who undergo complete CRS.[157,158]

The question of whether a PCI limit by itself should be used to select patients for cytoreduction remains to be fully elucidated. Although various studies have established different PCI thresholds, what is clear is that a high PCI (potentially above 20, based on the maximum PCI score limit defined, when considering all the studies included) is associated with significantly lower benefit from CRS/HIPEC. This is particularly true for patients who have other adverse prognostic factors. Nomograms such as the Colorectal Peritoneal Metastases Prognostic Surgical Score, which incorporates age, locoregional lymph node status, and presence of signet ring cell histology in addition to PCI score, have been developed to supplement the PCI score as a marker of therapeutic futility and merit further investigation.[135]

PCI limit in PSD associated with appendiceal cancer/pseudomyxoma peritonei

Several studies have examined the PCI of patients with PSD associated with appendiceal tumors. Although PCI predicts the ability to achieve a complete cytoreduction in patients with low-grade tumors, PCI is not associated with long-term OS when complete cytoreduction is obtained.[159–163] Additionally, although the goal of surgery should be to obtain a CC0/1 cytoreduction, incomplete cytoreduction may still confer a survival benefit for patients with low-grade tumors and a high PCI.[136,164,165] Recurrence- and progression-free survival are associated with PCI, but even in patients in whom there is recurrence, iterative procedures may lead to long-term survival benefit.[166–169] Therefore, the decision to proceed with surgery should not be made on the basis of PCI alone.

In patients with high-grade tumors, PCI may be more important. In a retrospective analysis of 125 patients with high-grade disease, Jimenez et al.[163] noted PCI 20 or above as an adverse prognostic indicator even after adjusting for CC score. Similarly, Elias et al.,[170] in a retrospective analysis of 301 patients with pseudomyxoma peritonei, noted PCI to be a significant factor in patients with high-grade tumors treated with complete cytoreduction. In contrast, in the largest multi-institutional study of patients with high-grade disease performed to date, Votanopoulos et al.[171] noted that PCI correlated with the ability to obtain a complete CRS, which correlated with survival. A PCI of 21 or above was associated with a 30% CC0 rate. Among patients in whom complete CRS (250 of 521 patients) was achieved, PCI was not associated with survival. At multiple PCI thresholds from below 5 to above 25, OS was greater than 4.5 years.[171] It should be noted that in this study, complete CRS was defined as the ability to obtain a CC0 resection because survival of CC1 patients (traditionally considered as optimally cytoreduced in the setting of low-grade disease) was significantly inferior to that of CC0 patients, as observed in prior studies.[172,173] PCI also correlated with perioperative morbidity as noted in other studies.[170,174] Therefore, in patients with high-grade tumors, the ability to obtain a CC0 resection rather than a PCI limit should be considered in determining oncological benefit of CRS/HIPEC. Table 4-5 summarizes studies that have described a PCI limit for appendiceal PSD.

PCI limit in PSD associated with gastric cancer

Metastatic gastric cancer with peritoneal dissemination is clinically aggressive and universally fatal. Most patients are treated with systemic therapy and best supportive care. However, CRS/HIPEC has emerged as a potential option in well-selected patients with peritoneal metastatic disease in whom complete cytoreduction can be anticipated.[33,175] Glehen et al.,[176] in a French multicenter retrospective analysis, demonstrated that survival improves in patients with low-volume disease in whom a CC0 cytoreduction is possible. The association between the PCI and ability to obtain a complete cytoreduction has been demonstrated in multiple other studies.[2,177,178] Given poor survival when any macroscopic disease is left in situ following resection, many studies have underscored the importance of a CC0 cytoreduction.[176,179,180] To achieve this, some series have used a neoadjuvant intraperitoneal/systemic or bidirectional intraperitoneal/systemic chemotherapy-based approach to maximize response and decrease tumor burden prior to surgery.[177,181] Additionally, because the PCI correlates with perioperative morbidity and mortality, proper patient selection, even when a complete cytoreduction is achievable, is critical.[182] Whereas earlier studies established this cutoff based on historical definitions of extensive carcinomatosis (PCI $\geq$20), more modern series have suggested a PCI of below 7, based on the finding that survival is improved to between 15 and 18 months, with acceptable perioperative morbidity, when a CC0 resection is achieved.[179,181,183,184] Table 4-6 summarizes studies attempting to define a PCI cutoff in patients with gastric PSD who undergo CRS/HIPEC.

CONCLUSION

CRS/HIPEC provides a survival benefit with acceptable perioperative morbidity in patients with PSD from colon, appendiceal, and gastric primary cancers treated at high-volume/experienced peritoneal malignancy centers. Because long-term benefit is associated with complete cytoreduction, the goal of surgery should be to achieve a CC0/1 cytoreduction.

In patients with colon cancer–associated PSD, CRS/HIPEC should be offered to patients with a low PCI (<20) in whom complete cytoreduction can be achieved. In patients with appendiceal cancer–associated PSD, CRS/HIPEC should be offered to all patients in whom a complete cytoreduction can be anticipated, irrespective of PCI. In patients with gastric cancer–associated PSD, CRS/HIPEC may be offered to patients with low PCI (<7) in whom complete cytoreduction can be anticipated.

Peritoneal Key Question 2

In patients with gastric or colorectal adenocarcinoma metastatic to the peritoneum, does cytoreductive surgery (CRS) plus hyperthermic intraperitoneal perfusion with chemotherapy (HIPEC) prolong survival or increase the risk of complications compared with CRS alone?

INTRODUCTION

The peritoneum is a common site of metastatic disease and recurrence in patients with colonic and gastric adenocarcinoma. Among patients with these cancers, those with peritoneal metastases generally live for a shorter duration than do patients with either liver or lung metastases. The etiology for the relatively poor survival of patients with peritoneal disease is unknown but may be related to diminished penetration of chemotherapy into the peritoneum or the propensity of peritoneal disease to cause gastrointestinal obstruction or malignant ascites.

Data support the use of HIPEC for appendiceal tumors, mesothelioma, and, most recently, ovarian cancer. Based on the existing evidence in these histologies, HIPEC has been increasingly studied and used for patients with other cancers. Current National Comprehensive Cancer Network guidelines for colon cancer state that complete CRS and/or intraperitoneal chemotherapy can be considered in select patients but that the conflicting data regarding clinical efficacy make this approach controversial.[185] In addition, adding HIPEC to CRS may increase the complications of surgery. Current guidelines for gastric cancer do not comment on either CRS or HIPEC.[186] There are several recent trials and large registry reports of HIPEC both in gastric and colorectal cancer, that are attempting to clarify the role of this modality for patients with peritoneal carcinomatosis or patients at high risk of developing peritoneal disease. The purpose of this work was to evaluate whether CRS plus HIPEC prolongs survival or increases the risk of complications in patients with gastric or colorectal adenocarcinoma metastatic to the peritoneum, compared with CRS alone.

METHODOLOGY

A systematic search of PubMed was performed to screen all articles from 1990 to 2019. Medical Subject Headings (MeSH) terms included "Cytoreductive Surgery," "Hyperthermic Intraperitoneal Perfusion with Chemotherapy," and "HIPEC." Searches were restricted to the English language and human subjects. Findings are reported in accordance with the Preferred Reporting Items for Systematic Reviews and Meta-Analyses (PRISMA).[144]

The initial search yielded 1,291 abstracts (Fig. 4-20). Of those 1,291 abstracts, 1,049 were not relevant to the disease site or surgical key question and were excluded. Ultimately, 242 abstracts were reviewed. For the colorectal cancer disease site, only randomized clinical trials were included. Owing to the paucity of randomized trials

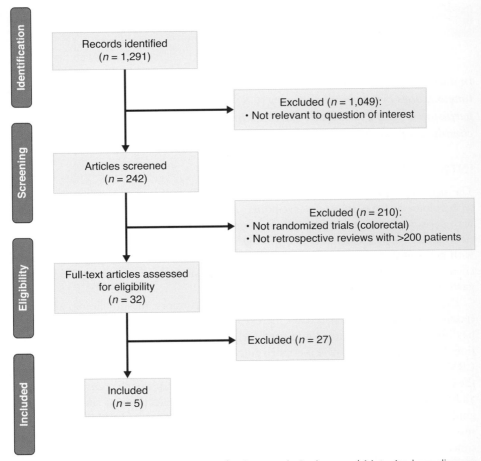

FIGURE 4-20 Preferred Reporting Items for Systematic Reviews and Meta-Analyses diagram for cytoreductive surgery plus hyperthermic intraperitoneal perfusion with chemotherapy in patients with gastric or colorectal adenocarcinoma metastatic to the peritoneum, compared with cytoreduction surgery alone.

for the gastric cancer disease site, only retrospective reviews with greater than 200 patients were included. Thirty-two full-text manuscripts were reviewed and of these, an additional 27 manuscripts were excluded as retrospective reviews with less than 200 evaluable patients.

Five studies met all the criteria for inclusion in this systematic review (Table 4-7).[12,33,107,187,188] Outcome measures of overall survival (OS) and complications were identified. Each article was reviewed and assigned a quality of evidence based on the Grading of Recommendations, Assessment, Development, and Evaluation (GRADE) system.[145] Of these five full-text articles, there were four randomized clinical trials and one retrospective review of a large registry. Overall, the quality of evidence ranged from moderate to high.

TABLE 4-7 Selected Randomized Controlled Trials and Large Prospective Registry Studies of Hyperthermic Intraperitoneal Perfusion with Chemotherapy for Colorectal and Gastric Cancer

Author, Year	Study Type	Study Group	Control Group	Intervention	CRS and HIPEC Complication Rate	CRS Complication Rate	Outcome	Grade of Evidence*
Bonnot et al. (CYTO-CHIP),[187] 2018	RCR	Gastric carcinomatosis	CRS	CRS, HIPEC	54% grade 3–5 morbidity, 7.4% mortality	55.3% grade 3–5 morbidity, 10.1% mortality	Median OS, 12.1 mo for CRS vs. 18.8 mo for CRS and HIPEC	+++
Goéré et al. (PROPHYLOCHIP),[188] 2018	RCT	Colorectal, perforated tumor, ovarian metastases, or isolated peritoneal disease resected with primary	Surveillance	Second-look surgery and HIPEC	41% grade 3 or 4 morbidity, 0% mortality rate	NA	3-y OS, 80% surveillance vs. 79% HIPEC	++++
Quenet at al. (PRODIGE 7),[13] 2018	RCT	Colorectal carcinomatosis	CRS	CRS, HIPEC	24.1% grade 3–5 morbidity	13.6% grade 3–5 morbidity	Median OS, 41.2 mo for CRS vs. 41.7 mo for CRS and HIPEC	++++
Verwaal et al.,[107] 2003	RCT	Colorectal carcinomatosis	Systemic chemotherapy	CRS, HIPEC	8% mortality rate, unclear morbidity rate	NA	Median OS, 12.6 mo for systemic vs. 22.3 mo for HIPEC	++++
Yang et al.,[33] 2011	RCT	Gastric carcinomatosis	CRS	CRS, HIPEC	14.7% serious adverse events	11.7% serious adverse events	Median OS, 6.5 mo for CRS vs. 11 mo for CRS and HIPEC	++++

CRS: cytoreduction surgery; HIPEC: hyperthermic intraperitoneal chemotherapy; NA: not available; OS: overall survival; RCR: retrospective chart review; RCT: randomized clinical trial.
*Grade: +++ moderate; ++++ high.

FINDINGS

The study by Verwaal et al.,[107] the only completed randomized clinical trial that compared CRS/HIPEC to systemic chemotherapy, established this treatment as an option for patients with colorectal carcinomatosis. Although this trial did not specifically address the benefit of HIPEC to CRS alone, the data generated from the trial stand as the primary justification for inclusion of CRS plus HIPEC in current national guidelines and provide an early report of OS and perioperative mortality rates. The limitations of this study have been frequently outlined but include the small number of patients ($N = 105$) and the inclusion of appendiceal tumors (17% of trial participants).[107] Another consideration is that chemotherapy efficacy has improved greatly since this trial, raising questions about the out-of-date systemic chemotherapy control arm.

In the recently reported PROPHYLOCHIP study, the benefit of prophylactic HIPEC after 6 months of adjuvant chemotherapy was investigated in a population of patients with colorectal cancer at high risk of peritoneal disease.[188] The high-risk population was defined as patients with perforated tumor, minimal resected carcinomatosis, and ovarian metastases. Although the study supported the role of a peritoneal-centered surveillance strategy for these high-risk patients, a proactive strategy of second-look surgery with HIPEC failed to improve survival.[188]

In another recently reported trial, the French PRODIGE 7 trial, patients with colorectal peritoneal carcinomatosis were randomized to either CRS alone or CRS plus HIPEC with oxaliplatin.[12] The median OS of patients who received CRS alone did not differ from that of patients who received CRS plus HIPEC (41.2 vs. 41.7 months; $P = .995$). Although the results from this trial have not yet been published, there are several notable aspects deserving of comment as this is the only completed randomized controlled trial to address the benefit of HIPEC over CRS alone in this population. Sixteen patients crossed over from the non-HIPEC to the HIPEC arm; however, there was no significant difference in OS with exclusion of the crossover patients. The median length of stay was increased in the CRS plus HIPEC arm by 5 days, and 60-day morbidity was also increased in the CRS plus HIPEC arm (24% vs. 14%; $P = .03$). In subset analysis of the group with a peritoneal cancer index (a classification system used to categorize disease based on size and location within the abdomen) of 11 to 15, a statistically significant increase in OS was associated with HIPEC.[12] As this subgroup analysis was not planned and the finding is not easily explainable, it should not be viewed as a clear indication for treatment in this subgroup of patients. The protocol included a 30-minute perfusion with oxaliplatin, which differs from the practice of most centers in the United States that perform a perfusion of 90 to 120 minutes with mitomycin.

In the only published randomized controlled trial of HIPEC in gastric cancer, Yang et al.[33] randomized 68 patients with peritoneal carcinomatosis to CRS versus CRS plus HIPEC. The perfusion regimen included flat doses of cisplatin (120 mg) and mitomycin (30 mg) for 60 to 90 minutes. The median OS of patients in the CRS arm was 6.5 months and that of patients in the CRS plus HIPEC arm was 11 months ($P = .046$). Serious adverse event rates were not significantly different between the two arms. The trial was relatively small, and the administration of systemic chemotherapy was not clearly defined or reported. In addition, the peritoneal cancer index of patients enrolled in the trial was generally high; approximately one-third of the patients had a score above 20.[33] Further randomized trials will therefore be required to confirm these findings and clearly identify the morbidity associated with CRS with HIPEC in patients requiring subtotal or total gastrectomy. There is also a recently presented retrospective review of a prospective registry from France of 277 patients (CYTO-CHIP) with peritoneal metastases from gastric cancer who underwent either CRS or CRS plus HIPEC.[187] Although the significant selection bias of this study, which accrued patients from 19 centers over 25 years (<1 patient per center per year) must be acknowledged, this study provides additional support for the benefit of HIPEC for gastric cancer–associated carcinomatosis. Median OS durations of patients who underwent CRS plus HIPEC and CRS alone were 18.8 and 12.1 months, respectively ($P = .002$). The 5-year OS rate of patients who underwent CRS plus HIPEC was also surprisingly high at 20%, compared with 6% in the CRS-alone arm. There was no difference in the rate of major complications between the groups.[187]

CONCLUSION

Current evidence does not support the addition of a 30-minute HIPEC with oxaliplatin to CRS for patients with colorectal cancer–associated carcinomatosis, and further studies are required to clarify the role of other HIPEC regimens in this population. Data from a randomized clinical trial do support CRS plus HIPEC in patients with gastric cancer–associated carcinomatosis. Enthusiasm is increasing for the initiation of a cooperative group trial investigating the benefit of HIPEC for patients undergoing CRS for gastric and colorectal cancer in the United States.

Although the quality of data from completed randomized clinical trials and large prospective registry studies of HIPEC is high, the limited number of trials makes definitive recommendations for the treatment of peritoneal disease difficult in controversial disease sites such as gastric and colorectal cancer. Current evidence does support HIPEC in patients undergoing CRS for gastric cancer metastatic to the peritoneum. Although there is evidence to support the use of CRS/HIPEC in patients with colorectal cancer metastatic to the peritoneum, the benefit of HIPEC relative to CRS alone is unclear. Most studies do not demonstrate an increased risk of complications with HIPEC, but oxaliplatin-containing regimens remain a concern.

REFERENCES

1. Jacquet P, Sugarbaker PH. Clinical research methodologies in diagnosis and staging of patients with peritoneal carcinomatosis. *Cancer Treat Res.* 1996;82:359-374. doi:10.1007/978-1-4613-1247-5_23
2. Glehen O, Gilly FN, Boutitie F, et al. Toward curative treatment of peritoneal carcinomatosis from nonovarian origin by cytoreductive surgery combined with perioperative intraperitoneal chemotherapy: a multi-institutional study of 1,290 patients. *Cancer.* 2010;116(24):5608-5618. doi:10.1002/cncr.25356
3. Faron M, Macovei R, Goéré D, Honoré C, Benhaim L, Elias D. Linear relationship of peritoneal cancer index and survival in patients with peritoneal metastases from colorectal cancer. *Ann Surg Oncol.* 2016;23(1):114-119. doi:10.1245/s10434-015-4627-8
4. Klaver CEL, Groenen H, Morton DG, et al. Recommendations and consensus on the treatment of peritoneal metastases of colorectal origin: a systematic review of national and international guidelines. *Colorectal Dis.* 2017;19(3):224-236. doi:10.1111/codi.13593

5. Carr NJ, Cecil TD, Mohamed F, et al. A consensus for classification and pathologic reporting of pseudomyxoma peritonei and associated appendiceal neoplasia: the results of the Peritoneal Surface Oncology Group International (PSOGI) modified Delphi process. *Am J Surg Pathol.* 2016;40(1):14-26. doi:10.1097/PAS.0000000000000535

6. Amin MB, Edge SB, Greene F, et al, eds. *AJCC Cancer Staging Manual.* 8th ed. Springer; 2017.

7. Yan TD, Deraco M, Elias D, et al. A novel tumor-node-metastasis (TNM) staging system of diffuse malignant peritoneal mesothelioma using outcome analysis of a multi-institutional database. *Cancer.* 2011;117(9):1855-1863. doi:10.1002/cncr.25640

8. Sadeghi B, Arvieux C, Glehen O, et al. Peritoneal carcinomatosis from non-gynecologic malignancies: results of the EVOCAPE 1 multicentric prospective study. *Cancer.* 2000;88(2):358-363. doi:10.1002/(sici)1097-0142(20000115)88:2<358::aid-cncr16>3.0.co;2-o

9. Levine EA, Stewart JH IV, Shen P, Russell GB, Loggie BL, Votanopoulos KI. Intraperitoneal chemotherapy for peritoneal surface malignancy: experience with 1,000 patients. *J Am Coll Surg.* 2014;218(4):573-585. doi:10.1016/j.jamcollsurg.2013.12.013

10. Verwaal VJ, Bruin S, Boot H, van Slooten G, van Tinteren H. 8-Year follow-up of randomized trial: cytoreduction and hyperthermic intraperitoneal chemotherapy versus systemic chemotherapy in patients with peritoneal carcinomatosis of colorectal cancer. *Ann Surg Oncol.* 2008;15(9):2426-2432. doi:10.1245/s10434-008-9966-2

11. Blackham AU, Swett K, Eng C, et al. Perioperative systemic chemotherapy for appendiceal mucinous carcinoma peritonei treated with cytoreductive surgery and hyperthermic intraperitoneal chemotherapy. *J Surg Oncol.* 2014;109(7):740-745. doi:10.1002/jso.23547

12. Quenet F, Elias D, Roca L, et al. A UNICANCER phase III trial of hyperthermic intra-peritoneal chemotherapy (HIPEC) for colorectal peritoneal carcinomatosis (PC): PRODIGE 7. *J Clin Oncol.* 2018;36(18):LBA3503-LBA3503. doi:10.1200/JCO.2018.36.18_suppl.LBA3503

13. Esquivel J, Sugarbaker PH. Clinical presentation of the pseudomyxoma peritonei syndrome. *Br J Surg.* 2000;87(10):1414-1418. doi:10.1046/j.1365-2168.2000.01553.x

14. Acherman YI, Welch LS, Bromley CM, Sugarbaker PH. Clinical presentation of peritoneal mesothelioma. *Tumori.* 2003;89(3):269-273. doi:10.1177/030089160308900307

15. Sugarbaker PH, Welch LS, Mohamed F, Glehen O. A review of peritoneal mesothelioma at the Washington Cancer Institute. *Surg Oncol Clin N Am.* 2003;12(3):605-621, xi. doi:10.1016/s1055-3207(03)00045-0

16. Gupta JP, Jain AK, Agrawal BK, Gupta S. Gastroscopic cytology and biopsies in diagnosis of gastric malignancies. *J Surg Oncol.* 1983;22(1):62-64. doi:10.1002/jso.2930220117

17. Stell DA, Carter CR, Stewart I, Anderson JR. Prospective comparison of laparoscopy, ultrasonography and computed tomography in the staging of gastric cancer. *Br J Surg.* 1996;83(9):1260-1262.

18. Aoyagi T, Terracina KP, Raza A, Takabe K. Current treatment options for colon cancer peritoneal carcinomatosis. *World J Gastroenterol.* 2014;20(35):12493-12500. doi:10.3748/wjg.v20.i35.12493

19. Wagner PL, Austin F, Sathaiah M, et al. Significance of serum tumor marker levels in peritoneal carcinomatosis of appendiceal origin. *Ann Surg Oncol.* 2013;20(2):506-514. doi:10.1245/s10434-012-2627-5

20. Verwaal VJ, Kusamura S, Baratti D, Deraco M. The eligibility for local-regional treatment of peritoneal surface malignancy. *J Surg Oncol.* 2008;98(4):220-223. doi:10.1002/jso.21060

21. Valle M, Federici O, Garofalo A. Patient selection for cytoreductive surgery and hyperthermic intraperitoneal chemotherapy, and role of laparoscopy in diagnosis, staging, and treatment. *Surg Oncol Clin N Am.* 2012;21(4):515-531. doi:10.1016/j.soc.2012.07.005

22. Jacquet P, Jelinek JS, Steves MA, Sugarbaker PH. Evaluation of computed tomography in patients with peritoneal carcinomatosis. *Cancer.* 1993;72(5):1631-1636. doi:10.1016/j.soc.2012.07.005

23. Levy AD, Arnáiz J, Shaw JC, Sobin LH. Primary peritoneal tumors: imaging features with pathologic correlation. *Radiographics.* 2008;28(2):583-607, 621-622. doi:10.1148/rg.282075175

24. Rajeev R, Klooster B, Turaga KK. Impact of surgical volume of centers on post-operative outcomes from cytoreductive surgery and hyperthermic intra-peritoneal chemoperfusion. *J Gastrointest Oncol.* 2016;7(1):122-128. doi:10.3978/j.issn.2078-6891.2015.099

25. Bao P, Bartlett D. Surgical techniques in visceral resection and peritonectomy procedures. *Cancer J.* 2009;15(3):204-211. doi:10.1097/PPO.0b013e3181a9c6f0

26. Sugarbaker PH. Peritonectomy procedures. *Surg Oncol Clin N Am.* 2003;12(3):703-727, xiii. doi:10.1016/s1055-3207(03)00048-6

27. Jafari MD, Halabi WJ, Stamos MJ, et al. Surgical outcomes of hyperthermic intraperitoneal chemotherapy: analysis of the American College of Surgeons National Surgical Quality Improvement Program. *JAMA Surg.* 2014;149(2):170-175. doi:10.1001/jamasurg.2013.3640

28. Foster JM, Sleightholm R, Patel A, et al. Morbidity and mortality rates following cytoreductive surgery combined with hyperthermic intraperitoneal chemotherapy compared with other high-risk surgical oncology procedures. *JAMA Netw Open*. 2019;2(1):e186847. doi:10.1001/jamanetworkopen.2018.6847

29. Birkmeyer JD, Siewers AE, Finlayson EV, et al. Hospital volume and surgical mortality in the United States. *N Engl J Med*. 2002;346(15):1128-1137. doi:10.1056/NEJMsa012337

30. Meza-Perez S, Randall TD. Immunological functions of the omentum. *Trends Immunol*. 2017;38(7):526-536. doi:10.1016/j.it.2017.03.002

31. Koppe MJ, Nagtegaal ID, de Wilt JH, Ceelen WP. Recent insights into the pathophysiology of omental metastases. *J Surg Oncol*. 2014;110(6):670-675. doi 10.1002/jso.23681

32. Carmignani CP, Sugarbaker TA, Bromley CM, Sugarbaker PH. Intraperitoneal cancer dissemination: mechanisms of the patterns of spread. *Cancer Metastasis Rev*. 2003;22(4):465-472. doi:10.1023/a:1023791229361

33. Yang X-J, Huang C-Q, Suo T, et al. Cytoreductive surgery and hyperthermic intraperitoneal chemotherapy improves survival of patients with peritoneal carcinomatosis from gastric cancer: final results of a phase III randomized clinical trial. *Ann Surg Oncol*. 2011;18(6):1575-1581. doi:10.1245/s10434-011-1631-5

34. Glehen O, Kwiatkowski F, Sugarbaker PH, et al. Cytoreductive surgery combined with perioperative intraperitoneal chemotherapy for the management of peritoneal carcinomatosis from colorectal cancer: a multi-institutional study. *J Clin Oncol*. 2004;22(16):3284-3292. doi:10.1200/JCO.2004.10.012

35. Elias D, Glehen O, Pocard M, et al. A comparative study of complete cytoreductive surgery plus intraperitoneal chemotherapy to treat peritoneal dissemination from colon, rectum, small bowel, and nonpseudomyxoma appendix. *Ann Surg*. 2010;251(5):896-901. doi:10.1097/SLA.0b013e3181d9765d

36. Sugarbaker PH. Peritonectomy procedures. *Cancer Treat Res*. 2007;134:247-264. doi:10.1007/978-0-387-48993-3_15

37. Mehta SS, Bhatt A, Glehen O. Cytoreductive surgery and peritonectomy procedures. *Indian J Surg Oncol*. 2016;7(2):139-151. doi:10.1007/s13193-016-0505-5

38. Mercier F, Mohamed F, Cazauran JB, et al. An update of peritonectomy procedures used in cytoreductive surgery for peritoneal malignancy. *Int J Hyperthermia*. 2019;36(1):744-752. doi:10.1080/02656736.2019.1635717

39. Deraco M, Glehen O, Helm CW, Morris DL, van der Speeten K, Sugarbaker PH. *Cytoreductive Surgery & Perioperative Chemotherapy for Peritoneal Surface Malignancy*. Ciné-Med Publishing; 2013.

40. Sugarbaker PH. Cytoreductive surgery and perioperative intraperitoneal chemotherapy as a curative approach to pseudomyxoma peritonei syndrome. *Tumori*. 2001;87(4):S3-S5.

41. Bijelic L, Sugarbaker PH. Cytoreduction of the small bowel surfaces. *J Surg Oncol*. 2008;97(2):176-179. doi:10.1002/jso.20912

42. van Oudheusden TR, Braam HJ, Luyer MD, et al. Peritoneal cancer patients not suitable for cytoreductive surgery and HIPEC during explorative surgery: risk factors, treatment options, and prognosis. *Ann Surg Oncol*. 2015;22(4):1236-1242. doi:10.1245/s10434-014-4148-x

43. Jayakrishnan TT, Zacharias AJ, Sharma A, Pappas SG, Gamb in TC, Turaga KK. Role of laparoscopy in patients with peritoneal metastases considered for cytoreductive surgery and hyperthermic intraperitoneal chemotherapy (HIPEC). *World J Surg Oncol*. 2014;12:270. doi:10.1186/1477-7819-12-270

44. Esquivel J, Chua TC, Stojadinovic A, et al. Accuracy and clinical relevance of computed tomography scan interpretation of peritoneal cancer index in colorectal cancer peritoneal carcinomatosis: a multi-institutional study. *J Surg Oncol*. 2010;102(6):565-570. doi:10.1002/jso.21601

45. von Breitenbuch P, Boerner T, Jeiter T, Piso P, Schlitt HJ. Laparoscopy as a useful selection tool for patients with prior surgery and peritoneal metastases suitable for multimodality treatment strategies. *Surg Endosc*. 2018;32(5):2288-2294. doi:10.1007/s00464-017-5923-0

46. Deraco M, Baratti D, Kusamura S, Laterza B, Balestra MR. Surgical technique of parietal and visceral peritonectomy for peritoneal surface malignancies. *J Surg Oncol*. 2009;100(4):321-328. doi:10.1002/jso.21388

47. Sugarbaker PH. Pseudomyxoma peritonei. A cancer whose biology is characterized by a redistribution phenomenon. *Ann Surg*. 1994;219(2):109-111.

48. Mittal R, Chandramohan A, Moran B. Pseudomyxoma peritonei: natural history and treatment. *Int J Hyperthermia*. 2017;33(5):511-519. doi:10.1080/02656736.2017.1310938

49. Raptopoulos V, Gourtsoyiannis N. Peritoneal carcinomatosis. *Eur Radiol*. 2001;11(11):2195-2206. doi:10.1007/s003300100998

50. Sugarbaker PH. Parietal peritonectomy. *Ann Surg Oncol.* 2012;19(4):1250. doi:10.1245/s10434 -012-2229-2

51. Hallam S, Tyler R, Price M, Beggs A, Youssef H. Meta-analysis of prognostic factors for patients with colorectal peritoneal metastasis undergoing cytoreductive surgery and heated intraperitoneal chemotherapy. *BJS Open.* 2019;3(5):585-594. doi:10.1002/bjs5.50179

52. Ahmed S, Levine EA, Randle RW, et al. Significance of diaphragmatic resections and thoracic chemoperfusion on outcomes of peritoneal surface disease treated with cytoreductive surgery (CRS) and hyperthermic intraperitoneal chemotherapy (HIPEC). *Ann Surg Oncol.* 2014;21(13):4226-4231. doi:10.1245/s10434-014-3891-3

53. Franssen B, Tabrizian P, Weinberg A, et al. Outcome of cytoreductive surgery and hyperthermic intraperitoneal chemotherapy on patients with diaphragmatic involvement. *Ann Surg Oncol.* 2015;22(5):1639-1644. doi:10.1245/s10434-014-4083-x

54. Grotz TE, Mansfield PF, Royal RE, et al. Intrathoracic chemoperfusion decreases recurrences in patients with full-thickness diaphragm involvement with mucinous appendiceal adenocarcinoma. *Ann Surg Oncol.* 2016;23(9):2914-2919. doi:10.1245/s10434-016-5209-0

55. Sullivan BJ, Bekhor EY, Carpiniello M, et al. Diaphragmatic peritoneal stripping versus full-thickness resection in CRS/HIPEC: is there a difference? *Ann Surg Oncol.* 2020;27(1):250-258. doi:10.1245/s10434-019-07797-8

56. Lampl B, Leebmann H, Mayr M, Piso P. Rare diaphragmatic complications following cytoreductive surgery and HIPEC: report of two cases. *Surg Today.* 2014;44(2):383-386. doi:10.1007 /s00595-012-0445-9

57. Halkia E, Efstathiou E, Spiliotis J, Romanidis K, Salmas M. Management of diaphragmatic peritoneal carcinomatosis: surgical anatomy guidelines and results. *J BUON.* 2014;19(1):29-33.

58. Healy JC, Reznek RH. The peritoneum, mesenteries and omenta: normal anatomy and pathological processes. *Eur Radiol.* 1998;8(6):886-900. doi:10.1007/s003300050485

59. Meyers MA, Oliphant M, Berne AS, Feldberg MA. The peritoneal ligaments and mesenteries: pathways of intraabdominal spread of disease. *Radiology.* 1987;163(3):593-604. doi:10.1148 /radiology.163.3.3575702

60. Bhatt A, Glehen O. Extent of peritoneal resection for peritoneal metastases: looking beyond a complete cytoreduction. *Ann Surg Oncol.* 2020;27(5):1458-1470. doi:10.1245/s10434-020-08208-z

61. Sugarbaker PH. Management of peritoneal metastases—basic concepts. *J BUON.* 2015;20(suppl 1): S2-S11.

62. Hertel H, Diebolder H, Herrmann J, et al. Is the decision for colorectal resection justified by histopathologic findings: a prospective study of 100 patients with advanced ovarian cancer. *Gynecol Oncol.* 2001;83(3):481-484. doi:10.1006/gyno.2001.6338

63. Sakakura C, Hagiwara A, Yamazaki J, et al. Management of postoperative follow-up and surgical treatment for Krukenberg tumor from colorectal cancers. *Hepatogastroenterology.* 2004;51(59):1350-1353.

64. Banerjee S, Kapur S, Moran BJ. The role of prophylactic oophorectomy in women undergoing surgery for colorectal cancer. *Colorectal Dis.* 2005;7(3):214-217. doi:10.1111/j.1463-1318.2005.00770.x

65. Yada-Hashimoto N, Yamamoto T, Kamiura S, et al. Metastatic ovarian tumors: a review of 64 cases. *Gynecol Oncol.* 2003;89(2):314-317. doi:10.1016/s0090-8258(03)00075-1

66. Evers DJ, Verwaal VJ. Indication for oophorectomy during cytoreduction for intraperitoneal metastatic spread of colorectal or appendiceal origin. *Br J Surg.* 2011;98(2):287-292. doi:10.1002/bjs.7303

67. Braam HJ, van Oudheusden TR, de Hingh IH, et al. Urological procedures in patients with peritoneal carcinomatosis of colorectal cancer treated with HIPEC: morbidity and survival analysis. *Anticancer Res.* 2015;35(1):295-300.

68. Tan GHC, Shannon NB, Chia CS, Lee LS, Soo KC, Teo MCC. The impact of urological resection and reconstruction on patients undergoing cytoreductive surgery (CRS) and hyperthermic intraperitoneal chemotherapy (HIPEC). *Asian J Urol.* 2018;5(3):194-198. doi:10.1016/j.ajur.2017.09.003

69. Coccolini F, Lotti M, Manfredi R, et al. Ureteral stenting in cytoreductive surgery plus hyperthermic intraperitoneal chemotherapy as a routine procedure: evidence and necessity. *Urol Int.* 2012;89(3):307-310. doi:10.1159/000339920

70. Abu-Zaid A, Abou Al-Shaar H, Azzam A, et al. Routine ureteric stenting before cytoreductive surgery plus hyperthermic intraperitoneal chemotherapy in managing peritoneal carcinomatosis from gynecologic malignancies: a single-center experience. *Ir J Med Sci.* 2017;186(2):269-273. doi:10.1007/s11845-016-1452-4

71. Pinar U, Tremblay J-F, Passot G, et al. Reconstruction after ureteral resection during HIPEC surgery: re-implantation with uretero-neocystostomy seems safer than end-to-end anastomosis. *J Visc Surg.* 2017;154(4):227-230. doi:10.1016/j.jviscsurg.2017.01.002

72. Dhar P, Chattopadhyay K, Bhattacharyya D, Roychoudhury A, Biswas A, Ghosh S. Antioxidative effect of conjugated linolenic acid in diabetic and non-diabetic blood: an in vitro study. *J Oleo Sci.* 2006;56(1):19-24. doi:10.5650/jos.56.19

73. Bhatt A, Bhamre R, Rohila J, Kalikar V, Desouza A, Saklani A. Patients with extensive regional lymph node involvement (pN2) following potentially curative surgery for colorectal cancer are at increased risk for developing peritoneal metastases: a retrospective single-institution study. *Colorectal Dis.* 2019;21(3):287-296. doi:10.1111/codi.14481

74. Enblad M, Graf W, Birgisson H. Risk factors for appendiceal and colorectal peritoneal metastases. *Eur J Surg Oncol.* 2018;44(7):997-1005. doi:10.1016/j.ejso.2018.02.245

75. Spelt L, Sasor A, Ansari D, Andersson R. Pattern of tumour growth of the primary colon cancer predicts long-term outcome after resection of liver metastases. *Scand J Gastroenterol.* 2016;51(10):1233-1238. doi:10.1080/00365521.2016.1190400

76. Pelz JO, Stojadinovic A, Nissan A, Hohenberger W, Esquivel J. Evaluation of a peritoneal surface disease severity score in patients with colon cancer with peritoneal carcinomatosis. *J Surg Oncol.* 2009;99(1):9-15. doi:10.1002/jso.21169

77. Yoon W, Alame A, Berri R. Peritoneal Surface Disease Severity Score as a predictor of resectability in the treatment of peritoneal surface malignancies. *Am J Surg.* 2014;207(3):403-407. doi:10.1016/j.amjsurg.2013.09.021

78. Furuhata T, Okita K, Nishidate T, et al. Oncological benefit of primary tumor resection with high tie lymph node dissection in unresectable colorectal cancer with synchronous peritoneal metastasis: a propensity score analysis of data from a multi-institute database. *Int J Clin Oncol.* 2015;20(5):922-927. doi:10.1007/s10147-015-0815-6

79. Sato H, Kotake K, Sugihara K, et al. Clinicopathological factors associated with recurrence and prognosis after R0 resection for stage IV colorectal cancer with peritoneal metastasis. *Dig Surg.* 2016;33(5):382-391. doi:10.1159/000444097

80. Bonnot PE, Piessen G, Kepenekian V, et al. Cytoreductive surgery with or without hyperthermic intraperitoneal chemotherapy for gastric cancer with peritoneal metastases (CYTO-CHIP study): a propensity score analysis. *J Clin Oncol.* 2019;37(23):2028-2040. doi:10.1200/JCO .18.01688

81. van der Kaaij RT, Wassenaar ECE, Koemans WJ, et al. Treatment of PERItoneal disease in Stomach Cancer with cytOreductive surgery and hyperthermic intraPEritoneal chemotherapy: PERI-SCOPE I initial results. *Br J Surg.* 2020;107(11):1520-1528. doi:10.1002/bjs.11588

82. Kusamura S, O'Dwyer ST, Baratti D, Younan R, Deraco M. Technical aspects of cytoreductive surgery. *J Surg Oncol.* 2008;98(4):232-236. doi:10.1002/jso.21058

83. Wiseman JT, Kimbrough C, Beal EW, et al. Predictors of anastomotic failure after cytoreductive surgery and hyperthermic intraperitoneal chemotherapy: does technique matter? *Ann Surg Oncol.* 2020;27(3):783-792. doi:10.1245/s10434-019-07964-x

84. Saxena A, Valle SJ, Liauw W, Morris DL. Limited synchronous hepatic resection does not compromise peri-operative outcomes or survival after cytoreductive surgery and hyperthermic intraperitoneal chemotherapy. *J Surg Oncol.* 2017;115(4):417-424. doi:10.1002/jso.24543

85. Delhorme J-B, Dupont-Kazma L, Addeo P, et al. Peritoneal carcinomatosis with synchronous liver metastases from colorectal cancer: who will benefit from complete cytoreductive surgery? *Int J Surg.* 2016;25:98-105. doi:10.1016/j.ijsu.2015.11.025

86. Lorimier G, Linot B, Paillocher N, et al. Curative cytoreductive surgery followed by hyperthermic intraperitoneal chemotherapy in patients with peritoneal carcinomatosis and synchronous resectable liver metastases arising from colorectal cancer. *Eur J Surg Oncol.* 2017;43(1):150-158. doi:10.1016/j.ejso.2016.09.010

87. Maggiori L, Goéré D, Viana B, et al. Should patients with peritoneal carcinomatosis of colorectal origin with synchronous liver metastases be treated with a curative intent? A case-control study. *Ann Surg.* 2013;258(1):116-121. doi:10.1097/SLA.0b013e3182778089

88. Cloyd JM, Abdel-Misih S, Hays J, Dillhoff ME, Pawlik TM, Schmidt C. Impact of synchronous liver resection on the perioperative outcomes of patients undergoing CRS-HIPEC. *J Gastrointest Surg.* 2018;22(9):1576-1584. doi:10.1007/s11605-018-3784-z

89. Mouw TJ, Lu J, Woody-Fowler M, et al. Morbidity and mortality of synchronous hepatectomy with cytoreductive surgery/hyperthermic intraperitoneal chemotherapy (CRS/HIPEC). *J Gastrointest Oncol.* 2018;9(5):828-832. doi:10.21037/jgo.2018.06.04

90. Navez J, Remue C, Leonard D, et al. Surgical treatment of colorectal cancer with peritoneal and liver metastases using combined liver and cytoreductive surgery and hyperthermic intraperitoneal chemotherapy: report from a single-centre experience. *Ann Surg Oncol.* 2016;23(suppl 5):666-673. doi:10.1245/s10434-016-5543-2

91. Abreu de Carvalho LF, Scuderi V, Maes H, et al. Simultaneous parenchyma-preserving liver resection, cytoreductive surgery and intraperitoneal chemotherapy for stage IV colorectal cancer. *Acta Chir Belg.* 2015;115(4):261-267. doi:10.1080/00015458.2015.11681109

92. Saxena A, Liauw W, Morris DL. Splenectomy is an independent risk factor for poorer perioperative outcomes after cytoreductive surgery and hyperthermic intraperitoneal chemotherapy: an analysis of 936 procedures. *J Gastrointest Oncol.* 2017;8(4):737-746. doi:10.21037/jgo.2017.07.09

93. Dagbert F, Thievenaz R, Decullier E, et al. Splenectomy increases postoperative complications following cytoreductive surgery and hyperthermic intraperitoneal chemotherapy. *Ann Surg Oncol.* 2016;23(6):1980-1985. doi:10.1245/s10434-016-5147-x

94. Votanopoulos K, Ihemelandu C, Shen P, Stewart J, Russell G, Levine EA. A comparison of hematologic toxicity profiles after heated intraperitoneal chemotherapy with oxaliplatin and mitomycin C. *J Surg Res.* 2013;179(1):e133-e139. doi:10.1016/j.jss.2012.01.015

95. Dagbert F, Passot G, Glehen O, Bakrin N. Glisson capsulectomy for extensive superficial liver involvement in peritoneal carcinomatosis (with video). *J Visc Surg.* 2015;152(5):332-333. doi:10.1016/j.jviscsurg.2015.08.002

96. Sugarbaker PH. The hepatic bridge. *Eur J Surg Oncol.* 2018;44(7):1083-1086. doi:10.1016/j.ejso.2018.03.031

97. Sugarbaker PH. Pont hepatique (hepatic bridge), an important anatomic structure in cytoreductive surgery. *J Surg Oncol.* 2010;101(3):251-252. doi:10.1002/jso.21478

98. Veerapong J, Solomon H, Helm CW. Division of the pont hepatique of the liver in cytoreductive surgery for peritoneal malignancy. *Gynecol Oncol.* 2013;128(1):133. doi:10.1016/j.ygyno.2012.09.018

99. Gold JS, Are C, Kornprat P, et al. Increased use of parenchymal-sparing surgery for bilateral liver metastases from colorectal cancer is associated with improved mortality without change in oncologic outcome: trends in treatment over time in 440 patients. *Ann Surg.* 2008;247(1):109-117. doi:10.1097/SLA.0b013e3181557e47

100. Hata S, Imamura H, Aoki T, et al. Value of visual inspection, bimanual palpation, and intraoperative ultrasonography during hepatic resection for liver metastases of colorectal carcinoma. *World J Surg.* 2011;35(12):2779-2787. doi:10.1007/s00268-011-1264-7

101. Gurusamy KS, Pamecha V, Sharma D, Davidson BR. Techniques for liver parenchymal transection in liver resection. *Cochrane Database Syst Rev.* 2009;(1):CD006880. doi:10.1002/14651858.CD006880.pub2

102. Spratt JS, Adcock RA, Muskovin M, Sherrill W, McKeown J. Clinical delivery system for intraperitoneal hyperthermic chemotherapy. *Cancer Res.* 1980;40(2):256-260.

103. Sticca RP, Dach BW. Rationale for hyperthermia with intraoperative intraperitoneal chemotherapy agents. *Surg Oncol Clin N Am.* 2003;12(3):689-701. doi:10.1002/14651858.CD006880.pub2

104. Schaaf L, Schwab M, Ulmer C, et al. Hyperthermia synergizes with chemotherapy by inhibiting PARP1-dependent DNA replication arrest. *Cancer Res.* 2016;76(10):2868-2875. doi:10.1158/0008-5472.CAN-15-2908

105. Elias D, Lefevre JH, Chevalier J, et al. Complete cytoreductive surgery plus intraperitoneal chemohyperthermia with oxaliplatin for peritoneal carcinomatosis of colorectal origin. *J Clin Oncol.* 2009;27(5):681-685. doi:10.1200/JCO.2008.19.7160

106. Franko J, Ibrahim Z, Gusani NJ, Holtzman MP, Bartlett DL, Zeh HJ III. Cytoreductive surgery and hyperthermic intraperitoneal chemoperfusion versus systemic chemotherapy alone for colorectal peritoneal carcinomatosis. *Cancer.* 2010;116(16):3756-3762. doi:10.1002/cncr.25116

107. Verwaal VJ, van Ruth S, de Bree E, et al. Randomized trial of cytoreduction and hyperthermic intraperitoneal chemotherapy versus systemic chemotherapy and palliative surgery in patients with peritoneal carcinomatosis of colorectal cancer. *J Clin Oncol.* 2003;21(20):3737-3743. doi:10.1200/JCO.2003.04.187

108. van Driel WJ, Koole SN, Sikorska K, et al. Hyperthermic intraperitoneal chemotherapy in ovarian cancer. *N Engl J Med.* 2018;378(3):230-240. doi:10.1056/NEJMoa1708618

109. Sugarbaker PH. Successful management of microscopic residual disease in large bowel cancer. *Cancer Chemother Pharmacol.* 1999;43 suppl:S15-S25. doi:10.1007/s002800051093

110. Levine EA, Votanopoulos KI, Shen P, et al. A multicenter randomized trial to evaluate hematologic toxicities after hyperthermic intraperitoneal chemotherapy with oxaliplatin or mitomycin in patients with appendiceal tumors. *J Am Coll Surg.* 2018;226(4):434-443. doi:10.1016/j.jamcollsurg.2017.12.027

111. Gouy S, Ferron G, Glehen O, et al. Results of a multicenter phase I dose-finding trial of hyperthermic intraperitoneal cisplatin after neoadjuvant chemotherapy and complete cytoreductive surgery and followed by maintenance bevacizumab in initially unresectable ovarian cancer. *Gynecol Oncol.* 2016;142(2):237-242. doi:10.1016/j.ygyno.2016.05.032

112. Badrudin D, Sideris L, Perrault-Mercier C, Hubert J, Leblond FA, Dubé P. Comparison of open and closed abdomen techniques for the delivery of intraperitoneal pemetrexed using a murine model. *J Surg Oncol*. 2018;117(6):1318-1322. doi:10.1002/jso.24960

113. Halkia E, Tsochrinis A, Vassiliadou DT, et al. Peritoneal carcinomatosis: intraoperative parameters in open (coliseum) versus closed abdomen HIPEC. *Int J Surg Oncol*. 2015;2015:610597. doi:10.1155/2015/610597

114. Rodríguez Silva C, Moreno Ruiz FJ, Bellido Estévez I, et al. Are there intra-operative hemodynamic differences between the coliseum and closed HIPEC techniques in the treatment of peritoneal metastasis? A retrospective cohort study. *World J Surg Oncol*. 2017;15(1):51. doi:10.1186/s12957-017-1119-2

115. Sugarbaker PH. Comprehensive management of peritoneal surface malignancy using cytoreductive surgery and perioperative intraperitoneal chemotherapy: the Washington Cancer Institute approach. *Expert Opin Pharmacother*. 2009;10(12):1965-1977. doi:10.1517/14656560903044974

116. Neuss MN, Gilmore TR, Belderson KM, et al. 2016 Updated American Society of Clinical Oncology/Oncology Nursing Society Chemotherapy Administration Safety Standards, including standards for pediatric oncology. *Oncol Nurs Forum*. 2017;44(1):31-43. doi:10.1188/17.ONF.31-43

117. Turaga K, Levine E, Barone R, et al. Consensus guidelines from the American Society of Peritoneal Surface Malignancies on standardizing the delivery of hyperthermic intraperitoneal chemotherapy (HIPEC) in colorectal cancer patients in the United States. *Ann Surg Oncol*. 2014;21(5):1501-1505. doi:10.1245/s10434-013-3061-z

118. Dodson RM, Kuncewitch M, Votanopoulos KI, Shen P, Levine EA. Techniques for cytoreductive surgery with hyperthermic intraperitoneal chemotherapy. *Ann Surg Oncol*. 2018;25(8):2152-2158. doi:10.1245/s10434-018-6336-6

119. Baumgartner JM, Kelly KJ, Lowy AM. Safety considerations and occupational hazards. In: Ceelen WP, Levine EA, eds. *Intraperitoneal Cancer Therapy: Principles and Practice*. CRC Press; 2016:317-324.

120. Goldenshluger M, Zippel D, Ben-Yaacov A, et al. Core body temperature but not intraabdominal pressure predicts postoperative complications following closed-system hyperthermic intraperitoneal chemotherapy (HIPEC) administration. *Ann Surg Oncol*. 2018;25(3):660-666. doi:10.1245/s10434-017-6279-3

121. Howell SB, Pfeifle CL, Wung WE, et al. Intraperitoneal cisplatin with systemic thiosulfate protection. *Ann Intern Med*. 1982;97(6):845-851. doi:10.7326/0003-4819-97-6-845

122. Bartlett DL, Buell JF, Libutti SK, et al. A phase I trial of continuous hyperthermic peritoneal perfusion with tumor necrosis factor and cisplatin in the treatment of peritoneal carcinomatosis. *Cancer*. 1998;83(6):1251-1261. doi:10.1002/(SICI)1097-0142(19980915)83:6<1251::AID-CNCR27>3.0.CO;2-3

123. Mehta AM, Van den Hoven JM, Rosing H, et al. Stability of oxaliplatin in chloride-containing carrier solutions used in hyperthermic intraperitoneal chemotherapy. *Int J Pharm*. 2015;479(1):23-27. doi:10.1016/j.ijpharm.2014.12.025

124. da Silva RG, Sugarbaker PH. Analysis of prognostic factors in seventy patients having a complete cytoreduction plus perioperative intraperitoneal chemotherapy for carcinomatosis from colorectal cancer. *J Am Coll Surg*. 2006;203(6):878-886. doi:10.1016/j.jamcollsurg.2006.08.024

125. Elias D, Gilly F, Boutitie F, et al. Peritoneal colorectal carcinomatosis treated with surgery and perioperative intraperitoneal chemotherapy: retrospective analysis of 523 patients from a multicentric French study. *J Clin Oncol*. 2010;28(1):63-68. doi:10.1200/JCO.2009.23.9285

126. Verwaal VJ, van Tinteren H, van Ruth S, Zoetmulder FA. Predicting the survival of patients with peritoneal carcinomatosis of colorectal origin treated by aggressive cytoreduction and hyperthermic intraperitoneal chemotherapy. *Br J Surg*. 2004;91(6):739-746. doi:10.1002/bjs.4516

127. Sugarbaker PH. Intraperitoneal chemotherapy and cytoreductive surgery for the prevention and treatment of peritoneal carcinomatosis and sarcomatosis. *Semin Surg Oncol*. 1998;14(3):254-261. doi:10.1002/(sici)1098-2388(199804/05)14:3<254::aid-ssu10>3.0.co;2-u

128. Elias D, Souadka A, Fayard F, et al. Variation in the peritoneal cancer index scores between surgeons and according to when they are determined (before or after cytoreductive surgery). *Eur J Surg Oncol*. 2012;38(6):503-508. doi:10.1016/j.ejso.2012.01.001

129. Esquivel J, Sticca R, Sugarbaker P, et al. Cytoreductive surgery and hyperthermic intraperitoneal chemotherapy in the management of peritoneal surface malignancies of colonic origin: a consensus statement. Society of Surgical Oncology. *Ann Surg Oncol*. 2007;14(1):128-133. doi:10.1245/s10434-006-9185-7

130. Portilla AG, Shigeki K, Dario B, Marcello D. The intraoperative staging systems in the management of peritoneal surface malignancy. *J Surg Oncol*. 2008;98(4):228-231. doi:10.1002/jso.21068

131. Gilly FN, Beaujard A, Glehen O, et al. Peritonectomy combined with intraperitoneal chemohyperthermia in abdominal cancer with peritoneal carcinomatosis: phase I-II study. *Anticancer Res.* 1999;19(3B):2317-2321.

132. Gilly FN, Carry PY, Sayag AC, et al. Regional chemotherapy (with mitomycin C) and intraoperative hyperthermia for digestive cancers with peritoneal carcinomatosis. *Hepatogastroenterology.* 1994;41(2):124-129.

133. Harmon RL, Sugarbaker PH. Prognostic indicators in peritoneal carcinomatosis from gastrointestinal cancer. *Int Semin Surg Oncol.* 2005;2(1):3. doi:10.1186/1477-7800-2-3

134. Prada-Villaverde A, Esquivel J, Lowy AM, et al. The American Society of Peritoneal Surface Malignancies evaluation of HIPEC with mitomycin C versus oxaliplatin in 539 patients with colon cancer undergoing a complete cytoreductive surgery. *J Surg Oncol.* 2014;110(7):779-785. doi:10.1002/jso.23728

135. Simkens GA, van Oudheusden TR, Nieboer D, et al. Development of a prognostic nomogram for patients with peritoneally metastasized colorectal cancer treated with cytoreductive surgery and HIPEC. *Ann Surg Oncol.* 2016;23(13):4214-4221. doi:10.1245/s10434-016-5211-6

136. Chua TC, Moran BJ, Sugarbaker PH, et al. Early- and long-term outcome data of patients with pseudomyxoma peritonei from appendiceal origin treated by a strategy of cytoreductive surgery and hyperthermic intraperitoneal chemotherapy. *J Clin Oncol.* 2012;30(20):2449-2456. doi:10.1200/JCO.2011.39.7166

137. Kusamura S, Baratti D, Deraco M. Multidimensional analysis of the learning curve for cytoreductive surgery and hyperthermic intraperitoneal chemotherapy in peritoneal surface malignancies. *Ann Surg.* 2012;255(2):348-356. doi:10.1097/SLA.0b013e3182436c28

138. Fichmann D, Roth L, Raptis DA, et al. Standard operating procedures for anesthesia management in cytoreductive surgery and hyperthermic intraperitoneal chemotherapy improve patient outcomes: a patient cohort analysis. *Ann Surg Oncol.* 2019;26(11):3652-3662. doi:10.1245/s10434-019-07644-w

139. Baratti D, Kusamura S, Iusco D, et al. Postoperative complications after cytoreductive surgery and hyperthermic intraperitoneal chemotherapy affect long-term outcome of patients with peritoneal metastases from colorectal cancer: a two-center study of 101 patients. *Dis Colon Rectum.* 2014;57(7):858-868. doi:10.1097/DCR.0000000000000149

140. Choudry MHA, Shuai Y, Jones HL, et al. Postoperative complications independently predict cancer-related survival in peritoneal malignancies. *Ann Surg Oncol.* 2018;25(13):3950-3959. doi:10.1245/s10434-018-6823-9

141. Sugarbaker PH. Management of peritoneal-surface malignancy: the surgeon's role. *Langenbecks Arch Surg.* 1999;384(6):576-587. doi:10.1007/s004230050246

142. Yonemura Y, Canbay E, Ishibashi H. Prognostic factors of peritoneal metastases from colorectal cancer following cytoreductive surgery and perioperative chemotherapy. *ScientificWorldJournal.* 2013;2013:978394. doi:10.1155/2013/978394

143. Goéré D, Souadka A, Faron M, et al. Extent of colorectal peritoneal carcinomatosis: attempt to define a threshold above which HIPEC does not offer survival benefit: a comparative study. *Ann Surg Oncol.* 2015;22(9):2958-2964. doi:10.1245/s10434-015-4387-5

144. Moher D, Liberati A, Tetzlaff J, Altman DG, PRISMA Group. Preferred reporting items for systematic reviews and meta-analyses: the PRISMA statement. *PLoS Med.* 2009;6(7):e1000097. doi:10.1371/journal.pmed.1000097

145. Guyatt GH, Oxman AD, Vist GE, et al. GRADE: an emerging consensus on rating quality of evidence and strength of recommendations. *BMJ.* 2008;336(7650):924-926. doi:10.1136/bmj.39489.470347.AD

146. Cashin PH, Dranichnikov F, Mahteme H. Cytoreductive surgery and hyperthermic intra-peritoneal chemotherapy treatment of colorectal peritoneal metastases: cohort analysis of high volume disease and cure rate. *J Surg Oncol.* 2014;110(2):203-206. doi:10.1002/jso.23610

147. Huang C-Q, Yang X-J, Yu Y, et al. Cytoreductive surgery plus hyperthermic intraperitoneal chemotherapy improves survival for patients with peritoneal carcinomatosis from colorectal cancer: a phase II study from a Chinese center. *PloS One.* 2014;9(9):e108509. doi:10.1371/journal.pone.0108509

148. Robella M, Vaira M, Marsanic P, et al. Treatment of peritoneal carcinomatosis from colonic cancer by cytoreduction, peritonectomy and HIPEC: preliminary results in highly selected patients. *Minerva Chir.* 2013;68(6):551-558.

149. Brandl A, Weiss S, von Winterfeld M, et al. Predictive value of peritoneal cancer index for survival in patients with mucinous peritoneal malignancies treated with cytoreductive surgery and hyperthermic intraperitoneal chemotherapy: a single centre experience. *Int J Hyperthermia.* 2018;34(5):512-517. doi:10.1080/02656736.2017.1351627

150. Elias D, Blot F, El Otmany A, et al. Curative treatment of peritoneal carcinomatosis arising from colorectal cancer by complete resection and intraperitoneal chemotherapy. *Cancer.* 2001;92(1):71-76. doi:10.1002/1097-0142(20010701)92:1<71::aid-cncr1293>3.0.co;2-9

151. Elias D, Mariani A, Cloutier A-S, et al. Modified selection criteria for complete cytoreductive surgery plus HIPEC based on peritoneal cancer index and small bowel involvement for peritoneal carcinomatosis of colorectal origin. *Eur J Surg Oncol.* 2014;40(11):1467-1473. doi:10.1016/j.ejso.2014.06.006

152. Goéré D, Malka D, Tzanis D, et al. Is there a possibility of a cure in patients with colorectal peritoneal carcinomatosis amenable to complete cytoreductive surgery and intraperitoneal chemotherapy? *Ann Surg.* 2013;257(6):1065-1071. doi:10.1097/SLA.0b013e31827e9289

153. Hompes D, D'Hoore A, Van Cutsem E, et al. The treatment of peritoneal carcinomatosis of colorectal cancer with complete cytoreductive surgery and hyperthermic intraperitoneal peroperative chemotherapy (HIPEC) with oxaliplatin: a Belgian multicentre prospective phase II clinical study. *Ann Surg Oncol.* 2012;19(7):2186-2194. doi:10.1245/s10434-012-2264-z

154. Tabrizian P, Shrager B, Jibara G, et al. Cytoreductive surgery and hyperthermic intraperitoneal chemotherapy for peritoneal carcinomatosis: outcomes from a single tertiary institution. *J Gastrointest Surg.* 2014;18(5):1024-1031. doi:10.1007/s11605-014-2477-5

155. Yan TD, Morris DL. Cytoreductive surgery and perioperative intraperitoneal chemotherapy for isolated colorectal peritoneal carcinomatosis: experimental therapy or standard of care? *Ann Surg.* 2008;248(5):829-835. doi:10.1097/SLA.0b013e31818a15b5

156. Quénet F, Elias D, Roca L, et al. Cytoreductive surgery plus hyperthermic intraperitoneal chemotherapy versus cytoreductive surgery alone for colorectal peritoneal metastases (PRODIGE 7): a multicentre, randomised, open-label, phase 3 trial. *Lancet Oncol.* 2021;22(2):256-266. doi:10.1016/S1470-2045(20)30599-4

157. Ceelen W. HIPEC with oxaliplatin for colorectal peritoneal metastasis: the end of the road? *Eur J Surg Oncol.* 2019;45(3):400-402. doi:10.1016/j.ejso.2018.10.542

158. Koh CE, Ansari N, Morris D, Moran B, Australian and New Zealand Peritoneal Malignancy Collaborative. Beware mis-representation of PRODIGE 7: danger of throwing out the cytoreductive surgery baby with the hyperthermic intraperitoneal chemotherapy bathwater. *ANZ J Surg.* 2019;89(9):992-994. doi:10.1111/ans.15424

159. Polanco PM, Ding Y, Knox JM, et al. Outcomes of cytoreductive surgery and hyperthermic intraperitoneal chemoperfusion in patients with high-grade, high-volume disseminated mucinous appendiceal neoplasms. *Ann Surg Oncol.* 2016;23(2):382-390. doi:10.1245/s10434-015-4838-z

160. El Halabi H, Gushchin V, Francis J, et al. The role of cytoreductive surgery and heated intraperitoneal chemotherapy (CRS/HIPEC) in patients with high-grade appendiceal carcinoma and extensive peritoneal carcinomatosis. *Ann Surg Oncol.* 2012;19(1):110-114. doi:10.1245/s10434-011-1840-y

161. Yan TD, Bijelic L, Sugarbaker PH. Critical analysis of treatment failure after complete cytoreductive surgery and perioperative intraperitoneal chemotherapy for peritoneal dissemination from appendiceal mucinous neoplasms. *Ann Surg Oncol.* 2007;14(8):2289-2299. doi:10.1245/s10434-007-9462-0

162. Chua TC, Yan TD, Smigielski ME, et al. Long-term survival in patients with pseudomyxoma peritonei treated with cytoreductive surgery and perioperative intraperitoneal chemotherapy: 10 years of experience from a single institution. *Ann Surg Oncol.* 2009;16(7):1903-1911. doi:10.1245/s10434-009-0341-8

163. Jimenez W, Sardi A, Nieroda C, et al. Predictive and prognostic survival factors in peritoneal carcinomatosis from appendiceal cancer after cytoreductive surgery with hyperthermic intraperitoneal chemotherapy. *Ann Surg Oncol.* 2014;21(13):4218-4225. doi:10.1245/s10434-014-3869-1

164. Votanopoulos KI, Russell G, Randle RW, Shen P, Stewart JH, Levine EA. Peritoneal surface disease (PSD) from appendiceal cancer treated with cytoreductive surgery (CRS) and hyperthermic intraperitoneal chemotherapy (HIPEC): overview of 481 cases. *Ann Surg Oncol.* 2015;22(4):1274-1279. doi:10.1245/s10434-014-4147-y

165. Benhaim L, Faron M, Gelli M, et al. Survival after complete cytoreductive surgery and HIPEC for extensive pseudomyxoma peritonei. *Surg Oncol.* 2019;29:78-83. doi:10.1016/j.suronc.2019.03.004

166. Bekhor E, Carr J, Hofstedt M, et al. The safety of iterative cytoreductive surgery and HIPEC for peritoneal carcinomatosis: a high volume center prospectively maintained database analysis. *Ann Surg Oncol.* 2019;27(5):1448-1455. doi:10.1245/s10434-019-08141-w

167. Chua TC, Quinn LE, Zhao J, Morris DL. Iterative cytoreductive surgery and hyperthermic intraperitoneal chemotherapy for recurrent peritoneal metastases. *J Surg Oncol.* 2013;108(2):81-88. doi:10.1002/jso.23356

168. Choudry HA, Bednar F, Shuai Y, et al. Repeat cytoreductive surgery-hyperthermic intraperitoneal chemoperfusion is feasible and offers survival benefit in select patients with peritoneal metastases. *Ann Surg Oncol.* 2019;26(5):1445-1453. doi:10.1245/s10434-019-07218-w

169. Kitai T, Yamanaka K, Sugimoto N, Inamoto O. Surgical management for peritoneal carcinomatosis of appendiceal origin with a high-tumor burden. *Surg Today*. 2020;50(2):171-177. doi:10.1007/s00595-019-01856-z

170. Elias D, Gilly F, Quenet F, et al. Pseudomyxoma peritonei: a French multicentric study of 301 patients treated with cytoreductive surgery and intraperitoneal chemotherapy. *Eur J Surg Oncol*. 2010;36(5):456-462. doi:10.1016/j.ejso.2010.01.006

171. Votanopoulos KI, Bartlett D, Moran B, et al. PCI is not predictive of survival after complete CRS/HIPEC in peritoneal dissemination from high-grade appendiceal primaries. *Ann Surg Oncol*. 2018;25(3):674-678. doi:10.1245/s10434-017-6315-3

172. Aziz O, Jaradat I, Chakrabarty B, et al. Predicting survival after cytoreductive surgery and hyperthermic intraperitoneal chemotherapy for appendix adenocarcinoma. *Dis Colon Rectum*. 2018;61(7):795-802. doi:10.1097/DCR.0000000000001076

173. Lieu CH, Lambert LA, Wolff RA, et al. Systemic chemotherapy and surgical cytoreduction for poorly differentiated and signet ring cell adenocarcinomas of the appendix. *Ann Oncol*. 2012;23(3):652-658. doi:10.1093/annonc/mdr279

174. Cioppa T, Vaira M, Bing C, D'Amico S, Bruscino A, De Simone M. Cytoreduction and hyperthermic intraperitoneal chemotherapy in the treatment of peritoneal carcinomatosis from pseudomyxoma peritonei. *World J Gastroenterol*. 2008;14(44):6817-6823. doi:10.3748/wjg.14.6817

175. Di Vita M, Cappellani A, Piccolo G, et al. The role of HIPEC in the treatment of peritoneal carcinomatosis from gastric cancer: between lights and shadows. *Anticancer Drugs*. 2015;26(2):123-138. doi:10.1097/CAD.0000000000000179

176. Glehen O, Gilly FN, Arvieux C, et al. Peritoneal carcinomatosis from gastric cancer: a multi-institutional study of 159 patients treated by cytoreductive surgery combined with perioperative intraperitoneal chemotherapy. *Ann Surg Oncol*. 2010;17(9):2370-2377. doi:10.1245/s10434-010-1039-7

177. Yonemura Y, Elnemr A, Endou Y, et al. Multidisciplinary therapy for treatment of patients with peritoneal carcinomatosis from gastric cancer. *World J Gastrointest Oncol*. 2010;2(2):85-97. doi:10.4251/wjgo.v2.i2.85

178. Rau B, Brandl A, Piso P, et al. Peritoneal metastasis in gastric cancer: results from the German database. *Gastric Cancer*. 2020;23(1):11-22. doi:10.1007/s10120-019-00978-0

179. Chia CS, You B, Decullier E, et al. Patients with peritoneal carcinomatosis from gastric cancer treated with cytoreductive surgery and hyperthermic intraperitoneal chemotherapy: is cure a possibility? *Ann Surg Oncol*. 2016;23(6):1971-1979. doi:10.1245/s10434-015-5081-3

180. Yang X-J, Li Y, Yonemura Y. Cytoreductive surgery plus hyperthermic intraperitoneal chemotherapy to treat gastric cancer with ascites and/or peritoneal carcinomatosis: results from a Chinese center. *J Surg Oncol*. 2010;101(6):457-464. doi:10.1002/jso.21519

181. Canbay E, Mizumoto A, Ichinose M, et al. Outcome data of patients with peritoneal carcinomatosis from gastric origin treated by a strategy of bidirectional chemotherapy prior to cytoreductive surgery and hyperthermic intraperitoneal chemotherapy in a single specialized center in Japan. *Ann Surg Oncol*. 2014;21(4):1147-1152. doi:10.1245/s10434-013-3443-2

182. Hotopp T. HIPEC and CRS in peritoneal metastatic gastric cancer—who really benefits? *Surg Oncol*. 2019;28:159-166. doi:10.1016/j.suronc.2019.01.005

183. Manzanedo I, Pereira F, Rihuete Caro C, et al. Cytoreductive surgery and hyperthermic intraperitoneal chemotherapy (HIPEC) for gastric cancer with peritoneal carcinomatosis: multicenter study of Spanish Group of Peritoneal Oncologic Surgery (GECOP). *Ann Surg Oncol*. 2019;26(8):2615-2621. doi:10.1245/s10434-019-07450-4

184. Kimbrough CW, Beal E, Abdel-Misih S, Pawlik TM, Cloyd JM. Survival outcomes among patients with gastric adenocarcinoma who received hyperthermic intraperitoneal chemotherapy with cytoreductive surgery. *JAMA Surg*. 2019;154(8):780-782. doi:10.1001/jamasurg.2019.1698

185. National Comprehensive Cancer Network Guidelines Version 4.2018. Colon cancer. Accessed March 1, 2019. http://www.nccn.org

186. National Comprehensive Cancer Network Guidelines Version 2.2018. Gastric cancer. Accessed March 1, 2019. http://www.nccn.org

187. Bonnot PE, Piessen G, Pocard M, et al. CYTO-CHIP: cytoreductive surgery versus cytoreductive surgery and hyperthermic intraperitoneal chemotherapy for gastric cancer with peritoneal metastasis: a propensity-score analysis from BIG RENAPE and FREGAT working groups. *J Clin Oncol*. 2018;36(4 suppl):8. doi:10.1200/JCO.2018.36.4_suppl.8

188. Goéré D, Glehen O, Quenet F, et al. Results of a randomized phase 3 study evaluating the potential benefit of a second-look surgery plus HIPEC in patients at high risk of developing colorectal peritoneal metastases (PROPHYLOCHIP-NTC01226394). *J Clin Oncol*. 2018;36(15 suppl):3531. doi:10.1200/JCO.2018.36.15_suppl.3531

Synoptic Operative Report: Peritoneal

Date of procedure _____ Surgeon(s) _____

_____

Preoperative Details

Primary origin of carcinomatosis
☐ Appendix
☐ Colon
☐ Ovary
☐ Gastric mesothelioma
☐ Other _____

Presentation
☐ Synchronous
☐ Metachronous carcinomatosis

Preoperative imaging
☐ CT
☐ MRI
☐ PET
☐ Other _____

Preoperative chemotherapy
☐ Yes
☐ No

ECOG performance status
☐ 0
☐ 1
☐ 2
☐ 3
☐ 4

ASA class
☐ 1
☐ 2
☐ 3
☐ 4
☐ 5

Anesthesia
☐ General
☐ General with epidural
☐ Other _____

Preoperative DVT prophylaxis _____

Synoptic Operative Report: Peritoneal

Date of procedure _____   Surgeon(s) _____

_____

Preoperative antibiotics
☐ Yes
Type _____
☐ No

Preoperative ureteral stents
☐ Yes
☐ No

Bowel prep
☐ Yes
☐ No

Exploration and Resection

Laparoscopy before exploration
☐ Yes
☐ No

PCI index/distribution/lesions size
range locations (0–39)
_____

Ascites present
☐ Yes
Volume _____
☐ No

Peritonectomy sites
☐ RUQ
☐ Pelvis
☐ LUQ
☐ RLQ
☐ LLQ

Organs resected
_____

Number of anastomosis
_____

Stoma
☐ Small bowel
☐ Colon
☐ Loop
☐ End stoma

CCR (0–2) and/or
R score (R0/R1, R2a, R2b, R2c)
_____

Synoptic Operative Report: Peritoneal

Date of procedure _____ Surgeon(s) _____

_____

Intraperitoneal Chemotherapy

Technique
☐ Open
☐ Closed

Type and dose of chemotherapy _____

Inflow/outflow temperature probes _____

Perfusate temperature at outflow _____

Perfusate fluid volume and flow rate _____

Perfusion time _____

Disposition

Extubated in OR
☐ Yes
☐ No

Intubated
☐ Yes
☐ No

Estimated blood loss _____

Fluids administered _____

Drains _____

Disposition
☐ ICU
☐ Floor

COMMENTARY: PERITONEAL SECTION

H. Richard Alexander Jr., MD
Chief Surgical Officer, Rutgers Cancer Institute of New Jersey
Professor and Head, Surgical Oncology
Department of Surgery, Rutgers Robert Wood Johnson Medical School

The peritoneal section of the American College of Surgeons' *Operative Standards for Cancer Surgery*, Volume 3, provides a comprehensive review of the technical aspects of cytoreduction and hyperthermic intraperitoneal chemotherapy (HIPEC) for patients with peritoneal metastases from various intra-abdominal malignancies.[1] Just 40 years ago, patients with peritoneal carcinomatosis were almost always treated with limited measures and primarily with palliative intent. It is important to appreciate that once peritoneal metastases develop from colorectal, appendiceal, gastric, or ovarian cancers or from malignant peritoneal mesothelioma, patient morbidity and mortality almost always result from intra-abdominal disease progression.[2] Therefore, treatment strategies designed to control disease in the abdomen should translate to meaningful clinical benefit. Currently, many patients are offered integrated multimodal therapy that includes systemic chemotherapy, operative cytoreduction, and some type of regional intraperitoneal chemotherapy with or without hyperthermia. The authors should be complimented for their comprehensive review of this subject. The technical aspects of operative cytoreduction and, in particular, the description of the various technical options for cytoreduction in problematic areas of the abdomen such as the porta hepatis, lesser sac, small bowel mesentery, and pelvis are nicely detailed. The authors also provide a thoughtful overview of the technical considerations of HIPEC including drug administration in the operating room environment, the open versus closed perfusion techniques, the choice of chemotherapy agents, and the use of hyperthermia. The topics of patient selection, morbidity, and long-term patient outcomes are weaved into the section nicely.

Over the past 30 years, improvements in patient selection, technical aspects of the procedure, and the use of more standardized perioperative management pathways have contributed to decreased morbidity and mortality from cytoreduction and HIPEC to the point that they are now comparable to other commonly performed operative procedures to resect primary or metastatic cancers arising in the gastrointestinal tract.[3] However, despite numerous prospective randomized controlled trials (RCTs) evaluating the role of HIPEC in selected patients with peritoneal metastases from ovarian, colorectal, appendiceal, or gastric cancer, there is still no widely accepted indication for cytoreductive surgery and HIPEC in patients with most of these conditions. On the other hand, there is fairly broad consensus that in selected patients with malignant peritoneal mesothelioma or peritoneal metastases from low-grade mucinous appendiceal neoplasms or well-differentiated appendiceal adenocarcinoma, cytoreduction and HIPEC should be considered as first-line therapy, although no prospective random assignment trials have been conducted specifically in patients with these conditions.[4,5] This is due to the rarity of these conditions and the fact that there are limited other effective treatment options. It is worth a brief review of the results of these RCTs to better understand what we know and what we don't know about the use of cytoreduction and HIPEC in the management of patients with peritoneal metastases.

Two RCTs, one in the first-line and one in the recurrent disease setting, have been reported in patients with peritoneal metastases (stage IIIc or IV) from epithelial ovarian cancer. A multicenter study in newly diagnosed patients with stage IIIc epithelial ovarian cancer who had stable or responding disease after three cycles of carboplatin and paclitaxel were randomized intraoperatively after optimal cytoreduction to receive or not receive 100 mg of cisplatin/m^2 via a 120-minute HIPEC with administration of systemic sodium thiosulfate to mitigate potential systemic cis-platinum toxicity.[6] Adverse events were similar between the two groups, and the use of HIPEC resulted in a significant improvement in overall survival (approximately 34 vs. 46 months median overall survival, respectively). A second smaller random assignment study evaluated HIPEC after optimal cytoreduction using various chemotherapy regimens based on tumor platinum sensitivity in patients with recurrent epithelial ovarian cancer.[7] Although there have been some criticisms of this study related to design and data analysis, the study showed a significant improvement in mean overall survival with HIPEC (13.4 vs. 26.7 months, respectively). However, despite the results of these two studies, HIPEC has not been widely adopted as a standard practice in these clinical settings. This phenomenon is reminiscent of previous RCTs which showed that in patients with optimally cytoreduced epithelial ovarian cancer, postoperative intraperitoneal cis-platinum resulted in improved overall survival compared to patients receiving systemic cis-platinum.[8,9] Despite the demonstrated improvement in overall survival in these well-conducted RCTs, the practice of intraperitoneal administration of cis-platinum was never widely adopted because of practical challenges with intraperitoneal drug administration and in the long-term management of the intraperitoneal catheters.

In patients with peritoneal metastases from gastric cancer, there have been two RCTs that reported benefit from treatment regimens which included cytoreduction and HIPEC but have had limited impact on the use of HIPEC in this patient population. A small RCT with fewer than 20 patients, RCT comparing systemic chemotherapy alone to cytoreduction, HIPEC, and systemic chemotherapy (GYMSSA) showed a significant improvement in overall survival with multimodal therapy (4.3 vs. 11.1 months, respectively).[10] The criticisms of this study were the considerable morbidity associated with multimodal treatment and that survival in both groups was very short, suggesting that the data might not be relevant to the general population of patients with peritoneal metastases from gastric cancer. A second RCT compared cytoreduction alone to cytoreduction with HIPEC using a combination of cisplatin and mitomycin C administered for between 60 and 90 minutes.[11] In the overall patient cohort, the burden of peritoneal disease was quite high— median peritoneal cancer index was 15—and approximately one-third of patients had a peritoneal cancer index greater than 20. As in the other RCT, median overall survival was short in both groups, as one would anticipate with such a high disease burden, but was significantly longer with HIPEC (6.5 vs. 11 months, respectively). On multivariate analysis of factors independently associated with outcome, the use of systemic chemotherapy for 6 months or more was associated with significantly improved survival. In fact, use of chemotherapy for 6 months or more (generally a surrogate for chemotherapy-sensitive disease because patients do not continue therapy when disease progresses) had a more significant effect on outcome than HIPEC. However, in the manuscript, there is no description as to the type of chemotherapy used and which patients received it, so it is impossible to know whether the two treatment groups were balanced with respect to that parameter.

The results of three RCTs that have evaluated the use of HIPEC in patients with peritoneal metastases from colorectal or appendiceal cancers have been used by both advocates and critics of HIPEC to support their respective positions. The first reported RCT assigned patients with colorectal or appendiceal cancer peritoneal metastases to systemic chemotherapy using 5-fluorouracil and leucovorin and palliative surgical intervention versus cytoreduction and HIPEC followed by the same systemic chemotherapy.[12,13] Although median overall survival was significantly prolonged with the use of cytoreduction and HIPEC (12.6 vs. 22.3 months, respectively), the study has been criticized for the high treatment-related mortality rate (8%) in the cytoreduction and HIPEC group and the fact that the chemotherapy regimen used is now antiquated. The results of the PRODIGE 7 trial were recently reported; this study randomly assigned patients with colorectal peritoneal metastases to cytoreduction alone or cytoreduction with HIPEC.[14] Of note, almost all patients received perioperative chemotherapy. The median overall survival was 41.7 months and not different between the groups. In this trial, HIPEC was administered for 30 minutes with either 360 or 460 mg/m^2 of oxaliplatin (depending on whether the open or closed technique was used) and concomitant intravenous 5-fluorouracil was administered. Whereas critics would argue these data definitively demonstrate that HIPEC has no salutary effect in this clinical setting, proponents would argue that the HIPEC treatment parameters used in the study are different than what is routinely employed in other countries (oxaliplatin for 30 minutes vs. mitomycin C for 90 to 120 minutes). Several retrospective uncontrolled studies provide conflicting information regarding the comparative efficacy of oxaliplatin administered for 30 minutes compared to mitomycin C administered for 90 to 120 minutes via HIPEC.[15–17] There is one RCT evaluating the role of HIPEC (the only RCT evaluating HIPEC that has been completed in North America) which may shed some meaningful information on this question. Patients with peritoneal metastases from appendiceal cancer were randomly assigned to undergo cytoreduction and HIPEC using either 200 mg/m^2 oxaliplatin or 40 mg of mitomycin C.[18] There was no difference in progression-free or overall survival between the groups; whether or not these data can be extrapolated to patients with colorectal cancer is a topic of debate.

In summary, the utility of cytoreduction and HIPEC across the landscape of peritoneal metastases from various abdominal cancers remains complex. With respect to patient selection, the extent of peritoneal disease and the ability to achieve a complete cytoreduction (both of which reflect disease burden, favorable disease distribution, and lack of tumor infiltration) are universally important factors to achieve a good outcome. The preponderance of data from most RCTs (and other retrospective studies) also show that outcomes after cytoreduction and HIPEC are optimal in patients with chemotherapy-sensitive disease. Conversely, the data suggest that in patients with colorectal, high-grade appendiceal, or gastric cancers with progressive disease while on chemotherapy, salvage cytoreduction and HIPEC has limited clinical utility. Other RCTs have shown no clinical benefit of HIPEC administered in the prophylactic setting in high-risk colorectal cancer patients.[19,20] Additional RCTs will be required to define the clinical benefit of cytoreduction and HIPEC in patients with gastric and colorectal cancers, and until then, the practice of thoughtful multidisciplinary clinical decision-making for individual patients will continue.

REFERENCES

1. Alexander HR Jr. Hyperthermia and its modern use in cancer treatment. *Cancer*. 2003;98(2):219-221. doi:10.1002/cncr.11471
2. Sadeghi B, Arvieux C, Glehen O, et al. Peritoneal carcinomatosis from non-gynecologic malignancies: results of the EVOCAPE 1 multicentric prospective study. *Cancer*. 2000;88(2):358-363. doi:10.1002/(sici)1097-0142 (20000115)88:2<358::aid-cncr16>3.0.co;2-o
3. Foster JM, Sleightholm R, Patel A, et al. Morbidity and mortality rates following cytoreductive surgery combined with hyperthermic intraperitoneal chemotherapy compared with other high-risk surgical oncology procedures. *JAMA Netw Open*. 2019;2(1):e186847. doi:10.1001/jamanetworkopen.2018.6847
4. Chicago Consensus Working Group. The Chicago consensus on peritoneal surface malignancies: management of peritoneal mesothelioma. *Ann Surg Oncol*. 2020;27(6):1774-1779. doi:10.1245/s10434-020-08324-w
5. Chicago Consensus Working Group. The Chicago consensus on peritoneal surface malignancies: management of appendiceal neoplasms. *Ann Surg Oncol*. 2020;27(6):1753-1760. doi:10.1245/s10434-020-08316-w
6. van Driel WJ, Koole SN, Sikorska K, et al. Hyperthermic intraperitoneal chemotherapy in ovarian cancer. *N Engl J Med*. 2018;378(3):230-240. doi:10.1056/NEJMoa1708618
7. Spiliotis J, Halkia E, Lianos E, et al. Cytoreductive surgery and HIPEC in recurrent epithelial ovarian cancer: a prospective randomized phase III study. *Ann Surg Oncol*. 2015;22(5):1570-1575. doi:10.1245/s10434-014-4157-9
8. Armstrong DK, Bundy B, Wenzel L, et al. Intraperitoneal cisplatin and paclitaxel in ovarian cancer. *N Engl J Med*. 2006;354(1):34-43. doi:10.1056/NEJMoa052985
9. Alberts DS, Liu PY, Hannigan EV, et al. Intraperitoneal cisplatin plus intravenous cyclophosphamide versus intravenous cisplatin plus intravenous cyclophosphamide for stage III ovarian cancer. *N Engl J Med*. 1996;335(26):1950-1955. doi:10.1056/NEJM199612263352603
10. Rudloff U, Langan RC, Mullinax JE, et al. Impact of maximal cytoreductive surgery plus regional heated intraperitoneal chemotherapy (HIPEC) on outcome of patients with peritoneal carcinomatosis of gastric origin: results of the GYMSSA trial. *J Surg Oncol*. 2014;110(3):275-284. doi:10.1002/jso.23633
11. Yang X-J, Huang C-Q, Suo T, et al. Cytoreductive surgery and hyperthermic intraperitoneal chemotherapy improves survival of patients with peritoneal carcinomatosis from gastric cancer: final results of a phase III randomized clinical trial. *Ann Surg Oncol*. 2011;18(6):1575-1581. doi:10.1245/s10434-011-1631-5
12. Verwaal VJ, van Ruth S, de Bree E, et al. Randomized trial of cytoreduction and hyperthermic intraperitoneal chemotherapy versus systemic chemotherapy and palliative surgery in patients with peritoneal carcinomatosis of colorectal cancer. *J Clin Oncol*. 2003;21(20):3737-3743. doi:10.1200/JCO.2003.04.187
13. Verwaal VJ, Bruin S, Boot H, van Slooten G, van Tinteren H. 8-Year follow-up of randomized trial: cytoreduction and hyperthermic intraperitoneal chemotherapy versus systemic chemotherapy in patients with peritoneal carcinomatosis of colorectal cancer. *Ann Surg Oncol*. 2008;15(9):2426-2432. doi:10.1245/s10434-008-9966-2
14. Quénet F, Elias D, Roca L, et al. Cytoreductive surgery plus hyperthermic intraperitoneal chemotherapy versus cytoreductive surgery alone for colorectal peritoneal metastases (PRODIGE 7): a multicentre, randomised, open-label, phase 3 trial. *Lancet Oncol*. 2021;22(2):256-266. doi:10.1016/S1470-2045(20)30599-4
15. van Eden WJ, Kok NFM, Woensdregt K, Huitema ADR, Boot H, Aalbers AGJ. Safety of intraperitoneal mitomycin C versus intraperitoneal oxaliplatin in patients with peritoneal carcinomatosis of colorectal cancer undergoing cytoreductive surgery and HIPEC. *Eur J Surg Oncol*. 2018;44(2):220-227. doi:10.1016/j.ejso.2017.10.216
16. Prada-Villaverde A, Esquivel J, Lowy AM, et al. The American Society of Peritoneal Surface Malignancies evaluation of HIPEC with mitomycin C versus oxaliplatin in 539 patients with colon cancer undergoing a complete cytoreductive surgery. *J Surg Oncol*. 2014;110(7):779-785. doi:10.1002/jso.23728
17. Leung V, Huo YR, Liauw W, Morris DL. Oxaliplatin versus mitomycin C for HIPEC in colorectal cancer peritoneal carcinomatosis. *Eur J Surg Oncol*. 2017;43(1):144-149. doi:10.1016/j.ejso.2016.09.015
18. Levine EA, Votanopoulos KI, Shen P, et al. A multicenter randomized trial to evaluate hematologic toxicities after hyperthermic intraperitoneal chemotherapy with oxaliplatin or mitomycin in patients with appendiceal tumors. *J Am Coll Surg*. 2018;226(4):434-443. doi:10.1016/j.jamcollsurg.2017.12.027
19. Goéré D, Glehen O, Quenet F, et al. Second-look surgery plus hyperthermic intraperitoneal chemotherapy versus surveillance in patients at high risk of developing colorectal peritoneal metastases (PROPHYLOCHIP-PRODIGE 15): a randomised, phase 3 study. *Lancet Oncol*. 2020;21(9):1147-1154. doi:10.1016/S1470-2045(20)30322-3
20. Klaver CEL, Wisselink DD, Punt CJA, et al. Adjuvant hyperthermic intraperitoneal chemotherapy in patients with locally advanced colon cancer (COLOPEC): a multicentre, open-label, randomised trial. *Lancet Gastroenterol Hepatol*. 2019;4(10):761-770. doi:10.1016/S2468-1253(19)30239-0

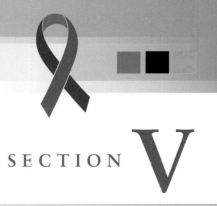

SECTION V

UROTHELIAL

INTRODUCTION

Urothelial carcinoma encompasses cancers of the pelvicalyceal system, ureter, bladder, and part of the urethra. In the United States, urothelial carcinoma of the bladder is the second most common malignancy of the genitourinary tract and the second most common cause of death among all genitourinary tumors. An estimated 80,470 new cases of bladder cancer and over 18,770 deaths from bladder cancer were expected in 2018 in the United States.[1] Approximately three-fourths of patients with bladder tumors present with non-muscle-invasive bladder cancer (NMIBC), whereas 20% to 40% will either present with or progress to high-grade muscle-invasive bladder cancer (MIBC). Left untreated, MIBCs are highly lethal and lead to significant risk of morbidity and mortality. Median survival is less than 1 year, even among patients with tumors that are confined to the bladder.[2] Upper tract urothelial carcinomas (UTUCs) account for only about 5% of all urothelial carcinomas, and primary prostatic urothelial carcinoma without concomitant bladder urothelial carcinoma is quite rare. At the time of diagnosis, approximately 25% of patients with UTUCs have a history of previous NMIBC.[3] Recurrent bladder carcinomas following treatment for UTUCs are very common and occur in up to 50% of patients.[4]

Radical cystectomy (RC) and thorough, meticulous pelvic lymph node dissection is the standard management for MIBC and high-grade NMIBCs, which are considered at high risk of progression. Although low-grade UTUCs may be managed endoscopically, high-grade tumors generally require radical surgery given limitations of biopsy, staging inaccuracies, and inability to adequately treat with adjuvant local therapy. In addition, although surgical techniques may vary owing to patient factors, the urologist's preferences and training background also has an impact on management. And although much of the variability is to be expected and is reasonable, there are some basic surgical tenets based on broad and published evidence that should be considered critical elements to the management of urothelial carcinoma. This section outlines the available evidence and consensus of topical experts on these critical elements for the management of urothelial carcinoma.

CLINICAL STAGING

Accurate diagnosis and staging are critical to assuring optimal outcomes with bladder cancer. Management begins with transurethral resection of bladder tumor (TURBT) with careful attention to histopathologic details such as the depth of invasion, presence of carcinoma in situ, lymphovascular invasion, and/or histologic variants. Subsequent management heavily relies on findings at initial and/or repeat TURBT. Patients with high-grade T1 disease should undergo a re-resection for better risk stratification.[5] In those who have persistent high-grade T1 disease on repeat resection or T1 tumors with associated carcinoma in situ, lymphovascular invasion, or variant histology, upfront RC should be considered owing to the high risk of progression.[6] Staging workup should include chest imaging and cross-sectional imaging of the abdomen and pelvis with intravenous (IV) contrast whenever feasible. Positron emission tomography (PET) scans and bone scans should not be routinely used for initial staging workup.

Magnetic resonance imaging (MRI) has also been used to assess clinical stage prior to RC, but its accuracy ranges from 50% to 90% and is highly dependent on imaging technique. Dynamic gadolinium-enhanced MRI helps better differentiate the tumor from surrounding tissues because of the earlier enhancement of tumor by contrast, but it still suffers from nodal understaging.[7]

As with many other cancers, urothelial cancer is staged according to the tumor-node-metastasis (TNM) staging classifications. The staging is specific to urethral, bladder, or upper tract location of the tumor (Tables 5-1, 5-2, and 5-3).[8] Urothelial cancers are primarily staged by the depth of invasion through the urinary tract structure walls from which they derive (Figs. 5-1 and 5-2). Other important histologic factors include the presence of variant histology, lymphovascular invasion, number of lymph nodes involved, presence of extracapsular nodal extension, and size of the largest tumor deposit in the lymph nodes.[9,10] Notably, patients with bladder cancer in whom the tumor extends into the prostatic stroma would have a T4a designation regardless of the route of spread despite the poorer prognosis seen in those with direct invasion through the bladder.[10] However, patients with urothelial carcinoma arising from the prostatic urethra alone (without spread from the bladder) are staged according to the urethral cancer staging system, in which prostatic stromal invasion would be staged as T2. This is an important distinction when considering systemic therapy. Although not formally in the staging system, extension of tumor into the seminal vesicles has been shown to be associated with a very poor prognosis.[11]

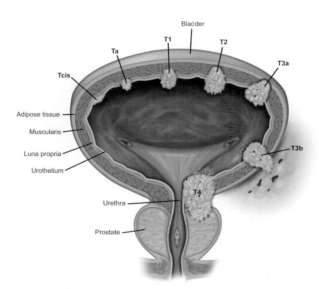

FIGURE 5-1   Staging of invasion for bladder urothelial carcinoma (UC): UC of the bladder is staged by depth of invasion as illustrated here from superficial noninvasive and cancer in situ to invasive of the subepithelial connective tissue (T1), muscularis layer (T2), fat layer (T3), and surrounding structures (T4).

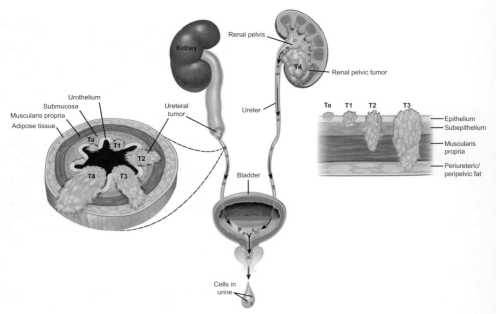

FIGURE 5-2 Staging of invasion for upper tract urothelial carcinoma (UTUC): UTUC of the ureter or renal pelvis is staged by depth of invasion as illustrated here from superficial noninvasive to invasive of the subepithelial connective tissue (T1), muscularis propria layer (T2), fat layer (T3), and renal parenchyma or surrounding structures (T4).

MULTIDISCIPLINARY CARE

Bladder cancer and UTUC share many characteristics in common, but there is mounting evidence that molecular differences exist between the two.[12] Although urothelial carcinomas respond to systemic therapy regardless of their site of origin, surgical management varies widely. Invasive primary prostatic urethral carcinomas should be treated with radical cystoprostatectomy, whereas invasive UTUC of the upper ureter and pelvicalyceal system should be treated with nephroureterectomy with excision of a bladder cuff. High-grade distal ureter tumors may be managed with distal ureterectomy and ureteral reimplantation with particular attention to surveillance of the remnant urothelium. Adequate and meticulous map-based lymph node dissection should accompany any surgical management of urothelial carcinomas.

Generally, MIBCs and some of the high-grade NMIBCs are managed by RC as the standard therapy, which in men entails the removal of the bladder, prostate, and seminal vesicles. Although prostate-sparing surgery has been reported in some series with excellent functional results, concern for the development of recurrent urothelial carcinoma within the remnant prostatic urethra has hampered its widespread acceptance.[13–15] In females, traditional RC (otherwise known as an anterior pelvic exenteration) entails the removal of the bladder, anterior vagina, uterus, and adnexa. In recent years, female organ–preservation surgery has gained more acceptance given the low

TABLE 5-1 American Joint Committee on Cancer Staging Criteria for Bladder Cancer, Eighth Edition

TABLE 5-1A Definition of Primary Tumor (T)

T Category	T Criteria
TX	Primary tumor cannot be assessed
T0	No evidence of primary tumor
Ta	Noninvasive papillary carcinoma
Tis	Carcinoma in situ: "flat tumor"
T1	Tumor invades subepithelial connective tissue
T2	Tumor invades muscularis propria
pT2a	Tumor invades superficial muscularis propria (inner half)
pT2b	Tumor invades deep muscularis propria (outer half)
T3	Tumor invades perivesical tissue
pT3a	Microscopically
pT3b	Macroscopically (extravesical mass)
T4	Extravesical tumor invades any of the following: prostatic stroma, seminal vesicles, uterus, vagina, pelvic wall, abdominal wall
T4a	Extravesical tumor invades directly into prostatic stroma, seminal vesicles, uterus, vagina
T4b	Extravesical tumor invades pelvic wall, abdominal wall

TABLE 5-1B Definition of Regional Lymph Node (N)

N Category	N Criteria
NX	Lymph nodes cannot be assessed
N0	No lymph node metastasis
N1	Single regional lymph node metastasis in the true pelvis (hypogastric, obturator, external iliac, or presacral lymph node)
N2	Multiple regional lymph node metastasis in the true pelvis (hypogastric, obturator, external iliac, or presacral lymph node metastasis)
N3	Lymph node metastasis to the common iliac lymph nodes

Note: Regional lymph nodes include both primary and secondary drainage regions. All other nodes above the aortic bifurcation are considered distant lymph nodes.

TABLE 5-1C Definition of Distant Metastasis (M)

M Category	M Criteria
M0	No distant metastasis
M1	Distant metastasis
M1a	Distant metastases limited to lymph nodes beyond the common iliacs
M1b	Nonlymph node distant metastases

TABLE 5-1D American Joint Committee on Cancer Prognostic Stage Groups

T Stage	N Stage	M Stage	Group Stage
Ta	N0	M0	0a
Tis	N0	M0	is
T1	N0	M0	I
T2a	N0	M0	II
T2b	N0	M0	II
T3a	N0	M0	IIIA
T3b	N0	M0	IIIA
T4a	N0	M0	IIIA
T1–T4a	N1	M0	IIIA
T1–T4a	N2, N3	M0	IIIB
T4b	Any N	M0	IVA
Any T	Any N	M1a	IVA
Any T	Any N	M1b	IVB

Note: American Joint Committee on Cancer staging and TNM classification for bladder cancer.[8] Used with permission of the American Joint Committee on Cancer (AJCC), Chicago, Illinois. The original and primary source for this information is the *AJCC Cancer Staging Manual*, Eighth Edition (2017) published by Springer International Publishing.

TABLE 5-2 American Joint Committee on Cancer Staging Criteria for Upper Urinary Tract Cancer, Eighth Edition

TABLE 5-2A Definition of Primary Tumor (T)

T Category	T Criteria
TX	Primary tumor cannot be assessed
T0	No evidence of primary tumor
Ta	Noninvasive papillary carcinoma
Tis	Carcinoma in situ: "flat tumor"
T1	Tumor invades subepithelial connective tissue
T2	Tumor invades muscularis propria
T3 (renal pelvis)	Tumor invades beyond muscularis into peripelvic fat or renal parenchyma
pT3 (ureter)	Tumor invades beyond muscularis into periureteric fat
T4	Tumor invades adjacent organs or through the kidney into perinephric fat

TABLE 5-2B Definition of Regional Lymph Node (N)

N Category	N Criteria
NX	Lymph nodes cannot be assessed
N0	No lymph node metastasis
N1	Metastasis in a single lymph node, ≤2 cm in greatest dimension
N2	Metastasis in a single lymph node, >2 cm or multiple lymph nodes
NX	Lymph nodes cannot be assessed

Note: Regional lymph nodes include both primary and secondary drainage regions. All other nodes above the aortic bifurcation are considered distant lymph nodes.

TABLE 5-2C Definition of Distant Metastasis (M)

M Category	M Criteria
M0	No distant metastasis
M1	Distant metastasis

TABLE 5-2D American Joint Committee on Cancer Prognostic Stage Groups

T Stage	N Stage	M Stage	Group Stage
Ta	N0	M0	0a
Tis	N0	M0	is
T1	N0	M0	I
T2	N0	M0	II
T3	N0	M0	III
T4	N0	M0	IV
Any T	N1–N2	M0	IV
Any T	Any N	M1	IV

Note: American Joint Committee on Cancer staging and TNM classification for upper urinary tract cancer.[8] Used with permission of the American Joint Committee on Cancer (AJCC), Chicago, Illinois. The original and primary source for this information is the AJCC Cancer Staging Manual, Eighth Edition (2017) published by Springer International Publishing.

TABLE 5-3 American Joint Committee on Cancer Staging Criteria for Primary Urethral Cancer

TABLE 5-3A Definition of Primary Tumor (T)

Prostatic Urethra

T Category	T Criteria
TX	Primary tumor cannot be assessed
T0	No evidence of primary tumor
Ta	Noninvasive papillary carcinoma
Tis	Carcinoma in situ involving the prostatic urethra or periurethral or prostatic ducts without stromal invasion
T1	Invasion of prostatic urethral subepithelial connective tissue
T2	Invasion of prostatic stroma
T3	Invasion of periprostatic fat
T4	Invasion of adjacent organs (i.e., bladder, rectum)

TABLE 5-3A Definition of Primary Tumor (T) *(Continued)*

Penile Urethra

T Category	T Criteria
TX	Primary tumor cannot be assessed
T0	No evidence of primary tumor
Ta	Noninvasive papillary carcinoma
Tis	Carcinoma in situ
T1	Invasion of urethral subepithelial connective tissue
T2	Invasion of corpus spongiosum
T3	Invasion of corpus cavernosum
T4	Invasion of adjacent organs (i.e., bladder, rectum)

TABLE 5-3B Definition of Regional Lymph Node (N)

N Category	N Criteria
NX	Lymph nodes cannot be assessed
N0	No lymph node metastasis
N1	Metastasis in one regional lymph node
N2	Metastasis in greater than one regional lymph node

Note: Regional lymph nodes include both primary and secondary drainage regions. All other nodes above the aortic bifurcation are considered distant lymph nodes.

TABLE 5-3C Definition of Distant Metastasis (M)

M Category	M Criteria
M0	No distant metastasis
M1	Distant metastasis

TABLE 5-3D   American Joint Committee on Cancer Prognostic Stage Groups

T Stage	N Stage	M Stage	Group Stage
Ta	N0	M0	0a
Tis	N0	M0	0is
T1	N0	M0	I
T2	N0	M0	II
T3	N0	M0	III
T1, T2, T3	N1	M0	III
T4	N0–N2	M0	IV
Any T	N2	M0	IV
Any T	Any N	M1	IV

Note: American Joint Committee on Cancer staging and TNM classification for primary urethral cancer.[8] Used with permission of the American Joint Committee on Cancer (AJCC), Chicago, Illinois. The original and primary source for this information is the *AJCC Cancer Staging Manual*, Eighth Edition (2017) published by Springer International Publishing.

rate of involvement of these adjacent organs.[16] Caution must be exercised, however, in performing vaginal-sparing procedures in patients with tumors at the base of the bladder because a positive margin in this area can have poor prognosis. As mentioned previously, surgery for urothelial carcinoma should be accompanied by extensive and meticulous lymph node dissection, which are described in later chapters.

Clinicians should have a detailed and balanced discussion with patients about the different options for urinary diversion following RC. The ultimate choice, however, should rely on the patients' desires and priorities as well as the surgeon's experience. Those who refuse an RC and urinary diversion do have other options. Partial cystectomy is an option in very select cases such as isolated disease in the dome of the bladder without concomitant carcinoma in situ, but very few patients qualify. Other bladder-sparing protocols such as "radical TURBT" should only be used in patients who refuse curative options or are not candidates for any other therapy.

Surgery holds a critical role in the management of urothelial carcinoma, but multidisciplinary care is ultimately necessary in many cases for optimal management of the disease. There is ample data and level I evidence that cisplatin-based neoadjuvant chemotherapy prior to RC improves survival.[17,18] Cisplatin-based adjuvant chemotherapy should be offered to patients with extravesical disease (i.e., T3 to T4) or with positive lymph nodes. Although the same level of evidence does not exist for adjuvant chemotherapy, meta-analyses of the several trials in this space have shown an overall benefit.[19,20] The American Urological Association (AUA) guidelines recommend that eligible patients who have not received cisplatin-based neoadjuvant chemotherapy and have non–organ-confined (pT3/T4 and/or N+) disease at RC should be offered cisplatin-based adjuvant chemotherapy.[21] Although robust data are lacking for perioperative use of cisplatin-based chemotherapy for urethral cancer and UTUC, extrapolation from the management of high-grade MIBC may lead to improved outcomes. Neoadjuvant treatment should be favored over adjuvant chemotherapy, particularly for the upper tract, given that surgery may render the patient ineligible for cisplatin owing to compromised renal function. There are also a number of ongoing clinical trials assessing the value of alternative systemic treatment such as immunotherapy in the neoadjuvant as well as the adjuvant setting for patients who are not cisplatin eligible.

In select patients with MIBC, bladder-sparing chemoradiation is a suitable alternative to RC.[22–24] However, population-based studies have reported underutilization of this treatment.[25,26] Data from the National Cancer Database showed that only 7.6% of the MIBC patients received bladder-sparing chemoradiation or radiation; up to 25% of that population received no treatment but observation only.[25] Currently, the AUA/American Society of Clinical Oncology/American Society for Radiation Oncology/Society of Urologic Oncology guideline recommends that bladder preservation is best achieved with "trimodal" therapy, which entails a grossly complete TURBT followed by concurrent chemoradiation,[21] and the National Comprehensive Cancer Network guidelines provide more details on patient selection for those with smaller solitary tumors, negative nodes, no carcinoma in situ, no tumor-related hydronephrosis, and good pretreatment bladder function.[27] Radiation combined with chemotherapy is considered superior to radiation alone; however, many patients who are unfit for radical surgery usually have poor renal function and performance status.[28] It is important to differentiate palliative chemoradiation designed to slow disease progression and alleviate symptoms such as intractable hematuria versus trimodal therapy for curative intent. In particular, trimodal therapy entails frequent surveillance cystoscopy and a plan for salvage RC if there is tumor progression through the chemoradiation treatments, whereas salvage cystectomy is not the plan typically for palliative treatment.[28] In addition, radiation-induced genitourinary and gastrointestinal tract toxicities should be carefully controlled and managed because it is meaningless to preserve a bladder without function.[29]

PERIOPERATIVE CARE

RC remains a formidable operation with significant potential for perioperative complications and impact on the quality of life. Recent improvements in perioperative management and, in particular, Enhanced Recovery After Surgery (ERAS) protocols have greatly decreased gastrointestinal complication rates as well as the length of hospital stay while improving the patient experience.[30,31] Deep venous thromboembolism (DVT) and subsequent pulmonary embolism remain a common culprit of morbidity and mortality after RC. Smoking, hypercoagulation status of malignancy, pelvic surgery, and extended postoperative immobility are all risk factors for DVT.[32] Currently, the AUA Best Practice Statement recommends the use of mechanical (pneumatic compression devices) or pharmacologic (unfractionated heparin or low molecular weight

TABLE 5-4   Surveillance Measures for Bladder Cancer from Commission on Cancer

Measure	Measure Description	Initial Release
1	At least two lymph nodes are removed in patients under 80 y undergoing partial or radical cystectomy	Spring 2016
2	Radical or partial cystectomy; or trimodal therapy (local tumor destruction/excision with chemotherapy and radiation) for clinical T234N0M0 patients, first treatment within 90 d of diagnosis	Spring 2017
3	Neoadjuvant or adjuvant chemotherapy offered or administered for patients with muscle-invasive cancer undergoing radical cystectomy	Spring 2017

heparins) prophylaxis based on different patient risk stratification.[33] However, the use of pharmacologic prophylaxis after RC is still controversial because of the concern of possible postoperative bleeding.[32]

QUALITY MEASURES

Efforts are ongoing to develop quality measures for surgical intervention that use objective data and identify reasonable minimal standards that should take place in typical patients with urothelial cancer.[34] Currently, the Commission on Cancer includes several measurements developed from the National Cancer Database for bladder cancer. There are three such measures listed by the Commission on Cancer as "surveillance" measures. These measures are shown in Table 5-4.[35] There are currently no Commission on Cancer quality measures for UTUC or NMIBC, although some research studies have investigated the potential of such measures for these tumor types. A recent multicenter study reported the real-world experience of implementing evidence-based quality indicators for TURBT, which included using a bladder diagram, single post-TURBT instillation of mitomycin C, detrusor muscle in the specimen, and early re-TURBT in high-risk NMIBC. With a 3-year follow-up, these standardized steps significantly lower the early recurrence rate and residual cancer.[36]

CHAPTER 10

Endoscopic Management

CRITICAL ELEMENTS

- Endoscopic Evaluation of Urethra and Bladder
- Transurethral Resection of Bladder Tumor
- Endoscopic Evaluation and Treatment of Upper Tract Disease
- Postoperative Instillation of Intravesical Chemotherapy

1. ENDOSCOPIC EVALUATION OF URETHRA AND BLADDER

Recommendation: All patients with a suspected urothelial cancer should undergo endoscopic evaluation that includes visualization of the urethra and bladder. Bimanual examination of the bladder should be performed before and after endoscopic resection to assess for tumor palpability and tumor invasion into adjacent structures. The use of white light–enhanced technologies, including photodynamic cystoscopy and narrow band imaging (NBI), should be considered to improve tumor detection. A second endoscopic evaluation performed 2 to 6 weeks following the initial resection should be performed for all high-grade Ta and any T1 lesions.

Type of Data: Retrospective reports, case series, or case-control studies; prospective clinical trials

Strength of Recommendation: Strong recommendation, low-quality evidence

Rationale

Staging of urothelial bladder cancer is primarily based on the presence or absence of invasion of the bladder wall. If the tumor is noninvasive, lesions should be characterized as flat or papillary. If tumor invasion of the bladder wall is present, depth of involvement serves to further stage the disease. Although imaging studies are required

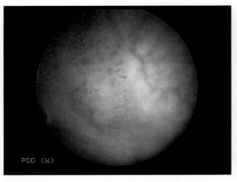
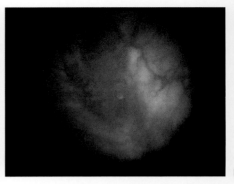

A   B

FIGURE 5-3   Cystoscopic view of a urothelial tumor under white light (**A**) and blue light (**B**) evaluation demonstrate abnormal-appearing tissue. The addition of adjunct imaging modalities can make tumors more easily noticed.

to determine stage precisely, understaging and overstaging are common with sole reliance on imaging alone.[37] Therefore, retrieval of tissue from a properly performed transurethral endoscopic resection is recommended for all patients with bladder cancer. Endoscopic resection performed with rigid electrocautery equipment allows for synchronous removal of any intraluminal component as well as excision of a section of bladder wall underlying the region of tumor growth to provide tissue for pathologic characterization of invasion and depth of involvement.

Although endoscopic evaluation is initiated under white light, white light enhancement technologies improve the ability to detect urothelial tumors endoscopically. Photodynamic diagnostic cystoscopy (also sometimes referred to as "blue light cystoscopy") relies on the relative selective accumulation of protoporphyrin IX in neoplastic cells. Two protoporphyrin IX–inducing agents, aminolevulinic acid and hexyl aminolevulinate, are instilled intravesically prior to photodynamic diagnostic cystoscopy procedures. The photosensitizing agent selectively concentrated in neoplastic cells emits a red fluorescence when excited selectively with a blue-violet light projected via the scope (Fig. 5-3). Meta-analyses of multiple studies have demonstrated that an additional tumor detection rate of 20% (95% confidence interval [CI], 8% to 35%) is achieved with photodynamic diagnostic techniques at the time of transurethral resection (TUR).[38] The additional tumor-detected rate of carcinoma in situ appears to be even higher (39%; 95% CI, 23% to 57%). Prospective studies have also demonstrated an improved recurrence-free survival at 12 and 24 months when resection of disease is performed with blue light enhancement.[39–41]

NBI technology relies on optical filters to project a limited bandwidth of light in the green and blue spectrums corresponding to the light-absorptive properties of hemoglobin (Fig. 5-4). NBI-equipped endoscopes are thus able to enhance the display of blood vessels in the mucosa and submucosa of the bladder without the need for dyes. The resulting dark green and black vessels projected on a white normal mucosal surface provides an alternative detection scheme for highlighting hypervascular lesions. The enhanced vascular regions may represent tumor vascularity or inflammation.

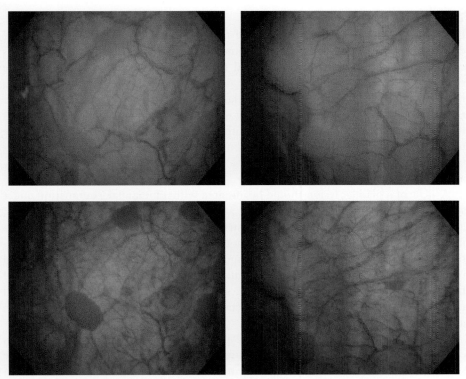

FIGURE 5-4 White light cystoscopy (*top panel*) and narrow band imaging (*bottom panel*) of bladder lesions demonstrate how adjunct imaging technology may make abnormal areas that could otherwise be overlooked easier to identify.

Multiple systematic reviews and meta-analyses have found an improved ability to detect papillary and flat disease using NBI over white light cystoscopy alone.[42–44] Early reports suggest that NBI-assisted TUR may improve subsequent tumor recurrence outcomes in patients at low risk of developing recurrent disease,[45] but additional prospective trials are needed to further clarify the cancer-control benefits across all noninvasive lesions.

A single TUR may be adequate for the diagnosis, staging, and complete removal of many lower risk, noninvasive bladder tumors. However, studies have documented that high-grade Ta and T1 non-muscle-invasive bladder cancers (NMIBCs) are often understaged and incompletely removed by an initial resection.[46] A second endoscopic resection performed 2 to 6 weeks following the initial resection improves complete resection rates and optimizes tumor staging[47] and is, therefore, recommended for all high-grade Ta and any T1 lesions.[48] The rates of detecting muscle invasion (T2 disease) on a restaging resection following an initial T1 diagnosis ranges from 4% to 25% but may be as high as 45% if muscle tissue was not present in the initial resection specimen.[47] More recent data suggest that the risk of understaging of T1 urothelial cancer may be related to the depth of invasion identified on the initial resection.[49]

Technical Aspects

Prior to the initiating the resection, the type and depth of anesthetic should be discussed with both the patient and the anesthesia provider. Although most lesions can be safely removed without the need for paralysis, some lesions may require these agents. Paralysis decreases patient motion and abdominal excursion during breathing and facilitates the resection of larger tumors, tumors on the more mobile regions of the bladder, or tumors laterally near the obturator nerve. Paralysis allows for easier manipulation of the bladder with suprapubic pressure in order to be able to reach tumors in difficult locations. Finally, full paralysis decreases the likelihood of inducing an obturator reflex, which can inadvertently cause bladder injury and bleeding.[50]

A TUR of a bladder lesion should be initiated with a bimanual examination under sedation/anesthesia to determine whether a mass is palpable, the size of any masses, and their mobility or fixation to adjacent structures. This information is used for staging and treatment planning. Performed both before and after the endoscopic resection has been completed, a bimanual exam assesses for a palpable residual mass and provides important information on clinical staging (cT3 if mass is mobile and cT4 if fixed to surrounding organs or the pelvic sidewall) and resectability. The bimanual examination is performed via a digital rectal examination in a male and vaginally in a female.

The endoscopic evaluation should be initiated under white light and includes careful evaluation of the urethra, including the prostatic portion in the male. The status of the urethra is critical in determining treatment options, estimating the ability to respond to subsequent topical therapy, and determining possible reconstructive options should radical cystectomy be required. The urethra should undergo separate staging as recommended in the *American Joint Committee on Cancer (AJCC) Cancer Staging Manual*, Eighth Edition.[8] Complete examination of the bladder lining using the 30- and 70-lens systems to identify the presence, size, location, configuration, and number of any intravesical lesions should then be completed. The proximity to the ureteral orifices should be noted and documented. Areas of abnormal mucosal changes, including surrounding erythema, should be noted as these may represent regions of carcinoma in situ.

2. TRANSURETHRAL RESECTION OF BLADDER TUMOR

Recommendation: The surgeon should aim to resect the entire bladder tumor, including sampling of underlying muscle layer and tumor edges, in order to adequately stage the disease and decrease the risk of recurrence. Suspicious mucosal areas should be biopsied. In the setting of abnormal urinary biomarkers, random bladder biopsies should be considered but are otherwise unnecessary.

Type of Data: Retrospective reports, case series, or case-control studies

Strength of Recommendation: Strong recommendation, low-quality evidence

Rationale

Transurethral resection of bladder tumor (TURBT) is both a diagnostic and therapeutic operation. The goals of surgery include removing all visible tumors and providing pathologic material in order to determine the histologic type, grade, and depth of invasion. These findings will determine the need for additional therapy, surveillance strategies, and prognostic outcomes.[51]

Technical Aspects

The resection should proceed in an orderly fashion, beginning at one edge of the tumor and progressing to the other, from superficial to deep.[52] The exophytic or intravesical portion of the tumor should be resected first, followed by a deep resection of the detrusor muscle, and then the tumor edges. Layer-by-layer resection should be favored over deep resection in any one specific location in order to provide a clear view of the entire resection site. In cases of known or suspected invasive disease, it is advisable to resect down to deep muscle or normal glistening fat, with caution to avoid inadvertent perforation of the transmural bladder wall (Fig. 5-5).[47] Notably, one should always try to minimize charring of the pathologic specimen in order not to hinder pathologic evaluation. After the tumor has been completely resected, it is recommended to fulgurate the base and edges of the tumor resection bed for hemostasis.[53]

Occasionally, tumor will cover or grow into/from a ureteral orifice. In this case, resection of the orifice should be performed with pure cutting current; no coagulation current should be used over the ureteral orifice to avoid stricture. Placement of a temporary ureteral stent while awaiting resolution of postoperative edema to resolve is optional in cases in which there is potential concern for ureteral obstruction.[54]

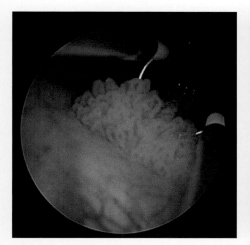 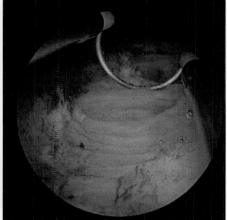

FIGURE 5-5 Demonstration of transurethral resection of bladder tumor during resection. The resection in progress is notable for visible muscle fibers of the bladder wall as part of the resection.

In addition to the formal tumor resection, at least a biopsy with a cold cup forceps, if not a formal resection, should be performed on any suspicious mucosal areas, and each should be sent for pathologic evaluation as separate specimens.[5] Furthermore, in the setting of abnormal urinary biomarker (cytology, fluorescence in situ hybridization [FISH], etc.) without macroscopic evidence of disease, random bladder biopsies should be performed. Otherwise, random bladder biopsies are not routinely necessary.[54]

Resection can be carried out with monopolar energy, requiring external patient grounding and the use of nonconductive irrigation solution (water, glycine, or sorbitol), which carries a risk of TUR syndrome (hypervolemic hyponatremia). Newer technologies using bipolar electrocautery allow the resection to be performed in isotonic saline, which minimizes the risk of TUR syndrome.[55] Other advantages associated with bipolar technology include lower risk of overall complications, minimized risk of bleeding, shorter operative times, lower risk of obturator reflex, and less cautery artifact in the specimen. Finally, the use of bipolar energy is associated with a lower risk of recurrent tumor.[56,57]

The conventional resection should be performed in a staged fashion in which the tumor is removed in multiple different sections proceeding sequentially until the base is reached. Then, the base should be resected deeply to include muscle to provide adequate staging information.[52] This technique is the most common and accepted method of resection. The alternative technique of an en bloc resection can be performed using loop modifications, lasers, and water jet–based enucleation. This technique includes the incision of surrounding normal mucosa with a wide margin in order to remove the tumor in one piece. The tumor is then pulled away and removed from the underlying tissue with blunt dissection.[58–61] The advantage of this technique is that it allows conservation of the three-dimensional architecture of the tumor; however, this technique should be reserved for tumors 3 cm or less.[58,62]

Complete and thorough TUR of bladder tumor(s) represents the criterion standard for the treatment of urothelial cancer, as it both is used to establish the clinical stage of disease and has therapeutic value itself. However, in patients with obvious low-grade papillary noninvasive tumors, muscle is not necessary in the specimen. Moreover, electrocautery alone may not yield tumor sampling; however, it is safe and efficacious in properly selected patients.[53,63] There is no difference in disease-specific survival or disease progression in patients with superficial low-grade recurrences when electrocautery alone is used.[63] Nevertheless, electrocautery with or without biopsy alone should not replace TUR in the setting of primary treatment for the initial tumor or for a recurrence suspected with a change in tumor grade or stage.

At the conclusion of any resection and/or biopsy, hemostasis should be obtained. All actively bleeding sites should be cauterized. The bladder tumor chips should be evacuated out and sent for pathologic evaluation. Bladder drainage should be considered with a catheter to avoid postoperative overdistension, particularly in cases of suspected or known perforation. If hematuria is persistent, continuous bladder irrigation can be considered adjunctively but not as a replacement for meticulous hemostasis.

3. ENDOSCOPIC EVALUATION AND TREATMENT OF UPPER TRACT DISEASE

Recommendation: When upper tract urothelial cancer is suspected, endoscopy of the upper genitourinary tract should be performed to accurately describe the anatomic location and volume of the disease involving the pelvicalyceal system and ureteral segments, as well as to obtain acceptable biopsy and cytology samples, to accurately grade and stage the tumor for surgical planning. For select patients with low-grade, noninvasive cancer, tumor ablation can adequately control disease.

Type of Data: Retrospective reports, case series, or case-control studies

Strength of Recommendation: Strong recommendation, low-quality evidence

Rationale

Although cystoscopy, dedicated upper tract imaging, and urine cytology have long been considered standard in the diagnostic evaluation of upper tract urothelial carcinoma (UTUC), advancements in upper tract endoscopy have established ureteroscopy as an important adjunctive procedure in the management of this disease.[64] Endoscopic evaluation of upper tract malignancy is both safe and necessary for optimal disease-risk stratification. Careful evaluation of the entire upper tract is associated with more accurate tumor grading, staging, and characterization. Ureteroscopic biopsy specimens have been shown to have a greater than 90% concordance with final pathologic grade on nephroureterectomy.[65] The data obtained from a diagnostic ureteroscopy help dictate surgical planning and guide management decisions. The data allow for appropriate patient selection, particularly when considering kidney-sparing treatments.[66]

Endoscopic ablative techniques can, in carefully selected cases, provide acceptable oncologic control while sparing the patient excess perioperative morbidity. Retrospective data support the safety and efficacy of endoscopic tumor ablation in low-grade, noninvasive UTUC. Caution should be used in cases of high-grade disease, given an increased risk of local recurrence and progression in this population.[67]

Use of percutaneous renal access can be considered for tumors inaccessible from a retrograde ureteroscopic approach. Limited retrospective studies have demonstrated good cancer-specific survival in the management of properly selected low-grade, noninvasive tumors without the need for radical nephroureterectomy. However, this approach is associated with increased perioperative morbidity over standard ureteroscopy and a potential risk of tumor seeding in the percutaneous access tract.[63]

Technical Aspects

A distinction should be made between diagnostic endoscopy and therapeutic procedures. Diagnostic endoscopy is intended to carefully evaluate upper tract pathology, whereas procedures with therapeutic intent are typically more complex and technically challenging. Optimizing outcomes with either approach requires attention to key principles to achieve the defined goals of the procedure with minimal trauma.

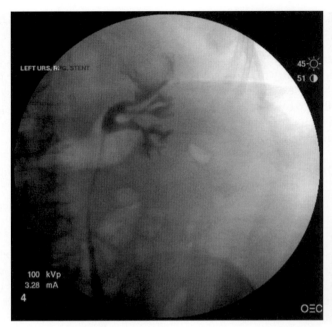

FIGURE 5-6 Retrograde pyeloureterogram demonstrating filling defects along the ureter and in the renal pelvis from upper tract urothelial carcinoma.

Initially, the ureter is intubated with a safety wire that should be coiled in the renal pelvis under fluoroscopic guidance; this can serve to assist with ureteral stent placement in the case of ureteral injury or false-passage creation. A retrograde pyelo-ureterogram can demonstrate filling defects along the ureter and renal pelvis as areas of concern (Fig. 5-6). Ureteroscopy should include careful inspection of the entire ureter and pelvicalyceal system. A systematic evaluation with close, direct inspection of each individual calyx is essential. Tumor number, approximate size, location, and gross morphology (papillary, pedunculated, or sessile architecture) should be noted to aid in risk stratification and treatment decision-making. In cases in which an endoscope cannot be safely or easily advanced into the ureter, placement of a temporary stent can be used to passively dilate the ureter over 2 to 3 weeks before reattempting the procedure.

Biopsy samples should be obtained when indicated, using ureteroscopic forceps, brushes, or wire baskets. Brushes may be favored for flat lesions and forceps for sessile tumors, whereas the wire basket allows for larger tissue yield from papillary or pedunculated tumors. When possible, multiple biopsy samples should be obtained to improve diagnostic accuracy. Larger tumors can be processed as standard cell-block specimens, but smaller tumors are often better preserved when processed as cytology specimens.[69] Following biopsy, hemostasis can be obtained by Bugbee cautery or defocused laser fulguration. Gentle aspiration washings of the renal pelvis through the ureteroscope working channel can improve yield of tumor cells for cytologic diagnosis.

This kidney-sparing approach should be strongly considered in patients with low-risk tumors, solitary kidneys, severe renal insufficiency, and bilateral tumors.[70] Tumors that are papillary, unifocal, low grade, and less than 1.5 cm should be considered for endoscopic treatment in lieu of radical nephroureterectomy when technically feasible.[71] Radical nephroureterectomy is typically recommended for tumors larger than 2 cm but can be used in select cases for smaller tumors.[72] Ureteroscopic ablation can also play a palliative role in the treatment of severely comorbid or elderly patients who are not candidates for radical nephroureterectomy.

In patients deemed candidates for kidney-sparing endoscopic management of their disease, laser ablation can be performed using rigid or flexible ureteroscopy (Fig. 5-6). Holmium:YAG and neodymium:YAG lasers are both effective and widely available laser energy sources. The holmium laser causes coagulation at low energies and tissue ablation at higher energies with effects that are a function of pulse duration, energy, and frequency. Its lower tissue penetration makes it ideal for superficial lesions and ureteral tumors. The neodymium laser, which destroys tissues through thermal coagulation, has a higher depth of penetration (2 to 4 mm) and can be more effective with larger lesions in the pelvis or calyces. When ablating ureteral tumors, circumferential coagulation of the ureteral lumen should be avoided, as this puts the patient at significant risk of stricture formation. Optional placement of a double-J ureteral stent following ureteral ablation is typical to help avoid postoperative obstruction complications. Laser fibers of up to 550 microns can be used for ablation of ureteral tumors, whereas fibers 200 microns and smaller are preferred for calyceal tumors, allowing for improved flexion of the ureteroscope within the kidney. Any attempt at definitive management with endoscopic ablative techniques requires rigorous follow-up, especially for common sites of urothelial recurrence in the bladder and upper tracts, which can be monitored with endoscopy and imaging. Periodic cross-sectional imaging with computed tomography (CT) or magnetic resonance imaging (MRI) can be used to monitor for signs of progression locally and in nodal and distant sites.

4. POSTOPERATIVE INSTILLATION OF INTRAVESICAL CHEMOTHERAPY

Recommendation: Chemotherapy (gemcitabine or mitomycin) should be instilled into the bladder within 24 hours (but ideally within 6 hours) following endoscopic resection of NMIBC.

Type of Data: Prospective clinical trials, systematic reviews, and meta-analyses

Strength of Recommendation: Strong recommendation, high-quality evidence

Rationale
Microscopic tumor cells at the site of resection and reimplantation of "free-floating" tumor cells in the bladder may contribute to increased cancer recurrence. Immediate postoperative instillation with intravesical chemotherapy has been shown to decrease recurrence in select patients with suspected NMIBCs who undergo endoscopic resection.

A systematic review and meta-analysis of 11 studies that randomized 2,278 patients with NMIBC demonstrated that a single instillation of chemotherapy following resection reduced the risk of 5-year recurrence by 35% (hazard ratio [HR], 0.65; 95% CI, 0.58 to 0.74; $P < .001$); 5-year recurrence rates were 59% versus 45%. The risk of progression to a higher stage or cancer mortality, however, was not improved with a single dose of intravesical therapy.[73]

The ideal patients for postoperative instillation with intravesical chemotherapy are those with low-risk or selected intermediate-risk disease. A single dose of intravesical therapy may have limited effect in patients with an elevated European Organisation for Research and Treatment of Cancer (EORTC) recurrence risk score (EORTC recurrence risk score ≥5; patients with eight or more tumors and those with one or more recurrence per year).[74] In addition, intravesical therapy should not be administered when bladder perforation occurs, extensive resections are performed, there is considerable hematuria, or patients have had previous adverse reactions.

In the past, mitomycin was most commonly used in the immediate postoperative setting for patients with superficial bladder tumors. However, concerns for toxicity, including cystitis (up to 30%), dermatologic rash (10%), and even contracted bladder (5%), limited widespread adoption.[75] A recently published randomized trial of 406 patients with suspected low-grade NMIBC demonstrated that immediate postoperative intravesical instillation of gemcitabine was superior to instillation of saline in reducing the risk of cancer recurrence. Patients received 2 g of gemcitabine in 100 mL of saline within 3 hours after TURBT. In the intention-to-treat analysis, patients treated with gemcitabine had a 35% risk of recurrence over 4 years, as compared with 47% of patients treated with saline (HR, 0.66; 95% CI, 0.48 to 0.90; $P < .001$). This translated to an absolute reduction in recurrence of 12% at 4 years. For patients with confirmed low-grade NMIBC on initial TURBT who received gemcitabine postoperatively, this translated to an absolute reduction in recurrence of 20% at 4 years. Importantly, there was no difference in adverse effects or progression between the two cohorts.[76] Although no head-to-head study has been performed, the combination of mitomycin's toxicity profile coupled with data demonstrating better tolerability, much lower cost, and effectiveness of gemcitabine suggests gemcitabine as the more practical option.[71]

Technical Aspects

Intravesical treatment should be initiated within 24 hours of the initial resection, but ideally, it should be administered within 6 hours of the procedure. Multiple intravesical agents have been studied, including epirubicin, pirarubicin, and thiotepa; however, mitomycin C and gemcitabine are the two agents most commonly used in the United States.

Intravesical chemotherapy is contraindicated in patients with an allergy or history of adverse reaction to that chemotherapy and if perforation of the bladder occurred or is potentially suspected. The typical dose for mitomycin is 40 mg in 20 mL. The bladder should otherwise be empty, and alkalization of the urine with sodium bicarbonate can be considered. Gemcitabine has typically been given as 2,000 mg in 50 to 100 mL. After the chemotherapy is instilled in the bladder via foley catheter, the catheter should be held clamped for 1 to 2 hours as tolerated by the patient, and then the bladder should be emptied.[77]

CHAPTER 11

Partial Cystectomy

CRITICAL ELEMENTS

- Intraoperative Localization of Tumor
- Resection to Adequate Margins

1. INTRAOPERATIVE LOCALIZATION OF TUMOR

Recommendation: All candidates for partial cystectomy should undergo a systematic intraoperative evaluation to confirm the safety and feasibility of complete tumor resection with partial cystectomy. Intraoperative evaluation may include cystoscopy, histologic confirmation, consideration for cystoscopic bladder mapping biopsies, and intraoperative palpation following bladder distention.

Type of Data: Retrospective reports, case series, or case-control studies

Strength of Recommendation: Strong recommendation, low-quality evidence

Rationale

Partial cystectomy may be considered in highly select patients who have tumors that are amenable to complete resection with preservation of an amount of bladder sufficient to maintain renal function.[78,79] Preoperative imaging with computed tomography (CT) or magnetic resonance imaging (MRI) may assist with tumor localization, particularly to evaluate lesion size and location. In addition, for bladder paragangliomas, traditional characterization of disease extent has been with [131]iodine metaiodobenzylguanidine (MIBG) scanning, although functional imaging modalities including [18F]-fluoro-2-deoxy-d-glucose ([18F]-FDG) and now [68Ga]-DOTA(0)-Tyr(3)-octreotate ([68Ga]-DOTATATE) positron emission tomography (PET)/CT have recently shown potentially superior sensitivity and specificity.[80]

Urine or serum catecholamines should also be obtained preoperatively for these patients, as management for catecholamine-secreting tumors includes preoperative alpha-blockade.

Following this preoperative workup, cystoscopic assessment is critical to document the size and location of the primary tumor and to establish the absence of synchronous multifocal disease.[71] The ideal location of a tumor for partial cystectomy is the dome of the bladder, as this is anatomically away from other structures and allows resection with optimal maintenance of bladder capacity.[71] Conversely, tumors located at the bladder trigone are poorly suited to partial cystectomy because they are close to the bladder neck and ureteral orifices; maintenance of urinary function following resection is, therefore, challenging. In cases of tumor in a bladder diverticulum, the proximity of the ureteral orifices to the neck of the diverticulum should be noted in order to facilitate patient counseling and operative planning regarding potential need for ureteral reimplantation. Examination under anesthesia at the time of cystoscopy should be performed as well to palpate for a three-dimensional tumor mass and assess for tumor fixation to adjacent organs (e.g., prostate, anterior vaginal wall, pelvic sidewall).

Tumor histology should be confirmed to guide further surgical management. For urachal adenocarcinoma, en bloc resection of the umbilicus should be performed with partial cystectomy, given the potential for tumor involvement.[81] When partial cystectomy is being considered for urothelial histology, preoperative "mapping" should be obtained to rule out the presence of occult concomitant carcinoma in situ (CIS) elsewhere in the bladder. In male patients, prostatic urethral biopsies should also be considered in this situation.

Technical Aspects

To facilitate intraoperative localization, the bladder should be distended through a urethral catheter. For larger tumors, particularly at the bladder dome or anterior bladder wall, manual external palpation after bladder distention may allow the tumor to be localized.

Intraoperative cystoscopy should be used to assist with localization.[82] This technique entails performing intraoperative cystoscopy and positioning the cystoscope close to the tumor, dimming the operating room lights to visualize the cystoscope light through the bladder wall, and marking the resection margins externally on the bladder (Fig. 5-7). During this process, external palpation, along with cystoscopic visualization, can confirm that the correct resection margin is being marked with the intent of achieving clinically and microscopically negative margins.

For tumors in a bladder diverticulum, circumferential dissection of the diverticulum outside the bladder prior to bladder entry should be performed when feasible. In cases in which the extent of the diverticulum cannot be sufficiently established, umbilical tape may be packed into the diverticulum on bladder entry to distend the diverticulum and allow identification of the structure's borders. The goal of resection is to achieve clinically and microscopically negative margins.

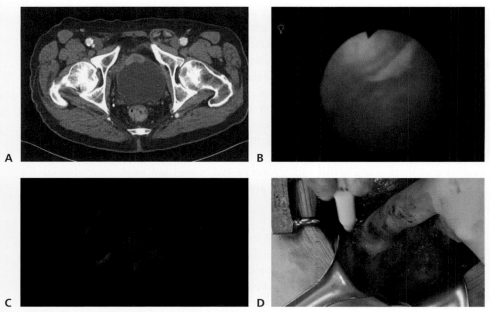

FIGURE 5-7 Preoperative imaging and intraoperative tumor localization for partial cystectomy. **A:** Axial CT image of pelvis showing the tumor on the bladder dome. **B:** Cystoscopic view of the tumor is helpful to aim the cystoscope and provide reference external to the bladder for resection. **C:** External view of bladder with cystoscope positioned at the tumor with the operating room lights dimmed allows for determination of safe margins of resection. **D:** Marking of resection margins on outer surface of bladder to achieve adequate resection on partial cystectomy.

2. RESECTION TO ADEQUATE MARGINS

Recommendation: Partial cystectomy should be performed to gross resection margins of 2 cm whenever possible. Intraoperatively, the status of the resection margins should be confirmed histopathologically with frozen section analysis. Partial cystectomy should not be considered in patients in whom a gross complete resection with a negative margin cannot be anticipated or in those who carry a concurrent diagnosis of CIS.

Type of Data: Retrospective reports, case series, or case-control studies

Strength of Recommendation: Strong recommendation, low-quality evidence

Rationale

Aggressive curative treatments are used for only 50% of patients with muscle-invasive bladder cancer today because of factors such as advanced age at diagnosis, social disparities, and restricted access to tertiary care centers.[25] Although the standard treatment for muscle-invasive bladder cancer is radical cystectomy with pelvic lymph node dissection, recent efforts are being made to identify patients for bladder-sparing partial cystectomy. The low frequency with which partial cystectomy has been used historically for patients with urothelial bladder cancer resulted from the small proportion of patients who are considered favorable candidates for this approach. In fact, a recent population-based study showed that partial cystectomy represented only 7% to 10% of all cystectomies and 3.7% of all operations for muscle-invasive bladder cancer in the United States between 2004 and 2008.[83]

High rates of local recurrences of up to 78% were reported in early series of partial cystectomy for invasive urothelial carcinoma in the late 1970s, which led to low utilization of the procedure in the years to follow.[84] More recently, however, high-volume centers have demonstrated that radical and partial cystectomy might have comparable oncologic outcomes when patients are carefully selected.[78,79,85–89]

Margin status

The proportion of patients with positive surgical margins in partial cystectomy specimens has been increasing, according to data from the National Cancer Database.[90] Following partial cystectomy, positive surgical margins have been shown to be a strong prognostic factor, reducing 5-year cancer-specific survival from 72% to 32%.[91] Similarly, recurrence-free survival and overall survival are both significantly shorter among patients with positive surgical margins despite use of adjuvant chemotherapy or radiation therapy.[92]

Intraoperatively, a complete and wide tumor excision should be performed to 2-cm gross surgical margins of healthy bladder mucosa when possible and to a minimum of 1 cm.[87] These numbers are arbitrary and based on past oncologic concepts taken from previous single-center reports rather than higher level of evidence. Nevertheless, these should be used as guidelines to select patients for partial cystectomy; when that is not possible, radical cystectomy should be strongly considered.[93]

Systematic intraoperative frozen section evaluation of the surgical margins is also recommended. Pathologic assessment of the edges of the resected specimen or from normal-appearing tissue surrounding this specimen should be performed.[94] Although the benefit of frozen sections for urologic malignancies is still debated, this strategy should be routine at partial cystectomy as it appears to reduce rates of positive margins and recurrence.[95–97]

Ureteral implantation

The need for ureteral reimplantation during partial cystectomy has also been associated with improved outcomes if it is able to achieve negative margins.[98] Tumors located at the bladder trigone and ureteral orifice may increase the risk of contralateral ureteral injury and thus limit the extent of possible resection, which may compromise outcomes.[89] These patients may be best guided toward radical cystectomy (Fig. 5-8).

Carcinoma in situ

Whether diagnosed concomitantly with muscle-invasive bladder cancer before curative treatment on initial transurethral resection or later within the cystectomy specimen,

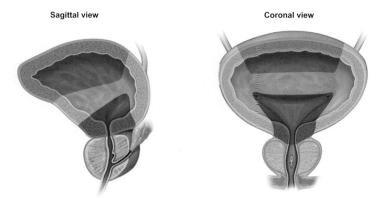

Sagittal view   Coronal view

FIGURE 5-8 Sagittal and coronal views of location of tumors that are absolute contraindications for partial cystectomy (*red zone*: within bladder neck and trigone), relative contraindications (*yellow zone*: within 2 cm of trigone), and amenable to partial cystectomy (*green zone*: dome and posterior tumors in particular).

CIS is associated with poor outcome.[99] CIS is typically multifocal and is considered representative of a field disease that promotes carcinogenesis even in surrounding apparent normal mucosa.[99–101] A correlation between preoperative CIS and positive surgical margins in partial cystectomy specimens has also been demonstrated; both were associated with higher rates of recurrence after surgery.[78] Therefore, partial cystectomy should be avoided in patients who have a concurrent diagnosis of CIS.[21,102]

Technical Aspects

Partial cystectomy is initiated through an open infraumbilical midline incision using a pre- or transperitoneal approach, although minimally invasive surgery through laparoscopic or robotic techniques are also suitable.[96] Once the Retzius space is accessed, blunt dissection and detachment of the bladder from the pelvic wall and sustaining surrounding structures (urachus, peritoneum lateral to the medial umbilical ligament) should be performed to ensure maximum mobility of the bladder.[103]

Once the bladder wall is exposed, intraoperative transurethral cystoscopy with transillumination helps demarcate surgical margins. A cystostomy should be created at least 1 to 2 cm away from the tumor (Fig. 5-9).[87,94] Alternatively, when cystoscopy light does not clearly elucidate the ideal location for cystotomy, a needle placed through the bladder wall can be used to indicate the best area to start the tumor resection at the desired area.

Following complete en bloc removal of the tumor, surgical margins should be assessed. Any area containing evidence of microscopic residual disease should be managed with additional resection. According to surgical oncologic principles, after suturing the bladder defect, copious warm water irrigation is recommended to reduce possible pelvic seeding of tumor cells.[104,105]

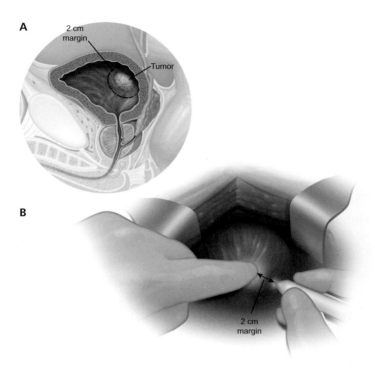

FIGURE 5-9   Identification of margin or partial cystectomy. **A:** A 2-cm margin should be scored circumferentially via cystoscopic view. **B:** Concurrently, transillumination from the cystoscopy can help identify the tumor site so that a 2-cm margin can be marked on the outside of the bladder as well.

Currently, partial cystectomy should be considered as a suitable organ-sparing alternative only in highly selected patients with localized bladder urothelial cancer. The development of new minimally invasive techniques as well pathologic and genetic understanding of this disease will help surgeons to determine the ideal patient for this approach and perhaps refine its use in the future.

CHAPTER 12

Radical Cystectomy

CRITICAL ELEMENTS

- Removal of Bladder to Negative Resection Margins
- Concomitant Pelvic Organ Management in Men and Women
- Pelvic Lymph Node Dissection
- Selection of a Urinary Diversion Procedure

1. REMOVAL OF BLADDER TO NEGATIVE RESECTION MARGINS

Recommendation: Removal of the bladder should occur with an effort to minimize the risks of tumor spillage or positive tumor margins. Intraoperative histopathologic evaluation of the distal ureteral margin need not be performed routinely at the time of radical cystectomy in the absence of cystoscopic suspicion of tumor at the trigone or urethra. Intraoperative histopathologic evaluation of the distal urethral margin should be performed when bladder neck, prostatic (in men), or urethral invasion is suspected based on cystoscopy or when considering candidacy for orthotopic urinary diversion but is otherwise unnecessary for urethral-sparing surgery when no nearby tumor involvement is suspected.

Type of Data: Retrospective reports, case series, or case-control studies; prospective clinical trials

Strength of Recommendation: Strong recommendation, moderate-quality evidence

Rationale

Radical Cystectomy (RC)—removal of the bladder, perivesical tissues, prostate, and seminal vesicles in men and the ovaries, uterus with cervix, and anterior vagina in women—together with bilateral pelvic lymph node dissection (PLND) is the treatment of choice for patients with muscle-invasive and high-risk bladder cancer.[106] Five-year disease-specific survival approaches 80% in patients with pathologic node-negative disease after cystectomy.[107,108] Lymph node status appears to be the single greatest predictor of disease outcome, with 5-year disease-specific survival of patients with node-positive disease approximately 30% in the same series. Positive soft tissue margin status is also an independent predictor of recurrence and disease-specific survival.[109] For these reasons, extirpation with a negative surgical margin and avoidance of any tumor spillage must be prioritized.

The incidence of a positive distal ureteral margin on final pathology has been reported to be between 6% and 8%.[110] Upper tract recurrence rates are generally low: between 2% and 8%.[111] In a contemporary study, the sensitivity of intraoperative histopathologic assessment for final pathology margin status was only 59%, and upper tract recurrence did not develop in upward of 64% of patients who had adverse pathologic features on frozen section evaluation of the margin.[111] These data suggest that intraoperative analysis of the distal ureteral margin inconsistently provides accurate information and is costly, and its results may affect surgical decision-making with little impact on outcomes.[112] Therefore, although there may be some situations in which frank tumor invasion needs to be ruled out and intraoperative histopathologic assessment is of use, the routine use of intraoperative ureteral margins should not be mandated.

The incidence of urethral recurrence after RC ranges from 4% to 8% in men and 12% in women. Urethral recurrence is very low in patients with no suspicion of urethral, prostatic, or bladder neck involvement on cystoscopy.[113] Therefore, routine urethral intraoperative histopathologic assessment is not necessary with low risk of urethral involvement preoperatively. The presence of non-muscle-invasive disease at the margin and the presence and extent of prostatic urethral involvement are predictors of urethral recurrence that can have devastating impact on orthotopic urinary diversion.[113] Orthotopic neobladder should not be considered for patients with a positive intraoperative frozen section. Furthermore, in cases of positive intraoperative histopathologic assessment of the urethral margin for tumor involvement, resection to a clear margin should be attempted, and completion urethrectomy should be considered concurrently or in follow-up.

Technical Aspects

The dissection should be initiated by bluntly developing the space of Retzius and establishing the potential space between the bladder and pelvic sidewall. The perivesical fat should be maximized on the specimen to mitigate the risk of positive margin in the case of T3 disease. The peritoneum should then be opened widely and the urachus ligated and divided. Consideration of en bloc resection of the urachal remnant should occur in cases of adenocarcinoma of the bladder and when tumors are located at the dome to maximize the likelihood of complete tumor resection (Fig. 5-10). On entering the abdomen, it is good practice to systematically inspect the abdomen for evidence of metastatic disease, specifically by palpating the liver and omentum. The mobility of the bladder and the tumor should be assessed. The preaortic and iliac lymph nodes should be inspected and palpated. This inspection should clarify clinical staging and the possibility of an R0 resection.

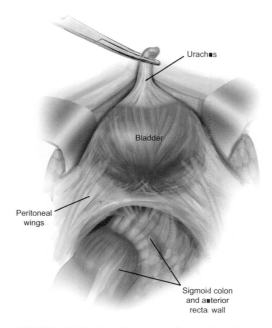

Urachus

Bladder

Peritoneal wings

Sigmoid colon and anterior rectal wall

FIGURE 5-10 Development of lateral and posterior bladder planes of resection should be performed by incision of the peritoneum overlaying these regions and dissection in these planes of resection. The urachus should be ligated high near the umbilicus and removed with the bladder specimen.

Ureteral dissection should be carried down to the hiatus and then doubly clipped to prevent spillage of urine prior to transection (Fig. 5-11). Distal ureteral frozen section is not routinely indicated but may be necessary on a case-specific basis for high suspicion or concern of tumor involvement.

Appropriate exposure and identification of the posterior plane between the bladder/prostate and rectum is essential for an R0 resection, especially in the setting of T2 or higher disease. Once the posterior peritoneum is incised, this plane should be developed with blunt finger dissection with the palm facing upward and carried anteriorly, ideally posterior to Denonvilliers fascia. The rectum should be swept downward away from the prostate and bladder (Fig. 5-12).

Female patients with tumors at the bladder neck and trigone and those with tumors involving the anterior vaginal wall are at greatest risk of urethral involvement.[114] For female patients who have chosen an alternative urinary diversion in which an intact urethra is not necessary, urethrectomy en bloc with cystectomy should be performed to minimize the risk of recurrence or positive surgical margin.[21] In women in whom orthotopic diversion is being attempted, an intraoperative histopathologic assessment of the urethral margin is desired before proceeding to the neobladder. In men, total en bloc resection including urethrectomy during cystoprostatectomy was considered

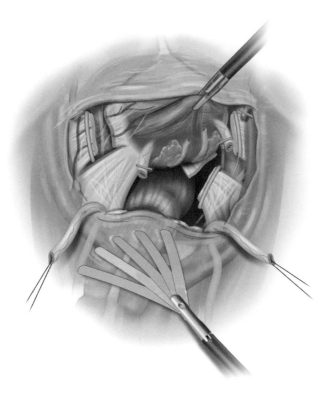

FIGURE 5-11 Dissection of the posterior-lateral planes around the bladder require clipping and transection of the ureter near the bladder to prevent any urine spillage as well as transection of the vascular pedicles of the bladder and, in males as illustrated here, the vas deferens.

standard of care historically; however, in more contemporary practice, routine urethrectomy (distal to the prostatic urethra) is not necessarily indicated. Routine urethral margins are not necessary in patients with no suspicion of urethral, prostatic, or bladder neck involvement on cystoscopy; however, if such involvement is noted, then margins should be considered. Involvement of the prostate and tumor grade and stage are predictive of urethral recurrence.[14] Even in patients with prostatic urethral involvement (ductal and not stromal), contemporary standard of care includes sending an intraoperative urethral margin for frozen section analysis; if negative, one can proceed with urethra sparing in concordance with patient's preoperative wishes.

Minimally invasive surgical techniques have become an accepted alternative to conventional open RC with the promise of reduced perioperative morbidity, reduced pain, and faster recovery. Robot-assisted radical cystectomy is being performed more often, and retrospective studies have reported lower rates of complications, faster recovery, and oncologic outcomes similar to open RC.[115,116] Five randomized controlled trials have shown similar oncologic results and rates of major complications with lower blood transfusion rates.[109] However, robot-assisted radical cystectomy has been associated with

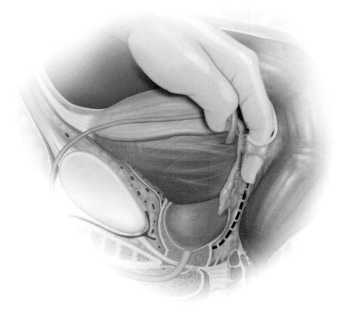

FIGURE 5-12 The posterior dissection in a male radical cystoprostatectomy requires identification and separation of the plane between the rectum and the bladder/prostate/seminal vesicles as shown by the dashed line. The rectum should be swept away from the bladder, ideally posterior to the Denonvilliers fascia.

lower intraoperative blood loss but with significantly longer operative time and higher cost. Some adaptations specific to minimally invasive surgery have been suggested to optimize oncologic outcomes with these techniques. These include starting the dissection in the posterior plane to maintain optimal visualization and resection margins (Fig. 5-13). Furthermore, cases of carcinomatosis due to possible urine spillage from the bladder neck have been reported, and clip or suture closure of the urethral margin prior to transection of the specimen is recommended to avoid urine spillage and potential seeding events.

2. CONCOMITANT PELVIC ORGAN MANAGEMENT IN MEN AND WOMEN

Recommendation: Organ preservation with organ-sparing cystectomy (OSC) is the favored approach to cystectomy for selected men and women with urothelial carcinomas T2 or less that are located away from the trigone or bladder neck and that do not involve the urethra.

Type of Data: Retrospective reports, case series, case-control studies

Strength of Recommendation: Strong recommendation, low-quality evidence

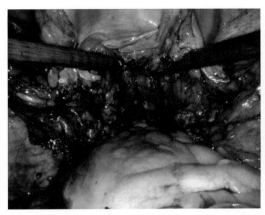

FIGURE 5-13 Adaptations of resection using minimally invasive surgery involve initial posterior plane of resection, which is typically performed before releasing the bladder in minimally invasive robotic surgery. Demonstrated here is the elevation of the bladder, prostate, and seminal vesicles off of the rectum, allowing exposure of the vascular pedicles and maintenance of surrounding tissue around bladder to optimize the likelihood of negative margins of resection.

Rationale

Women

Although urothelial carcinoma is more prevalent in men, women are also at risk of the disease, and women often present with advanced cancer.[117] RC is the standard treatment for women with muscle-invasive bladder cancer. Historically, RC was conducted concurrent with en bloc removal of the bladder, uterus, fallopian tubes, ovaries, anterior vaginal wall, and urethra (anterior pelvic exenteration) to achieve negative surgical margins and to ensure complete oncologic control (Fig. 5-14). However, in properly chosen patients, an organ-preserving approach (Fig. 5-15) may safely remove the tumor and avoid morbidity from removal of the reproductive organs, which can damage the neurovascular bundles located on the lateral vaginal walls, resulting in decreased vaginal sensation and lubrication. Surgical menopause secondary to oophorectomy has been associated with an increased risk of cardiovascular disease and osteoporosis and can also contribute to vaginal atrophy and dryness.[118] Devascularization of the clitoris can occur as paired pudendal arterial blood supply courses lateral to the urethra along the anterior vaginal wall.[119] The reproductive organs also provide suspensory support for the pelvic floor and orthotopic urinary diversions (Fig. 5-16).[120]

Contemporary series report reproductive organ involvement in 2.7% to 7.5% of women, and the vagina is the most common site of direct cancer extension.[120] Pelvic organ preservation with OSC appears to improve sexual function, continence (with construction of an orthotopic neobladder), and quality of life.[121-123] Oncologic outcomes

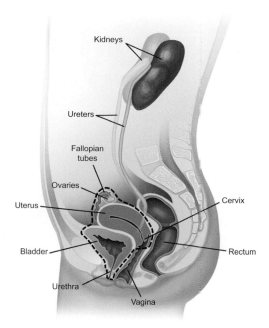

Kidneys

Ureters

Fallopian
tubes

Ovaries

Uterus

Cervix

Bladder

Rectum

Urethra

Vagina

FIGURE 5-14 Organs removed historically in complete female anterior pelvic exenteration include the urethra, bladder, uterus, portion of the anterior vaginal wall, fallopian tubes, and ovaries en bloc (*dotted black line*). Although this may be necessary for cancer control with some aggressive tumors, such extensive resection may not always be required.

appear equivalent between OSC in properly selected patients and anterior pelvic exenteration with respect to recurrence-free survival, cancer-specific survival, and overall survival.[122]

Patient selection is critical in balancing oncologic control with functional outcomes.[120,124] Organ-sparing procedures should be considered for women at particularly low risk of involvement of the adjacent reproductive organs: those with localized disease (T2 or less, absence of palpable mass after resection), a tumor located away from the trigone or the bladder neck, and absence of urethral involvement by tumor. These factors can be assessed at time of transurethral resection of bladder tumor (TURBT) or examination under anesthesia and with contemporary pelvic magnetic resonance imaging (MRI).[122,125] Patient characteristics such as functional status (including age and performance status), baseline sexual function, menopausal status, and family or personal history of gynecologic malignancies should also be considered; patient counseling is instrumental in determining the risks and benefits of pelvic organ preservation in each individual.

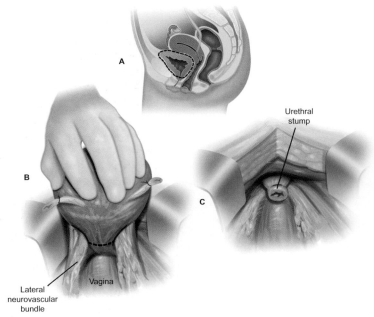

FIGURE 5-15 Most critical parts for the anatomy of women in terms of sparing sexual function. Broken lines designate desired planes of incision and dissection for organ sparing approaches. **A:** Preservation of the ovaries (estrogen-mediated vascularization of clitoris and vagina). **B:** Preservation of lateral neurovascular bundles on the vagina (and anterior vaginal wall). **C:** Preservation of urethra and, therefore, clitoral blood flow.

Men

Historically, RC in men included removal of the prostate and seminal vesicles. However, this radical procedure can damage structures important for both erectile and ejaculatory function as well as the continence mechanism of the distal urinary sphincter. An increased focus on survivorship and preservation of sexual function has motivated surgeons and patients to pursue OSC with reconstruction using an orthotopic neobladder. Although initially demonstrated for non-urothelial indications, these procedures have been associated with oncologic and functional outcomes comparable to RC in properly selected patients and may improve both continence and sexual function.[14,15,126]

Proper patient selection for OSC should balance oncologic risk with potential benefits.[124] Generally, men appropriate for an organ-sparing procedure include those with the following characteristics: tumor is located away from the trigone or the bladder neck, no involvement of the prostatic urethra, no evidence of locally advanced disease (T2 or less), and prostate cancer screening without concerning features.[124] Prostate urethral biopsies should be obtained if there is any visual suspicion of disease (either preoperative or intraoperative at time of cystectomy), prostate-specific antigen and screening direct rectal examination (and prostate biopsy when indicated) should be performed, and there should be careful notation of tumor location on cystoscopic

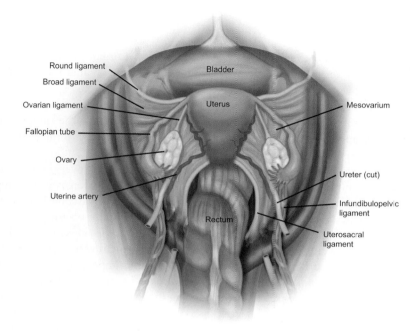

Round ligament

Broad ligament

Ovarian ligament

Fallopian tube

Ovary

Uterine artery

Bladder

Uterus

Rectum

Mesovarium

Ureter (cut)

Infundibulopelvic ligament

Uterosacral ligament

FIGURE 5-16 Transection of the ureter above the uterine artery to preserve uterine blood supply and support ligaments.

evaluation to ensure these criteria are met. Multiparametric pelvic MRI may have an emerging role in patient selection as well.[125] Age, baseline sexual function, urinary function, and personal desires should be considered because OSC should be avoided in patients who would not benefit from its purported advantages. Careful discussion with candidate patients is essential for managing expectations and improving quality of life after surgery while balancing cancer control. Multiple studies demonstrate comparable oncologic outcomes; however, confirmatory, high-level data are limited. To date, there is no oncologic evidence to exclude patients with muscle-invasive bladder cancer from OSC if they express their wishes in maintaining adequate sexual and urinary function.[127]

Minor differences in surgical technique have been described. As long as the prostate capsule is preserved, the external urinary sphincter is not damaged, and the neurovascular bundles and pelvic plexus are left intact, functional outcomes associated with OSC are favorable.[128,129] The literature reports 75% to 100% potency rates following OSC. Daytime continence rate is 95% to 100%, and the nighttime continence rate is 31% to 100%.[130]

Most prospective studies to date have been underpowered, owing mostly to poor patient accrual. Larger randomized trials are necessary to validate the aforementioned results and draw firm conclusions about the adequacy of this procedure, but the outcomes from single-institution series are compelling.

Technical Aspects

Women

OSC in women includes varying degrees of reproductive organ preservation and is described for both open and robotic operations based on known anatomic landmarks and considerations.[131-134]

For uterine preservation, the ureters can be divided at the level of the uterine arteries, thereby preserving not only the uterine blood supply but also the round, broad, and infundibulopelvic ligaments. Ovarian vessels can be identified adjacent to the ureters and preserved (Fig. 5-16).

For complete vaginal preservation, incision of the peritoneum over the vesicouterine pouch with blunt and sharp dissection in the midline location is a key step to identify the plane between the bladder and vagina. As the neurovascular bundles containing autonomic fibers from the pelvic plexus travel laterally on the vagina, care must be taken to ligate the posterior-medial and distal pedicles close to the bladder once this plane is developed (Fig. 5-15). The cranial and caudal vesicle pedicles can be taken as usual at their origin at the hypogastric vessels. It is important to note anterior vaginal wall thickness and blood supply and evaluate for potential involvement or extension of tumor past the perivesical fat during dissection and ligation of pedicles. If orthotopic diversion is planned, as the dissection is taken to the proximal urethra, care should be taken to preserve endopelvic fascia and pubourethral attachments (Fig. 5-15). Disruption of the levator muscles, periurethral tissues, and urethral sphincter (located ventrally) should be minimized to improve urinary function and continence. Care should be taken to avoid disruption of the pudendal blood supply to the clitoris to prevent atrophy.

Men

Several approaches to OSC exist, but they all share a common goal: selective partial removal of the prostate so as to leave vital structures unharmed for future recovery of potency and preservation of continence. Prostate-sparing cystectomy involves excision of the prostate central adenoma with preservation of the peripheral zone and prostatic capsule. To achieve this objective, a plane must be developed between the posterior bladder wall and the seminal vesicles and ampullae of the vas deferens. Sharp supra-ampullary dissection should be performed until the ejaculatory ducts are exposed.[135] The neurovascular pelvic plexus located posterior to the seminal vesicles should remain untouched (Fig. 5-17). When the prostate is exposed, the endopelvic fascia should be preserved on either side of the prostate. The prostate capsule should be incised using a transverse incision on the anterior surface of the prostate, and the adenoma should be removed while the capsule is preserved (Fig. 5-18).[136] Care should be taken to avoid dissection and cauterization close to the pedicles that course posterolateral to the prostate as those are preserved as well. Preservation of the posterior pelvic plexus, neurovascular bundles coursing laterally, and prostate capsule are thought to be the reasons behind potency and continence preservation in OSC.[137]

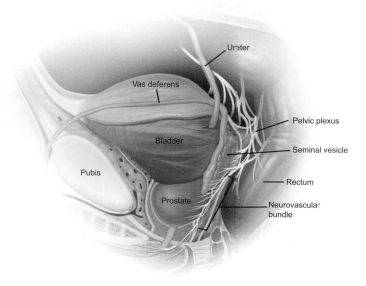

FIGURE 5-17   The neurovascular bundle runs adjacent to the prostate and passes at the tips of the seminal vesicle. Awareness of the path of the neurovascular bundle and avoidance of disturbing adjacent structures can optimize functional recovery.

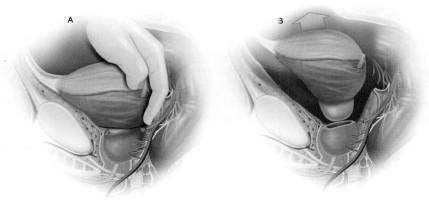

FIGURE 5-18   A: Prostate-sparing cystectomy can be performed in select cases for potentially improved postoperative sexual and urinary function. **B:** Prostate capsulotomy followed by en bloc removal of prostate adenoma with the bladder. Distal blood flow and innervation of the pelvic floor is left untouched to optimize outcomes.

3. PELVIC LYMPH NODE DISSECTION

Recommendation: A PLND using a standard template should accompany RC for urothelial carcinoma of the bladder.

Type of Data: Retrospective reports, case series, or case-control studies; prospective clinical trials

Strength of Recommendation: Strong recommendation, moderate-quality evidence

Rationale

PLND is currently accepted as a standard component for all radical cystectomies for urothelial carcinoma. No head-to-head trials directly comparing RC with or without PLND have been published. However, consensus exists that the potential for added morbidity from PLND is outweighed by its putative diagnostic—and perhaps therapeutic—benefits, even among lymph node–negative patients.

Several retrospective studies using data from single institutions and national registries have shown prolonged survival as a function of increasing lymph node yield among patients with pN0 tumors.[138–145] These data suggest that PLND may eradicate micrometastatic disease undetectable to the pathologist. Data also suggests that the extent of lymph node harvest may serve as a marker of the overall quality of oncologic care. Some authors have reported that a minimum lymph node yield (ranging from 4 to 16)[138–142] is required for oncologic benefit; however, given the high likelihood of unaccounted variables within the retrospective literature (e.g., quality of pathologic assessment, confounding by indication, whether nodes are sent in packets or en bloc), it seems unlikely that any strict numerical cutoff is sufficient.[145–147]

Recent focus has shifted from the number of lymph nodes removed to the anatomic extent of nodal dissection. In one retrospective study of over 1,200 patients, no cutoff point could be established because the authors observed a continuous overall survival benefit with increasing lymph node yield. Given that an extended dissection netted more nodes than a limited one (23 vs. 8, respectively), the authors concluded that an extended PLND should lead to better overall survival. This view has been shared based on many years of retrospective data, but inconsistent definitions of PLND templates (limited, standard, extended, and superextended) has contributed to the uncertainty surrounding this question and has hampered attempts to compare data between publications.[148]

Although no "official" borders for PLND templates exist, they can be extrapolated from the literature (Fig. 5-19).[149–151] A standard PLND template includes the lymph node chains from the external iliac vessels, internal iliac vessels, and obturator fossa. The boundaries include the genitofemoral nerve laterally, the bladder wall medially, the inguinal ligament distally, and the bifurcation of the common iliac artery (up to where the ureter crosses) proximally. A limited PLND would include lymph nodes from the external iliac vessels and obturator fossa. The extended PLND includes the standard boundaries plus the presacral lymph nodes medially and a proximal (cranial) border that terminates at the bifurcation of the aorta.

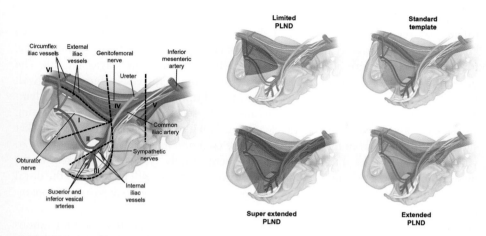

FIGURE 5-19 Left panel: Various nodal stations as numbered in the pelvis, which are involved with pelvic lymph node dissection. Right panel: Various extents of pelvic lymph node dissections (PLNDs) for cystectomy.

The first prospective data to evaluate the anatomic extent of PLND were reported in 2018 by the Association for Urologic Oncology of the German Cancer Society. In a multicenter randomized phase 3 trial, extended PLND was not superior to a limited template with respect to recurrence-free survival (hazard ratio [HR], 0.84; P = .36), cancer-specific survival (HR, 0.70; P = .10), or overall survival (HR, 0.78; P = .12).[152] At 90 days, Clavien-Dindo grade 3 or higher lymphoceles were more common among patients in the extended PLND group (3.4% vs. 8.6%; P = .04). This trial has been criticized for using nonstandard nomenclature in describing the templates: the limited dissection included internal iliac, external iliac, and obturator fields (which many consider a "standard" template). Further, the limited dissection yielded a median of 19 nodes (the extended dissection yielded 31 nodes). The high number of lymph nodes removed in both groups could have blunted any differential benefit of the extended dissection. The ongoing randomized phase 3 Southwest Oncology Group (SWOG S1011) trial compares standard to extended PLND and should have data available in the near future.

In the absence of definitive evidence to support one template over another, the current recommendation is the use of the standard template (as described in Fig. 5-19) for all patients undergoing RC for bladder cancer, which offers the best balance of oncologic efficacy and morbidity. This is, however, an area of active research and is described in greater detail in Urothelial Key Question 1.

Technical Aspects

The timing of PLND relative to the actual removal of the bladder is a matter of preference. From a technical perspective, removing the bladder first may allow for easier visualization of and access to the pelvic lymph nodes. However, there are also occasions in which removing the lymph nodes first allows better visualization of the pelvic vascular anatomy and facilitates the subsequent cystectomy (e.g., after prior pelvic surgery, in situ transplant).

For a standard template dissection, the lateral border of the dissection at the genitofemoral nerve should be defined at the start, with careful retraction of the nerve laterally away from the lymph node packet medially. This dissection should be performed along the length of the external iliac artery, revealing the pelvic sidewall. The dissection should encompass the space lateral to the iliac vessels and the sidewall toward the external iliac vein and down to the obturator nerve, separating the lymphatic tissue off the pelvic sidewall. This allows the surgeon to control the perforating vessels early and obtain good lateral clearance. Along the iliac artery, the nodal packet should be removed from the bifurcation of the common iliac artery proximally (up to where the ureter crosses) to the inguinal ligament distally. At the lateral extent of the dissection, lymphatic channels draining the lower extremity will be found at the distal aspect of the packet, so carefully placed clips are recommended to decrease postoperative lymphatic leakage.

Over the external iliac vein, extra care must be taken to identify aberrant venous anatomy that is common in this region, especially involving drainage from the obturator canal. Preemptively identified small venous branches can be controlled with small metal clips or bipolar diathermy. Larger branches should be preserved, if possible. The Cloquet node is encountered distally, overlying or immediately medial to the external iliac vein as it enters the femoral canal, and it can serve as a good landmark for ensuring the most distal extent has been reached (and should be removed).

4. SELECTION OF A URINARY DIVERSION PROCEDURE

Recommendation: Intraoperatively, the tumor extent, quality of the bowel to be used, and status of the urethra should all be evaluated to inform the final selection of a urinary diversion procedure at cystectomy.

Type of Data: Retrospective reports, case series, or case-control studies

Strength of Recommendation: Strong recommendation, low-quality evidence

Rationale

Most of the decision-making regarding the type of urinary diversion used for a patient undergoing cystectomy should be completed prior to surgery, with full involvement of the patient and family. However, findings at surgery may require a change in the planned procedure. It is critical that patients and families who are hoping for a continent diversion understand the potential for these intraoperative findings to preclude proceeding with a continent diversion. Intraoperatively, the tumor extent, quality of the bowel, and status of the urethra all inform the final decision with respect to diversion.

Three options for urinary diversion exist: ileal conduit, orthotopic diversion (neobladder), and continent cutaneous diversion.[21] Each patient must understand the advantages and disadvantages of each diversion procedure in the context of their own priorities.[153] Although only three absolute contraindications to continent diversion exist—poor renal function; lack of available bowel; and, for orthotopic diversion, lack of adequate urethra (poor sphincter function or stricture disease, or tumor at the urethral margin)—other relative contraindications must also be considered. These include poor performance status, a significant comorbidity profile, dementia, poor motivation, and prior high-dose pelvic radiation, especially to the prostate or cervix.[154]

In males, the only preoperative tumor-related relative contraindication to orthotopic diversion is involvement of the prostatic urethra by cancer. Carcinoma in situ of the prostatic urethra, most commonly seen in patients with a long history of carcinoma in situ of the bladder treated with multiple courses of intravesical therapy, may increase the risk of postoperative urethral recurrence from 5% to 12% and prostatic stroma invasion to 18% at 5 years.[135,155] Invasive tumor at the bladder neck is not a contraindication if the final urethral margin is negative. A patient with a history of prior radical prostatectomy may be considered for orthotopic diversion as long as the tumor is away from the urethral anastomosis and he has excellent continence.

For females, tumor at the bladder neck or palpable involvement of the cervix or anterior vaginal wall is associated with a high risk of urethral involvement, and the patient should be counseled away from orthotopic diversion.[156]

Technical Aspects

Ileal conduit

When an ileal conduit is planned, the primary intraoperative findings affecting the diversion relate to the segment of bowel being used. Patients who have a history of prior abdominal surgery or abdominal or pelvic radiation may pose a challenge, owing to extensive adhesions or radiation damage to the bowel. The distal ileum is usually chosen for an ileal conduit because of maximum mobility. However, more proximal ileal segments can be chosen with care to keep a wide vascular pedicle to the segment. Discarding a short segment of bowel on the proximal end can help to increase mobility between the butt end of the conduit and the bowel anastomosis. A basic tenet is to avoid using the jejunum for any diversion because of the active reabsorption that can result in electrolyte disturbance.[154]

Tumor involvement of the distal ureters may require excision of a long segment of distal ureter and thus may require a longer segment of bowel to create the conduit. There is controversy about the benefit of a frozen section of the cut ureteral ends. If the decision is made to send a frozen section from the margin involved with carcinoma in situ, as much ureter should be excised as possible without compromising ureteral length for the ureteral-to-intestinal anastomosis.[157] Similarly, extra bowel length should be taken in very obese patients to account for the extra length in the abdominal wall, with often a foreshortened mesentery in these patients.

Occasionally, there is direct tumor invasion into a loop of small bowel that requires a small bowel resection. If possible, the adjacent bowel should be used for the conduit to avoid having more than one bowel anastomosis. More problematic is the patient who is found to have carcinomatosis involving the serosa of multiple loops of bowel. Although it would be ideal to look for a loop without obvious tumor, these patients have a short life expectancy unless they have a good response to systemic therapy, so the choice of bowel is probably not critical.

Orthotopic diversion

Patients undergoing planned neobladder reconstruction have the same issues as those described earlier regarding bowel segment choice plus specific issues related to the integrity of the proximal urethral segment. A frozen section of the urethral margin should be obtained. The primary tumor finding at surgery that would require an alternative diversion is a positive frozen section of the urethral margin. This may occur in approximately 10% of males and somewhat higher percentage of females. Thus, it is critical to have a preoperative discussion of all options should that be the case.

The presence of grossly positive lymph nodes is not a contraindication to continent diversion. Pelvic recurrences rarely invade the neobladder directly but, of course, are associated with poor prognosis.[158] Clear invasion of the pelvic floor or symphysis pubis that is likely to lead to a margin-positive resection may make an orthotopic diversion unwise. Fiducial markers may be placed around the site of positive margin for postoperative radiation planning in this setting when appropriate. Adjuvant radiation can safely be applied to the neobladder if necessary.[159] Tumor involvement of the rectum or vagina that mandates wide en bloc resection is a relative contraindication to orthotopic diversion owing to the significant risk of fistula formation. Interposition of an omental flap may help decrease that risk.

Continent cutaneous diversion

Continent cutaneous diversions are much less commonly performed today than conduit or orthotopic diversions. The most popular is a pouch made out of the right colon with various types of catheterizable channels. In this case, intraoperative findings related to the extent of cancer rarely cause an issue other than those mentioned earlier. The surgeon undertaking construction of a continent cutaneous diversion should be familiar with several possible types of construction. If the appendix is planned to be used, an alternative must be available because the appendix in the typically older aged population undergoing these procedures may be scarred, short, or too narrow. Rarely, unexpected prior colon resection, unexpected colon cancer (ideally obviated by prior colonoscopy), or direct bladder cancer invasion of the ileocecal segment will require a change of plans.

Urothelial Key Question 1

In patients with muscle-invasive bladder cancer (MIBC) and high-risk bacillus Calmette-Guérin (BCG)–unresponsive non-muscle-invasive bladder cancer (NMIBC), what is the effect of performing an extended pelvic lymphadenectomy during radical cystectomy on oncologic outcomes (recurrence-free [RFS], cancer-specific [CSS], and overall survival [OS]), perioperative outcomes, and complication rates when compared with a standard pelvic lymphadenectomy?

INTRODUCTION

Although most bladder cancers are low grade and noninvasive, 20% are found to invade the detrusor muscle on diagnosis, and an additional 20% to 25% of noninvasive cancers will progress to a higher stage over time.[1] The standard-of-care treatment for MIBC is radical cystectomy with urinary diversion.[21] Radical cystectomy is also recommended to patients with high-risk NMIBC that does not respond to BCG therapy.[160] At the time of radical cystectomy, pathologic lymph node (LN) metastases are identified in approximately 23% of patients with MIBC and 8% with high-risk NMIBC. Therefore, a thorough anatomic lymph node dissection (LND) is essential, and the procedure is believed to be both therapeutic and diagnostically useful to guide adjuvant systemic treatment following radical cystectomy.[107,161]

A consistent definition of a standard lymph node dissection (sLND) for patients undergoing radical cystectomy for bladder cancer is provided by the American Urological Association (AUA) and the European Association of Urology (EAU) and includes the obturator, internal, and external iliac LNs (Fig. 5-19).[21,162] The utility of a more aggressive cranial extent to this dissection, however, has been vehemently debated. Adding to the uncertainty is the inconsistency with which the terms *limited*, *standard*, *extended*, and *superextended* LND have been used throughout the literature and in practice. The EAU guideline provides a definition of the more aggressive dissections: an extended lymph node dissection (eLND) includes the common iliac LNs to the aortic bifurcation, including the presacral nodes; and a superextended lymph node dissection (seLND) includes the retroperitoneal nodes to the inferior mesenteric artery.[162] Regardless of the exact definitions used, the key question of whether an sLND or a more aggressive LND should be performed, and in which patients, remains of clinical importance.

The purpose of this work was to provide a systematic review of the literature with the aim of evaluating the effect of eLND templates on oncologic outcomes, specifically local and distant RFS, CSS, and OS as well as perioperative outcomes and complications, in patients with MIBC and high-risk BCG-unresponsive NMIBC, compared with sLND. These data will be placed into context through a review of the factors that may affect the yield, oncologic benefit, and outcomes from an LND for patients with bladder cancer.

METHODOLOGY

A systematic search of PubMed was performed from inception through April 1, 2020. Medical Subject Headings (MeSH) terms included "Urinary Bladder Neoplasms" and "Lymph Node Excision." Searches were restricted to English language. All narrative reviews, systematic reviews, meta-analyses, editorials, and commentaries were excluded. Original articles were selected based on a priori inclusion criteria. Studies must have reported on oncologic outcomes (local or distant RFS, CSS, or OS), perioperative outcomes (estimated blood loss, operative time, length of stay), and/or complications. Prospective phase 2 or 3 studies and any retrospective studies that compared two or more extents of LND and attempted to control for confounding using multivariable or matched statistical analyses were selected. Studies that evaluated lymph node count (LNC) and correlated this with the outcomes of interest were included if they also attempted to control for confounding. Studies that only used no LND as the referent control were excluded, as this does not address the key question of how an eLND compares with an sLND. Further, any studies that reported the outcomes of increasing LNC using only a referent count of 0 were excluded for similar reasons.[163] Findings are reported in accordance with the Preferred Reporting Items for Systematic Reviews and Meta-Analyses (PRISMA).[163]

A total of 991 studies were identified via the search terms (Fig. 5-20). After exclusion of non-English language articles, 826 studies remained. After review of the titles and abstracts for relevance of those studies to the topic of this analysis, 113 studies were selected for full-text review, of which 80 were excluded. A total of 33 studies met all the criteria for inclusion in this systematic review. Consensus agreements were made by discussion when necessary. Tables 5-5A to 5-5C list the included studies that reported oncologic outcomes categorized by template dissection type (sLND, eLND, or seLND) (Table 5-5A), LNC (Table 5-5B), or both (Table 5-5C). The template dissection type of the reviewed studies are summarized in Table 5-5C within the "Study Group" and "Control Group" columns, and LNC is subcategorized in the "Outcomes" column. Table 5-6 lists the included studies that reported perioperative outcomes and complications.

Data were extracted from individual articles and independently reviewed by a single researcher. Each study was reviewed and assigned a quality of evidence based on the Grading of Recommendations, Assessment, Development, and Evaluation (GRADE) system.[191] Because of the statistical heterogeneity of various results reported, a meta-analysis was not conducted.

FINDINGS

RFS or disease-free survival was an outcome in 14 of the 33 included studies.[150,152,164–166,172,173,175,179,183–186,188] Of these 14 studies, 4 compared templates, 5 compared LNC, and 5 compared both templates and LNC. In total, 9 of 14 studies reported a benefit on multivariable analysis. The highest level data comes from the LEA AUO AB25/02 trial, whose primary outcome was RFS. At a median follow-up of 43 months, no significant difference in RFS was found at 5 years (64.6% vs. 59.2% in the extended and limited dissection group, respectively; hazard ratio [HR], 0.84;

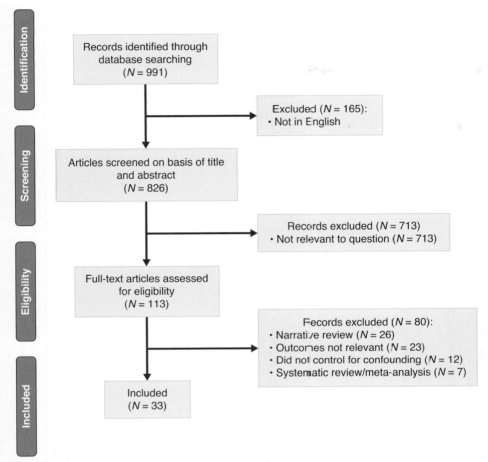

FIGURE 5-20 Preferred Reporting Items for Systematic Reviews and Meta-Analyses diagram for literature regarding extended pelvic lymphadenectomy during radical cystectomy.

$P = .36$).[152] However, the median RFS was not reached in either arm. More detailed data on the location of recurrence observed during follow-up was provided in the supplementary tables, and no differences in rates of local recurrence (6.6% vs. 8.9%; $P = .50$) or metastatic recurrence (23% vs. 20%; $P = .40$) were observed in the extended and limited dissection cohorts, respectively. The limitation with RFS, especially local recurrence, in this trial specifically was the relatively high LNC in both the seLND and the "limited" cohorts, which was a median 31 (interquartile range [IQR], 22 to 47) and 19 (IQR, 12 to 26) nodes, respectively, potentially skewing the result to the null. Local control of the pelvis and retroperitoneum is perhaps the most obvious benefit of a more extensive LND, and, indeed, two studies looking specifically at local control after surgery found improvements in the eLND (versus sLND) and higher LNC (≥10 vs. <10 nodes) cohorts.[164,166]

TABLE 5-5 Summary of Studies Related to Lymphadenectomy for Urothelial Cancer Surgery

TABLE 5-5A Studies Correlating Dissection Template with Oncologic Outcomes

Authors, Year	Type of Study	Patients, N	Study Population	NAC, %	Study Group	Control Group	Follow-up	Outcomes	Grade of Evidence*
Abdi et al.,[164] 2016	Retrospective, single institution	314	cTis–T4a cN1–cN3 cM0	25.7	eLND	sLND, matched cohort	Median, 19 (9–38) and 18 (8–36) mo in eLND and sLND	Local RFS: Referent: sLND eLND: HR, 0.63; 95% CI, 0.56–0.73 OS: no difference	++
Abol-Enein et al.,[165] 2011	Prospective, single institution	400	≥ cT2 Histology: 44.5% SCC	0	seLND	sLND	Median, 50.2 (IQR, 69) mo	DFS: Referent: sLND seLND: HR, 1.45; 95% CI, 1.06–1.98 In UCC-only subgroup, seLND improved DFS only in pN+	+++
Gschwend et al.,[152] 2019	Prospective phase 3 randomized study	401	cT1 G3 cT2–cT4a cN0 cM0	0	seLND	sLND	Median, 43 mo	Template: RFS: no difference CSS: no difference OS: no difference	++++
Jensen et al.,[150] 2012	Retrospective, two historical cohorts based on LND template	469	cTany cM0	0	seLND	Limited LND (obturator fossa only)	Median 113 (range, 86–143) and 45 (24–84) mo in seLND and limited	DFS: Referent: limited seLND: HR, 0.71; 95% CI, 0.50–1.01 OS: seLND: HR, 0.60; 95% CI, 0.45–0.81	++

CI: confidence interval; CSS, cancer-specific survival; DFS: disease-free survival; eLND: extended lymph node dissection; HR: hazard ratio; IQR: interquartile range; LND: lymph node dissection; NAC: neoadjuvant chemotherapy; OS: overall survival; RFS: recurrence-free survival; SCC: squamous cell carcinoma; seLND: superextended lymph node dissection; sLND: standard lymph node dissection; UCC: urothelial cell carcinoma.
*Grade: ++ low; +++ moderate; +++ + high.

TABLE 5-5B Studies Correlating Lymph Node Count with Oncologic Outcomes

Authors, Year	Type of Study	Patients, N	Study Population	NAC, %	Study Group	Control Group	Follow-up	Outcomes	Grade of Evidence*
Baumann et al.,[166] 2013	2° analysis of prospective data	442	cTany	29 (NAC + ADJ)	LNC ≥10	LNC <10	Median, 26.4 mo	Locoregional recurrence after cystectomy: Referent: ≥10 nodes <10 nodes: HR 2.37, 1.50–3.74	+++
Crozier et al.,[167] 2017	Retrospective, multi-institution	353	cTany cNany cM0	NA	LNC 6–15, ≥16	LNC 1–5	NR	CSS at 2 y: Referent: 1–5 nodes 6–15: HR, 0.78; 95% CI, 0.43–1.39 ≥16: HR, 0.31; 95% CI, 0.17–0.57 Increasing LNC improved CSS within template.	++
Fransen van de Putte et al.,[168] 2015	2° analysis of prospective data	274	cTany cN0–cN2	26.6	LNC (continuous)	NA	Median, 64.3 (IQR, 37.1–81.3) mo	CSS: no difference	+++
Froehner et al.,[169] 2014	Retrospective, single institution	735	cTany	5	LNC ≥17	LNC <17	Median, 7.8 y	CSS: no difference	++

(continued)

TABLE 5-5B Studies Correlating Lymph Node Count with Oncologic Outcomes (continued)

Authors, Year	Type of Study	Patients, N	Study Population	NAC, %	Study Group	Control Group	Follow-up	Outcomes	Grade of Evidence*
Herr,[170] 2003	Retrospective, single institution	667	cT2–cT4 N0 M0	NR	LNC continuous and quartiles	NA	Minimum, 5 y	CSS: pN0: LNC: RR, 0.87; $P = .001$ pN+: LNC: RR, 0.94; $P = .007$	++
Herr et al.,[146] 2004	2° analysis of prospective data	268	cT2–T4a cN0 cM0	50	LNC ≥10	LNC <10	Median, 8.9 y	OS: Referent: ≥10 nodes <10 nodes: HR, 2.0; 95% CI, 1.4–2.8	+++
Honma et al.,[171] 2006	Retrospective, single institution	146	cTany cNany	37	LNC ≥13	LNC <13	Median, 35 (3–169) mo	CSS, in pN+: pN+: ≥13 vs. <13 nodes: HR, 9.36; 95% CI, 2.52–34.70 pN0: no difference	++
Koppie et al.,[145] 2006	Retrospective, single institution	1,121; 1,042 with LN data	cTany	0	LNC (continuous)	NA	Median, 35 mo (for survivors, n = 596)	OS: Per node removed: HR, 0.97; 95% CI, 0.96–0.98	++
Lin et al.,[172] 2014	Retrospective, single institution	196	cTis/Ta/T1	1	LNC ≥10	LNC <10	Median, LNC <10: 75 mo ≥10: 54.6 mo	RFS: no difference	++

May et al.,[141] 2011	Retrospective, multi-institution	12	0	cTany pN0 only cM0	LNC ≥16	<16	Median, 45 (range, 2–240) mo	CSS: Referent: <16 nodes ≥16 nodes (HR, 0.74; 95% CI, 0.56–0.99) LNC as continuous variable: no difference	++
Morgan et al.,[142] 2012	SEER	3,170	4	cTany cN0 cM0	LNC 1–5, 6–13, ≥14	NA	NR	OS, pN0: Referent: ≥14 nodes 6–13 nodes: no difference 1–5 nodes: HR, 1.33; 95% CI, 1.12–1.58 CSS, pN0: 6–13 nodes: no difference 1–5 nodes: HR, 1.36; 95% CI, 1.11–1.67 OS/CSS, pN+: no difference	+++
Park et al.,[173] 2011	Retrospective, single institution	450	0	cTany	LNC ≥18	<18	Median, 26.8 (range, 2–204) mo	CSS: no difference RFS: no difference No difference in CSS or RFS when LNC analyzed in quartiles or continuous variable	++

(continued)

TABLE 5-5B Studies Correlating Lymph Node Count with Oncologic Outcomes *(continued)*

Authors, Year	Type of Study	Patients, N	Study Population	NAC, %	Study Group	Control Group	Follow-up	Outcomes	Grade of Evidence*
Ploussard et al.,[174] 2014	Retrospective, multi-institution	8,141	cTany	2.9	LNC ≥20	LNC <20	Median, 32 (IQR, 15–70) mo	OS: Referent: <20 nodes ≥20 nodes, baseline: HR, 0.90; 95% CI, 0.84–0.96 ≥20 nodes, 1 y: HR, 0.90; 95% CI, 0.83–0.97 ≥20 nodes, 2, 3, 4, 10 y: no difference	++
Rink et al.,[175] 2012	Retrospective, multi-institution	3,088	cTany pN0 only cM0	0	LNC tertiles, cutoffs ≥9 and ≥20 nodes, LNC continuous variable	NA	Median, 47 mo (IQR, 70)	CSS, pN0: no difference Recurrence, pN0: 1st vs. 3rd tertile: HR, 0.85; 95% CI, 0.71–0.99 1st vs. 2nd tertile: HR, 0.90; 95% CI, 0.76–1.07 LNC (continuous): HR, 0.99; 95% CI, 0.99–1.00	++

Study	Design	N	cT		LNC	LNC	Follow-up	Outcomes	
Shirotake et al.,[176] 2009	Retrospective, single institution	179	cTany	10.6	LNC ≥9	<9	Mean, 64 (range, 1–253) mo	CSS, pN0/N+: Referent: ≥9 nodes <9: HR, 3.48; 95% CI, 1.50–9.31 CSS, pN0: <9: HR, 6.94; 95% CI, 1.88–38.21	++
Siemens et al.,[177] 2015	Ontario Cancer Registry	2,802	≥ cT2	0	LNC quartiles: <5, 5–8, 9–13, >13	NA	NR	OS: Referent: >13 nodes <5 nodes: HR, 1.33; 95% CI, 1.12–1.57 5–8/9–13/>13 nodes: no difference CSS: <5 nodes: HR, 1.36; 95% CI, 1.12–1.64 5–8/9–13/>13 nodes: no difference	+++
Stein et al.,[178] 2003	Retrospective, single institution	1,054	HG, invasive	NR	LNC ≥15	<15	Median, 10.1 (range, 0–26) y	OS, pN+: Referent: <15 nodes ≥15: RR, 0.63; 95% CI, 0.40–0.99	++

(continued)

TABLE 5-5B Studies Correlating Lymph Node Count with Oncologic Outcomes *(continued)*

Authors, Year	Type of Study	Patients, N	Study Population	NAC, %	Study Group	Control Group	Follow-up	Outcomes	Grade of Evidence*
Ugurlu et al.,[179] 2015	Retrospective, single institution	85	cTany	0	LNC ≥20	LNC <20	Mean, 44.9 (± 27.4) mo	OS: no difference DFS: no difference	++
Von Landenberg et al.,[180] 2018	NCDB	16,505	cTany cN0 cM0	15	LNC ≥10	LNC <10	Median, 55.5 (IQR, 34.7–75.9) mo	OS, matched population: Referent: <10 nodes ≥10 nodes: HR, 0.85; 95% CI, 0.81–0.89 OS, matched population, −NAC: ≥10 nodes, cT1/a/is: HR, 0.85; 95% CI, 0.76–0.95 ≥10 nodes, cT2: HR, 0.85; 95% CI, 0.79–0.90 ≥10 nodes, cT3/4: HR, 0.85; 95% CI, 0.75–0.96 OS, matched population, +NAC: ≥10 nodes, cT1/a/is: HR, 0.49; 95% CI, 0.28–0.83	+++

	Database				LNC (quartiles)			Outcomes	Grade
						NA	NR	≥10 nodes, cT2: no difference ≥10 nodes, cT3/4: no difference	+++
Wright et al.,[181] 2008	SEER	1,260	pN+ pM0	NR	NR	NA	NR	OS: Referent: 1–5 nodes 6–9: HR, 0.71; 95% CI, 0.59–0.86 10–16: HR, 0.52; 95% CI, 0.43–0.64 >16: HR, 0.54; 95% CI, 0.45–0.65 CSS: 6–9: HR, 0.76; 95% CI, 0.62–0.94 10–16: HR, 0.53; 95% CI, 0.42–0.67 >16: IIR, 0.55; 95% CI, 0.44–0.69	+++

ADJ: adjuvant; CI: confidence interval; CSS: cancer-specific survival; DFS: disease-free survival; HG: high-grade; HR: hazard ratio; IQR: interquartile range; LN: lymph node; LNC: lymph node count; NA: not applicable; NAC: neoadjuvant chemotherapy; NCDB: National Cancer Database; NR: not reported; OS: overall survival; RFS: recurrence-free survival; RR: risk ratio; SEER: Surveillance Epidemiology, and End Results.

*Grade: ++ low; +++ moderate.

TABLE 5-5C Studies Correlating Both Dissection Template and Lymph Node Count with Oncologic Outcomes

Authors, Year	Type of Study	Patients, N	Study Population	NAC, %	Study Group	Control Group	Follow-up	Outcomes	Grade of Evidence*
Brunocilla et al.,[182] 2013	Retrospective, single institution	282	< cT2 if G3 ≥ cT2	0	seLND eLND sLND (lateral to the ureters on common)	Limited LND (external and obturator)	Mean, 59.2 (SD, 44.3; range, 1–171) mo	CSS: Referent: no or limited LND sLND: no benefit eLND/seLND: HR, 0.455; 95% CI, 0.365–0.894 Reference: <14 nodes ≥14: HR, 0.556; 95% CI, 0.282–0.995	++
Choi et al.,[183] 2019	Retrospective, single institution	448	cTany cNany	0	seLND eLND (lateral to the ureters on common)	sLND	Median, 41.6 (11.3–68.9) mo	Template not significant for DFS, CSS, or OS Distant RFS: LNC, HR, 0.981; 95% CI, 0.965–0.997 CSS: LNC, HR, 0.980; 95% CI, 0.967–0.993 OS: LNC, HR, 0.984; 95% CI, 0.974–0.995	++

Study	Design	N	Stage		Extended	Limited LND	Median (range) follow-up	Outcomes	
Holmer et al.,[184] 2009	Retrospective, single institution	170	< cT4b cM0	0	eLND	Limited LND (perivesical, obturator, laterally to external iliac vein)	Median (range), 94 (61–122) and 38 (13–70) mo in limited and eLND	CSS: Referent: limited LND eLND: HR, 0.47; 95% CI, 0.25–0.88 No difference with 16 cutoff RFS: eLND: HR, 0.42; 95% CI, 0.23–0.79 No difference with 16 cutoff	++
Mata et al.,[185] 2015	2° analysis of prospective data	440	cT1–cT2 pN0 only cM0	0	eLND	sLND	Median, 5.4 (95% CI, 5.1–5.9) y	No difference in DFS or OS based on template or LNC	+++
Park et al.,[186] 2011	Retrospective, single institution	155	cTany pN0 only	0	seLND	sLND	Mean, 36.6 (range, 12–141) mo	5-y RFS: Template: no difference LNC, HR, 1.087; 95% CI, 1.004–1.176 5-y OS: Template and LNC no difference	++

(continued)

TABLE 5-5C Studies Correlating Both Dissection Template and Lymph Node Count With Oncologic Outcomes *(continued)*

Authors, Year	Type of Study	Patients, N	Study Population	NAC, %	Study Group	Control Group	Follow-up	Outcomes	Grade of Evidence*
Simone et al.,[187] 2012	Retrospective analysis of prospective study data	Cohort A: 156 Cohort B: 154 (centers 1 and 2)	cTany pN1–pN3 cM0	0	eLND	sLND	Cohort A: mean, 28.9 (SD 28.7) y Cohort B: center 1 mean, 27.9 (SD 27.4) y Center 2 mean, 29.3 (SD 27.8) y	CSS: Referent LNC >30 10–30: HR, 1.46; 95% CI, 0.5–1.46 <10: HR, 2.09; 95% CI, 0.36–2.1 Referent sLND eLND: HR, 1.91; 95% CI, 1.12–3.23	++
Simone et al.,[188] 2013	2° analysis of prospective data	933	cTany cM0	0	eLND	sLND	NA	RFS: Referent eLND sLND: HR, 1.95; 95% CI, 1.56–2.47 LNC not significant CSS: sLND: HR, 1.76; 95% CI, 1.36–2.99 LNC not significant	+++

CI: confidence interval; CSS: cancer-specific survival; DFS: disease-free survival; eLND: extended lymph node dissection; HR: hazard ratio; LNC: lymph node count; LND: lymph node dissection; NAC: neoadjuvant chemotherapy; OS: overall survival; RFS: recurrence-free survival; SD: standard deviation; seLND: superextended lymph node dissection; sLND: standard lymph node dissection.
*Grade: ++ low; +++ moderate.

TABLE 5-6 Studies Reporting Perioperative Outcomes and Complications Associated with Pelvic Lymph Node Dissections

Authors, Year	Patients, N	Study Group	Control Group	Complication Outcomes	Grade of Evidence*
Abdi et al.,[164] 2016	314	eLND	sLND, matched cohort	No difference in length of stay or intraoperative or postoperative complications Mean EBL (mL): eLND vs. sLND (1,047 vs. 584; $P < .001$) Number of transfusions: eLND vs. sLND (2.4 ± 3.5 vs. 1.1 ± 2.1; $P = .03$) On multivariable analysis of matched cohort, eLND did not predict any complications.	++
Filson et al.,[189] 2016	4,975	6–10 nodes ≥11 nodes	1–5 nodes	OR time, defined as time from induction of anesthesia to reversal. Compared with removal of 1–5 nodes: +14.8 min with removal 6–10 nodes +24.9 min with removal of ≥11 nodes	+++
Gschwend et al.,[152] 2019	401	seLND	sLND	No difference in mortality and overall major (Clavien-Dindo ≥3) complications after 30 and 90 d Lymphoceles requiring intervention ≤90 d: seLND 8.6% vs. sLND 3.4% ($P = .04$)	++++
Kim et al.,[190] 2014	308	LNC as a continuous variable	NA	Early (<30 d) complications LNC (per node) odds ratio, 1.235; 95% confidence interval, 1.153–1.674 Late (30–90 d) complications LNC (per node) odds ratio, 1.054; 95% confidence interval, 1.005–1.106	++

EBL: estimated blood loss; eLND: extended lymph node dissection; LNC: lymph node count; NA: not applicable; OR: operating room; seLND: superextended lymph node dissection; sLND: standard lymph node dissection.
*Grade: ++ low; +++ moderate; ++++ high.

Cancer-specific survival was an outcome in 18 of the 33 included studies.[141,142,152,] [167–171,173,175–177,181–184,187,188] Of these 18 studies, 1 study compared templates, 12 compared LNC, and 5 compared both templates and LNC. In total, 13 of the 18 studies reported a benefit on multivariable analysis. In the LEA AUO AB25/02 trial, CSS was a secondary outcome, and no significant difference was observed at 5 years (64.5% vs. 75.9% in the limited and extended dissection cohorts, respectively; $P = .10$).[152] However, the HR was 0.78 and the 95% confidence interval (CI) was 0.46 to 1.07, nearly demonstrating a statistically significant difference. Most (8/12) of the retrospective LNC studies reported a benefit on CSS. In 2 negative studies, neoadjuvant chemotherapy (NAC) was used (albeit in a small percentage of patients—26% and 5%), potentially suggesting that systemic therapy may mitigate effects of a more extensive LND, a concept that formed the basis of a different study in a national cancer registry.[168,169,180] In the 5 studies that evaluated both templates and LNC, the template comparison was either not significant on multivariable analysis or used limited/no LND in 3. This could suggest that although CSS could be improved by an LND, the dissection should be complete and thorough and at least include the standard template.

OS was reported as an outcome in 15 out of the 33 included studies.[142,145,146,150,] [152,164,174,177–181,183,185,186] Of these 15 studies, 3 compared templates, 9 compared LNC, and 3 compared both templates and LNC. In total, 10 of the 15 studies reported a benefit on multivariable analysis. In the LEA AUO AB25/02 trial, OS was a secondary outcome, and there was no benefit observed in the extended dissection cohort (HR, 0.78; 95% CI, 0.57 to 1.07; $P = .12$).[152] Again, with respect to this outcome, the 95% CI of the HR (0.57 to 1.07) nearly demonstrated statistical significance in favor of a more extended LND. In the only positive retrospective study to compare templates, an seLND improved OS compared with a limited LND, which included the obturator only and was therefore biased to demonstrate a benefit in the seLND cohort.[150] Furthermore, 2 retrospective studies that found OS benefit to increasing LNC used 5 or fewer nodes as the comparator cohort, which may indicate substandard template extent or thoroughness of dissection.[142,177] In the 1 study to report a benefit in OS that evaluated both template extent and LNC, only LNC was significant on multivariable analysis.[183] Again, this suggests that the thoroughness of the dissection is potentially more important than the extent when an sLND is used as the comparator. In a National Cancer Database study by von Landenberg et al.,[180] the impact of NAC appeared to impact the benefit of LNC in terms of OS, with high LNC only improving the HR of OS in patients who did not receive NAC. Finally, 2 studies reported conflicting information regarding whether patients with pathologically negative or positive nodes experience an OS benefit from higher LNC.[142,178]

Only four of the included studies reported perioperative outcomes and/or complications.[152,164,189,190] Two of these studies compared templates, and two compared LNC. In the LEA AUO AB25/02 trial, one of the secondary outcomes was complications categorized in Clavien-Dindo grades reported at 30 and 90 days postoperatively.[152] Mortality and Clavien-Dindo grade 3 or higher toxicities were similar between the two arms. According to the supplementary tables, rates of postoperative bleeding, cardiopulmonary, gastrointestinal, genitourinary, infectious, thromboembolic, and wound dehiscence complications were similar between the two arms.

Lymphoceles requiring drainage occurred in 7 patients (3.4%) in the limited dissection group and in 17 patients (8.6%) in the extended dissection group ($P = .04$). Other perioperative outcomes that have clinical relevance include the finding that increasing LNC from a baseline of 1 to 5 nodes to 6 to 10 and 11 or more nodes resulted in an additional 15 and 25 minutes of operative time, respectively.[189] Further, an eLND template may increase estimated blood loss and transfusion rates compared with an sLND, as demonstrated in a matched cohort.[164] Finally, increasing LNC appears to be associated with both early and late perioperative complications.[190]

DISCUSSION

LND is undoubtedly an essential component in the surgical management of patients with bladder cancer. However, the degree to which a more extended LND improves oncologic outcomes continues to be debated. Further, the impact of an eLND on perioperative outcomes and complications is similarly understudied. The results of this systematic review suggest that some patients can derive benefit in the form of RFS, CSS, and/or OS from a more extended LND and that the perioperative outcomes and complications are manageable. However, the highest level data and the only randomized prospective study (the LEA AUO AB25/02 trial) demonstrates that an eLND should not be considered the standard for every patient at this time.[152] A second randomized study from the United States, the SWOG 1011, has completed accrual and is pending readout. Several notable differences exist between the LEA AUO AB25/02 trial and the SWOG 1011 trial: the SWOG study enrolled only patients with T2 or greater tumors, allowed patients who had received NAC, used a different power calculation, and allowed a less aggressive cranial limit in the more extended LND cohort (anywhere between the aortic bifurcation up to the inferior mediastinal artery).[192] To place current and future data in context, it is critical to understand the insights provided from classic LN mapping studies, the nontechnical factors that affect LN yield, and the influence of tumor biology and treatment pressures from neoadjuvant systemic chemotherapy on LND outcomes in patients with bladder cancer.

The understanding of the basic anatomy and drainage of cancer cells via the lymphatic system informs the debate on the role of an eLND in patients with bladder cancer. The first LN mapping study on pelvic lymphadenectomy and total cystectomy for carcinoma of the bladder was by Kerr and Colby[193] in the 1950s and relied on direct palpation of the "abdominal organs, the aorta, common iliac, external and internal iliac vessels"—a technique which was noted to be time honored but unreliable for the identification of metastases. Since then, several pathologic mapping studies and radiographic studies of sentinel LNs have demonstrated an orderly anatomic distribution of LN metastasis. Leissner et al.[194] demonstrated that the primary lymphatic drainage from the bladder is to the obturator, internal, and external iliac LNs.[194,195] Secondary sites of drainage are the presacral nodes and common iliac nodes. Additional studies have demonstrated that laterality of tumor within the bladder does not have a significant effect on the laterality of LN-positive disease; in one study, 15% of patients had a positive LN on the contralateral side.[196] Further, in this study, preoperative cystoscopic intramural injection of radioactive isotope demonstrated contralateral lymphatic drainage in 40% of cases. Although more than 90% of patients with pathologic node metastasis will be identified by a dissection up to the common iliac bifurcation, a more extended node dissection to the bifurcation of the aorta will identify additional nodal disease, resulting in a higher pathologic N stage in up to 40% of patients with nodal metastasis.[197]

Several technical and nontechnical factors are known to influence LNC and, therefore, influence the interpretability of results from any study evaluating outcomes of LND. First, completeness and thoroughness of LND are critical and likely more important than the numerical LN yield, regardless of the template used. As an example, Dorin et al.[197] reported on 646 patients from two high-volume treatment centers who were treated with radical cystectomy and nearly identical LND extents (by virtue of similar training experience). However, significantly different LN yields were obtained. Regardless, similar RFS and OS was noted between the cohorts, suggesting that anatomic completeness of the surgical dissection is more important than the LN yield measured histopathologically. This discrepancy in LN yield stems from differences in the method by which LN specimens are labeled and sent to pathology and/or handled for analysis. In one study, sending the specimens to pathology in individual packets (submission of LN specimen separated by anatomic location and side) compared with en bloc (submission of LN and radical cystectomy as a single specimen) resulted in a 3.5- and 1.6-fold increase in LN yield in sLND and eLND templates, respectively.[147] In another analysis of over 1,300 patients who underwent radical cystectomy, LN yield was significantly higher in the cohort sent as distinct nodal packets compared with the en bloc cohort (median 68 vs. 31 nodes; $P < .001$), and a trend toward more metastatic LN was also identified (median 3 vs. 2; $P = .06$).[198] Improved detection of nodal metastases, consequently, can result in improved staging, which will direct appropriate treatments and improve outcomes in all cohorts (Will Rogers phenomenon).

Finally, specific tumor biology and the treatment pressures applied by systemic chemotherapy before surgery can affect the utility of a more extensive LND in patients with bladder cancer. In one study comprising approximately 50% squamous cell carcinoma, an seLND improved disease-free survival, but in the urothelial cell carcinoma–only cohort, this effect was lost, underscoring the fact that disease biology should be considered.[165] The effect of NAC on the efficacy of LND has largely been unstudied but is of paramount importance considering contemporary practice patterns and guidelines that recommend its use in many patients with MIBC prior to radical cystectomy.[21,162] One study evaluated the National Cancer Database and identified nearly 8,700 patients who underwent radical cystectomy and lymphadenectomy between 2004 and 2012. They categorized LNC into adequate ($\geq$10 nodes) and inadequate (<10 nodes). Patients who did not receive NAC experienced an OS benefit from an adequate dissection. However, in those patients who did receive NAC, adequacy of the lymphadenectomy did not affect OS. The authors postulated, therefore, that micrometastatic disease may be effectively eradicated by NAC and that an adequate LND would, in turn, confer little additional benefit. Another possibility is that patients with residual disease after NAC harbor such aggressive disease that an adequate or even superextended dissection may not improve survival. Barring the known limitations of large registry-based analyses using the surrogate outcome of OS in a medically comorbid patient population, these findings are intriguing. Although the LEA AUO AB25/02 trial did not include patients who received NAC, SWOG 1011 does include this cohort of patients, which will provide insight into the role of lymphadenectomy in patients who may have lower risk of micrometastatic disease.

CONCLUSION

LND forms a critical component of the surgical management of high-risk and invasive bladder cancer. Adherence to the principles of thorough and complete dissections affects LN yield, diagnostic ability, and, likely, therapeutic efficacy. Using knowledge from early mapping studies, a bilateral standard lymphadenectomy of the obturator, internal, and external iliac nodes should be performed in all patients. This adheres to guidelines set forth by both the AUA and the EAU. A more extended node dissection including the common iliac, sciatic fossa, and presacral LNs up to the bifurcation of the aorta and even up to the inferior mesenteric artery likely benefits a subgroup of patients in terms of local and systemic RFS, CSS, and OS. Whether this benefit will extend to patients who received NAC prior to cystectomy has yet to be determined. The most extensive LNDs appeared to increase lymphoceles that require intervention in a randomized controlled study, and some retrospective data suggest higher perioperative complications. Ultimately, disease biology may dictate the potential for a thorough and extensive LND to confer a survival benefit, and, therefore, molecular subtypes or novel genomic signatures may be needed to help select these patients.

Urothelial Key Question 2

In patients with muscle-invasive and high-risk non-muscle-invasive bladder cancer, what is the effect of robotic-assisted radical cystectomy (RARC) on oncologic outcomes (progression-free survival [PFS] and surrogates), perioperative outcomes, and complication rates compared with open radical cystectomy (ORC)?

INTRODUCTION

Across surgical fields, the number of robotic surgical procedures performed each year has continued to increase both in the United States and abroad, despite relative stagnation in the number of urologic procedures performed each year.[199] In urologic oncology, robotic approaches are most widely used in radical prostatectomy. The diffusion of robotic approaches for both prostatectomy and nephrectomy has occurred in the absence of randomized data to support the superiority of this approach. Minimally invasive radical prostatectomy (predominately robotically assisted) became the most common approach to radical prostatectomy in the United States in 2008.[200] However, the first randomized data comparing open and robotic radical prostatectomy were not published until 2016.[201]

In contrast, diffusion of RARC has been slower. Additionally, randomized trials have been performed much earlier in the diffusion process, with Nix et al.[202] publishing a prospective randomized comparison of perioperative and pathologic outcomes for patients treated with RARC and ORC in 2010. Since that time, a number of small, single-center studies have been published. However, the next large advance in the evidence base in the question came with the publication of the robot-assisted radical cystectomy versus open radical cystectomy in patients with bladder cancer (RAZOR) trial,[203] a multicenter phase 3 trial with survival, rather than feasibility, outcomes.

For the most part, robotic-assisted surgery has been adopted with the assumption that the harms of such an approach are limited to the additional health system resources required for both platform acquisition and ongoing costs. However, specifically assessing recurrence patterns following open and RARC, Nguyen et al.[204] described an increased frequency of extrapelvic lymph node recurrence and peritoneal carcinomatosis in a retrospective review of patients treated with RARC. Perhaps more concerning is the recently published data in the use of minimally invasive (primarily robotic-assisted) radical hysterectomy for cervical cancer. In a trial of 631 patients randomized to minimally invasive or open abdominal hysterectomy for early cervical cancer, those undergoing minimally invasive surgery had significantly worse disease-free survival and overall survival.[205] An observational study published in parallel with this trial in the *New England Journal of Medicine* demonstrated similar results.[206] Further, these authors found that adoption of minimally invasive surgery was associated with a decline in 4-year relative survival at the population level,[206] a result which has been corroborated in other settings.[207]

Thus, there is both the need for critical evaluation of the role of robotic-assisted surgery in radical cystectomy and a relevant evidentiary base. A number of systematic reviews and meta-analyses have already been performed to summarize the available data comparing RARC and ORC. Therefore, the purpose of this work was to systematically review and summarize these systematic reviews to evaluate the effect of RARC on oncologic outcomes (PFS and surrogates), perioperative outcomes, and complication rates in patients with muscle-invasive and high-risk non-muscle-invasive bladder cancer, compared with ORC.

METHODOLOGY

A systematic search of PubMed from inception through July 21, 2019, was conducted. A combination of Medical Subject Headings (MeSH) terms and relevant free text keywords used included "Cystectomy," "Bladder Cancer," "Robotic," and "Systematic Review" or "Meta-analysis" and related terms. No language restrictions were applied. Following abstract review, a search of the bibliographies of included systematic reviews and major urologic and oncologic journals was conducted to ensure all relevant studies were captured. Findings are reported in accordance with the Preferred Reporting Items for Systematic Reviews and Meta-Analyses (PRISMA).[163]

The search and screening strategy was decided a priori. This included published systematic reviews in any language which evaluated the effects of RARC as compared with those of ORC on oncologic outcomes, perioperative outcomes, or complications rates among adult patients (aged 18 years and older) in the treatment of advanced bladder cancer (muscle-invasive or high-risk non-muscle-invasive). Systematic reviews were defined as those performed using a comprehensive, a priori–defined search strategy. Studies that performed quantitative analysis by pooling results from included studies were deemed to include meta-analysis. Systematic reviews and meta-analyses, which included nonrandomized study methodologies including cohort studies, case-control studies, and case series were excluded, owing to the risk of confounding and selection bias. Nonsystematic reviews, including narrative reviews and editorials, were excluded, as well as studies that failed to include the landmark RAZOR trial,[203] as this represents the only phase 3 multicenter study comparing RARC and ORC and was therefore felt to provide the most generalizable data on this question.

Titles and abstracts were reviewed independently in duplicate by the two authors. The initial plan was to resolve any conflicts by consensus; however, no conflicts were encountered. Once consensus was reached on the included studies, data abstraction in duplicate using a data abstraction form designed specifically for the purpose of this review was conducted. Given that the eligible systematic reviews included the same studies and cohorts, a meta-analysis was not repeated.

Outcomes of interest for review, and hence for included systematic reviews, included oncologic outcomes, perioperative outcomes, and complication rates. Oncologic outcomes included PFS as well as surrogates including margin status and lymph node yield. The literature was deemed immature for assessment of cancer-specific or overall survival. Because of previously identified uncertainty regarding the association between RARC and atypical sites of recurrence (e.g., port site recurrences), recurrence patterns according to operative approach were specifically assessed. Perioperative out-comes of interest included estimated blood loss, operative time, and hospital length of stay. Finally, complications included any complication (Clavien-Dindo grades 1 to 5) and severe complications (Clavien-Dindo grades 3 to 5).

The quality of identified systematic reviews were assessed using the Assessment of Multiple Systematic Reviews 2 (AMSTAR 2) checklist.[208] AMSTAR 2 is an up-dated version of AMSTAR, which was initially published in 2007.[209-211] To briefly summarize, AMSTAR was developed on the basis of a scoping review followed by factor analysis to identify key components in the quality assessment of systematic reviews. The original AMSTAR was limited to randomized controlled trials and assessed 11 domains including a priori protocol documentation, assessment of sci-entific quality, and risk of publication bias. Based on user feedback and critique, an expert group was convened, and a nominal group technique was used to propose and prioritize changes to the original AMSTAR instrument. The resulting AMSTAR 2 includes 16 items relating to the use of a population, intervention, comparison, and outcome (PICO) structure, a priori review methodology, selection of study designs (including nonrandomized designs), comprehensive literature search strategy, study selection in duplicate, data extraction in duplicate, list of excluded studies and justi-fication, description of included studies, assessment of risk of bias, sources of fund-ing, appropriate meta-analytic methodology, assessment of impact of risk of bias on meta-analytic results, appropriate accounting of risk of bias in primary studies on review results, explanation of heterogeneity, assessment of publication bias, and reporting of conflict of interest. Of these, 7 domains are deemed critical: protocol registration, adequacy of literature search, justification of exclusion, risk of bias of individual studies, appropriateness of meta-analytic methodology, consideration of risk of bias when interpreting review results, and assessment of publication bias. Unlike AMSTAR, in which results were summated with resulting categorization into tertiles, it is "strongly recommended"[208] that individual item ratings are not combined to give an overall score. However, overall confidence in the results of the review is provided using the following criteria: high confidence—no or one noncriti-cal weakness; moderate confidence—more than one noncritical weakness; low—one critical flaw, with or without noncritical weaknesses; and critically low—more than one critical flaw with or without noncritical weaknesses. The two authors indepen-dently performed quality assessment with disagreements resolved by consensus.

The initial search yielded 22 articles (Fig. 5-21). An additional systematic review was identified on the basis of hand searching, for a total of 23 articles identified for screening. Initial review of the titles and abstracts excluded 5 studies due to lack of relevance to the topic of this analysis. Therefore, 18 manuscripts underwent full-text review (Table 5-7). Three studies met all the criteria for inclusion in this systematic review (Table 5-8). The two authors independently performed quality assessment and resolved disagreements by consensus. Because the eligible systematic reviews included the same studies and cohorts, a meta-analysis was not repeated.

Each article was reviewed and assigned a quality of evidence based on the Grad-ing of Recommendations, Assessment, Development, and Evaluation (GRADE) sys-tem.[191] Overall, the evidence was moderate.

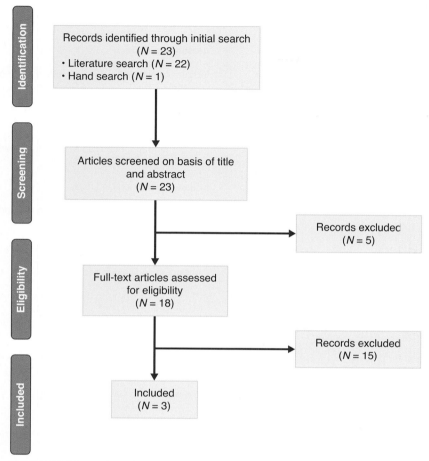

FIGURE 5-21   Preferred Reporting Items for Systematic Reviews and Meta-Analyses diagram for literature regarding robotic-assisted radical cystectomy.

FINDINGS

Rai et al.[227] performed a Cochrane systematic review and meta-analysis, identifying five randomized clinical trials (RCTs) (seven publications) that met the inclusion criteria.[202,203,230–234] Among 541 patients evaluable, there was no difference in time to recurrence or major complications between RARC and ORC (primary outcomes; Table 5-8). Furthermore, there was no difference between the groups regarding positive margin rates or quality of life. Compared with ORC, RARC was associated with an improvement in transfusion rates (risk ratio [RR], 0.58; 95% confidence interval [CI], 0.43 to 0.80) and decreased hospital length of stay (mean difference [MD], −0.67; 95% CI, −1.22 to −0.12). The authors noted that they were unable to conduct any of the preplanned subgroup analyses to assess the impact of patient age, pathologic stage, body habitus, or surgeon expertise on outcomes secondary to the

TABLE 5-7 Studies Excluded Following Full-Text Review

Authors, Year	Journal	Reason for Exclusion
Fonseka et al.,[212] 2015	*Arch Ital Urol Androl*	Includes nonrandomized data; does not include landmark trial
Ishii et al.,[213] 2014	*J Endourol*	Includes nonrandomized data; does not include landmark trial
Li et al.,[214] 2013	*Cancer Treat Rev*	Includes nonrandomized data; does not include landmark trial
Lobo et al.,[215] 2018	*Arab J Urol*	Includes nonrandomized data
Novara et al.,[216] 2015	*Eur Urol*	Includes nonrandomized data; does not include landmark trial
Palazzetti et al.,[217] 2017	*Actas Urol Esp*	Does not include landmark trial
Shen and Sun,[218] 2016	*BMC Urol*	Does not include landmark trial
Son et al.,[219] 2017	*J Laparoendosc Adv Surg Tech A*	Includes nonrandomized data; does not include landmark trial
Tan et al.,[220] 2016	*PLoS One*	Does not include landmark trial
Tang et al.,[221] 2014	*Eur J Surg Oncol*	Includes nonrandomized data; does not include landmark trial
Tang et al.,[222] 2018	*Int J Med Robot*	Does not include landmark trial
Tyritzis et al.,[223] 2018	*Int J Urol*	Nonsystematic review
Tyritzis et al.,[224] 2019	*Minerva Urol Nefrol*	Nonsystematic review
Tzelves et al.,[225] 2019	*J Endourol*	Includes nonrandomized data
Yuh et al.,[226] 2015	*Eur Urol*	Includes nonrandomized data; does not include landmark trial

small sample size for the analysis. The overall confidence in the review was moderate according to AMSTAR 2 criteria (Table 5-9). There were no major concerns with the methodology of this review; however, there were minor concerns as to whether the study adequately assessed the impact of bias on the meta-analysis outcomes and whether there was a satisfactory explanation for the observed heterogeneity.

Two other systematic reviews and meta-analyses of RCT data have also been published (all published within the same close time frame), using the same cohort of patients as Rai et al.[227] Sathianathen et al.[228] found comparable 90-day quality of life and Clavien-Dindo grades 3 to 5 complication rates between RARC and ORC patients, in addition to no difference in relative risk of disease recurrence (RR, 0.94; 95% CI, 0.69 to 1.29). Secondary outcome analysis confirmed the results of Rai et al.[227]

TABLE 5-8   Studies Included in Systematic Review of Robotic-Assisted Radical Cystectomy

Authors, Year	Included Studies, n	RARC, n	ORC, n	Meta-Analysis Primary Outcome(s) (RARC vs. ORC)	Meta-Analysis Secondary Outcome(s) (RARC vs. ORC)	Grade of Evidence*
Rai et al.,[227] 2019	5	271	270	Time to recurrence: HR, 1.05; 95% CI, 0.77–1.43 Major complications (Clavien-Dindo grades 3–5): RR, 1.06; 95% CI, 0.76–1.48	Transfusion rate: RR, 0.58; 95% CI, 0.43–0.80 Hospital stay: MD, −0.67; 95% CI, −1.22 to −0.12 Quality of life: SMD, 0.08; 95% CI, 0.32 lower to 0.16 higher Positive margin rates: RR, 1.16; 95% CI, 0.56–2.40	+++
Sathianathen et al.,[228] 2019	5	540		Disease recurrence: RR, 0.94; 95% CI, 0.69–1.29 90-d Clavien-Dindo grades 3–5: RR, 1.06; 95% CI, 0.75–1.49 90-d quality of life: SMD, −0.03; 95% CI, −0.27 to 0.21	Positive margin rates: RR, 1.16; 95% CI, 0.56–2.40 Perioperative transfusions: RR, 0.58; 95% CI, 0.43–0.80 Operative time: MD, 68.51 min; 95% CI, 30.55–105.48 Hospital stay: RR, −0.63 d; 95% CI, −1.21 to −0.05	+++
Satkunasivam et al.,[229] 2019	5	271	270	RFS/PFS: HR, 0.89; 95% CI, 0.64–1.24	Positive margin status: OR, 1.00; 95% CI, 0.48–2.11 Lymph node yield: MD, 1.98; 95% CI, −5.2 to 1.25 Local recurrence: OR, 2.41; 95% CI, 0.96–6.05 Abdominal/distant recurrence: OR, 0.60; 95% CI, 0.24–1.51 Estimated blood loss: MD, −280.50; 95% CI, −435.83 to −125.18 Operating room time: MD, 75.00; 95% CI, 26.39–123.61 Length of stay: MD, −0.50; 95% CI, −1.15–0.14 Any Clavien-Dindo grade complications: OR, 0.82; 95% CI, 0.53–1.25 Clavien Dindo ≥3 complications: OR, 1.08; 95% CI, 0.69–1.67	+++

CI: confidence interval; HR: hazard ratio; MD: mean difference; OR: odds ratio; ORC: open radical cystectomy; PFS: progression-free survival; RARC: robotic-assisted radical cystectomy; RFS: recurrence-free survival; RR: risk ratio; SMD: standard mean difference.
*Grade: +++ moderate

regarding perioperative transfusions, hospital stay, and positive margin findings. Furthermore, Sathianathen et al.[228] found that operative time was significantly longer for patients undergoing RARC compared with ORC (MD, 68.51 minutes; 95% CI, 30.55 to 105.48). The overall confidence in this review was low (Table 5-9). Several methodological concerns included the following: lack of a clear PICO statement, lack of a clear explanation of the selection of study inclusion/exclusion criteria, the impact of funding sources for the included studies, and lack of a clear assessment for the potential risk of bias on the results of the meta-analysis.

The third systematic review and meta-analysis, published by Satkunasivam et al.,[229] assessed several additional outcomes not previously addressed in the other analyses. They found no difference in recurrence- and PFS (hazard ratio, 0.89; 95% CI, 0.64 to 1.24) between RARC and ORC patients. Furthermore, there was no difference in lymph node yield (MD, 1.98; 95% CI, −5.2 to 1.25), odds of local recurrence (odds ratio [OR], 2.41; 95% CI, 0.96 to 6.05), or odds of abdominal/distant recurrence (OR, 0.60; 95% CI, 0.24 to 1.51). Patients undergoing RARC had a lower estimated blood loss (MD, −280.50; 95% CI, −435.83 to −125.18) compared with those undergoing ORC. According to AMSTAR 2 criteria, the overall confidence in this review was low (Table 5-9). Perhaps secondary to the shorter length of a brief correspondence, this systematic review did not explicitly mention a priori methodology, duplicate study selection or data extraction, study exclusion justification, or a comprehensive assessment/explanation of risk of bias.

DISCUSSION

Over the past decade, the advent of minimally invasive radical cystectomy has resulted in an uptake in RARC. To assess both perioperative and oncologic safety, several RCTs have recently been published, followed by three systematic reviews and meta-analyses of trial data.[227–229] Assessing data for more than 500 patients, these analyses generally found that there was no difference in perioperative complication rates (both minor and major), quality-of-life metrics, and oncologic outcomes. However, there is likely an advantage to RARC with regard to estimated blood loss/transfusion rates and hospital length of stay, at the cost of longer operative times. Certainly, long-term follow-up data are necessary to ensure oncologic safety equivalent to ORC.

The largest RCT to date comparing RARC with ORC is the RAZOR trial published in 2018.[203] For this noninferiority trial, there were 350 eligible participants (aged 18 years or older) with biopsy-proven clinical stage T1 to T4, N0 to N1, M0 bladder cancer, or refractory carcinoma in situ randomized to receive RARC or ORC with extracorporeal urinary diversion. The primary endpoint was 2-year PFS. Three hundred and two patients (150 in the RARC group and 152 in the ORC group) were included in the per-protocol analysis, and 2-year PFS was 72.3% (95% CI, 64.3% to 78.8%) in the RARC group and 71.6% (95% CI, 63.6% to 78.2%) in the ORC group (difference, 0.7%; 95% CI, −9.6% to 10.9%; $P_{noninferiority}$ = .001), indicating noninferiority of RARC. Furthermore, adverse events were comparable between the two groups (67% for RARC vs. 69% for ORC), with urinary tract infection and postoperative ileus as the most common. Given the noninferior PFS outcomes, the authors of this trial urged future RCTs to assess the value of robotic surgical intervention in a similar manner for patients with other cancer types.

TABLE 5-9 Critical Appraisal of Included Systematic Reviews Using the AMSTAR 2 Tool

AMSTAR 2 Question	Rai et al.[227]	Sathianathen et al.[228]	Satkunasivam et al.[229]
1. Did the research question and inclusion criteria include the PICO components?	Yes	No	Yes
2. Did the report explicitly state that methods were established a priori with justification of any deviations?	Yes	Yes	No
3. Did the authors explain selection of study designs for inclusion?	Yes	No	No
4. Did the authors use a comprehensive search strategy?	Yes	Yes	No
5. Did the authors perform study selection in duplicate?	Yes	Yes	No
6. Did the authors perform data extraction in duplicate?	Yes	Yes	No
7. Did the authors provide a list of excluded studies with justification?	Yes	No	No
8. Did the authors describe included studies in adequate detail?	Yes	No	Yes
9. Did the authors use a satisfactory technique for assessing risk of bias?	Yes	Yes	No
10. Did the authors report on sources of funding for included studies?	Yes	No	No
11. Did the authors use appropriate methods for meta-analysis?	Yes	Yes	Yes
12. Did the authors assess the potential effect of risk of bias on the results of the meta-analysis?	No	No	No
13. Did the authors account for risk of bias when interpreting results of the review?	Yes	No	No
14. Did the authors provide a satisfactory explanation heterogeneity observed?	No	No	No
15. Did the authors perform adequate assessment of publication bias?	No	No	No
16. Did the authors report any potential sources of conflict of interest, including any funding received for the review?	Yes	Yes	Yes
Overall confidence in the results of the review	Moderate	Low	Low

AMSTAR: Assessment of Multiple Systematic Reviews.
Note: Critical domains highlighted in bold.

For the current AMSTAR 2 review, strict criteria for study selection were used, which included only systematic reviews and meta-analyses assessing RCT data. As such, a large systematic review and meta-analysis that included the 5 published RCTs, as well as 49 observational studies, was excluded.[225] Tzelves et al.[225] assessed 29,697 patients, including 6,500 in the RARC group and 23,197 in the ORC group. They found that minor complications (grades 1 to 2) were fewer in the RARC group (OR, 0.54; 95% CI, 0.38 to 0.76), findings that persisted when analyzing complications after both 30 and 90 days postoperatively. Additionally, major complications (grades 3 to 5) were also fewer in the RARC group (OR, 0.78; 95% CI, 0.65 to 0.94); however, this finding did not remain when assessing complications within 30 days of surgery. Finally, RARC was associated with lower blood transfusion rates (OR, 0.19; 95% CI, 0.13 to 0.27) and lower postoperative mortality rates (OR, 0.69; 95% CI, 0.58 to 0.84), but there was no difference in readmission rates (OR, 1.00; 95% CI, 0.73 to 1.37). The results from this study, primarily based on observational data, highlight the inherent selection bias associated with choosing a surgical approach. These outcomes generally favor RARC in contrast to meta-analyses using only RCT data that demonstrate minimal differences between the two surgical approaches.

With improving comfort level among surgeons performing RARC, there has been an uptake in the use of RARC with intracorporeal urinary diversion.[235] Importantly, the RCTs to date, including the RAZOR trial, have exclusively used extracorporeal diversion. The ongoing Intracorporeal Robot-Assisted vs Open Radical Cystectomy (iROC) trial is set to compare differences between RARC with intracorporeal diversion versus ORC (NCT03049410). Patients will be randomized 1:1, with a target enrollment of 340 patients and a primary outcome of number of days alive and out of the hospital within 90 days of surgery. Secondary outcomes include difficulties due to health conditions measured using World Health Organization Disability Assessment Schedule Version 2.0 within 12 months of surgery and quality of life measured using EQ-5D-5L Health Questionnaire and European Organisation for Research and Treatment of Cancer (EORTC) QLQ-C30 Version 3 within 12 months of surgery. Key inclusion criteria include adult patients with carcinoma in situ or stage pTa or pT1 or greater/equal to pT2 and less than/equal to N1 on imaging. This study will compare optimal RARC (with intracorporeal urinary diversion) with optimal ORC (at high-volume institutions using an Enhanced Recovery After Surgery [ERAS] protocol), in addition to properly assessing rehabilitation after radical cystectomy.

Given the noninferiority of RARC to ORC, it is important to highlight that ERAS protocols may provide greater incremental benefits for patients undergoing radical cystectomy than robotic-assisted surgery. Any benefit of RARC (i.e., decreased blood loss, shorter length of stay) comes at the expense of higher direct costs. However, the use of ERAS protocols, accounting for surgical approach (ORC versus RARC), is associated with a significantly increased likelihood of length of stay less than 10 days. In a study assessing 304 radical cystectomies (54 ORC, 250 RARC with intracorporeal diversion) performed at a single institution, Tan et al.[236] identified 45 ORC cases performed without ERAS before the commencement of the RARC program, 50 RARC cases performed without ERAS, and 40 RARC cases with ERAS. They found that patients undergoing RARC with ERAS had a shorter median length of stay of 7 days (interquartile range [IQR], 6 to 10 days) compared with the RARC without ERAS group (median, 11 days; IQR, 8 to 15 days) and the ORC group (median, 17 days; IQR, 14 to 21 days). In a multinomial logistic regression model, the ERAS pathway (no versus yes; OR, 0.20; 95% CI, 0.07 to 0.57) and younger patients (continuous; OR, 1.10; 95% CI, 1.01 to 1.13) were independently associated with a length of stay of 10 days or less. These results suggest that the greatest patient-derived benefit and cost-effectiveness may be centralizing patients to centers proficient in RARC with standardized ERAS pathways.

There are several limitations with the current AMSTAR 2 review of systematic reviews/meta-analyses comparing RARC with ORC. First, most studies are under-powered for important survival outcomes. Second, reviews that did not assess unpublished literature were included. Thus, with potentially more data and updated reviews, this comparative review may need to be reassessed in the future. Finally, it was difficult to assess publication bias given the small number of studies that fit the inclusion criteria. Nonetheless, the first review of systematic reviews/meta-analyses on this topic using a comprehensive and validated tool was performed.

CONCLUSION

Patients undergoing RARC compared versus ORC may derive a perioperative blood transfusion benefit and decreased length of stay. However, long-term perioperative and oncologic outcomes are generally comparable between the two surgical modalities. Additional studies assessing the impact of intracorporeal urinary diversion and implementation of ERAS pathways will continue to delineate the optimal approach to surgically treating patients with muscle-invasive bladder cancer.

CHAPTER 13

Nephroureterectomy

CRITICAL ELEMENTS

- Removal of Kidney and Ureter
- Management of the Distal Ureter/Cuff
- Lymphadenectomy for Upper Tract Urothelial Cancer during Definitive Resection
- Perioperative Instillation of Intravesical Chemotherapy

1. REMOVAL OF KIDNEY AND URETER

Recommendation: Nephroureterectomy for upper tract urothelial carcinoma (UTUC) should generally include resection of the kidney and entire ureter. Segmental ureterectomy may be considered for patients with either low-grade urothelial cell carcinoma or noninvasive high-grade urothelial cell carcinoma of the upper urothelial tract.

Type of Data: Retrospective reports, case series, or case-control studies

Strength of Recommendation: Strong recommendation, low-quality evidence

Rationale

In the surgical management of UTUC, failure to completely resect the affected upper urothelial tract results in an increased risk of recurrence. Nephroureterectomy has long remained the gold standard for the treatment of upper tract urothelial cell carcinoma, with exceptions generally made for situations in which postnephrectomy renal function could be an issue.

Radical nephroureterectomy should be the treatment modality of choice for most patients with urothelial cell carcinoma of the upper urinary tract.[237] Surgical extirpation should include resection of the kidney, entire ureter, and bladder cuff (Fig. 5-22).[237,238] This critical element discusses the kidney and ureter. The bladder cuff is discussed in the next critical element in this chapter. Resection of the distal ureter and its ureteral

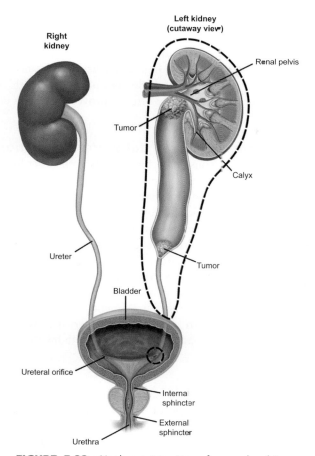

Right kidney

Left kidney (cutaway view)

Renal pelvis

Tumor

Calyx

Ureter

Tumor

Bladder

Ureteral orifice

Internal sphincter

External sphincter

Urethra

FIGURE 5-22 Nephroureterectomy for renal pelvis or ureteral tumor involves resection of the kidney and ureter up through a bladder cuff around the ureteral orifice, as shown by dashed line.

orifice should be performed regardless of stage, as this location harbors a high risk of future disease recurrence.[238–241] In all cases, uncontrolled entry into the urinary tract must be avoided, as this increases the risk of tumor spillage and local recurrence.[237]

The optimal surgical approach to nephroureterectomy remains contested. Despite adoption of newer approaches, oncologic outcomes have not changed substantially over time.[242] Although open radical nephroureterectomy is perhaps the best studied approach, there has been widespread adoption of the laparoscopic and, more recently, robotic-assisted laparoscopic approaches. Numerous retrospective studies have established comparable oncologic outcomes between the open and laparoscopic approaches.[243–251] Presently, only one prospective randomized trial has explored oncologic differences between the two. Findings from that trial demonstrated that laparoscopic nephroureterectomy was not inferior to open nephroureterectomy for patients with organ-confined disease.[252] More recently, there has been a rise in the use of robotic-assisted laparoscopic radical nephroureterectomy.[253] Although long-term outcomes are still scarce, several recent retrospective studies have demonstrated oncologic equivalency between the robotic approach and conventional open and laparoscopic techniques.[253–255] For patients with high-grade urothelial cancer invasive to the lamina propria or beyond, locally advanced disease, or locoregional lymphadenopathy, open radical nephroureterectomy may offer improved outcomes compared with the laparoscopic approach.[252,256]

Circumstances for segmental or distal ureteral resection

Segmental ureterectomy may be considered for patients with either low-grade urothelial cell carcinoma or noninvasive high-grade urothelial cell carcinoma of the upper tracts.[67,257–259] For patients in whom renal preservation is desirable or necessary, segmental ureteral resection may provide oncologic benefit similar to nephroureterectomy while preserving renal function in the ipsilateral kidney.[260,261] Patients with low-risk distal ureteral tumors are most likely to benefit from segmental resection and ureteroneocystostomy when preservation of renal function is necessary.[262–264] There may be circumstances in which appropriately selected patients with high-risk distal ureteral tumors may benefit from segmental ureterectomy when renal function is an imperative.[257] Segmental resection is generally discouraged for patients with tumors of the mid-ureter and proximal ureter. These patients are more likely to experience disease recurrence and less favorable oncologic outcomes, particularly patients with high-risk disease.[257,262]

Technical Aspects

Considerations

Advances in available technology allow for a variety of approaches to nephroureterectomy. Of particular benefit has been the application of laparoscopic and robotic-assisted laparoscopic platforms designed to reduce the morbidity of surgery. Although laparoscopic surgery has gained acceptance and adoption, not all patients or tumors are well suited for this approach. In cases of bulky tumors or regional lymphadenopathy, open nephroureterectomy remains an excellent option, but laparoscopic approaches could be considered based on surgeon experience. Because of the variety of available approaches, each approach are discussed separately, and special considerations are addressed.

Open nephroureterectomy

A single-incision approach may be used to perform nephroureterectomy. Although this does not necessarily provide improved exposure when compared with the two-incision approach, it is an option depending on surgeon comfort. Perhaps the most familiar approach to most surgeons is a midline transperitoneal laparotomy incision with intraperitoneal exposure. Alternatively, an extraperitoneal thoracoabdominal approach may be used. This may allow for improved exposure of the upper pole, particularly with bulky tumors. The two-incision approach is an appealing alternative to a single-incision approach as it allows for excellent exposure during both the radical nephrectomy portion of the case as well as dissection of the distal ureter.

Typically, with any open approach, the abdomen should be opened and sharp and blunt dissection should then be used to develop the space between the anterior aspect of the Gerota's fascia and the colonic mesentery. The colon may then be medialized to gain access to the retroperitoneum and expose the Gerota fascia, ureter, and renal hilum. Care should be taken to not violate the kidney or tumor in order to avoid any positive margin of resection.

Once adequate hilar control has been established and renal artery and vein transected, the posterior pararenal space may be developed bluntly and elevated off the psoas muscle posteriorly. The inferior pole of the kidney may now be easily identified as well as the ureter. The lateral attachments of the kidney may then be freed, and the kidney retracted caudally to allow exposure of the upper pole attachments and the adrenal gland. The upper pole attachments may then be divided laterally to medially. If there is no concern for adrenal gland involvement, this gland may be spared and dissected free from the upper pole attachments. If adrenalectomy is indicated, the gland should be removed en bloc with the specimen.

Further dissection of the ureter should then be performed down to its insertion into the bladder. Clipping of the ureter distal to the known tumor location may now be used to reduce the risk of tumor seeding within the urinary tract during manipulation of the kidney and ureter. Care should also be taken during this process not to avulse or violate the ureter, as this may result in spillage of urine containing tumor cells. Management of the distal ureter at this point should include excision of the entire distal ureter including the intramural ureter and the ureteral orifice. Strategies for managing the distal ureter are described later in this chapter.

Minimally invasive nephroureterectomy

Pure, hand-assisted, and robotic-assisted laparoscopic approaches to nephroureterectomy can be safely performed with equivalent oncologic outcomes and decreased morbidity from incision size in many cases. The techniques do present unique challenges that must be considered. In particular, technical challenges introduced by adapting minimally invasive techniques should not be accepted if they lead to inadequate ureteral resection. In such cases, completion of the procedure with limited open counterincision may be necessary. With each technique, methods involving strategic port placement or conversion of well-placed hand-ports for distal ureteral surgery can accomplish adequate resection for good oncologic outcomes.

Segmental ureterectomy

Although nephroureterectomy is the criterion standard for upper tract urothelial cell carcinoma, segmental ureterectomy may be considered for low-grade noninvasive urothelial cell carcinoma of the proximal and mid-ureter. This may be of use in patients with tumors that cannot be fully addressed via endoscopic means and in whom renal preservation is imperative.

The choice of incision may be influenced based on location of the tumor. A subcostal flank incision provides adequate exposure for proximal ureter tumors, whereas those of the mid-ureter may be best accessed through a modified Gibson incision.

The ureter may now be identified as it courses through the retroperitoneum and mobilized. Care should be taken not to skeletonize the ureter, as this may lead to devascularization of healthy segments and future ureteral stricture. Once the ureter has been mobilized proximally and distally to the location of the tumor, the ureter may be ligated at least 1 cm proximally and distally to the lesion. Frozen section should be used to ensure that the healthy margins remain free of tumor before proceeding with ureteroureterostomy. Ureteroscopy may also be used to ensure that there is no evidence of visible tumor proximal and distal to the excised segment. The ureter should then be widely spatulated, and ureteroureterostomy may be performed over an internal double-J stent. It is imperative that the anastomosis remains tension free. If additional length is required, the kidney may be mobilized downward to provide additional length. This is particularly helpful in more proximal ureter lesions. An omental or peritoneal flap should then be used if circumstances allow, and a closed-suction drain should be placed in the retroperitoneum.

2. MANAGEMENT OF THE DISTAL URETER/CUFF

Recommendation: During radical nephroureterectomy, the distal ureter must be excised in its entirety, inclusive of the full-thickness intramural segment and ureteral orifice ("bladder cuff"). Open transvesical and extravesical excision approaches offer comparable oncologic efficacy. Endoscopic or minimally invasive extravesical ligation methods of cuff excision have been associated with higher intravesical recurrence rates and should not be used.

Type of Data: Retrospective reports, case series, or case-control studies; systematic reviews and meta-analyses

Strength of Recommendation: Strong recommendation, weak evidence

Rationale

Appropriate management of the distal ureter during a radical nephroureterectomy requires removal of the entire distal ureter, including the intramural segment and ureteral orifice ("bladder cuff"), which, if done poorly, can be a source of local recurrence.

A number of methods have been described to accomplish proper management of the bladder cuff. These can be broadly categorized as extravesical, transvesical, or endoscopic approaches.

The extravesical and transvesical approaches to removal of the bladder cuff both involve careful mobilization of the distal ureter, with care taken to complete the ureteral dissection in its entirety to the ureteral hiatus. This can be challenging, given the posterolateral location of the ureter's entry into the bladder, and the length of the intramural segment of the ureter is often longer than expected.

A number of endoscopic techniques have been described. Three broad endoscopic techniques are noted. The "pluck" technique involves cystoscopic detachment of the intramural ureter by transurethral resection of the orifice to the level of perivesical fat.[265] A similar but separate approach is to cystoscopically detach the ureter by circumferentially incising and coring out the intramural segment using an endoscopic hook.[265] A third approach is to divide the ureter at the time of nephroureterectomy and intussuscept it using a catheter, after which the ureter is transected transurethrally ("ureteral stripping").[266] Additional modifications to these include partial cystoscopic incisions, either following or prior to extravesical ligation with a stapling device or similar instrument.[267]

No randomized controlled trials that compare distal ureteral/bladder cuff management options have been conducted. Xylinas et al.[240] retrospectively studied 2,681 patients in the largest multi-institutional series to date that compared the oncologic outcomes associated with each of the various cuff management approaches. The majority of patients in this series underwent transvesical removal of the distal bladder cuff (1,811 patients, 67.5%,), followed by the extravesical approach (785 patients, 29.3%) and endoscopic approach (85 patients, 3.2%).[240] The endoscopic technique used in this cohort was described as one in which the ipsilateral ureteral orifice was first coagulated, after which a hook electrode was used to incise a 10-mm cuff of bladder mucosa around the ureteral orifice down to the level of the perivesical fat. The endoscopic approach was more commonly used during laparoscopic nephroureterectomy ($P < .01$). Median follow-up was 57.5 months (range, 1 to 271 months), and in a multivariable analysis, the endoscopic approach was associated with a higher risk of intravesical disease recurrence (hazard ratio [HR], 1.74; 95% confidence interval [CI], 1.14 to 2.64; $P = .01$). This remained true even when excluding patients with a prior history of bladder cancer and when matching for tumor node metastasis (TNM) stage and lymph node status (HR, 10.8; 95% CI, 5.27 to 22.2; $P < .001$). There were no differences between the transvesical and extravesical approaches in this study, and there were no differences in recurrence-free survival, cancer-specific survival, or overall survival between the three groups.[240]

A narrative review of 42 publications comparing various endoscopic management techniques with the open approach found that there was no clear advantage to any single endoscopic modality, noting that recurrence rates at the ureteral resection scar were between 0% and 4% with the "pluck," ureteral stripping, cystoscopic detachment of the ureter and endoscopic ligation, and open techniques.[267] This review notably separated any intravesical recurrences from recurrences occurring at the resection scar alone. The highest scar recurrence rate reported in this review was 14% and was observed with the extravesical laparoscopic stapling technique. No formal risk of bias assessment or assessment of heterogeneity of the studies included was performed in this review. The type of open bladder cuff management (transvesical or extravesical) was also not clearly specified in this review.[3] The ureteral stripping procedure has separately been reported to be associated with a relatively high intravesical recurrence rate (any intravesical recurrence, not limited to the ureteral scar) of 35.7% of patients, with a 3-year recurrence-free rate of only 57.7%, compared with 75.0% using traditional open techniques ($P = .03$).[268]

A systematic review and meta-analysis of 8,275 patients found that intravesical recurrence occurred in 29% of cases overall, with patient-specific risk factors being male sex (HR, 1.37; $P < .0001$), previous bladder cancer (HR, 1.96; $P < .001$), and preoperative chronic kidney disease (HR, 1.87; $P = .002$).[239] Laparoscopic approaches

(HR, 1.62; $P = .003$), extravesical bladder cuff removal (HR, 1.22; $P = .02$), and positive surgical margins (HR, 1.90; $P = .004$) were also associated with risk of intravesical recurrence. In this analysis, only 405 patients (9%) reported in four prior studies underwent endoscopic bladder cuff removal. Two of these studies reported increased risk of intravesical recurrence with the technique, whereas two did not. In the meta-analysis, endoscopic cuff management was not significantly associated with worsened risk of intravesical recurrence (HR, 1.14; 95% CI, 0.55 to 2.37; $P = .72$). In contrast, the extravesical approach to bladder cuff removal was a significant predictor of intravesical recurrence (HR, 1.22; 95% CI, 1.03 to 1.45; $P = .02$). Extravesical cuff management in the included studies is believed to have primarily comprised blind extravesical stapling or clamping of the distal ureter with inadequate resection of the bladder cuff and intramural segment.[239]

With respect to sex-related outcomes after radical nephroureterectomy, the data are sparse and mixed. Fernández et al.[269] reported no association between sex and disease recurrence or disease-specific survival in an analysis of 1,363 patients from the UTUC Collaboration Group. However, a Japanese study of 502 patients found that predictors of intravesical recurrence following radical nephroureterectomy included male sex (HR, 3.22; $P = .002$), ureteral tumor location, and multifocality of tumor.[270]

Technical Aspects

Classically, in open techniques, a midline or lower quadrant incision is used to perform the transvesical and extravesical approaches.

For the extravesical approach, the distal ureter is first mobilized toward the bladder to the level of its intramural segment. Using a right angle or similar occlusive clamp to avoid uncontrolled intravesical entry and urine spillage, the ureter should be ligated en bloc, with care taken to include the portion of the bladder encircling the ureteral orifice. Mobilization of the ureter requires identification and ligation of the lateral vascular pedicles of the bladder. In women, additional blood supply emerging from the infundibulopelvic ligaments are usually encountered and must be controlled (Fig. 5-23).[271] A common concern with the extravesical approach is inadequate dissection of the intramural segment, resulting in remnant distal ureter within the trigone. To minimize this, tension should be maintained on the ureter as the dissection is carried toward the posterolateral bladder. As a component of an oncologically safe bladder cuff resection, the bladder should be filled prior to cystotomy with either sterile water or a chemotherapeutic agent and clamped. Instillation of either a hypotonic solution or cytotoxic agent for approximately 15 to 20 minutes can reduce the risk of local recurrence through lysis and minimization of the seeding of free-floating urothelial carcinoma cells.[272] The detrusor muscle surrounding the ureter should be carefully incised circumferentially, and the bladder emptied. To help with visualization, the bladder should be mobilized and rotated anteriorly; ligation of the superior vesical artery can help with mobility and visualization in some cases. The periureteral incision should be carried until bulging bladder mucosa is seen around the entirety of the ureteral hiatus. Once intravesical entry occurs, a 4-0 absorbable monofilament stay suture should be placed. The ureter should be freed completely and passed off the field with the specimen, and the mucosa can be closed in a running manner with

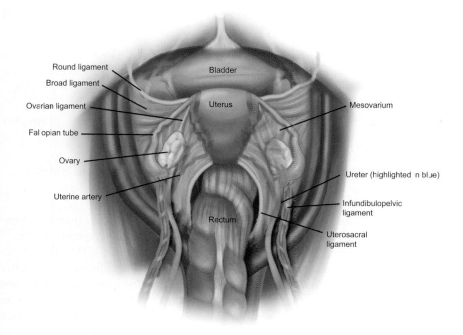

Round ligament

Bladder

Broad ligament

Ovarian ligament

Uterus

Mesovarium

Fallopian tube

Ovary

Ureter (highlighted in blue)

Uterine artery

Infundibulopelvic ligament

Rectum

Uterosacral ligament

FIGURE 5-23 Anatomic considerations of bladder cuff in female patients: blood supply arising within the infundibulopelvic ligaments may need to be controlled for adequate distal ureterectomy and resection of bladder cuff.

the 4-0 monofilament. The detrusor layer should be closed with a running 3-0 absorbable monofilament.

For the intravesical approach, mobilization of the ureter occurs as previously described. The detrusor is incised circumferentially around the ureteral entry point into the bladder, and a midline cystotomy is made, approximately 3 to 4 cm in length. Residual urine and instillation solution should be evacuated with suction and the ureteral orifice identified. A traction suture of 3-0 silk or similar should be placed to close the ureteral orifice, and a 0.5- to 1-cm cuff of bladder mucosa should be excised around the orifice. Additional dissection is often required to separate the intradetrusor component of the ureter before it is brought into continuity with the previous dissection posteriorly and extravesically. The urothelium around the ureteral hiatus and the cystotomy should then be closed as previously described in two layers using absorbable monofilament suture.

As noted earlier, endoscopic resection of the ureteral orifice is associated with higher rates of cancer recurrence and is considered inferior to either intravesical or extravesical approaches to bladder cuff management. The endoscopic resection should typically be carried out prior to nephroureterectomy with the patient in dorsal lithotomy. A transurethral resectoscope should be used to resect the intramural distal segment and ureteral orifice completely until extravesical fat is visualized. A catheter should then be placed and the nephroureterectomy completed in standard fashion.

3. LYMPHADENECTOMY FOR UPPER TRACT UROTHELIAL CANCER DURING DEFINITIVE RESECTION

Recommendation: A template-based lymphadenectomy based on laterality and location of the primary tumor should be considered at the time of nephroureterectomy or segmental ureterectomy for high-risk, high-grade, or suspected high-grade UTUC.

Type of Data: Retrospective reports, case series, case-control studies, prospective clinical trials

Strength of Recommendation: Strong recommendation, weak evidence

Rationale

Lymph node dissection at the time of nephroureterectomy or segmental ureterectomy for UTUC is controversial, and consensus does not exist as to its therapeutic benefit.[273] Much of the rationale for performing lymph node dissection for UTUC is extrapolated from the bladder cancer literature, retrospective data, and limited prospective observational studies. For patients with bladder cancer, pelvic lymph node dissection is an accepted standard based on high-quality evidence.[21,151] UTUC is relatively rare compared with urothelial carcinoma of the bladder, and the quality of the literature is correspondingly less robust, being mostly limited to a heterogenous collection of retrospective series lacking selection criteria.[274–277]

In general, there is believed to be staging and prognostic benefit to the performance of lymph node dissection for UTUC. However, whether a therapeutic or oncologic benefit exists is not known. Extrapolating from the bladder cancer literature has led many to believe that there is a patient population in which an oncologic benefit from lymph node dissection can be derived, and this is supported by a number of retrospective series. The Upper Tract Urothelial Carcinoma Collaboration was developed to provide the field a more robust base of evidence as to the therapeutic role of lymph node dissection for UTUC and has published some retrospective multicenter data.[278,279] In general, the literature does support the feasibility and safety of lymph node dissection for UTUC. Major complications as a direct result of lymph node dissection are uncommon.[280]

The lack of prespecified or, for that matter, any identifiable dissection templates based on primary tumor location/laterality is a significant limitation of the available literature, and further illumination of the benefits of lymph node dissection will require adoption and adherence to a template-based approach. Early mapping studies led to a general practice of performing a regional lymphadenectomy depending on the anatomic location of the tumor (renal pelvis, distal ureter, etc.) and laterality.[281,282] Further work by Kondo et al.[280,283] revealed considerably more extensive landing sites for lymph node metastasis, and most recently, Matin et al.[284] confirmed these widened templates but suggested significant cranial migration of distal and mid-ureteral tumors (Figs. 5-24, 5-25, and 5-26).

The available literature does suggest a staging advantage associated with lymph node dissection for UTUC.[285] The presence of lymph node metastasis portends a significant negative impact on oncologic outcomes,[286] and recent multi-institutional

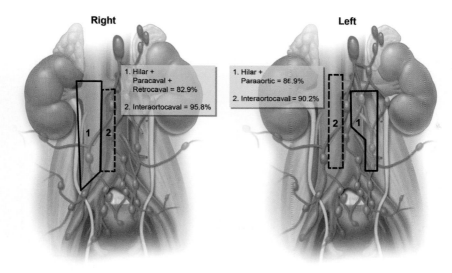

FIGURE 5-24   Drainage of ureteral and renal pelvic tumors vary based on tumor location on the side of the kidney and location of the tumor along the ureter. For proximal and renal pelvic tumors, perihilar dissection along with the below-designated regions of dissection capture the most likely sites of drainage for these tumors. Removal of region 1 on the right and left will capture 82.9% (*right*) and 86.9% (*left*) of the drainage. Removal of regions 1 and 2 will capture 95.8% (*right*) and 90.2% (*left*) of the tumor lymphatic drainage.

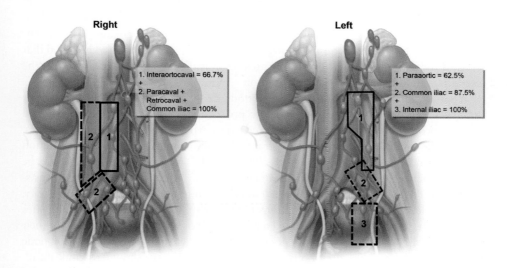

FIGURE 5-25   Drainage of ureteral and renal pelvic tumors vary based on tumor location on the side of the kidney and location of the tumor along the ureter. For mid-ureteral tumors, the below-designated regions of dissection capture the most likely sites of drainage for these tumors. Removal of region 1 on the right and left will capture 62.5% (*right*) and 62.5% (*left*) of the drainage. Extended resection to include all the regions shown will capture almost all tumor lymphatic drainage on both sides.

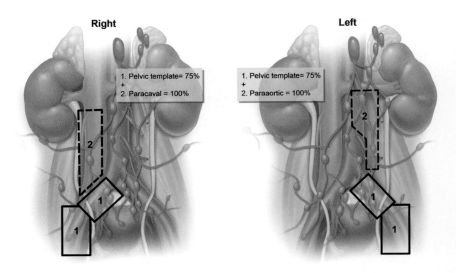

FIGURE 5-26 Drainage of ureteral and renal pelvic tumors vary based on tumor location on the side of the kidney and location of the tumor along the ureter. For distal ureteral tumors, the below-designated regions of dissection capture the most likely sites of drainage for these tumors. Removal of pelvic nodes on the right and left will capture 75% of the drainage on either side. Extended resection to include all the regions shown will capture almost all tumor lymphatic drainage on both sides.

series have demonstrated that patients with lymph node metastases have worse cancer-specific survival,[287–289] suggesting that accurate staging via lymph node dissection would improve the triage of postoperative patients into risk-adapted follow-up and adjuvant pathways. It is likely that patients who obtain the greatest staging benefit from lymph node dissection have higher risk disease,[278] and it should be noted that many of these studies did not prespecify an anatomic dissection template based on the laterality and location of the primary tumor.

Whether patients who undergo lymph node dissection for UTUC enjoy superior survival outcomes as a direct result of the procedure cannot be definitely answered without prospective randomized controlled trials with defined anatomic templates. Some of the available literature demonstrates that performing a lymph node dissection is an independent predictor of cancer-specific survival[276–278] and that this benefit may be most pronounced in cases of locally advanced disease.[278] These findings are not consistent across the available literature, which again is limited by significant heterogeneity, a lack of selection criteria, and limitations in the use of predefined anatomic templates of dissection. Kondo et al.[290] performed a prospective observational evaluation of their proposed templates and, based on their criteria of complete template-based lymph node dissection versus incomplete or no lymph node dissection, have shown a significant reduction of local recurrences and improved overall survival and cancer-specific survival in those with renal pelvis cancer but, interestingly, not ureteral tumors. The difference was most pronounced in patients with pathologic T2 disease. The absence of a benefit for ureteral tumors may be explained by the fact that their templates did not account for the potential cranial lymphatic migration of mid-ureteral and distal ureteral tumors. At the time of this writing, the Kondo prospective observational data showing a benefit for lymph node dissection in renal pelvis cancer represents the best quality evidence available showing a recurrence and survival advantage for template-based lymph node dissection according to the location and laterality of the primary tumor.

Technical Aspects

Performance of a lymph node dissection should be based on the templates described in Figures 5-24, 5-25, and 5-26. Prerequisites for performing an adequate lymph node dissection are a thorough knowledge of the retroperitoneal anatomy, especially with respect to the great vessels and their critical branches (renal vessels, superior and inferior mesenteric arteries/veins, gonadal arteries/veins, lumbar arteries/veins, and various variant branches); meticulous technique using a split-and-roll method over the inferior vena cava or aorta; and a clear understanding of the relationship of vital structures (pancreas, renal hilum, large and small bowel, and diaphragm) to the great vessels and the lymph node packets. Lumbar vessels should be identified and ligated as necessary. Great care should be taken to apply surgical clips and/or a vessel-sealing device in areas with heavy lymphatic flow (distal and proximal extent of the dissection).

4. PERIOPERATIVE INSTILLATION OF INTRAVESICAL CHEMOTHERAPY

Recommendation: Chemotherapy consisting of either mitomycin C (MMC) or pirarubicin should be instilled into the bladder of all patients undergoing nephroureterectomy for UTUC, during or immediately following surgery.

Type of Data: Prospective clinical trials; retrospective reports, case series, or case-control studies

Strength of Recommendation: Strong recommendation, moderate-quality evidence

Rationale

An estimated 22% to 47% of patients experience bladder tumor recurrence after undergoing nephroureterectomy for UTUC.[70] Perioperative intravesical instillation of chemotherapy has been proposed as a potential approach to mitigate this risk. To date, two prospective randomized trials have demonstrated that a single postoperative dose of intravesical chemotherapy after nephroureterectomy significantly reduces the risk of bladder tumor recurrence.[291,292] In the One Dose Mitomycin C (ODMIT-C) trial, use of a single dose of postoperative MMC led to a relative and absolute risk reduction of bladder tumor recurrence by 40% and 11%, respectively, at 1 year.[291] Likewise, in the phase 2 tetrahydropyranyladriamycin (THP Monotherapy Study Group Trial, which used a single intravesical instillation of pirarubicin within 48 hours of surgery, bladder tumor recurrences were reduced in the chemotherapy group, with 2-year absolute- and relative-risk reductions of 60% and 25%, respectively.[292]

Multiple meta-analyses have further supported these superior outcomes,[293,294] and a randomized phase 3 trial is currently underway to investigate this question across a larger cohort with longer follow-up.[295]

In other existing reports, the timing of instillation of chemotherapy has varied, but chemotherapy has generally been administered within 72 hours following resection. In a recent retrospective study, the timing of intravesical instillation was assessed by comparing bladder tumor recurrence rates following either intraoperative or postoperative (24 to 72 hours after nephroureterectomy) instillation of MMC.[296] Intraoperative instillation of chemotherapy was associated with a lower risk of bladder tumor recurrence at 1 year. However, the study is limited because of its small sample size of evaluated patients and its retrospective design.

Despite the compelling evidence that supports its routine use, intravesical chemotherapy is instilled in as few as 51% of patients undergoing nephroureterectomy.[297]

Technical Aspects

In the operating room, after anesthetic induction and intubation, a urethral catheter should be inserted, and 40 mL of 1 mg/mL MMC should be instilled intravesically immediately prior to commencing surgery. The catheter should then be clamped, and the catheter should be sterilely prepared into the surgical field. The MMC should be drained 1 hour into the operation, prior to making a cystotomy in order to prevent escape of MMC into the intraperitoneal space. A segment of the bladder cuff should be excised together with the ureter, and the cystotomy should be closed in two layers. This approach necessitates the exchange for a fresh catheter at the conclusion of the case.

REFERENCES

1. Siegel RL, Miller KD, Jemal A. Cancer statistics, 2019. *CA Cancer J Clin.* 2019;69(1):7-34. doi:10.3322/caac.21551
2. Westergren DO, Gårdmark T, Lindhagen L, Chau A, Malmström PU. A nationwide, population based analysis of patients with organ confined, muscle invasive bladder cancer not receiving curative intent therapy in Sweden from 1997 to 2014. *J Urol.* 2019;202(5):905-912. doi:10.1097/JU.0000000000000350
3. Cha EK, Shariat SF, Kormaksson M, et al. Predicting clinical outcomes after radical nephroureterectomy for upper tract urothelial carcinoma. *Eur Urol.* 2012;61(4):818-825. doi:10.1016/j.eururo.2012.01.021
4. Gakis G, Schubert T, Alemozaffar M, et al. Update of the ICUD-SIU consultation on upper tract urothelial carcinoma 2016: treatment of localized high-risk disease. *World J Urol.* 2017;35(3):327-335. doi:10.1007/s00345-016-1819-1
5. Klaassen Z, Kamat AM, Kassouf W, et al. Treatment strategy for newly diagnosed t1 high-grade bladder urothelial carcinoma: new insights and updated recommendations. *Eur Urol.* 2018;74(5):597-608. doi:10.1016/j.eururo.2018.06.024
6. Daneshmand S. Determining the role of cystectomy for high-grade T1 urothelial carcinoma. *Urol Clin North Am.* 2013;40(2):233-247. doi:10.1016/j.ucl.2013.01.003
7. Daneshmand S, Ahmadi H, Huynh LN, Dobos N. Preoperative staging of invasive bladder cancer with dynamic gadolinium-enhanced magnetic resonance imaging: results from a prospective study. *Urology.* 2012;80(6):1313-1318. doi:10.1016/j.urology.2012.07.056
8. Amin MB, Edge SB, Greene F, et al, eds. *AJCC Cancer Staging Manual.* 8th ed. Spring International Publishing; 2017.
9. Quek ML, Stein JP, Nichols PW, et al. Prognostic significance of lymphovascular invasion of bladder cancer treated with radical cystectomy. *J Urol.* 2005;174(1):103-106. doi:10.1097/01.ju.0000163267.93769.d8

10. May M, Herrmann E, Bolenz C, et al. Lymph node density affects cancer-specific survival in patients with lymph node-positive urothelial bladder cancer following radical cystectomy. *Eur Urol.* 2011;59(5):712-718. doi:10.1016/j.eururo.2011.01.030

11. Daneshmand S, Stein JP, Lesser T, et al. Prognosis of seminal vesicle involvement by transitional cell carcinoma of the bladder. *J Urol.* 2004;172(1):81-84. doi:10.1097/01.ju.0000132131.64727.ff

12. Green DA, Rink M, Xylinas E, et al. Urothelial carcinoma of the bladder and the upper tract: disparate twins. *J Urol.* 2013;189(4):1214-1221. doi:10.1016/j.juro.2012.05.079

13. Abdelaziz AY, Shaker H, Seifelnasr M, Elfol H, Nazim M, Mahmoued M. Early oncological and functional outcomes of prostate capsule sparing cystectomy compared with standard radical cystectomy. *Curr Urol.* 2019;13(1):37-45. doi:10.1159/000499296

14. Saad M, Moschini M, Stabile A, et al. Long-term functional and oncological outcomes of nerve-sparing and prostate capsule-sparing cystectomy: a single-centre experience. *BJU Int.* 2020;125(2):253-259. doi:10.1111/bju.14850

15. Voskuilen CS, Fransen van de Putte EE, Pérez-Reggeti JI, et al. Prostate sparing cystectomy for bladder cancer: a two-center study. *Eur J Surg Oncol.* 2018;44(9):1446-1452. doi:10.1016/j.ejso.2018.05.032

16. Niver BE, Daneshmand S, Satkunasivam R. Female reproductive organ-sparing radical cystectomy: contemporary indications, techniques and outcomes. *Curr Opin Urol.* 2015;25(2):105-110. doi:10.1097/MOU.0000000000000146

17. Grossman HB, Natale RB, Tangen CM, et al. Neoadjuvant chemotherapy plus cystectomy compared with cystectomy alone for locally advanced bladder cancer. *N Engl J Med.* 2003;349(9):859-866. doi:10.1056/NEJMoa022148

18. Meeks JJ, Bellmunt J, Bochner BH, et al. A systematic review of neoadjuvant and adjuvant chemotherapy for muscle-invasive bladder cancer. *Eur Urol.* 2012;62(3):523-533. doi:10.1016/j.eururo.2012.05.048

19. Vale CL. Adjuvant chemotherapy in invasive bladder cancer: a systematic review and meta-analysis of individual patient data: advanced bladder cancer (ABC) meta-analysis collaboration. *Eur Urol.* 2005;48(2):189-201. doi:10.1016/j.eururo.2005.04.005

20. Gakis G, Morgan TM, Daneshmand S, et al. Impact of perioperative chemotherapy on survival in patients with advanced primary urethral cancer: results of the international collaboration on primary urethral carcinoma. *Ann Oncol.* 2015;26(8):1754-1759. doi:10.1093/annonc/mdv230

21. Chang SS, Bochner BH, Chou R, et al. Treatment of non-metastatic muscle-invasive bladder cancer: AUA/ASCO/ASTRO/SUO guideline. *J Urol.* 2017;198(3):552-559. doi:10.1016/j.juro.2017.04.086

22. Mak RH, Hunt D, Shipley WU, et al. Long-term outcomes in patients with muscle-invasive bladder cancer after selective bladder-preserving combined-modality therapy: a pooled analysis of Radiation Therapy Oncology Group protocols 8802, 8903, 9506, 9706, 9906, and 0233. *J Clin Oncol.* 2014;32(34):3801-3809. doi:10.1200/JCO.2014.57.5548

23. Vashistha V, Wang H, Mazzone A, et al. Radical cystectomy compared to combined modality treatment for muscle-invasive bladder cancer: a systematic review and meta-analysis. *Int J Radiat Oncol Biol Phys.* 2017;97(5):1002-1020. doi:10.1016/j.ijrobp.2016.11.056

24. Efstathiou JA, Spiegel DY, Shipley WU, et al. Long-term outcomes of selective bladder preservation by combined-modality therapy for invasive bladder cancer: the MGH experience. *Eur Urol.* 2012;61(4):705-711. doi:10.1016/j.eururo.2011.11.010

25. Gray PJ, Fedewa SA, Shipley WU, et al. Use of potentially curative therapies for muscle-invasive bladder cancer in the United States: results from the National Cancer Data Base. *Eur Urol.* 2013;63(5):823-829. doi:10.1016/j.eururo.2012.11.015

26. Haque W, Verma V, Butler EB, Teh BS. National practice patterns and outcomes for T4b urothelial cancer of the bladder. *Clin Genitourin Cancer.* 2018;16(1):42.e41-49.e41. doi:10.1016/j.clgc.2017.08.013

27. Flaig TW, Spiess PE, Agarwal N, et al. NCCN guidelines insights: bladder cancer, version 5.2018. *J Natl Compr Canc Netw.* 2018;16(9):1041-1053. doi:10.6004/jnccn.2018.0072

28. James ND, Hussain SA, Hall E, et al. Radiotherapy with or without chemotherapy in muscle-invasive bladder cancer. *N Engl J Med.* 2012;366(16):1477-1488. doi:10.1056/NEJMoa1106106

29. Efstathiou JA, Bae K, Shipley WU, et al. Late pelvic toxicity after bladder-sparing therapy in patients with invasive bladder cancer: RTOG 89-03, 95-06, 97-06, 99-06. *J Clin Oncol.* 2009;27(25):4055-4061. doi:10.1200/JCO.2008.19.5776

30. Chen J, Djaladat H, Schuckman AK, et al. Surgical approach as a determinant factor of clinical outcome following radical cystectomy: does enhanced recovery after surgery (ERAS) level the playing field? *Urol Oncol.* 2019;37(10):765-773. doi:10.1016/j.urolonc.2019.06.001

31. Zainfeld D, Shah A, Daneshmand S. Enhanced recovery after surgery pathways: role and outcomes in the management of muscle invasive bladder cancer. *Urol Clin North Am*. 2018;45(2):229-239. doi:10.1016/j.ucl.2017.12.007

32. Rice KR, Brassell SA, McLeod DG. Venous thromboembolism in urologic surgery: prophylaxis, diagnosis, and treatment. *Rev Urol*. 2010;12(2-3):e111-e124.

33. Forrest JB, Clemens JQ, Finamore P, et al. AUA best practice statement for the prevention of deep vein thrombosis in patients undergoing urologic surgery. *J Urol*. 2009;181(3):1170-1177. doi:10.1016/j.juro.2008.12.027

34. Aquina CT, Truong M, Justiniano CF, et al. Variation in adequate lymph node yield for gastric, lung, and bladder cancer: attributable to the surgeon, pathologist, or hospital? *Ann Surg Oncol*. 2020;27(11):4093-4106. doi:10.1245/s10434-020-08509-3

35. American College of Surgeons. CoC Quality of Care Measures 2020 Surveys. Published 2020. Updated August 19, 2020. Accessed February 23, 2021. https://www.facs.org/Quality-Programs/Cancer/NCDB/qualitymeasurescocweb

36. Mariappan P, Johnston A, Padovani L, et al. Enhanced quality and effectiveness of transurethral resection of bladder tumour in non-muscle-invasive bladder cancer: a multicentre real-world experience from Scotland's Quality Performance Indicators programme. *Eur Urol*. 2020;78(4):520-530. doi:10.1016/j.eururo.2020.06.051

37. Shariat SF, Palapattu GS, Karakiewicz PI, et al. Discrepancy between clinical and pathologic stage: impact on prognosis after radical cystectomy. *Eur Urol*. 2007;51(1):137-151. doi:10.1016/j.eururo.2006.05.021

38. Kausch I, Sommerauer M, Montorsi F, et al. Photodynamic diagnosis in non-muscle-invasive bladder cancer: a systematic review and cumulative analysis of prospective studies. *Eur Urol*. 2010;57(4):595-606. doi:10.1016/j.eururo.2009.11.041

39. Babjuk M, Soukup V, Petrik R, Jirsa M, Dvoracek J. 5-Aminolaevulinic acid-induced fluorescence cystoscopy during transurethral resection reduces the risk of recurrence in stage Ta/T1 bladder cancer. *BJU Int*. 2005;96(6):798-802. doi:10.1111/j.1464-410X.2004.05715.x

40. Filbeck T, Pichlmeier U, Knuechel R, Wieland WF, Roessler W. Clinically relevant improvement of recurrence-free survival with 5-aminolevulinic acid induced fluorescence diagnosis in patients with superficial bladder tumors. *J Urol*. 2002;168(1):67-71.

41. Riedl CR, Daniltchenko D, Koenig F, Simak R, Loening SA, Pflueger H. Fluorescence endoscopy with 5-aminolevulinic acid reduces early recurrence rate in superficial bladder cancer. *J Urol*. 2001;165(4):1121-1123.

42. Li K, Lin T, Fan X, Duan Y, Huang J. Diagnosis of narrow-band imaging in non-muscle-invasive bladder cancer: a systematic review and meta-analysis. *Int J Urol*. 2013;20(6):602-609. doi:10.1111/j.1442-2042.2012.03211.x

43. Xiong Y, Li J, Ma S, et al. A meta-analysis of narrow band imaging for the diagnosis and therapeutic outcome of non-muscle invasive bladder cancer. *PLoS One*. 2017;12(2):e0170819. doi:10.1371/journal.pone.0170819

44. Zheng C, Lv Y, Zhong Q, Wang R, Jiang Q. Narrow band imaging diagnosis of bladder cancer: systematic review and meta-analysis. *BJU Int*. 2012;110(11 pt B):E680-E687. doi:10.1111/j.1464-1410X.2012.11500.x

45. Naito S, Algaba F, Babjuk M, et al. The Clinical Research Office of the Endourological Society (CROES) multicentre randomised trial of narrow band imaging-assisted transurethral resection of bladder tumour (TURBT) versus conventional white light imaging-assisted TURBT in primary non-muscle-invasive bladder cancer patients: trial protocol and 1-year results. *Eur Urol*. 2016;70(3):506-515. doi:10.1016/j.eururo.2016.03.053

46. Brausi M, Collette L, Kurth K, et al. Variability in the recurrence rate at first follow-up cystoscopy after TUR in stage Ta T1 transitional cell carcinoma of the bladder: a combined analysis of seven EORTC studies. *Eur Urol*. 2002;41(5):523-531. doi:10.1016/s0302-2838(02)00068-4

47. Herr HW, Donat SM. Quality control in transurethral resection of bladder tumours. *BJU Int*. 2008;102(9 pt B):1242-1246. doi:10.1111/j.1464-410X.2008.07966.x

48. Babjuk M, Böhle A, Burger M, et al. EAU guidelines on non-muscle-invasive urothelial carcinoma of the bladder: update 2016. *Eur Urol*. 2017;71(3):447-461. doi:10.1016/j.eururo.2016.1005.1041

49. Audenet F, Retinger C, Chien C, et al. Is restaging transurethral resection necessary in patients with non-muscle invasive bladder cancer and limited lamina propria invasion? *Urol Oncol*. 2017;35(10):603.e1-603.e5. doi:10.1016/j.urolonc.2017.1006.1042

50. Panagoda PI, Vasdev N, Gowrie-Mohan S. Avoiding the obturator jerk during TURBT. *Curr Urol*. 2018;12(1):1-5. doi:10.1159/000447223

51. Soloway MS, Sofer M, Vaidya A. Contemporary management of stage T1 transitional cell carcinoma of the bladder. *J Urol.* 2002;167(4):1573-1583.
52. Soloway MS, Patel J. Surgical techniques for endoscopic resection of bladder cancer. *Urol Clin North Am.* 1992;19(3):467-471.
53. Carmack AJ, Soloway MS. The diagnosis and staging of bladder cancer: from RBCs to TURs. *Urology.* 2006;67(3 suppl 1):3-10. doi:10.1016/j.urology.2006.01.026
54. Pan D, Soloway MS. The importance of transurethral resection in managing patients with urothelial cancer in the bladder: proposal for a transurethral resection of bladder tumor checklist. *Eur Urol.* 2012;61(6):1199-1203. doi:10.1016/j.eururo.2012.03.018
55. Avallone MA, Sack BS, El-Arabi A, et al. Ten-year review of perioperative complications after transurethral resection of bladder tumors: analysis of monopolar and plasmakinetic bipolar cases. *J Endourol.* 2017;31(8):767-773. doi:10.1089/end.2017.0056
56. Sugihara T, Yasunaga H, Horiguchi H, et al. Comparison of perioperative outcomes including severe bladder injury between monopolar and bipolar transurethral resection of bladder tumors: a population based comparison. *J Urol.* 2014;192(5):1355-1359. doi:10.1016/j.juro.2014.05.100
57. Zhao C, Tang K, Yang H, Xia D, Chen Z. Bipolar versus monopolar transurethral resection of nonmuscle-invasive bladder cancer: a meta-analysis. *J Endourol.* 2016;30(1):5-12. doi:10.1089/end.2015.0410
58. Ukai R, Hashimoto K, Iwasa T, Nakayama H. Transurethral resection in one piece (TURBO) is an accurate tool for pathological staging of bladder tumor. *Int J Urol.* 2010;17(8):708-714. doi:10.1111/j.1442-2042.2010.02571.x
59. Ukai R, Kawashita E, Ikeda H. A new technique for transurethral resection of superficial bladder tumor in 1 piece. *J Urol.* 2000;163(3):878-879.
60. Gao X, Ren S, Xu C, Sun Y. Thulium laser resection via a flexible cystoscope for recurrent non-muscle-invasive bladder cancer: initial clinical experience. *BJU Int.* 2008;102(9):1115-1118. doi:10.1111/j.1464-410X.2008.07814.x
61. Fritsche HM, Otto W, Eder F, et al. Water-jet-aided transurethral dissection of urothelial carcinoma: a prospective clinical study. *J Endourol.* 2011;25(10):1599-1603. doi:10.1089/end.2011.0042
62. Xishuang S, Deyong Y, Xiangyu C, et al. Comparing the safety and efficiency of conventional monopolar, plasmakinetic, and holmium laser transurethral resection of primary non-muscle invasive bladder cancer. *J Endourol.* 2010;24(1):69-73. doi:10.1089/end.2009.0171
63. Donat SM, North A, Dalbagni G, Herr HW. Efficacy of office fulguration for recurrent low grade papillary bladder tumors less than 0.5 cm. *J Urol.* 2004;171(2 pt 1):636-639. doi:10.1097/01.ju.0000103100.22951.5e
64. Guo RQ, Hong P, Xiong GY, et al. Impact of ureteroscopy before radical nephroureterectomy for upper tract urothelial carcinomas on oncological outcomes: a meta-analysis. *BJU Int.* 2018;121(2):184-193. doi:10.1111/bju.14053
65. Rojas CP, Castle SM, Llanos CA, et al. Low biopsy volume in ureteroscopy does not affect tumor biopsy grading in upper tract urothelial carcinoma. *Urol Oncol.* 2013;31(8):1696-1700. doi:10.1016/j.urolonc.2012.05.010
66. Tsivian A, Tsivian M, Stanevsky Y, Tavdy E, Sidi AA. Routine diagnostic ureteroscopy for suspected upper tract transitional-cell carcinoma. *J Endourol.* 2014;28(8):922-925. doi:10.1089/end.2013.0703
67. Seisen T, Peyronnet B, Dominguez-Escrig JL, et al. Oncologic outcomes of kidney-sparing surgery versus radical nephroureterectomy for upper tract urothelial carcinoma: a systematic review by the EAU Non-Muscle Invasive Bladder Cancer Guidelines Panel. *Eur Urol.* 2016;70(6):1052-1068. doi:10.1016/j.eururo.2016.07.014
68. Cutress ML, Stewart GD, Zakikhani P, Phipps S, Thomas BG, Tolley DA. Ureteroscopic and percutaneous management of upper tract urothelial carcinoma (UTUC): systematic review. *BJU Int.* 2012;110(5):614-628. doi:10.1111/j.1464-410X.2012.11068 x
69. Bagley DH, Grasso M III. Ureteroscopic laser treatment of upper urinary tract neoplasms. *World J Urol.* 2010;28(2):143-149. doi:10.1007/s00345-010-0525-7
70. Roupret M, Babjuk M, Comperat E, et al. European Association of Urology guidelines on upper urinary tract urothelial carcinoma: 2017 update. *Eur Urol.* 2018;73(1):111-122. doi:10.1016/j.eururo.2017.07.036
71. Flaig TW, Spiess PE, Agarwal N, et al. Bladder Cancer, version 3.2020, NCCN clinical practice guidelines in oncology. *J Natl Compr Canc Netw.* 2020;18(3):329-354. doi:10.6004/jnccn.2020.0011
72. Scotland KB, Kleinmann N, Cason D, et al. Ureteroscopic management of large ≥2 cm upper tract urothelial carcinoma: a comprehensive 23-year experience. *Urology.* 2018;121:66-73. doi:10.1016/j.urology.2018.05.042

73. Sylvester RJ, Oosterlinck W, Holmang S, et al. Systematic review and individual patient data meta-analysis of randomized trials comparing a single immediate instillation of chemotherapy after transurethral resection with transurethral resection alone in patients with stage pTa-pT1 urothelial carcinoma of the bladder: which patients benefit from the instillation? *Eur Urol.* 2016;69(2):231-244. doi:10.1016/j.eururo.2015.05.050

74. Babjuk M, Burger M, Comperat EM, et al. Indication for a single postoperative instillation of chemotherapy in non-muscle-invasive bladder cancer: what factors should be considered? *Eur Urol Focus.* 2018;4(4):525-528. doi:10.1016/j.euf.2018.07.023

75. O'Donnell MA. Practical applications of intravesical chemotherapy and immunotherapy in high-risk patients with superficial bladder cancer. *Urol Clin North Am.* 2005;32(2):121-131. doi:10.1016/j.ucl.2005.01.003

76. Messing EM, Tangen CM, Lerner SP, et al. Effect of intravesical instillation of gemcitabine vs saline immediately following resection of suspected low-grade non-muscle-invasive bladder cancer on tumor recurrence: SWOG S0337 randomized clinical trial. *JAMA.* 2018;319(18):1880-1888. doi:10.1001/jama.2018.4657

77. American Urological Association guideline: Intravesical Administration of Therapeutic Medication. https://www.auanet.org/guidelines/guidelines/intravesical-administration-of-therapeutic-medication

78. Holzbeierlein JM, Lopez-Corona E, Bochner BH, et al. Partial cystectomy: a contemporary review of the Memorial Sloan-Kettering Cancer Center experience and recommendations for patient selection. *J Urol.* 2004;172(3):878-881. doi:10.1097/01.ju.0000135530.59860.7d

79. Knoedler JJ, Boorjian SA, Kim SP, et al. Does partial cystectomy compromise oncologic outcomes for patients with bladder cancer compared to radical cystectomy? A matched case-control analysis. *J Urol.* 2012;188(4):1115-1119. doi:10.1016/j.juro.2012.06.029

80. Arora S, Kumar R, Passah A, et al. Prospective evaluation of ^{68}Ga-DOTANOC positron emission tomography/computed tomography and ^{131}I-meta-iodobenzylguanidine single-photon emission computed tomography/computed tomography in extra-adrenal paragangliomas, including uncommon primary sites and to define their diagnostic roles in current scenario. *Nucl Med Commun.* 2019;40(12):1230-1242. doi:10.1097/MNM.0000000000001096

81. Ashley RA, Inman BA, Sebo TJ, et al. Urachal carcinoma: clinicopathologic features and long-term outcomes of an aggressive malignancy. *Cancer.* 2006;107(4):712-720. doi:10.1002/cncr.22060

82. Gofrit ON, Shapiro A, Katz R, et al. Cystoscopic-assisted partial cystectomy: description of technique and results. *Res Rep Urol.* 2014;6:139-143. doi:10.2147/RRU.S66861

83. Fedeli U, Fedewa SA, Ward EM. Treatment of muscle invasive bladder cancer: evidence from the National Cancer Database, 2003 to 2007. *J Urol.* 2011;185(1):72-78. doi:10.1016/j.juro.2010.09.015

84. Brannan W, Ochsner MG, Fuselier HA Jr, Landry GR. Partial cystectomy in the treatment of transitional cell carcinoma of the bladder. *J Urol.* 1978;119(2):213-215. doi:10.1016/s0022-5347(17)57436-4

85. Kassouf W, Swanson D, Kamat AM, et al. Partial cystectomy for muscle invasive urothelial carcinoma of the bladder: a contemporary review of the M. D. Anderson Cancer Center experience. *J Urol.* 2006;175(6):2058-2062. doi:10.1016/S0022-5347(06)00322-3

86. Smaldone MC, Jacobs BL, Smaldone AM, Hrebinko RL Jr. Long-term results of selective partial cystectomy for invasive urothelial bladder carcinoma. *Urology.* 2008;72(3):613-616. doi:10.1016/j.urology.2008.04.052

87. Knoedler J, Frank I. Organ-sparing surgery in urology: partial cystectomy. *Curr Opin Urol.* 2015;25(2):111-115. doi:10.1097/MOU.0000000000000145

88. Capitanio U, Isbarn H, Shariat SF, et al. Partial cystectomy does not undermine cancer control in appropriately selected patients with urothelial carcinoma of the bladder: a population-based matched analysisst. *Urology.* 2009;74(4):858-864. doi:10.1016/j.urology.2009.03.052

89. Ma B, Li H, Zhang C, et al. Lymphovascular invasion, ureteral reimplantation and prior history of urothelial carcinoma are associated with poor prognosis after partial cystectomy for muscle-invasive bladder cancer with negative pelvic lymph nodes. *Eur J Surg Oncol.* 2013;39(10):1150-1156. doi:10.1016/j.ejso.2013.04.006

90. Orosco RK, Tapia VJ, Califano JA, et al. Positive surgical margins in the 10 most common solid cancers. *Sci Rep.* 2018;8(1):5686. doi:10.1038/s41598-018-23403-5

91. Dotan ZA, Kavanagh K, Yossepowitch O, et al. Positive surgical margins in soft tissue following radical cystectomy for bladder cancer and cancer specific survival. *J Urol.* 2007;178(6):2308-2313. doi:10.1016/j.juro.2007.08.023

92. Shao IH, Chang YH, Yu KJ, et al. Outcomes and prognostic factors of simple partial cystectomy for localized bladder urothelial cell carcinoma. *Kaohsiung J Med Sci.* 2016;32(4):191-195. doi:10.1016/j.kjms.2016.02.008

93. Fahmy N, Aprikian A, Tanguay S, et al. Practice patterns and recurrence after partial cystectomy for bladder cancer. *World J Urol.* 2010;28(4):419-423. do :10.1007/s00345-009-0478-x

94. Ebbing J, Heckmann RC, Collins JW, et al. Oncological outcomes, quality of life outcomes and complications of partial cystectomy for selected cases of muscle-invasive bladder cancer. *Sci Rep.* 2018;8(1):8360. doi:10.1038/s41598-018-26089-x

95. Dandekar NP, Tongaonkar HB, Dalal AV, Kulkarni JN, Kamat MR. Partial cystectomy for invasive bladder cancer. *J Surg Oncol.* 1995;60(1):24-29. doi:10.1002/jso.2930600106

96. Socd A, Klett DE, Abdollah F, et al. Robot-assisted partial cystectomy with intraoperative frozen section examination: evolution and evaluation of a novel technique. *Investig Clin Urol.* 2016;57(3):221-228. doi:10.4111/icu.2016.57.3.221

97. Miyamoto H. Clinical benefits of frozen section assessment during urological surgery: does it contribute to improving surgical margin status and patient outcomes as previously thought? *Int J Urol.* 2017;24(1):25-31. doi:10.1111/iju.13247

98. Zhang M, Tao R, Zhang C, Shen Z. Lymphovascular invasion and the presence of more than three tumors are associated with poor outcomes of muscle-invasive bladder cancer after bladder-conserving therapies. *Urology.* 2010;76(4):902-907. doi:10.1016/j.urology.2010.05.007

99. Subiela JD, Rodriguez Faba O, Guerrero Ramos F, et al. Carcinoma in situ of the urinary bladder: a systematic review of current knowledge regarding detection, treatment, and outcomes. *Eur Urol Focus.* 2020;6(4):674-682. doi:10.1016/j.euf.2019.03.012

100. Palmeira C, Lameiras C, Amaro T, et al. CIS is a surrogate marker of genetic instability and field carcinogenesis in the urothelial mucosa. *Urol Oncol.* 2011;29(2):205-211. doi:10.1016/j.urolonc.2009.07.022

101. Amin MB, McKenney JK. An approach to the diagnosis of flat intraepithelial lesions of the urinary bladder using the World Health Organization/International Society of Urological Pathology consensus classification system. *Adv Anat Pathol.* 2002;9(4):222-232. doi:10.1097/00125480-200207000-00002

102. Spiess PE, Agarwal N, Bangs R, et al. Bladder cancer, version 5.2017, NCCN clinical practice guidelines in oncology. *J Natl Compr Canc Netw.* 2017;15(10):1240-1267. doi:10.6004/jnccn.2017.0156

103. Smith JA Jr, Howards SS, Preminger GM, Dmochowski RR. *Hinman's Atlas of Urologic Surgery.* 4th ed. Elsevier Inc; 2018.

104. Wein AJ, Kavoussi LR, Partin AW, Peters CA, eds. *Campbell-Walsh Urology.* 11th. ed. Elsevier Inc; 2016.

105. Bailey GC, Frank I, Tollefson MK, Gettman MT, Knoedler JJ. Perioperative outcomes of robot-assisted laparoscopic partial cystectomy. *J Robot Surg.* 2018;12(2):223-228. doi:10.1007/s11701-017-0717-x

106. Morris DS, Weizer AZ, Ye Z, Dunn RL, Montie JE, Hollenbeck BK. Understanding bladder cancer death: tumor biology versus physician practice. *Cancer.* 2009;115(5):1011-1020. doi:10.1002/cncr.24136

107. Stein JP, Lieskovsky G, Cote R, et al. Radical cystectomy in the treatment of invasive bladder cancer: long-term results in 1,054 patients. *J Clin Oncol.* 2001;19(3):666-675. doi:10.1200/JCO.2001.19.3.666

108. Shariat SF, Karakiewicz PI, Palapattu GS, et al. Outcomes of radical cystectomy for transitional cell carcinoma of the bladder: a contemporary series from the Bladder Cancer Research Consortium. *J Urol.* 2006;176(6 pt 1):2414-2422. doi:10.1016/j.juro.2006.08.004

109. Novara G, Svatek RS, Karakiewicz PI, et al. Soft tissue surgical margin status is a powerful predictor of outcomes after radical cystectomy: a multicenter study of more than 4,400 patients. *J Urol.* 2010;183(6):2165-2170. doi:10.1016/j.juro.2010.02.021

110. Gakis G, Schilling D, Perner S, Schwentner C, Sievert K-D, Stenzl AJ. Sequential resection of malignant ureteral margins at radical cystectomy: a critical assessment of the value of frozen section analysis. *World J Urol.* 2011;29(4):451-456. doi:10.1007/s00345-010-0581-z

111. Satkunasivam R, Hu B, Metcalfe C, et al. Utility and significance of ureteric frozen section analysis during radical cystectomy. *BJU Int.* 2016;117(3):463-468. doi:10.1111/bju.13081

112. Chang SS. Re: utility and significance of ureteric frozen section analysis during radical cystectomy. *J Urol.* 2017;197(2):318-319. doi:10.1016/j.juro.2016.11.039

113. Huguet J, Monllau V, Sabaté S, et al. Diagnosis, risk factors, and outcome of urethral recurrences following radical cystectomy for bladder cancer in 729 male patients. *Eur Urol.* 2008;53(4): 785-793. doi:10.1016/j.eururo.2007.06.045

114. Stein JP, Penson DF, Wu SD, Skinner DG. Pathological guidelines for orthotopic urinary diversion in women with bladder cancer: a review of the literature. *J Urol.* 2007;178(3 pt 1):756-760. doi:10.1016/j.juro.2007.05.013

115. Guru KA, Kim HL, Piacente PM, Mohler JL. Robot-assisted radical cystectomy and pelvic lymph node dissection: initial experience at Roswell Park Cancer Institute. *Urology.* 2007;69(3): 469-474. doi:10.1016/j.urology.2006.10.037

116. Hanna N, Leow JJ, Sun M, et al. Comparative effectiveness of robot-assisted vs. open radical cystectomy. *Urol Oncol.* 2018;36(3):88.e1-88.e9. doi:10.1016/j.urolonc.2017.09.018

117. Shariat SF, Sfakianos JP, Droller MJ, Karakiewicz PI, Meryn S, Bochner BH. The effect of age and gender on bladder cancer: a critical review of the literature. *BJU Int.* 2010;105(3):300-308. doi:10.1111/j.1464-410X.2009.09076.x

118. Sussman RD, Han CJ, Marchalik D, et al. To oophorectomy or not to oophorectomy: practice patterns among urologists treating bladder cancer. *Urol Oncol.* 2018;36(3):90.e1-90.e7. doi:10.1016/j.urolonc.2017.11.018

119. O'Connell HE, Hutson JM, Anderson CR, Plenter RJ. Anatomical relationship between urethra and clitoris. *J Urol.* 1998;159(6):1892-1897. doi:10.1016/S0022-5347(01)63188-4

120. Djaladat H, Bruins HM, Miranda G, Cai J, Skinner EC, Daneshmand S. Reproductive organ involvement in female patients undergoing radical cystectomy for urothelial bladder cancer. *J Urol.* 2012;188(6):2134-2138. doi:10.1016/j.juro.2012.08.024

121. Gross T, Furrer M, Schorno P, et al. Reproductive organ-sparing cystectomy significantly improves continence in women after orthotopic bladder substitution without affecting oncological outcome. *BJU Int.* 2018;122(2):227-235. doi:10.1111/bju.14191

122. Veskimäe E, Neuzillet Y, Rouanne M, et al. Systematic review of the oncological and functional outcomes of pelvic organ-preserving radical cystectomy (RC) compared with standard RC in women who undergo curative surgery and orthotopic neobladder substitution for bladder cancer. *BJU Int.* 2017;120(1):12-24. doi:10.1111/bju.13819

123. Smith AB, Crowell K, Woods ME, et al. Functional outcomes following radical cystectomy in women with bladder cancer: a systematic review. *Eur Urol Focus.* 2017;3(1):136-143. doi:10.1016/j.euf.2016.05.005

124. Avulova S, Chang SS. Role and indications of organ-sparing "radical" cystectomy: the importance of careful patient selection and counseling. *Urol Clin North Am.* 2018;45(2):199-214. doi:10.1016/j.ucl.2017.12.005

125. Panebianco V, Narumi Y, Altun E, et al. Multiparametric magnetic resonance imaging for bladder cancer: development of VI-RADS (Vesical Imaging-Reporting And Data System). *Eur Urol.* 2018;74(3):294-306.

126. Colombo R, Pellucchi F, Moschini M, et al. Fifteen-year single-centre experience with three different surgical procedures of nerve-sparing cystectomy in selected organ-confined bladder cancer patients. *World J Urol.* 2015;33(10):1389-1395. doi:10.1007/s00345-015-1482-y

127. Nieuwenhuijzen JA, Meinhardt W, Horenblas S. Clinical outcomes after sexuality preserving cystectomy and neobladder (prostate sparing cystectomy) in 44 patients. *J Urol.* 2008;179(5 suppl): S35-S38. doi:10.1016/j.juro.2008.03.135

128. Koraitim M, Khalil R. Preservation of urosexual functions after radical cystectomy. *Urology.* 1992;39(2):117-121. doi:10.1016/0090-4295(92)90266-y

129. Spitz A, Stein JP, Lieskovsky G, Skinner DG. Orthotopic urinary diversion with preservation of erectile and ejaculatory function in men requiring radical cystectomy for nonurothelial malignancy: a new technique. *J Urol.* 1999;161(6):1761-1764.

130. Puppo P, Introini C, Bertolotto F, Naselli A. Potency preserving cystectomy with intrafascial prostatectomy for high risk superficial bladder cancer. *J Urol.* 2008;179(5):1727-1732. doi:10.1016/j.juro.2008.01.046

131. Colleselli K, Stenzl A, Eder R, Strasser H, Poisel S, Bartsch G. The female urethral sphincter: a morphological and topographical study. *J Urol.* 1998;160(1):49-54. doi:10.1016/s0022-5347(01)63025-8

132. Blank MA, Gu J, Allen JM, et al. The regional distribution of NPY-, PHM-, and VIP-containing nerves in the human female genital tract. *Int J Fertil.* 1986;31(3):218-222.

133. Menon M, Hemal AK, Tewari A, et al. Robot-assisted radical cystectomy and urinary diversion in female patients: technique with preservation of the uterus and vagina. *J Am Coll Surg.* 2004;198(3):386-393. doi:10.1016/j.jamcollsurg.2003.11.010

134. Koie T, Hatakeyama S, Yoneyama T, Hashimoto Y, Kamimura N, Ohyama C. Uterus-, fallopian tube-, ovary-, and vagina-sparing cystectomy followed by U-shaped ileal neobladder construction for female bladder cancer patients: oncological and functional outcomes. *Urology.* 2010;75(6):1499-1503. doi:10.1016/j.urology.2009.08.083

135. Stein JP, Clark P, Miranda G, Cai J, Groshen S, Skinner DG. Urethral tumor recurrence following cystectomy and urinary diversion: clinical and pathologica characteristics in 768 male patients. *J Urol.* 2005;173(4):1163-1168. doi:10.1097/01.ju.0000149679.56884.0f

136. Horenblas S, Meinhardt W, Ijzerman W, Moonen LF. Sexuality preserving cystectomy and neobladder: initial results. *J Urol.* 2001;166(3):837-840.

137. Colombo R, Bertini R, Salonia A, et al. Nerve and seminal sparing radical cystectomy with orthotopic urinary diversion for select patients with superficial bladder cancer: an innovative surgical approach. *J Urol.* 2001;165(1):51-55. doi:10.1097/00005392-200101000-00013

138. Herr HW, Bochner BH, Dalbagni G, Donat SM, Reuter VE, Bajorin DF. Impact of the number of lymph nodes retrieved on outcome in patients with muscle invasive bladder cancer. *J Urol.* 2002;167(3):1295-1298.

139. Konety BR, Joslyn SA, O'Donnell MA. Extent of pelvic lymphadenectomy and its impact on outcome in patients diagnosed with bladder cancer: analysis of data from the Surveillance, Epidemiology and End Results Program data base. *J Urol.* 2003;169(3):946-950. doi:10.1097/01.ju.0000052721.61645.a3

140. Leissner J, Hohenfellner R, Thuroff JW, Wolf HK. Lymphadenectomy in patients with transitional cell carcinoma of the urinary bladder; significance for staging and prognosis. *BJU Int.* 2000;85(7):817-823. doi:10.1046/j.1464-410x.2000.00614.x

141. May M, Herrmann E, Bolenz C, et al. Association between the number of dissected lymph nodes during pelvic lymphadenectomy and cancer-specific survival in patients with lymph node-negative urothelial carcinoma of the bladder undergoing radical cystectomy. *Ann Surg Oncol.* 2011;18(7):2018-2025.

142. Morgan TM, Barocas DA, Penson DF, et al. Lymph node yield at radical cystectomy predicts mortality in node-negative and not node-positive patients. *Urology.* 2012;80(3):632-640. doi:10.1016/j.urology.2012.03.070

143. Dhar NB, Klein EA, Reuther AM, Thalmann GN, Madersbacher S, Studer UE. Outcome after radical cystectomy with limited or extended pelvic lymph node dissection. *J Urol.* 2008;179(3):873-878. doi:10.1016/j.juro.2007.10.076

144. Fleischmann A, Thalmann GN, Markwalder R, Studer UE. Prognostic implications of extracapsular extension of pelvic lymph node metastases in urothelial carcinoma of the bladder. *Am J Surg Pathol.* 2005;29(1):89-95. doi:10.1097/01.pas.0000147396.08853.26

145. Koppie TM, Vickers AJ, Vora K, Dalbagni G, Bochner BH. Standardization of pelvic lymphadenectomy performed at radical cystectomy: can we establish a minimum number of lymph nodes that should be removed? *Cancer.* 2006;107(10):2368-2374. doi:10.1002/cncr.22250

146. Herr HW, Faulkner JR, Grossman HB, et al. Surgical factors influence bladder cancer outcomes: a cooperative group report. *J Clin Oncol.* 2004;22(14):2781-2789. doi:10.1200/JCO.2004.11.024

147. Bochner BH, Herr HW, Reuter VE. Impact of separate versus en bloc pelvic lymph node dissection on the number of lymph nodes retrieved in cystectomy specimens. *J Urol.* 2001;166(6):2295-2296.

148. Bi L, Huang H, Fan X, et al. Extended vs non-extended pelvic lymph node dissection and their influence on recurrence-free survival in patients undergoing radical cystectomy for bladder cancer: a systematic review and meta-analysis of comparative studies. *BJU Int.* 2014;113(5b):E39-E48. doi:10.1111/bju.12371

149. Herr H, Lee C, Chang S, Lerner S, Bladder Cancer Collaborative Group. Standardization of radical cystectomy and pelvic lymph node dissection for bladder cancer: a collaborative group report. *J Urol.* 2004;171(5):1823-1828. doi:10.1097/01.ju.0000120289.78049.0e

150. Jensen JB, Ulhøi BP, Jensen KME. Extended versus limited lymph node dissection in radical cystectomy: impact on recurrence pattern and survival. *Int J Urol.* 2012;19(1):39-47. doi:10.1111/j.1442-2042.2011.02887.x

151. Perera M, McGrath S, Sengupta S, Crozier J, Bolton D, Lawrentschuk N. Pelvic lymph node dissection during radical cystectomy for muscle-invasive bladder cancer. *Nat Rev Urol.* 2018;15(11):686-692. doi:10.1038/s41585-018-0066-1

152. Gschwend JE, Heck MM, Lehmann J, et al. Extended versus limited lymph node dissection in bladder cancer patients undergoing radical cystectomy: survival results from a prospective, randomized trial. *Eur Urol.* 2019;75(4):604-611. doi:10.1016/j.eururo.2018.09.047

153. Skinner EC. Choosing the right urinary diversion: patient's choice or surgeon's inclination? *Urol Oncol.* 2011;29(5):473-475. doi:10.1016/j.urolonc.2010.09.002

154. Faba OR, Tyson MD, Artibani W, et al. Update of the ICUD-SIU International Consultation on Bladder Cancer 2018: urinary diversion. *World J Urol.* 2019;37(1):85-93. doi:10.1007/s00345 -018-2484-3

155. Boorjian SA, Kim SP, Weight CJ, Cheville JC, Thapa P, Frank I. Risk factors and outcomes of urethral recurrence following radical cystectomy. *Eur Urol.* 2011;60(6):1266-1272. doi:10.1016 /j.eururo.2011.08.030

156. Stein JP, Cote RJ, Freeman JA, et al. Indications for lower urinary tract reconstruction in women after cystectomy for bladder cancer: a pathological review of female cystectomy specimens. *J Urol.* 1995;154(4):1329-1333.

157. Satkunasivam R, Hu B, Daneshmand S. Is frozen section analysis of ureteral margins at time of radical cystectomy useful? *Curr Urol Rep.* 2015;16(6):38. doi:10.1007/s11934-015 -0506-x

158. Hautmann RE, Simon J. Ileal neobladder and local recurrence of bladder cancer: patterns of failure and impact on function in men. *J Urol.* 1999;162(6):1963-1966. doi:10.1016 /s0022-5347(05)68079-2

159. Ballas L, Sargos P, Orre M, Bian SX, Daneshmand S, Eapen LJ. Tolerance of orthotopic ileal neobladders to radiotherapy: a multi-institutional retrospective study. *Clin Genitourin Cancer.* 2017;15(6):711-716. doi:10.1016/j.clgc.2017.05.007

160. Chang SS, Boorjian SA, Chou R, et al. Diagnosis and treatment of non-muscle invasive bladder cancer: AUA/SUO guideline. *J Urol.* 2016;196(4):1021-1029. doi:10.1016/j.juro.2016 .06.049

161. Bruins HM, Skinner EC, Dorin RP, et al. Incidence and location of lymph node metastases in patients undergoing radical cystectomy for clinical non-muscle invasive bladder cancer: results from a prospective lymph node mapping study. *Urol Oncol.* 2014;32(1):24.e13-24.e19. doi:10.1016/j.urolonc.2012.08.015.

162. Alfred Witjes J, Lebret T, Compérat EM, et al. Updated 2016 EAU guidelines on muscle-invasive and metastatic bladder cancer. *Eur Urol.* 2017;71(3):462-475. doi:10.1016/j.eururo.2016.06.020

163. Moher D, Liberati A, Tetzlaff J, Altman DG, PRIMA Group. Preferred reporting items for systematic reviews and meta-analyses: the PRISMA statement. *PLoS Med.* 2009;6(7):e1000097. doi:10.1371/journal.pmed.1000097

164. Abdi H, Pourmalek F, Gleave ME, So AI, Black PC. Balancing risk and benefit of extended pelvic lymph node dissection in patients undergoing radical cystectomy. *World J Urol.* 2016;34(1): 41-48. doi:10.1007/s00345-015-1734-x

165. Abol-Enein H, Tilki D, Mosbah A, et al. Does the extent of lymphadenectomy in radical cystectomy for bladder cancer influence disease-free survival? A prospective single-center study. *Eur Urol.* 2011;60(3):572-577. doi:10.1016/j.eururo.2011.05.062

166. Baumann BC, Guzzo TJ, He J, et al. A novel risk stratification to predict local-regional failures in urothelial carcinoma of the bladder after radical cystectomy. *Int J Radiat Oncol Biol Phys.* 2013;85(1):81-88. doi:10.1016/j.ijrobp.2012.03.007

167. Crozier J, Papa N, Perera M, et al. Lymph node yield in node-negative patients predicts cancer specific survival following radical cystectomy for transitional cell carcinoma. *Investig Clin Urol.* 2017;58(6):416-422. doi:10.4111/icu.2017.58.6.416

168. Fransen van de Putte EE, Hermans TJN, Werkhoven Ev, et al. Lymph node count at radical cystectomy does not influence long-term survival if surgeons adhere to a standardized template. *Urol Oncol.* 2015;33(12):504.e19-504.e24. doi:10.1016/j.urolonc.2015.08.001

169. Froehner M, Novotny V, Heberling U, et al. Relationship of the number of removed lymph nodes to bladder cancer and competing mortality after radical cystectomy. *Eur Urol.* 2014;66(6): 987-990. doi:10.1016/j.eururo.2014.07.046

170. Herr HW. Extent of surgery and pathology evaluation has an impact on bladder cancer outcomes after radical cystectomy. *Urology.* 2003;61(1):105-108. doi:10.1016/s0090-4295(02)02116-7

171. Honma I, Masumori N, Sato E, et al. Removal of more lymph nodes may provide better outcome, as well as more accurate pathologic findings, in patients with bladder cancer—analysis of role of pelvic lymph node dissection. *Urology.* 2006;68(3):543-548. doi:10.1016/j.urology.2006.03.049

172. Lin J, Deibert CM, Holder D, Benson MC, McKiernan JM. The role of pelvic lymphadenectomy in non-muscle invasive bladder cancer. *Can J Urol.* 2014;21(1):7108-7113.

173. Park J, Kim S, Jeong IG, et al. Does the greater number of lymph nodes removed during standard lymph node dissection predict better patient survival following radical cystectomy? *World J Urol.* 2011;29(4):443-449. doi:10.1007/s00345-011-0644-9

174. Ploussard G, Shariat SF, Dragomir A, et al. Conditional survival after radical cystectomy for bladder cancer: evidence for a patient changing risk profile over time. *European Urology.* 2014;66(2):361-370. doi:10.1016/j.eururo.2013.09.050

175. Rink M, Shariat SF, Xylinas E, et al. Does increasing the nodal yield improve outcomes in patients without nodal metastasis at radical cystectomy? *World J Urol.* 2012;30(6):807-814. doi:10.1007/s00345-012-0910-5

176. Shirotake S, Kikuchi E, Matsumoto K, et al. Role of pelvic lymph node dissection in lymph node-negative patients with invasive bladder cancer. *Jpn J Clin Oncol.* 2009;40(3):247-251. doi:10.1093/jjco/hyp147

177. Siemens DR, Mackillop WJ, Peng Y, Wei X, Berman D, Booth CM. Lymph node counts are valid indicators of the quality of surgical care in bladder cancer: a population-based study. *Urol Oncol.* 2015;33(10):425.e15-425.e23. doi:10.1016/j.urolonc.2015.06.005

178. Stein JP, Cai J, Groshen S, Skinner DG. Risk factors for patients with pelvic lymph node metastases following radical cystectomy with en bloc pelvic lymphadenectomy: the concept of lymph node density. *J Urol.* 2003;170(1):35-41. doi:10.1097/01.ju.0000072422.69286.0e

179. Ugurlu O, Baltaci S, Aslan G, et al. Does skip metastasis or other lymph node parameters have additional effects on survival of patients undergoing radical cystectomy for bladder cancer? *Korean J Urol.* 2015;56(5):357-364. doi:10.4111/kju.2015.56.5.357

180. von Landenberg N, Speed JM, Cole AP, et al. Impact of adequate pelvic lymph node dissection on overall survival after radical cystectomy: a stratified analysis by clinical stage and receipt of neoadjuvant chemotherapy. *Urol Oncol.* 2018;36(2):78.e13-78.e19. doi:10.1016/j.urolonc.2017.10.021

181. Wright JL, Lin DW, Porter MP. The association between extent of lymphadenectomy and survival among patients with lymph node metastases undergoing radical cystectomy. *Cancer.* 2008;112(11):2401-2408. doi:10.1002/cncr.23474

182. Brunocilla E, Pernetti R, Schiavina R, et al. The number of nodes removed as well as the template of the dissection is independently correlated to cancer-specific survival after radical cystectomy for muscle-invasive bladder cancer. *Int Urol Nephrol.* 2013;45(3):711-719. doi:10.1007/s11255-013-0461-8

183. Choi SY, You D, Hong B, Hong JH, Ahn H, Kim CS. Impact of lymph node dissection in radical cystectomy for bladder cancer: how many vs how far? *Surgical Oncology.* 2019;30(May):109-116. doi:10.1016/j.suronc.2019.06.008

184. Holmer M, Bendahl P-O, Davidsson T, Gudjonsson S, Månsson W, Liedberg F. Extended lymph node dissection in patients with urothelial cell carcinoma of the bladder: can it make a difference? *World J Urol.* 2009;27(4):521-526. doi:10.1007/s00345-008-0366-9

185. Mata DA, Groshen S, Von Rundstedt FC, et al. Variability in surgical quality in a phase III clinical trial of radical cystectomy in patients with organ-confined, node-negative urothelial carcinoma of the bladder. *J Surg Oncol.* 2015;111(7):923-928. doi:10.1002/jso.23903

186. Park E, Ha HK, Chung MK. Prediction of prognosis after radical cystectomy for pathologic node-negative bladder cancer. *Int Urol Nephrol.* 2011;43(4):1059-1065. doi:10.1007/s11255-011-9920-2

187. Simone G, Papalia R, Ferriero M, et al. Development and external validation of lymph node density cut-off points in prospective series of radical cystectomy and pelvic lymph node dissection. *Int J Urol.* 2012;19(12):1068-1074. doi:10.1111/j.1442-2042.2012.03103.x

188. Simone G, Papalia R, Ferriero M, et al. Stage-specific impact of extended versus standard pelvic lymph node dissection in radical cystectomy. *Int J Urol.* 2013;20(4):390-397. doi:10.1111/j.1442-2042.2012.03148.x

189. Filson CP, Tan HJ, Chamie K, Laviana AA, Hu JC. Determinants of radical cystectomy operative time. *Urol Oncol.* 2016;34(10):431.e17-431.e24. doi:10.1016/j.urolonc.2016.05.006

190. Kim SH, Yu A, Jung JH, Lee YJ, Lee ES. Incidence and risk factors of 30-day early and 90-day late morbidity and mortality of radical cystectomy during a 13-year follow-up: a comparative propensity-score matched analysis of complications between neobladder and ileal conduit. *Jpn J Clin Oncol.* 2014;44(7):667-685. doi:10.1093/jjco/hyu051

191. Balshem H, Helfand M, Schünemann HJ, et al. GRADE guidelines: 3. Rating the quality of evidence. *J Clin Epidemiol.* 2011;64(4):401-406. doi:10.1016/j.jclinepi.2010.07.015

192. Lerner SP, Svatek RS. What is the standard of care for pelvic lymphadenectomy performed at the time of radical cystectomy? *Eur Urol.* 2019;75(4):612-614. doi:10.1016/j.eururo.2018.12.028

193. Kerr WS, Colby FH. Pelvic lymphadenectomy and total cystectomy in the treatment of carcinoma of the bladder. *J Urol.* 1950;63(5):842-851. doi:10.1016/S0022-5347(17)68835-9

194. Leissner J, Ghoneim MA, Abol-Enein H, et al. Extended radical lymphadenectomy in patients with urothelial bladder cancer: results of a prospective multicenter study. *J Urol.* 2004;171(1): 139-144. doi:10.1097/01.ju.0000102302.26806.fb

195. Vazina A, Dugi D, Shariat SF, Evans J, Link R, Lerner SP. Stage specific lymph node metastasis mapping in radical cystectomy specimens. *J Urol.* 2004;171(5):1830-1834. doi:10.1097/01.ju.0000121604.58067.95

196. Roth B, Zehnder P, Birkhuser FD, Burkhard FC, Thalmann GN, Studer UE. Is bilateral extended pelvic lymphadenectomy necessary for strictly unilateral invasive bladder cancer? *J Urol.* 2012;187(5):1577-1582. doi:10.1016/j.juro.2011.12.106

197. Dorin RP, Daneshmand S, Eisenberg MS, et al. Lymph node dissection technique is more important than lymph node count in identifying nodal metastases in radical cystectomy patients: a comparative mapping study. *Eur Urol.* 2011;60(5):946-52. doi:10.1016/j.eururo.2011.07.012

198. Stein JP, Penson DF, Cai J, et al. Radical cystectomy with extended lymphadenectomy: evaluating separate package versus en bloc submission for node positive bladder cancer. *J Urol.* 2007;177(3):876-882. doi:10.1016/j.juro.2006.10.043

199. Childers CP, Maggard-Gibbons M. Estimation of the acquisition and operating costs for robotic surgery. *JAMA.* 2018;320(8):835-836. doi:10.1001/jama.2018.9219

200. Tyson MD II, Andrews PE, Ferrigni RF, Humphreys MR, Parker AS, Castle EP. Radical Prostatectomy Trends in the United States: 1998 to 2011. *Mayo Clin Proc.* 2016;91(1):10-16. doi:10.1016/j.mayocp.2015.09.018

201. Yaxley JW, Coughlin GD, Chambers SK, et al. Robot-assisted laparoscopic prostatectomy versus open radical retropubic prostatectomy: early outcomes from a randomised controlled phase 3 study. *Lancet.* 2016;388(10049):1057-1066. doi:10.1016/S0140-6736(16)30592-X

202. Nix J, Smith A, Kurpad R, Nielsen ME, Wallen EM, Pruthi RS. Prospective randomized controlled trial of robotic versus open radical cystectomy for bladder cancer: perioperative and pathologic results. *Eur Urol.* 2010;57(2):196-201. doi:10.1016/j.eururo.2009.10.024

203. Parekh DJ, Reis IM, Castle EP, et al. Robot-assisted radical cystectomy versus open radical cystectomy in patients with bladder cancer (RAZOR): an open-label, randomised, phase 3, non-inferiority trial. *Lancet.* 2018;391(10139):2525-2536. doi:10.1016/S0140-6736(18)30996-6

204. Nguyen DP, Al Hussein Al Awamlh B, Wu X, et al. Recurrence patterns after open and robot-assisted radical cystectomy for bladder cancer. *Eur Urol.* 2015;68(3):399-405. doi:10.1016/j.eururo.2015.02.003

205. Ramirez PT, Frumovitz M, Pareja R, et al. Minimally invasive versus abdominal radical hysterectomy for cervical cancer. *N Engl J Med.* 2018;379(20):1895-1904. doi:10.1056/NEJMoa1806395

206. Melamed A, Margul DJ, Chen L, et al. Survival after minimally invasive radical hysterectomy for early-stage cervical cancer. *N Engl J Med.* 2018;379(20):1905-1914. doi:10.1056/NEJMoa1804923

207. Cusimano MC, Baxter NN, Gien LT, et al. Impact of surgical approach on oncologic outcomes in women undergoing radical hysterectomy for cervical cancer. *Am J Obstet Gynecol.* 2019;221(6):619.e1-619.e24. doi:10.1016/j.ajog.2019.07.009

208. Shea BJ, Reeves BC, Wells G, et al. AMSTAR 2: a critical appraisal tool for systematic reviews that include randomised or non-randomised studies of healthcare interventions, or both. *BMJ.* 2017;358:j4008. doi:10.1136/bmj.j4008

209. Shea BJ, Hamel C, Wells GA, et al. AMSTAR is a reliable and valid measurement tool to assess the methodological quality of systematic reviews. *J Clin Epidemiol.* 2009;62(10):1013-1020. doi:10.1016/j.jclinepi.2008.10.009

210. Shea BJ, Grimshaw JM, Wells GA, et al. Development of AMSTAR: a measurement tool to assess the methodological quality of systematic reviews. *BMC Med Res Methodol.* 2007;7:10. doi:10.1186/1471-2288-7-10

211. Shea BJ, Bouter LM, Peterson J, et al. External validation of a measurement tool to assess systematic reviews (AMSTAR). *PLoS One.* 2007;2(12):e1350. doi:10.1371/journal.pone.0001350

212. Fonseka T, Ahmed K, Froghi S, Khan SA, Dasgupta P, Shamim Khan M. Comparing robotic, laparoscopic and open cystectomy: a systematic review and meta-analysis. *Arch Ital Urol Androl.* 2015;87(1):41-48. doi:10.4081/aiua.2015.1.41

213. Ishii H, Rai BP, Stolzenburg JU, et al. Robotic or open radical cystectomy, which is safer? A systematic review and meta-analysis of comparative studies. *J Endourol.* 2014;28(10):1215-1223. doi:10.1089/end.2014.0033

214. Li K, Lin T, Fan X, et al. Systematic review and meta-analysis of comparative studies reporting early outcomes after robot-assisted radical cystectomy versus open radical cystectomy. *Cancer Treat Rev.* 2013;39(6):551-560. doi:10.1016/j.ctrv.2012.11.007

215. Lobo N, Thurairaja R, Nair R, Dasgupta P, Khan MS. Robot-assisted radical cystectomy with intracorporeal urinary diversion—the new 'gold standard'? Evidence from a systematic review. *Arab J Urol.* 2018;16(3):307-313. doi:10.1016/j.aju.2018.01.006

216. Novara G, Catto JW, Wilson T, et al. Systematic review and cumulative analysis of perioperative outcomes and complications after robot-assisted radical cystectomy. *Eur Urol.* 2015;67(3): 376-401. doi:10.1016/j.eururo.2014.12.007

217. Palazzetti A, Sanchez-Salas R, Capogrosso P, et al. Systematic review of perioperative outcomes and complications after open, laparoscopic and robot-assisted radical cystectomy. *Actas Urol Esp.* 2017;41(7):416-425. doi:10.1016/j.acuro.2016.05.009

218. Shen Z, Sun Z. Systematic review and meta-analysis of randomised trials of perioperative outcomes comparing robot-assisted versus open radical cystectomy. *BMC Urol.* 2016;16(1):59. doi:10.1186/s12894-016-0177-z

219. Son SK, Lee NR, Kang SH, Lee SH. Safety and effectiveness of robot-assisted versus open radical cystectomy for bladder cancer: a systematic review and meta-analysis. *J Laparoendosc Adv Surg Tech A.* 2017;27(11):1109-1120. doi:10.1089/lap.2016.0437

220. Tan WS, Khetrapal P, Tan WP, Rodney S, Chau M, Kelly JD. Robotic assisted radical cystectomy with extracorporeal urinary diversion does not show a benefit over open radical cystectomy: a systematic review and meta-analysis of randomised controlled trials. *PLoS One.* 2016;11(11):e0166221. doi:10.1371/journal.pone.0166221

221. Tang K, Xia D, Li H, et al. Robotic vs. open radical cystectomy in bladder cancer: a systematic review and meta-analysis. *Eur J Surg Oncol.* 2014;40(11):1399-1411. doi:10.1016/j.ejso.2014.03.008

222. Tang JQ, Zhao Z, Liang Y, Liao G. Robotic-assisted versus open radical cystectomy in bladder cancer: a meta-analysis of four randomized controlled trails. *Int J Med Robot.* 2018;14(1). doi:10.1002/rcs.1867

223. Tyritzis SI, Wiklund NP. Is the open cystectomy era over? An update on the available evidence. *Int J Urol.* 2018;25(3):187-195. doi:10.1111/iju.13497

224. Tyritzis SI, Gaya JM, Wallestedt-Lantz A, et al. Current role of robotic bladder cancer surgery. *Minerva Urol Nefrol.* 2019;71(4):301-308. doi:10.23736/S0393-2249.19.03435-0

225. Tzelves L, Skolarikos A, Mourmouris P, et al. Does the use of the robot decrease the complication rate adherent to radical cystectomy? A systematic review and meta-analysis of studies comparing open to robotic counterparts. *J Endourol.* 2019;33(12):971-984. doi:10.1089/end.2019.0226

226. Yuh B, Wilson T, Bochner B, et al. Systematic review and cumulative analysis of oncologic and functional outcomes after robot-assisted radical cystectomy. *Eur Urol.* 2015;67(3):402-422. doi:10.1016/j.eururo.2014.12.008

227. Rai BP, Bondad J, Vasdev N, et al. Robotic versus open radical cystectomy for bladder cancer in adults. *Cochrane Database Syst Rev.* 2019;4(4):CD011903. doi:10.1002/14651858 .CD011903.pub2

228. Sathianathen NJ, Kalapara A, Frydenberg M, et al. Robotic assisted radical cystectomy vs open radical cystectomy: systematic review and meta-analysis. *J Urol.* 2019;201(4):715-720. doi:10.1016/j.juro.2018.10.006

229. Satkunasivam R, Tallman CT, Taylor JM, Miles BJ, Klaassen Z, Wallis CJD. Robot-assisted radical cystectomy versus open radical cystectomy: a meta-analysis of oncologic, perioperative, and complication-related outcomes. *Eur Urol Oncol.* 2019;2(4):443-447. doi:10.1016/j.euo.2018.10.008

230. Bochner BH, Dalbagni G, Sjoberg DD, et al. Comparing open radical cystectomy and robot-assisted laparoscopic radical cystectomy: a randomized clinical trial. *Eur Urol.* 2015;67(6):1042-1050. doi:10.1016/j.eururo.2014.11.043

231. Bochner BH, Dalbagni G, Marzouk KH, et al. Randomized trial comparing open radical cystectomy and robot-assisted laparoscopic radical cystectomy: oncologic outcomes. *Eur Urol.* 2018;74(4):465-471. doi:10.1016/j.eururo.2018.04.030

232. Khan MS, Gan C, Ahmed K, et al. A single-centre early phase randomised controlled three-arm trial of open, robotic, and laparoscopic radical cystectomy (CORAL). *Eur Urol.* 2016;69(4): 613-621. doi:10.1016/j.eururo.2015.07.038

233. Parekh DJ, Messer J, Fitzgerald J, Ercole B, Svatek R. Perioperative outcomes and oncologic efficacy from a pilot prospective randomized clinical trial of open versus robotic assisted radical cystectomy. *J Urol.* 2013;189(2):474-479. doi:10.1016/j.juro.2012.09.077

234. Messer JC, Punnen S, Fitzgerald J, Svatek R, Parekh DJ. Health-related quality of life from a prospective randomised clinical trial of robot-assisted laparoscopic vs open radical cystectomy. *BJU Int.* 2014;114(6):896-902. doi:10.1111/bju.12818

235. Patel HR, Santos PB, de Oliveira MC, Müller S. Is robotic-assisted radical cystectomy (RARC) with intracorporeal diversion becoming the new gold standard of care? *World J Urol.* 2016;34(1):25-32. doi:10.1007/s00345-015-1730-1

236. Tan WS, Tan MY, Lamb BW, et al. Intracorporeal robot-assisted radical cystectomy, together with an enhanced recovery programme, improves postoperative outcomes by aggregating marginal gains. *BJU Int.* 2018;121(4):632-639. doi:10.1111/bju.14073

237. Margulis V, Shariat SF, Matin SF, et al. Outcomes of radical nephroureterectomy: a series from the Upper Tract Urothelial Carcinoma Collaboration. *Cancer.* 2009;115(6):1224-1233. doi:10.1002/cncr.24135

238. Phé V, Cussenot O, Bitker MO, Rouprêt M. Does the surgical technique for management of the distal ureter influence the outcome after nephroureterectomy? *BJU Int.* 2011;108(1):130-138. doi:10.1111/j.1464-410X.2010.09835.x

239. Seisen T, Granger B, Colin P, et al. A systematic review and meta-analysis of clinicopathologic factors linked to intravesical recurrence after radical nephroureterectomy to treat upper tract urothelial carcinoma. *Eur Urol.* 2015;67(6):1122-1133. doi:10.1016/j.eururo.2014.11.035

240. Xylinas E, Rink M, Cha EK, et al. Impact of distal ureter management on oncologic outcomes following radical nephroureterectomy for upper tract urothelial carcinoma. *Eur Urol.* 2014;65(1):210-217. doi:10.1016/j.eururo.2012.04.052

241. Li WM, Shen JT, Li CC, et al. Oncologic outcomes following three different approaches to the distal ureter and bladder cuff in nephroureterectomy for primary upper urinary tract urothelial carcinoma. *Eur Urol.* 2010;57(6):963-969. doi:10.1016/j.eururo.2009.12.032

242. Adibi M, Youssef R, Shariat SF, et al. Oncological outcomes after radical nephroureterectomy for upper tract urothelial carcinoma: comparison over the three decades. *Int J Urol.* 2012;19(12):1060-1066. doi:10.1111/j.1442-2042.2012.03110.x

243. Ariane MM, Colin P, Ouzzane A, et al. Assessment of oncologic control obtained after open versus laparoscopic nephroureterectomy for upper urinary tract urothelial carcinomas (UUT-UCs): results from a large French multicenter collaborative study. *Ann Surg Oncol.* 2012;19(1):301-308. doi:10.1245/s10434-011-1841-x

244. Capitanio U, Shariat SF, Isbarn H, et al. Comparison of oncologic outcomes for open and laparoscopic nephroureterectomy: a multi-institutional analysis of 1249 cases. *Eur Urol.* 2009;56(1):1-9. doi:10.1016/j.eururo.2009.03.072

245. Fairey AS, Kassouf W, Estey E, et al. Comparison of oncological outcomes for open and laparoscopic radical nephroureterectomy: results from the Canadian Upper Tract Collaboration. *BJU Int.* 2013;112(6):791-797. doi:10.1111/j.1464-410X.2012.11474.x

246. Fang Z, Li L, Wang X, et al. Total retroperitoneal laparoscopic nephroureterectomy with bladder-cuff resection for upper urinary tract transitional cell carcinoma. *J Invest Surg.* 2014;27(6):354-359. doi:10.3109/08941939.2014.930214

247. Favaretto RL, Shariat SF, Chade DC, et al. Comparison between laparoscopic and open radical nephroureterectomy in a contemporary group of patients: are recurrence and disease-specific survival associated with surgical technique? *Eur Urol.* 2010;58(5):645-651. doi:10.1016/j.eururo.2010.08.005

248. Greco F, Wagner S, Hoda RM, Hamza A, Fornara P. Laparoscopic vs open radical nephroureterectomy for upper urinary tract urothelial cancer: oncological outcomes and 5-year follow-up. *BJU Int.* 2009;104(9):1274-1278. doi:10.1111/j.1464-410X.2009.08594.x

249. Kim TH, Hong B, Seo HK, Kang SH, Ku JH, Jeong BC. The comparison of oncologic outcomes between open and laparoscopic radical nephroureterectomy for the treatment of upper tract urothelial carcinoma: a Korean multicenter collaborative study. *Cancer Res Treat.* 2019;51(1):240-251. doi:10.4143/crt.2017.417

250. Liu JY, Dai YB, Zhou FJ, et al. Laparoscopic versus open nephroureterectomy to treat localized and/or locally advanced upper tract urothelial carcinoma: oncological outcomes from a multicenter study. *BMC Surg.* 2017;17(1):8. doi:10.1186/s12893-016-0202-x

251. Walton TJ, Novara G, Matsumoto K, et al. Oncological outcomes after laparoscopic and open radical nephroureterectomy: results from an international cohort. *BJU Int.* 2011;108(3):406-412. doi:10.1111/j.1464-410X.2010.09826.x

252. Simone G, Papalia R, Guaglianone S, et al. Laparoscopic versus open nephroureterectomy: perioperative and oncologic outcomes from a randomised prospective study. *Eur Urol.* 2009;56(3):520-526. doi:10.1016/j.eururo.2009.06.013

253. Rodriguez JF, Packiam VT, Boysen WR, et al. Utilization and outcomes of nephroureterectomy for upper tract urothelial carcinoma by surgical approach. *J Endourol.* 2017;31(7):661-665. doi:10.1089/end.2017.0086

254. Aboumohamed AA, Krane LS, Hemal AK. Oncologic outcomes following robot-assisted laparoscopic nephroureterectomy with bladder cuff excision for upper tract urothelial carcinoma. *J Urol.* 2015;194(6):1561-1566. doi:10.1016/j.juro.2015.07.081

255. Clements MB, Krupski TL, Culp SH. Robotic-assisted surgery for upper tract urothelial carcinoma: a comparative survival analysis. *Ann Surg Oncol.* 2018;25(9):2550-2562. doi:10.1245/s10434-018-6557-8

256. Kim HS, Ku JH, Jeong CW, Kwak C, Kim HH. Laparoscopic radical nephroureterectomy is associated with worse survival outcomes than open radical nephroureterectomy in patients with locally advanced upper tract urothelial carcinoma. *World J Urol.* 2016;34(6):859-869. doi:10.1007/s00345-015-1712-3

257. Jeldres C, Lughezzani G, Sun M, et al. Segmental ureterectomy can safely be performed in patients with transitional cell carcinoma of the ureter. *J Urol.* 2010;183(4):1324-1329. doi:10.1016/j.juro.2009.12.018

258. Bagrodia A, Kuehhas FE, Gayed BA, et al. Comparative analysis of oncologic outcomes of partial ureterectomy vs radical nephroureterectomy in upper tract urothelial carcinoma. *Urology.* 2013;81(5):972-977. doi:10.1016/j.urology.2012.12.059

259. Simonato A, Varca V, Gregori A, et al. Elective segmental ureterectomy for transitional cell carcinoma of the ureter: long-term follow-up in a series of 73 patients. *BJU Int.* 2012;110(11 pt B):E744-E749. doi:10.1111/j.1464-410X.2012.11554.x

260. Silberstein JL, Power NE, Savage C, et al. Renal function and oncologic outcomes of parenchymal sparing ureteral resection versus radical nephroureterectomy for upper tract urothelial carcinoma. *J Urol.* 2012;187(2):429-434. doi:10.1016/j.juro.2011.09.150

261. Zhang J, Yang F, Wang M, Niu Y, Chen W, Xing N. Comparison of radical nephroureterectomy and partial ureterectomy for the treatment of upper tract urothelial carcinoma. *Biomed Res Int.* 2018;2018:2793172. doi:10.1155/2018/2793172

262. Colin P, Ouzzane A, Pignot G, et al. Comparison of oncological outcomes after segmental ureterectomy or radical nephroureterectomy in urothelial carcinomas of the upper urinary tract: results from a large French multicentre study. *BJU Int.* 2012;110(8):1134-1141. doi:10.1111/j.1464-410X.2012.10960.x

263. Lehmann J, Suttmann H, Kovac I, et al. Transitional cell carcinoma of the ureter: prognostic factors influencing progression and survival. *Eur Urol.* 2007;51(5):1281-1288. doi:10.1016/j.eururo.2006.11.021

264. Lughezzani G, Jeldres C, Isbarn H, et al. Nephroureterectomy and segmental ureterectomy in the treatment of invasive upper tract urothelial carcinoma: a population-based study of 2299 patients. *Eur J Cancer.* 2009;45(18):3291-3297. doi:10.1016/j.ejca.2009.06.016

265. Walton TJ, Sherwood BT, Parkinson RJ, et al. Comparative outcomes following endoscopic ureteral detachment and formal bladder cuff excision in open nephroureterectomy for upper urinary tract transitional cell carcinoma. *J Urol.* 2009;181(2):532-539. doi:10.1016/j.juro.2008.10.032

266. Giovansili B, Peyromaure M, Saighi D, Dayma T, Zerbib M, Debre B. Stripping technique for endoscopic management of distal ureter during nephroureterectomy: experience of 32 procedures. *Urology.* 2004;64(3):448-452. doi:10.1016/j.urology.2004.04.080

267. Gkougkousis EG, Mellon JK, Griffiths TR. Management of the distal ureter during nephroureterectomy for upper urinary tract transitional cell carcinoma: a review. *Urol Int.* 2010;85(3):249-256. doi:10.1159/000302715

268. Saika T, Nishiguchi J, Tsushima T, et al. Comparative study of ureteral stripping versus open ureterectomy for nephroureterectomy in patients with transitional carcinoma of the renal pelvis. *Urology.* 2004;63(5):848-852. doi:10.1016/j.urology.2003.12.003

269. Fernández MI, Shariat SF, Margulis V, et al. Evidence-based sex-related outcomes after radical nephroureterectomy for upper tract urothelial carcinoma: results of large multicenter study. *Urology.* 2009;73(1):142-146. doi:10.1016/j.urology.2008.07.042

270. Kusuda Y, Miyake H, Terakawa T, Kondo Y, Miura T, Fujisawa M. Gender as a significant predictor of intravesical recurrence in patients with urothelial carcinoma of the upper urinary tract following nephroureterectomy. *Urol Oncol.* 2013;31(6):899-903. doi:10.1016/j.urolonc.2011.06.014

271. Kurpad R, Woods M. Robot-assisted radical cystectomy. *J Surg Oncol.* 2015;112(7):728-735. doi:10.1002/jso.24009

272. Hwang EC, Sathianathen NJ, Jung JH, Kim MH, Dahm P, Risk MC. Single-dose intravesical chemotherapy after nephroureterectomy for upper tract urothelial carcinoma. *Cochrane Database Syst Rev.* 2019;5(5):CD013160. doi:10.1002/14651858.CD013160.pub2

273. Rouprêt M, Babjuk M, Compérat E, et al. European Association of Urology guidelines on upper urinary tract urothelial cell carcinoma: 2015 update. *Eur Urol.* 2015;68(5):868-879. doi:10.1016/j.eururo.2015.06.044

274. Miyake H, Hara I, Gohji K, Arakawa S, Kamidono S. The significance of lymphadenectomy in transitional cell carcinoma of the upper urinary tract. *Br J Urol.* 1998;82(4):494-498. doi:10.1046/j.1464-410x.1998.00800.x

275. Kondo T, Nakazawa H, Ito F, Hashimoto Y, Toma H, Tanabe K. Impact of the extent of regional lymphadenectomy on the survival of patients with urothelial carcinoma of the upper urinary tract. *J Urol.* 2007;178(4 pt 1):1212-1217. doi:10.1016/j.juro.2007.05.158

276. Brausi MA, Gavioli M, De Luca G, et al. Retroperitoneal lymph node dissection (RPLD) in conjunction with nephroureterectomy in the treatment of infiltrative transitional cell carcinoma (TCC) of the upper urinary tract: impact on survival. *Eur Urol.* 2007;52(5):1414-1418. doi:10.1016/j.eururo.2007.04.070

277. Roscigno M, Cozzarini C, Bertini R, et al. Prognostic value of lymph node dissection in patients with muscle-invasive transitional cell carcinoma of the upper urinary tract. *Eur Urol.* 2008;53(4):794-802. doi:10.1016/j.eururo.2008.01.008

278. Roscigno M, Shariat SF, Margulis V, et al. Impact of lymph node dissection on cancer specific survival in patients with upper tract urothelial carcinoma treated with radical nephroureterectomy. *J Urol.* 2009;181(6):2482-2489. doi:10.1016/j.juro.2009.02.021

279. Roscigno M, Shariat SF, Margulis V, et al. The extent of lymphadenectomy seems to be associated with better survival in patients with nonmetastatic upper-tract urothelial carcinoma: how many lymph nodes should be removed? *Eur Urol.* 2009;56(3):512-518. doi:10.1016/j.eururo.2009.06.004

280. Kondo T, Tanabe K. Role of lymphadenectomy in the management of urothelial carcinoma of the bladder and the upper urinary tract. *Int J Urol.* 2012;19(8):710-721. doi:10.1111/j.1442-2042.2012.03009.x

281. McCarron JP Jr, Chasko SB, Gray GF Jr. Systematic mapping of nephroureterectomy specimens removed for urothelial cancer: pathological findings and clinical correlations. *J Urol.* 1982;128(2):243-246. doi:10.1016/s0022-5347(17)52871-2

282. Akaza H, Koiso K, Niijima T. Clinical evaluation of urothelial tumors of the renal pelvis and ureter based on a new classification system. *Cancer.* 1987;59(7):1369-1375. doi:10.1002/1097-0142(19870401)59:7<1369::aid-cncr2820590724>3.0.co;2-a

283. Kondo T, Nakazawa H, Ito F, Hashimoto Y, Toma H, Tanabe K. Primary site and incidence of lymph node metastases in urothelial carcinoma of upper urinary tract. *Urology.* 2007;69(2):265-269. doi:10.1016/j.urology.2006.10.014

284. Matin SF, Sfakianos JP, Espiritu PN, Coleman JA, Spiess PE. Patterns of lymphatic metastases in upper tract urothelial carcinoma and proposed dissection templates. *J Urol.* 2015;194(6):1567-1574. doi:10.1016/j.juro.2015.06.077

285. Seisen T, Shariat SF, Cussenot O, et al. Contemporary role of lymph node dissection at the time of radical nephroureterectomy for upper tract urothelial carcinoma. *World J Urol.* 2017;35(4):535-548. doi:10.1007/s00345-016-1764-z

286. Novara G, De Marco V, Gottardo F, et al. Independent predictors of cancer-specific survival in transitional cell carcinoma of the upper urinary tract: multi-institutional dataset from 3 European centers. *Cancer.* 2007;110(8):1715-1722. doi:10.1002/cncr.22970

287. Ouzzane A, Colin P, Ghoneim TP, et al. The impact of lymph node status and features on oncological outcomes in urothelial carcinoma of the upper urinary tract (UTUC) treated by nephroureterectomy. *World J Urol.* 2013;31(1):189-197. doi:10.1007/s00345-012-0983-1

288. Burger M, Shariat SF, Fritsche HM, et al. No overt influence of lymphadenectomy on cancer-specific survival in organ-confined versus locally advanced upper urinary tract urothelial carcinoma undergoing radical nephroureterectomy: a retrospective international, multi-institutional study. *World J Urol.* 2011;29(4):465-472. doi:10.1007/s00345-012-0983-1

289. Mason RJ, Kassouf W, Bell DG, et al. The contemporary role of lymph node dissection during nephroureterectomy in the management of upper urinary tract urothelial carcinoma: the Canadian experience. *Urology.* 2012;79(4):840-845. doi:10.1016/j.urology.2011.11.058

290. Kondo T, Hara I, Takagi T, et al. Template-based lymphadenectomy in urothelial carcinoma of the renal pelvis: a prospective study. *Int J Urol.* 2014;21(5):453-459. doi:10.1111/iju.12417

291. O'Brien T, Ray E, Singh R, Coker B, Beard R, British Association of Urological Surgeons Section of Oncology. Prevention of bladder tumours after nephroureterectomy for primary upper urinary tract urothelial carcinoma: a prospective, multicentre, randomised clinical trial of a single postoperative intravesical dose of mitomycin C (the ODMIT-C Trial). *Eur Urol.* 2011;60(4):703-710.

292. Ito A, Shintaku I, Satoh M, et al. Prospective randomized phase II trial of a single early intravesical instillation of pirarubicin (THP) in the prevention of bladder recurrence after nephroureterectomy for upper urinary tract urothelial carcinoma: the THP Monotherapy Study Group Trial. *J Clin Oncol.* 2013;31(11):1422-1427. doi:10.1200/JCO.2012.45.2128

293. Fang D, Li XS, Xiong GY, Yao L, He ZS, Zhou LQ. Prophylactic intravesical chemotherapy to prevent bladder tumors after nephroureterectomy for primary upper urinary tract urothelial carcinomas: a systematic review and meta-analysis. *Urol Int.* 2013;91(3):291-296. doi:10.1159/000350508

294. Deng X, Yang X, Cheng Y, et al. Prognostic value and efficacy valuation of postoperative intravesical instillation in primary urothelial carcinomas of upper urinary tract. *Int J Clin Exp Med.* 2014;7(12):4734-4746.

295. Miyamoto K, Ito A, Wakabayashi M, et al. A phase III trial of a single early intravesical instillation of pirarubicin to prevent bladder recurrence after radical nephroureterectomy for upper tract urothelial carcinoma (JCOG1403, UTUC THP Phase III). *Jpn J Clin Oncol.* 2018;48(1): 94-97. doi:10.1093/jjco/hyx158

296. Noennig B, Bozorgmehri S, Terry R, Otto B, Su LM, Crispen PL. Evaluation of intraoperative versus postoperative adjuvant mitomycin c with nephroureterectomy for urothelial carcinoma of the upper urinary tract. *Bladder Cancer.* 2018;4(4):389-394. doi:10.3233/BLC-180174

297. Lu DD, Boorjian SA, Raman JD. Intravesical chemotherapy use after radical nephroureterectomy: a national survey of urologic oncologists. *Urol Oncol.* 2017;35(3):113.e1-113.e7. doi:10.1016/j.urolonc.2016.10.016

Synoptic Operative Report: TURBT

Date of procedure _____   Surgeon(s) _____

_____

Clinical Information

Prior history of bladder cancer
☐ No
☐ Yes
Prior grade and stage

_____

Prior intravesical therapies
☐ No
☐ Yes
Therapy name and course

_____

Interoperative Findings

Bimanual Exam

Palpable tumor
☐ No
☐ Yes
Size _____

Bladder
☐ Mobile
☐ Fixed

Prostate exam (males)
☐ Normal
☐ Abnormal

Vaginal wall involvement (females)
☐ No
☐ Yes

Cervical involvement (females)
☐ No
☐ Yes

Tumor characterization

Estimated size
_____

Location
_____

Synoptic Operative Report: TURBT

Date of procedure _____ Surgeon(s) _____

_____

Multifocality
- ☐ No
- ☐ Yes

Gross appearance
- ☐ Papillary
- ☐ Sessile
- ☐ Flat
- ☐ Pedunculated

Estimated depth of invasion
- ☐ No visible tumor
- ☐ Tis
- ☐ Ta
- ☐ T1
- ☐ T2
- ☐ T3
- ☐ T4
- ☐ Tx

Appearance on white light–enhanced technologies (as applicable)
_____

Urinary Tract Assessment

Prostate hypertrophy (males)
- ☐ No
- ☐ Yes

Urethral anatomy
- ☐ Normal
- ☐ Abnormal _____

Presence of bladder diverticulum
- ☐ No
- ☐ Yes
  - Number _____
  - Location _____

Synoptic Operative Report: TURBT

Date of procedure _____ Surgeon(s) _____

_____

Ureteral orifice location
- ☐ Normal
- ☐ Abnormal _____

Presence of any anatomic variants of GU tract
- ☐ No
- ☐ Yes _____

Tumor involvement
- ☐ Involvement of ureteral orifices
  - ☐ Left
  - ☐ Right
  - ☐ Both
- ☐ Trigone
- ☐ Prostatic urethra
- ☐ Potential involvement of upper tract
- ☐ No other involvement

Procedure Summary

Extent of resection
- ☐ Complete
- ☐ Incomplete

Estimated blood loss _____

Depth of resection
- ☐ Muscle layer
- ☐ Fat layer
- ☐ Resection of ureteral orifice

Method of resection
- ☐ Bipolar
- ☐ Monopolar
- ☐ Cold cup biopsy
- ☐ Fulguration
- ☐ Other _____

Synoptic Operative Report: TURBT

Date of procedure _____   Surgeon(s) _____

_____

Type of resection
☐ En bloc resection
☐ Chip resection

Deep biopsies sent separately
☐ No
☐ Yes

Postresection

Potential residual disease
☐ No
☐ Yes
Location _____

Bladder perforation
☐ No
☐ Yes
Management _____

Placement of ureteral stent
  (if necessary)
☐ No
☐ Yes

Placement of urethral catheter
☐ No
☐ Yes

Postprocedure intravesical chemo
☐ No
☐ Yes
Drug _____
Dosage _____

Instilled in the OR
☐ Yes
☐ No

Synoptic Operative Report: Radical Cystectomy

Date of procedure _____   Surgeon(s) _____

_____

Clinical Information

Neoadjuvant chemotherapy
☐ No
☐ Yes
Drug _____
Cycle _____

Pelvic radiation history
☐ No
☐ Yes
Total dose _____

Prior abdominal/pelvic surgery
☐ No
☐ Yes _____

Prior intravesical therapy
☐ No
☐ Yes
Drug _____
Cycle _____

Preoperative clinical grade
☐ Low grade
☐ High grade
☐ Not available

Preoperative clinical stage
T stage _____

Imaging-evidence of enlarged
  or suspicious nodes
☐ No
☐ Yes

Hydronephrosis
☐ No
☐ Yes
      ☐ Left
      ☐ Right
      ☐ Both

Synoptic Operative Report: Radical Cystectomy

Date of procedure _____   Surgeon(s) _____

_____

Intraoperative Findings

Tumor

- ☐ Gross extension beyond bladder
- ☐ Adjacent organ extension

_____

- ☐ Pelvic wall adherence
- ☐ Metastatic disease _____
- ☐ No tumor extension

Ureter

Extent of ureteral resection   _____

Ureteral appearance

- ☐ Normal
- ☐ Hydronephrotic

Ureteral viability

- ☐ Good
- ☐ Ischemic
- ☐ Not evaluated

Intraoperative margin evaluation

- ☐ Visualization
- ☐ Frozen section
  - ☐ Negative
  - ☐ Positive
- ☐ Other _____

Urethra

Extent of urethral resection   _____

Intraoperative margin

- ☐ Visualization
- ☐ Frozen section
  - ☐ Negative
  - ☐ Positive
- ☐ Other _____

Synoptic Operative Report: Radical Cystectomy

Date of procedure _____   Surgeon(s) _____

_____

Lymphadenectomy

Extent of lymphadenectomy

☐ Limited template
☐ Standard template
☐ Extended template
☐ Superextended template
☐ Not performed

Lymph nodes appearance

☐ Grossly normal
☐ Grossly enlarged
☐ Adherence to adjacent anatomic structures
☐ No lymph nodes identified

Ability to complete lymphadenectomy

☐ Complete excision
☐ Incomplete excision

Procedure Summary

Surgical approach

☐ Open
☐ Laparoscopic assisted
  ☐ Intracorporeal
  ☐ Extracorporeal diversion
☐ Robotic assisted
  ☐ Intracorporeal
  ☐ Extracorporeal diversion

Estimated blood loss

_____

Concomitant prostatectomy (men)

☐ No
☐ Yes
  ☐ Nerve sparing
  ☐ Non–nerve sparing

Synoptic Operative Report: Radical Cystectomy

Date of procedure _____   Surgeon(s) _____

_____

Concomitant hysterectomy (women)
☐ No
☐ Yes
    ☐ With cervix
    ☐ Without cervix

Concomitant salpingo-oophorectomy (women)
☐ No
☐ Yes

Concomitant vaginectomy (women)
☐ No
☐ Yes

Specimen Removal
Method of specimen retrieval
_____

Any gross tumor spillage
☐ No
☐ Yes

Urinary Diversion
Choice of diversion
_____

Intestinal segment used
Name _____
Length _____

Ureteral anastomosis
☐ Refluxing
☐ Nonrefluxing

Location of urostomy
☐ Not applicable
☐ Right side
☐ Left side

Ureteral stents placed
☐ No
☐ Yes

Synoptic Operative Report: Nephroureterectomy

Date of procedure _____   Surgeon(s) _____

_____

Clinical Information

Preop assessment of renal function

Hydronephrosis
- ☐ No
- ☐ Yes
  - ☐ Left
  - ☐ Right
  - ☐ Both

Serum creatinine level
_____

eGFR
_____

Renal split function if available
_____

Tumor location
- ☐ Ureter
- ☐ Renal pelvis

Tumor laterality
- ☐ Left
- ☐ Right
- ☐ Both
- ☐ Not visible on imaging

Stage
- ☐ Ta
- ☐ Tis
- ☐ T1
- ☐ T2
- ☐ T3
- ☐ T4
- ☐ Tx

Synoptic Operative Report: Nephroureterectomy

Date of procedure _____   Surgeon(s) _____

_____

Enlarged or suspicious nodes
- ☐ No
- ☐ Yes

Neoadjuvant chemotherapy
- ☐ No
- ☐ Yes
  Drug _____
  Cycle _____

Prior endoscopic management
- ☐ No
- ☐ Yes
  Procedure name _____

Any complications from prior endoscopic management
- ☐ No
- ☐ Yes
  Complication name _____

Existence of ureteral stent
- ☐ No
- ☐ Yes
  - ☐ Left
  - ☐ Right
  - ☐ Both

Intraoperative Findings

Tumor involvement
- ☐ Limited to ureter or renal pelvis
- ☐ Gross extension beyond ureter or renal pelvis
- ☐ Bladder
- ☐ Metastatic lesions _____

Synoptic Operative Report: Nephroureterectomy

Date of procedure _____   Surgeon(s) _____

_____

Bladder

Concurrent cystoscopy
☐ No
☐ Yes
Tumor in bladder
☐ Yes
☐ No

Concurrent TURBT
☐ No
☐ Yes; Details _____

Lymphadenectomy

Extent of lymphadenectomy
☐ Limited
☐ Standard template by tumor location
☐ Extended RPLND template
☐ Not performed

Lymph nodes appearance
☐ Grossly normal
☐ Grossly enlarged
☐ Adherence to adjacent anatomic structures
☐ No lymph nodes identified

Ability to complete lymphadenectomy
☐ Complete excision
☐ Incomplete excision

Ipsilateral adrenal
☐ Spared
☐ Taken
☐ Unknown

Synoptic Operative Report: Nephroureterectomy

Date of procedure _____   Surgeon(s) _____

_____

Procedure Summary

Operative approach
- ☐ Open
- ☐ Laparoscopic/hand assist
- ☐ Robotic assisted

Operative scope
- ☐ Segmental resection (including segment and reanastomosis approach)
- ☐ Nephroureterectomy

Estimated blood loss   _____

Bladder tumor
- ☐ No concomitant bladder tumor
- ☐ TURBT
- ☐ Intravesical chemotherapy

_____

- ☐ Other management _____

Distal Ureter

Dissection approach
- ☐ Same incision as NU
- ☐ Counterincision

Ureter clipped prior to nephrectomy
- ☐ Yes
- ☐ No

Level of ureteral transection   _____

Method of resection
- ☐ Transvesical
- ☐ Extravesical

Synoptic Operative Report: Nephroureterectomy

Date of procedure _____   Surgeon(s) _____

_____

Ureteral margin evaluation
☐ Visualization
☐ Frozen section
☐ Other _____

Ureteral margin status
☐ Negative
☐ Positive
☐ Not available

Bladder closure
☐ No
☐ Yes

Specimen Removal
Method of specimen retrieval   _____

Any gross tumor or urine spillage
☐ No
☐ Yes

Synoptic Operative Report: Partial Cystectomy

Date of procedure _____   Surgeon(s) _____

_____

Clinical Information

Tumor location   _____

Pathology/histology (if available)   _____

Clinical stage

☐ Tis
☐ Ta
☐ T1
☐ T2
☐ T3
☐ T4
☐ Tx

Clinical grade

☐ Low grade
☐ High grade
☐ Not available

Preoperative "mapping" biopsy

☐ No
☐ Yes
Location
☐ Bladder
☐ Prostatic
☐ Urethra

Prior intravesical therapy

☐ No
☐ Yes
Therapy name

_____

Therapy course

_____

Synoptic Operative Report: Partial Cystectomy

Date of procedure _____   Surgeon(s) _____

_____

Prior chemotherapy
- ☐ No
- ☐ Yes
  - Drug _____
  - Cycle _____

Prior radiation
- ☐ No
- ☐ Yes
  - Total dose _____

Intraoperative Findings

Tumor involvement
- ☐ Gross extension beyond bladder
- ☐ Trigone
- ☐ Ureteral orifice
  - ☐ Left
  - ☐ Right
  - ☐ Both
- ☐ Urethra
- ☐ Diverticulum
- ☐ Urachus
- ☐ Other _____

Margin assessment
- ☐ Visualization
- ☐ Cystoscopic demarcation
- ☐ Palpation
- ☐ Frozen section
- ☐ Other _____

Synoptic Operative Report: Partial Cystectomy

Date of procedure _____   Surgeon(s) _____

_____

Lymphadenectomy

Extent of lymphadenectomy
- ☐ Limited
- ☐ Standard template
- ☐ Extended template
- ☐ Not performed

Lymph nodes appearance
- ☐ Grossly normal
- ☐ Grossly enlarged
- ☐ Adherence to adjacent anatomic structures
- ☐ No lymph nodes identified

Ability to complete lymphadenectomy
- ☐ Complete excision
- ☐ Incomplete excision

Procedure Summary

Operative approach
- ☐ Open
- ☐ Laparoscopic/hand assisted
- ☐ Robotic assisted

Estimated blood loss   _____

Bladder Resection

Extent of bladder resection   _____

Involvement of ureter and need for reimplant
- ☐ No
- ☐ Yes

Estimated margin of resection
- ☐ Negative
- ☐ Positive

Synoptic Operative Report: Partial Cystectomy

Date of procedure _____   Surgeon(s) _____

_____

Method and testing of
   bladder closure   _____

Estimated residual bladder capacity   _____

Specimen Removal
Method of specimen retrieval   _____

Any gross tumor or urine spillage   ☐   No
                                       ☐   Yes

COMMENTARY: UROTHELIAL CANCER

Anirban P. Mitra, MD, PhD
Tanner S. Miest, MD, PhD
Colin P. N. Dinney, MD
Department of Urology
The University of Texas MD Anderson Cancer Center

Surgical management for urothelial carcinoma can be complex and varied and depends on a multitude of factors, including location of primary tumor, stage, grade, and other clinicopathologic and patient characteristics. Although there is evidence to support the field-cancerization hypothesis for urothelial carcinomas,[1] operative principles are clearly directed toward the organ that is primarily affected. To rationally to address this, the authors of the urothelial cancer section of *Operative Standards for Cancer Surgery*, Volume 3, have proffered a series of standards and recommendations to help define appropriate quality surgery. Several of these are based on consensus guidelines from major international urological and oncologic societies, which in turn are based on randomized clinical trials. However, a majority of recommendations are based on retrospective observational studies, clinical judgment, and standard practice patterns.

The foundation for appropriate management of urothelial carcinoma rests on accurate clinical staging. The authors highlight the differences in tumor node metastasis (TNM) staging for tumors of the bladder, urethra, and upper tracts as well as the importance of other factors including histologic variants and lymphovascular invasion. The importance of adequate transurethral resection of bladder tumors and re-resection for patients with high-grade T1 disease for staging and risk stratification is highlighted. For upper tract tumors, thoroughness of endoscopic evaluation and judicious use of cytology and biopsy is important. Use of white light–enhanced cystoscopic modalities is helpful in identifying early lesions and carcinoma in situ, but it is not available universally. Importantly, these adjunct techniques do not substitute for a thorough resection, restaging, and examination under anesthesia. As discussed by the authors, postoperative intravesical chemotherapy instillation is appropriate and standard for patients with superficial bladder tumors undergoing endoscopic resection with no obvious evidence of bladder perforation. However, concerns for mitomycin-related toxicity and improved tolerability and cost-effectiveness of gemcitabine have led to a broader adoption of the latter in our practice.[2]

Preoperative planning and management of patients with invasive urothelial carcinoma are often best performed in a multidisciplinary setting, although access to this may be limited in some nonacademic and community settings. In appropriately selected patients, use of cisplatin-based neoadjuvant chemotherapy is associated with survival benefit in patients with invasive urothelial carcinomas of the bladder.[3] Adherence to surgical and oncologic guidelines when performing radical cystectomy at high-volume and academic centers may be associated with improved outcomes.[4,5] In addition to preoperative optimization in the context of enhanced recovery protocols, perioperative use of peripherally acting μ-opioid receptor antagonists can accelerate gastrointestinal recovery and decrease length of hospital stay following radical cystectomy with urinary diversion.[6,7]

As recommended by the authors, partial cystectomy for urothelial cancer of the bladder has limited role in oncologic management. This requires careful patient selection and adjunctive intraoperative use of endoscopic techniques to visualize the bladder lumen. In our experience, this may be best suited for patients with urachal adenocarcinoma involving the bladder dome. Radical cystectomy with urinary diversion remains the mainstay surgical approach for patients with invasive bladder cancer who are not candidates for or have failed organ-preserving approaches. In addition to highlighting the importance of negative surgical margins, the authors discuss the oncologic importance of pelvic lymphadenectomy. Although the only randomized prospective trial in this space currently does not support the use of extended pelvic lymphadenectomy in every patient, results of the SWOG 1011 trial addressing this question are pending.[8]

There are several options regarding urinary diversion following radical cystectomy as discussed in this section. Individual choice is ultimately a shared decision based on preoperative counseling, patient and disease characteristics, lifestyle, priorities, and other intangible preferences. Use of robotic surgery presents a new approach for cystectomy with the largest randomized controlled trial indicating noninferiority to open cystectomy with comparable rates of adverse events.[9] However, additional factors including implementation of intracorporeal urinary diversion and enhanced postoperative recovery pathways should be considered when making these choices.

This section also summarizes salient topics related to surgical management of upper tract urothelial carcinoma (UTUC) by radical nephroureterectomy (RNU). Of the topics discussed, surgical approach (especially as it relates to distal ureteral/bladder cuff management), use of intravesical chemotherapy, and the need for improved understanding of the role of lymph node dissection deserve to be highlighted. A diverse array of surgical approaches can be employed to perform an RNU, with the complexity of the surgical approach owing to the necessary retroperitoneal and pelvic exposure. Although surgeon comfort and experience should drive operative decision-making, the existing data suggests oncologic outcomes are similar for open versus laparoscopic approaches as long as bladder cuff management is via intra- or extravesical approaches rather than endoscopic. Robotic-assisted RNU has gained in popularity in recent years and offers the advantage of improved pelvic visualization to ensure complete excision of the distal ureter and bladder cuff via an extravesical approach. Pelvic access can also be optimized in challenging cases by swapping port locations of the camera and working arms after the nephrectomy in preparation for pelvic dissection.

Existing evidence supports the use of intravesical chemotherapy instillation perioperatively during or after RNU.[10,11] Although evidence is less robust defining the optimal timing of intravesical instillation, our practice is to ensure chemotherapy is indwelling while the kidney and ureter are being actively manipulated intraoperatively, with the logic being that this is the time of highest risk of distal urinary tract seeding. Ideally, 1.5 to 2 hours of dwell time should be targeted, which can be achieved by minimizing intraoperative IV fluids to avoid bladder overdistention. Additionally, early distal ureteral control with a surgical clip or tie can be used to further decrease the theoretical risk of antegrade tumor cell seeding.

Finally, the authors appropriately highlight the paucity of high-level evidence supporting lymph node dissection at the time of RNU or the appropriate extent of dissection when performed. Although logistical challenges of performing large prospective trials in comparatively rare disease types such as UTUC pose a challenge, future prospective trials should be prioritized to both define the prognostic and possible oncologic benefit of lymph node dissection and improve our understanding of optimal surgical templates based on tumor location. In addition to careful consideration of surgical approach and consistent use of perioperative intravesical chemotherapy, optimizing the application and extent of lymph node dissection for UTUC holds promise to improve disease outcomes.

In conclusion, this section summarizes the diversity, evidence levels, oncologic recommendations, and technical considerations for management of urothelial carcinomas of the upper and lower tracts. Although significant strides regarding perioperative topical and systemic therapeutic strategies and postoperative enhanced recovery protocols are being made, optimal treatment for these cancers will ultimately depend on surgical thoroughness and adherence to sound oncologic principles.

REFERENCES

1. Hafner C, Knuechel R, Stoehr R, Hartmann A. Clonality of multifocal urothelial carcinomas: 10 years of molecular genetic studies. *Int J Cancer*. 2002;101(1):1-6. doi:10.1002/ijc.10544
2. Koya MP, Simon MA, Soloway MS. Complications of intravesical therapy for urothelial cancer of the bladder. *J Urol*. 2006;175(6):2004-2010. doi:10.1016/S0022-5347(06)00264-3
3. Advanced Bladder Cancer Meta-analysis Collaboration. Neoadjuvant chemotherapy in invasive bladder cancer: update of a systematic review and meta-analysis of individual patient data. *Eur Urol*. 2005;48(2):202-206. doi:10.1016/j.eururo.2005.04.006
4. Morgan TM, Barocas DA, Keegan KA, et al. Volume outcomes of cystectomy—is it the surgeon or the setting? *J Urol*. 2012;188(6):2139-2144. doi:10.1016/j.juro.2012.08.042
5. Scarberry K, Berger NG, Scarberry KB, et al. Improved surgical outcomes following radical cystectomy at high-volume centers influence overall survival. *Urol Oncol*. 2018;36(6):308.e11-308.e17. doi:10.1016/j.urolonc.2018.03.007
6. Daneshmand S, Ahmadi H, Schuckman AK, et al. Enhanced recovery protocol after radical cystectomy for bladder cancer. *J Urol*. 2014;192(1):50-55. doi:10.1016/j.juro.2014.01.097
7. Kamat AM, Chang SS, Lee C, et al. Alvimopan, a peripherally acting mu-opioid receptor antagonist, accelerates gastrointestinal recovery and decreases length of hospital stay after radical cystectomy. *J Urol*. 2013;189(4S):e767. doi:10.1016/j.juro.2013.02.2289
8. Gschwend JE, Heck MM, Lehmann J, et al. Extended versus limited lymph node dissection in bladder cancer patients undergoing radical cystectomy: survival results from a prospective, randomized trial. *Eur Urol*. 2019;75(4):604-611. doi:10.1016/j.eururo.2018.09.047
9. Parekh DJ, Reis IM, Castle EP, et al. Robot-assisted radical cystectomy versus open radical cystectomy in patients with bladder cancer (RAZOR): an open-label, randomised, phase 3, non-inferiority trial. *Lancet*. 2018;391(10139):2525-2536. doi:10.1016/S0140-6736(18)30996-6
10. O'Brien T, Ray E, Singh R, British Association of Urological Surgeons Section of Oncology. Prevention of bladder tumours after nephroureterectomy for primary upper urinary tract urothelial carcinoma: a prospective, multicentre, randomised clinical trial of a single postoperative intravesical dose of mitomycin C (the ODMIT-C Trial). *Eur Urol*. 2011;60(4):703-710. doi:10.1016/j.eururo.2011.05.064
11. Ito A, Shintaku I, Satoh M, et al. Prospective randomized phase II trial of a single early intravesical instillation of pirarubicin (THP) in the prevention of bladder recurrence after nephroureterectomy for upper urinary tract urothelial carcinoma: the THP Monotherapy Study Group Trial. *J Clin Oncol*. 2013;31(11):1422-1427. doi:10.1200/JCO.2012.45.2128

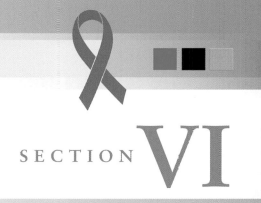

SECTION VI

HEPATOBILIARY

INTRODUCTION

Hepatectomy is performed for several common cancer processes, including primary hepatic tumors as well as metastases from other organs. This section includes standards for five of the most common hepatobiliary malignancies: colorectal liver metastases (CLM), hepatocellular cancer (HCC), perihilar and intrahepatic cholangiocarcinoma (PHC and ICC), and gallbladder cancer (GBC). For each of these, surgical resection is a central component of multidisciplinary care provided to patients with localized disease. Although the technique used to divide the liver parenchyma is similar irrespective of the underlying pathology, the technical aspects used at hepatectomy vary according to the biology of the specific diagnosis.

CLINICAL STAGING

Colorectal Liver Metastases

CLM represent the most common cancer found in the liver. Nearly 50% of patients with colorectal cancer present with synchronous tumors in the liver.[1,2] By definition, any patient who presents synchronously (at presentation or within 1 year of the primary) or metachronously (after 1 year from primary diagnosis) with CLM has stage IV disease.[3] The purpose of staging is to identify sites of extrahepatic disease to differentiate M1a (single site such as liver), M1b (two or more organs without peritoneal disease), and M1c (peritoneal disease) disease, according to the eighth edition of the American Joint Commission on Cancer (AJCC) *Staging Manual*. Table 6-1 shows the AJCC *Cancer Staging Manual*, Eighth Edition, staging for metastatic colorectal cancer. Unlike most stage IV gastrointestinal cancers, the optimal treatment for resectable CLM includes surgical resection.[4]

Hepatocellular Cancer

The sixth most common cancer worldwide, HCC is the most common primary liver cancer. The care of patients with these cancers is uniquely challenging given that underlying liver disease is present in up to 80% of patients with HCC.[5] Therefore, treatment depends on the presence and degree of underlying liver disease, the tumor's morphology, and the patient's comorbidities and psychosocial risk factors. Because a large percentage of patients have underlying liver disease, the risk of recurrence with resection alone is high (50% to 70%). Because liver transplantation confers 5-year overall survival rates above 70% as compared with 50% for surgical resection of patients with early-stage HCC meeting Milan transplant criteria (e.g., solitary tumor <5 cm in size or two to three tumors with each <3 cm in size), transplant is often pursued as first-line treatment in patients with cirrhosis.[6] However, comorbidities and/or psychosocial limitations, including access to a transplant center and organ shortage, are common barriers to transplantation. The AJCC *Cancer Staging Manual*, Eighth Edition, staging (Table 6-2) stratifies patient prognosis based on tumor-related factors of size, vascular invasion, number of tumors, nodes, and distant sites, but it does not fully capture the implications of multidisciplinary decision-making because so many patients with primary liver cancer have inhibited performance status or intrinsic liver disease, which are both more important than simple tumor anatomy.[3]

TABLE 6-1   American Joint Committee on Cancer Staging Criteria for Metastatic Colorectal Cancer, Eighth Edition

AJCC Stage	Tumor-Node-Metastasis Staging	Stage Findings
IVA	Any T	Any T stage
	Any N	Any N stage
	M1a	Metastasis to one site or organ is identified without peritoneal metastasis
IVB	Any T	Any T stage
	Any N	Any N stage
	M1b	Metastasis to two or more sites or organs is identified without peritoneal metastasis
IVC	Any T	Any T stage
	Any N	Any N stage
	M1c	Metastasis to the peritoneal surface is identified alone or with other site or organ metastases

Note: American Joint Committee on Cancer staging and TNM classification for metastatic colon cancer.[3] Used with permission of the American Joint Committee on Cancer (AJCC), Chicago, Illinois. The original and primary source for this information is the *AJCC Cancer Staging Manual*, Eighth Edition (2017) published by Springer International Publishing.

Perihilar Cholangiocarcinoma

Hilar cholangiocarcinoma, also referred to as PHC or Klatskin tumor, represents the most common type of bile duct cancers and accounts for nearly 60% of all cholangiocarcinomas. By definition, PHC is a tumor that originates from the confluence of the right and left hepatic ducts or its immediate vicinity. The anatomic constraints of this area, combined with the generally infiltrative nature of PHC (the vast majority of which are of the periductal infiltrative or sclerosing variety), present a unique set of challenges for the diagnosis and treatment of these aggressive tumors. As such, early engagement of a multidisciplinary team is highly recommended. Given that the common hepatic duct and its bifurcation are located in close proximity to the hepatic artery and portal vein, tumor involvement of one or more of these structures at the time of diagnosis is common. The location and degree of infiltration of the tumor longitudinally along the biliary tree and the extent to which it radially involves and affects the surrounding structures, especially as it relates to portal vein invasion and associated hepatic lobar atrophy, determine the potential for surgical resectability. Accurate ascertainment of these characteristics is, therefore, a critical aspect of preoperative planning. To this end, proper cross-sectional and biliary imaging must be pursued. Importantly, this must be accomplished before any attempt at instrumenting

TABLE 6-2 American Joint Committee on Cancer Staging Criteria for Primary Liver (Hepatocellular) Cancer, Eighth Edition

AJCC Stage	Tumor-Node-Metastasis Staging	Stage Findings
IA	T1a	Solitary tumor ≤2 cm
	N0	No regional lymph node metastasis
	M0	No distant metastasis
IB	T1b	Solitary tumor >2 cm without vascular invasion
	N0	No regional lymph node metastasis
	M0	No distant metastasis
II	T2	Solitary tumor >2 cm with vascular invasion, or multiple tumors, none >5 cm
	N0	No regional lymph node metastasis
	M0	No distant metastasis
IIIA	T3	Multiple tumors, at least one of which is >5 cm
	N0	No regional lymph node metastasis
	M0	No distant metastasis
IIIB	T4	Single tumor or multiple tumors of any size involving a major branch of the portal vein or hepatic vein, or tumor(s) with direct invasion of adjacent organs other than the gallbladder or with perforation of visceral peritoneum
	N0	No regional lymph node metastasis
	M0	No distant metastasis
IVA	Any T	Any T stage
	N1	Regional lymph node metastasis
	M0	No distant metastasis
IVB	Any T	Any T stage
	Any N	Any N stage
	M1	Distant metastasis

Note: American Joint Committee on Cancer staging and TNM classification for primary liver cancer.[3] Used with permission of the American Joint Committee on Cancer (AJCC), Chicago, Illinois. The original and primary source for this information is the *AJCC Cancer Staging Manual*, Eighth Edition (2017) published by Springer International Publishing.

or stenting the biliary tree, so as not to obscure the anatomic details of the study and contribute to cholangitis. High-quality contrast-enhanced multidetector computed tomography (CT), preferably protocoled for biliary evaluation, is a good initial study that offers excellent anatomic evaluation, especially in determining involvement of vascular structures. Magnetic resonance imaging (MRI), especially magnetic resonance cholangiopancreatography (MRCP), improves visualization of the biliary tree with its anatomic variants and appreciation of the extent of tumor infiltration and its relationship to surrounding structures. Moreover, MRCP has been demonstrated to have superior sensitivity, specificity, and accuracy compared with both endoscopic retrograde cholangiopancreatography and percutaneous transhepatic cholangiography and has largely come to replace direct cholangiography in the diagnostic workup and staging of PHC.[7] Table 6-3 details the *AJCC Cancer Staging Manual*, Eighth Edition, staging for PHC.[3]

Intrahepatic Cholangiocarcinoma

ICC constitutes the second most commonly diagnosed primary malignancy arising from the liver.[8] Males have a slightly higher risk of developing ICC compared with females (relative risk, 1:1.2 to 1.5), and the incidence of ICC is rising.[9] Chronic inflammation is one of the major risk factors for ICCs. Inflammatory conditions of the biliary tract (primary sclerosing cholangitis), choledochal cysts, infection with liver flukes, cirrhosis induced by viral hepatitis and nonalcoholic fatty liver disease, thorotrast, hepatolithiasis, and biliary papillomatosis have all been linked to development of ICC. Of these, primary sclerosing cholangitis is perhaps the most well-characterized risk factor. However, most patients with ICC will present without any identifiable risk factors. Unlike PHC, ICCs commonly do not cause biliary obstruction. Thus, most patients with ICC are diagnosed through imaging performed for nonspecific abdominal pain, elevated liver enzymes, or other unrelated symptoms. Therefore, it is not uncommon for patients with ICC to have a large unresectable mass in the liver or metastatic disease at the time of diagnosis. When patients do present with symptoms, abdominal pain without jaundice is usually the most common concern.

Liver protocol (i.e., noncontrast, arterial phase, venous phases, with thin cuts) CT scan and MRI are useful in ruling out benign liver lesions and identifying certain distinct characteristics of ICC. Next, metastases from primary organs like breast, endometrium, lung, pancreas, stomach, and large bowel should be ruled out. This includes endoscopy and appropriate screening to rule out other adenocarcinoma primaries. If the above workup is negative and the lesion is potentially resectable, patients may not need a biopsy. Table 6-4 shows the *AJCC Cancer Staging Manual*, Eighth Edition, staging for ICC.[3]

Gallbladder Cancer

A number of risk factors have been associated with the development of GBC, including gallstone disease, polyps, autoimmune disease, chronic infection, and anatomic abnormalities.[10] Chronic inflammation of the gallbladder seems to be a commonality among all these risk factors. Nearly one-half of GBC cases are incidentally diagnosed during or after routine cholecystectomy. These incidental GBCs tend to be found at

TABLE 6-3 American Joint Committee on Cancer Staging Criteria for Perihilar Cholangiocarcinoma, Eighth Edition

AJCC Stage	Tumor-Node-Metastasis Staging	Stage Findings
0	Tis	Carcinoma *in situ*/high-grade dysplasia
	N0	Not in nodes
	M0	Not in distant sites
I	T1	Invaded into bile duct wall muscle or fibrous tissue
	N0	Not in nodes
	M0	Not in distant sites
II	T2a or T2b	Invaded through bile duct wall into fatty tissue (T2a) or adjacent liver parenchyma (T2b)
	N0	Not in nodes
	M0	Not in distant sites
IIIA	T3	Unilateral branches of the portal vein or hepatic artery
	N0	Not in nodes
	M0	Not in distant sites
IIIB	T4	Tumor invades the main portal vein or its branches bilaterally, or the common hepatic artery; or unilateral second-order biliary radicals with contralateral portal vein or hepatic artery involvement
	N0	Not in nodes
	M0	Not in distant sites
IIIC	Any T	Any T stage
	N1	Spread to 1–3 regional nodes
	M0	Not in distant sites
IVA	Any T	Any T stage
	N2	Spread to ≥4 regional nodes
	M0	Not in distant sites
IVB	Any T	Any T stage
	Any N	Any N stage
	M1	Spread to distant (nonadjacent) sites including distant liver

Note: American Joint Committee on Cancer staging and TNM classification for perihilar cholangiocarcinoma.[3] Used with permission of the American Joint Committee on Cancer (AJCC), Chicago, Illinois. The original and primary source for this information is the *AJCC Cancer Staging Manual*, Eighth Edition (2017) published by Springer International Publishing.

TABLE 6-4   American Joint Committee on Cancer Staging Criteria for Intrahepatic Cholangiocarcinoma, Eighth Edition

AJCC Stage	Tumor-Node-Metastasis Staging	Stage Findings
0	Tis	Carcinoma *in situ* (intraductal tumor)
	N0	Not in nodes
	M0	Not in distant sites
IA	T1a	Solitary tumor ≤5 cm without vascular invasion
	N0	Not in nodes
	M0	Not in distant sites
IB	T1b	Solitary tumor >5 cm without vascular invasion
	N0	Not in nodes
	M0	Not in distant sites
II	T2	Solitary tumor with intrahepatic vascular invasion or multiple tumors, with or without vascular invasion
	N0	Not in nodes
	M0	Not in distant sites
IIIA	T3	Tumor perforating the visceral peritoneum
	N0	Not in nodes
	M0	Not in distant sites
IIIB	T4	Tumor involving local extrahepatic structures by direct invasion
	N0	Not in nodes
	M0	Not in distant sites
	—or—	—or—
	Any T	Any T
	N1	Spread to nearby nodes
	M0	Not in distant sites
IV	Any T	Any T stage
	Any N	Any N stage
	M1	Distant metastasis

Note: American Joint Committee on Cancer staging and TNM classification for intrahepatic cholangiocarcinoma.[3] Used with permission of the American Joint Committee on Cancer (AJCC), Chicago, Illinois. The original and primary source for this information is the *AJCC Cancer Staging Manual*, Eighth Edition (2017) published by Springer International Publishing.

earlier stages, with approximately one-third having disease confined to the lamina propria (stage T1a). Patients with de novo GBC tend to present at a more advanced stage, with 70% of these patients having metastatic disease.[11] Patients presenting with jaundice are rarely curable.

Radiographic staging includes axial imaging via CT or MRI. Staging laparoscopy may identify radiographically occult metastatic disease and is recommended before re-resection of incidental GBC.[12] For incidentally discovered GBC, the recommendation is for re-resection for patients with T stages greater than T1a (beyond the lamina propria into the muscularis, which is T1b) if a margin-negative resection is possible and if free of distant metastases. Table 6-5 details the *AJCC Cancer Staging Manual*, Eighth Edition, staging for GBC.[3]

MULTIDISCIPLINARY CARE

Colorectal Liver Metastases

Patient selection for surgery, and optimization prior to it, continues to evolve. Factors such as the clinical risk score and the modified clinical risk score (which incorporates KRAS mutation status) can be used to identify appropriate tumor biology for resection.[13,14] Increasing use of effective systemic chemotherapy has increased the proportion of patients who can benefit from surgery, even those with M1b (e.g., liver plus lung metastases or liver plus nodes).[15] Although controversy remains regarding whether chemotherapy should be delivered perioperatively (before and after resection) or simply after resection, the European Organisation for Research and Treatment of Cancer Intergroup Trial 40983 showed improvement in progression-free survival, especially in patients with carcinoembryonic antigen levels above 5 ng/ml. For example, the 3-year progression-free survival increased from 20% for surgery alone to 35% with perioperative FOLFOX in these medium- to high-risk patients.[16,17] Technical advancements that have expanded the proportion of patients considered resectable include techniques that allow larger resection volumes (including portal vein embolization to preoperatively grow the future remnant)[18,19] as well as advanced venous detachment techniques that allow multiple parenchymal-sparing resections to avoid hemihepatectomies and extended hepatectomies.[20]

Hepatocellular Cancer

Unlike for CLM, traditional cytotoxic chemotherapy agents are not used for HCC. Tyrosine kinase inhibitors such as sorafenib and lenvatinib and immunotherapy such as nivolumab[21] are the current standards for patients with advanced, unresectable HCC but are not typically used in surgical patients.[22] Currently, enrolling perioperative trials are integrating immunotherapies such as atezolizumab, nivolumab, and ipilimumab along with antiangiogenesis drugs such as bevacizumab.[23]

Perihilar Cholangiocarcinoma

If tissue sampling is desired to confirm diagnosis or to consider preoperative therapy such as the "Mayo protocol" of neoadjuvant chemoradiation for node-negative PHC up to 3 cm in size,[24] percutaneous biopsy should be avoided, especially if liver transplantation is an alternative for resection. Instead, endoscopic approaches, including

TABLE 6-5   American Joint Committee on Cancer Staging Criteria for Gallbladder Cancer, Eighth Edition

AJCC Stage	Tumor-Node-Metastasis Staging	Stage Findings
0	Tis	Carcinoma *in situ*
	N0	Not in nodes
	M0	Not in distant sites
I	T1a or T1b	Invades lamina propria (T1a) or muscularis
	N0	Not in nodes
	M0	Not in distant sites
IIA	T2a	Invades through muscularis into perimuscular connective tissue on peritoneal side without involving serosa
	N0	Not in nodes
	M0	Not in distant sites
IIB	T2b	Invades through muscularis into fibrous tissue of liver side (but not into liver parenchyma)
	N0	Not in nodes
	M0	Not in distant sites
IIIA	T3	Invades through serosa into peritoneum or liver and/or into another organ (omentum, liver, stomach, duodenum, colon, pancreas, extrahepatic bile duct)
	N0	Not in nodes
	M0	Not in distant sites
IIIB	T1–T3	T1–T3
	N1	Spread to 1–3 regional nodes
	M0	Not in distant sites
IVA	T4	Invades main portal vein or hepatic artery or two structures organs outside liver
	N0–N1	Spread to 0–3 regional nodes
	M0	Not in distant sites
IVB	Any T	Any T stage
	N2	Spread to ≥4 nodes
	M0	Not in distant sites
	—or—	—or—
	Any T	Any T stage
	Any N	Any N stage
	M1	Distant metastasis

Note: American Joint Committee on Cancer staging and TNM classification for gallbladder cancer.[3] Used with permission of the American Joint Committee on Cancer (AJCC), Chicago, Illinois. The original and primary source for this information is the *AJCC Cancer Staging Manual*, Eighth Edition (2017) published by Springer International Publishing.

SpyGlass biopsies, are preferred and have been reported to result in equivalent diagnostic yield for primary tumors while also allowing for nodal sampling if lymph nodes appear suspicious on imaging or endoscopic ultrasound. The application of fluorescence in situ hybridization has significantly improved the diagnostic yield of biliary brushings over standard cytologic evaluation.[25] Importantly, however, a negative or nondiagnostic biopsy does not rule out PHC. Because tissue diagnosis is not always achieved, with appropriate multidisciplinary review, treatment can be initiated without tissue confirmation.[26]

Intrahepatic Cholangiocarcinoma

Recent evidence has demonstrated that roughly 50% of ICCs have actionable mutations that may affect their prognosis and management, including targeted therapies for *IDH1/2* and *FGFR2*, the two most common mutations.[27] Therefore, ICC is best managed in a multidisciplinary setting. Next-generation sequencing is now part of standard of care.[28] Metastatic disease should be ruled out, and a measurement of the future liver remnant (FLR) should be performed as with other liver tumors before tumor board decisions. Neoadjuvant chemotherapy may be considered in patients with locally advanced or borderline resectable ICC to downsize the tumor, treat micrometastatic disease, and test the tumor biology.[29] Lymphovascular and perineural invasion, lymph node involvement, and tumor size of 5 cm or greater are poor prognostic features, which trigger discussions for adjuvant therapy, even with successfully cleared margins at the time of resection.[30]

Gallbladder Cancer

If an incidental node was already positive or if the patient has locally advanced disease (invading two organs or the portal vein), multidisciplinary tumor boards can consider the role of neoadjuvant therapy to test the tumor biology because the positive node placed the patient into stage IIIB and invasion of two organs is equivalent to stage IV disease, regardless of how "localized" the tumor seems. The BILCAP trial has the best (although mixed with other biliary tract cancers) data supporting adjuvant therapy for GBC with adjuvant capecitabine over observation alone.[30] Another adjuvant therapy option, from the SWOG S0809 trial, is with gemcitabine followed by capecitabine-sensitizing radiation to the resection bed and regional nodal basin.[31]

PERIOPERATIVE CARE

Preoperative Decision-Making for Resectability

The nuances of resection for each disease site are discussed in the individual chapters, but there are some common themes across all hepatectomies. Perhaps the most important concept of resectability is the need to save an FLR of adequate size with adequate regenerative capacity, biliary drainage, vascular inflow and outflow, and at least two contiguous segments. High-resolution liver protocol imaging with thin cuts is required to both understand the anatomy and to ensure that all lesions can be documented to the limits of our current technology.

Colorectal Liver Metastases

In the preoperative assessment of patients for hepatectomy, several factors should be considered, which follow the A-B-C clinical classification that has been conceptualized for other malignancies.[32,33] A represents anatomy, or the concept that the tumor (or tumors) has to be technically resectable with an adequate standardized FLR that is measured with volumetry software.[34,35] In patients with a history of extensive systemic chemotherapy and potential chemotherapy-associated liver injury (steatosis or steatohepatitis),[36] careful assessment of platelet count, splenomegaly, and liver dysfunction is required. B represents tumor biology, in that the burden of extrahepatic disease affects survival and should be taken into consideration prior to embarking on liver resection.[37] Finally, C represents the patient's condition or comorbidities, in that the patient has to be otherwise a physiologic candidate for the planned extent of liver resection.

Hepatocellular Cancer and Intrahepatic Cholangiocarcinoma

Because most HCC occurs in patients with cirrhosis, preoperative evaluation must include assessment of the degree of underlying liver disease, presence of portal hypertension, and carefully measured FLR. Similarly, ICC can also, although not as commonly as HCC, occur in the setting of an unhealthy liver. A high index of suspicion for portal hypertension (e.g., thrombocytopenia, ascites, varices, splenomegaly, or previous liver decompensation) should prompt evaluation with transjugular liver biopsy and measurements of a hepatic vein–portal vein pressure gradient. It is generally accepted that a gradient between the portal pressure minus the hepatic vein pressure greater than 10 mm Hg is a contraindication for resection secondary to increased operative morbidity and risk of life-threatening postoperative liver failure.[38]

In the setting of normal liver parenchyma, up to 80% of the liver can be removed safely when standardized to a patient's body size. In the setting of cirrhosis, most surgeons recommend sparing 40% to 60% of the patient's standardized total liver volume. Although volumetry is the reference standard in the United States for preventing postoperative hepatic insufficiency or even liver failure–related death, one potential shortcoming is the inability to measure actual liver function. Outside the United States, indocyanine green clearance (to measure biliary excretion and thus liver function) is commonly used to complement CT volumetry.

Perihilar Cholangiocarcinoma

Because PHCs directly abut or invade the central portion of the liver, an extended hepatectomy with biliary reconstruction is almost always required to achieve margin-negative resection. This type of complex and morbid operation is not suitable for patients with limited performance status. Equally critical is the need to ensure an adequate FLR. Size and quality of the FLR must be assessed in a similar method to other disease sites. If the FLR is estimated to be under 30%, which is largely the case with extended right hepatectomies, portal vein embolization should be considered to induce FLR hypertrophy and minimize the risk of postoperative liver insufficiency and even liver failure–related death.[39,40]

General consensus exists that patients with a small FLR, including those in need of portal vein embolization, benefit from preoperative biliary drainage, as bile stasis in the FLR is thought to limit adequate hypertrophy. Beyond this, the utility of routine preoperative biliary drainage remains debatable. Series have demonstrated that this practice was associated with greater rates of postoperative infectious complications without improving postoperative outcomes.[41,42] In addition, preoperative percutaneous biliary drainage has been reported to lead to tumor tract seeding in as many as 5% to 10% of patients.[43] Instead, selective preoperative biliary drainage is recommended for patients with cholangitis, significant hyperbilirubinemia (and its sequelae on patient performance status), or severe symptoms including malnutrition. An added benefit of biliary drainage is the ability to obtain direct cholangiography, which may provide accessory information for surgical planning.

Gallbladder Cancer

Surgeons considering re-resection must pay special attention to the depth of invasion on pathology, and if any question revolves around this, the pathology should be re-reviewed. Additional attention should be paid to the involvement of the cystic duct, sidedness of the tumor (hepatic vs. peritoneal side), and lymph node positivity if a node (often the Calot node) was incidentally resected. Technical aspects of the original cholecystectomy that may increase the risk of peritoneal spread should also be noted, such as perforation of the gallbladder, bile spillage, and failure to use an extraction bag for specimen retrieval. These high-risk features of the conduct of the original cholecystectomy may direct the tumor board to consider chemotherapy before re-resection. Otherwise, if there are no overt reasons to wait, locoregional clearance with re-resection after cholecystectomy within 4 to 8 weeks of the index operation is associated with improved overall survival compared with reoperation at earlier or later time points.[44] For de novo GBC, recommendation is for staging laparoscopy followed by margin-negative oncologic resection, including portal lymph node dissection and partial hepatectomy.

The improvement in postoperative mortality in liver surgery in the past two to three decades can be attributed to improved anatomic knowledge (avoiding intraoperative hemorrhage through improved preoperative imaging and intraoperative ultrasound guidance[45] and leaving adequate FLR based on preoperative volumetry measurements),[40] surgical technology (energy devices and hemostatic agents),[46,47] and anesthetic techniques (low central venous pressure fluid strategy and goal-direct fluid therapy).[48,49] Additional advancements include strategies for FLR optimization such as portal vein embolization[18,19] and techniques to reduce bile leaks and organ space infections.[50]

QUALITY MEASURES

Perhaps reflecting the wide variety of liver parenchyma transection techniques, formal quality measures of appropriate liver surgery remain undefined. Quality metrics regarding margins also are lacking owing to changing definitions of "acceptable" margins, especially with CLM. As more is learned about tumor biology with circulating tumor DNA, routine next-generation sequencing, and the role of combination procedures (resecting CLM with primary and/or with peritoneum), the importance of a liver parenchymal margin becomes even more diminished.

Perhaps the most closely studied oncologic metric in gastrointestinal cancer is lymph node resection number. These are the most appropriate for future quality metrics for GBC, PHC, and ICC but not for HCC, in which lymphadenectomy is not routinely required.[51] For example, although the *AJCC Cancer Staging Manual*, Eighth Edition, recommends six nodes to be resected for GBC, zero nodes are sampled in up to one-half of GBC patients, and thus, the most important quality metric is perhaps to start requiring *any* regional node sampling first.[52,53] For ICC, the *AJCC Cancer Staging Manual*, Eighth Edition, recommends six regional nodes as well; like in GBC, approximately one-half of patients do not have any nodes harvested, in a disease in which approximately 20% of patients are node positive.[54] And like in GBC, node positivity dramatically affects (negatively) survival in ICC.[55] For PHC, no study has formally defined what is adequate nodal harvest, although getting zero nodes in the specimen is less likely by anatomy (compared with ICC and GBC).[56] If the hepatoduodenal ligament is cleared for PHC, it is likely that all specimens should have at least the station 12 nodes. Because of the anatomic nuances of where each of these biliary tract and primary liver cancers are located, future AJCC recommendations for nodal harvest and pathology template should include both number *and* station because simply reaching a nodal threshold in the wrong nodal station would be a false assurance of any node-count metric.

CHAPTER **14**

Liver Resection for Colorectal Liver Metastases

CRITICAL ELEMENTS

- Systematic Abdominal Inspection and Intraoperative Ultrasound
- Resection of Planned Lesions to Macroscopically Negative Margins

1. SYSTEMATIC ABDOMINAL INSPECTION AND INTRAOPERATIVE ULTRASOUND

Recommendation: A systematic inspection of the abdomen should be routinely performed to exclude extrahepatic cancer and assess the health of the liver at the time of operation. Systematic intraoperative ultrasound of the liver should also be routinely performed to confirm technical resectability of the tumor(s), to detect radiographically occult disease, and to confirm the operative plan.

Type of Data: Retrospective reports, case series, or case-control studies

Strength of Recommendation: Strong recommendation, low-level evidence

Rationale

Systematic abdominal inspection

Three-phase contrasted thin-slice computed tomography (CT) and/or hepatobiliary-contrasted (gadoxetate) thin-slice magnetic resonance imaging (MRI) are mandatory components of the preoperative assessment of patients with colorectal liver metastases (CLM). These "liver protocol" scans reduce the likelihood of intraoperative surprises (e.g., additional lesions) and nontherapeutic laparotomy. Although these modalities typically detect extrahepatic and peritoneal disease that might preclude liver resection prior to entering the operating room, up to 10% of patients with potentially resectable CLM are found to have radiographically occult peritoneal disease, extraregional nodal disease, or additional intrahepatic disease at the time of planned resection.[57,58] A systematic approach to the intraoperative staging of patients with radiographically resectable CLM is therefore paramount.

The extent and burden of any unexpected peritoneal disease should be quantified. If direct peritoneal extension is limited (e.g., liver capsular lesion directly onto diaphragmatic peritoneum), a limited en bloc peritonectomy can be performed concurrent with the planned CLM resection. However, peritoneal disease beyond the direct area of extracapsular extension warrants a change in plan, including a multidisciplinary discussion with consideration of multimodality treatment. This may include systemic chemotherapy and future cytoreductive surgery in select cases.[59,60]

Extraregional nodal involvement of para-aortic, aortocaval, retropancreatic, or celiac nodal stations (i.e., regions beyond the stations of the hepatoduodenal ligament and common hepatic artery) is associated with a poor prognosis.[61,62] If identified on preoperative imaging, extraregional lymphadenopathy should be fully characterized via positron emission tomography (PET) imaging and/or percutaneous or endoscopic biopsy prior to entering the operating room. If positive, liver resection is contraindicated. Similarly, if extraregional lymphadenopathy is identified via operative inspection, intraoperative biopsy should be performed prior to liver resection. Metastatic lymphadenopathy in these basins represents a strong rationale to abort the planned hepatectomy and to discuss the most appropriate treatment and sequencing within a multidisciplinary consensus conference.

Although portal (hepatoduodenal ligament and common hepatic artery) lymphadenopathy is also associated with a worse prognosis relative to node-negative disease, the prognosis of patients with disease in these lymph nodes is generally better than that of patients with extraregional nodal disease. Liver resection with portal lymphadenectomy may be indicated in highly selected patients after careful consideration in a multidisciplinary format.[63]

The liver quality should be evaluated for the presence of steatosis, fibrosis, and/or chemotherapy-associated liver injury. If there is significant concern regarding the quality of the liver parenchyma, core needle biopsy of the liver parenchyma can be obtained to quantify the severity of fibrosis and/or chemotherapy-associated liver injury, particularly if the allowable extent of planned hepatectomy would be affected. However, because preoperative liver function can be accurately assessed preoperatively based on laboratory values and cross-sectional imaging findings, aborted cases due to unexpected intraoperative findings related to liver quality should be uncommon.

Staging laparoscopy

Staging laparoscopy is not recommended for all patients owing to the low yield in the detection of radiographically occult disease following modern imaging.[57,58] However, selective use of laparoscopy before laparotomy is appropriate if preoperative imaging and/or clinical history (T4 perforated colon cancer) suggests peritoneal lesions suspicious for metastasis or if concern exists for underlying intrinsic liver disease such as fibrosis, cirrhosis, and/or chemotherapy-associated liver injury, which would preclude the planned parenchymal resection.

Systematic intraoperative liver ultrasound

Radiographically occult hepatic metastases are identified in the operating room in up to 10% of patients.[64,65] Systematic intraoperative ultrasound of the liver is, therefore, recommended to confirm the number, size, and anatomic extent of any lesions identified on preoperative imaging; to identify or rule out radiographically occult disease; to determine the relationship of metastases to vascular and biliary pedicles; and to guide parenchymal transection (and/or intraoperative ablation) (Figs. 6-1 and 6-2). If occult intraparenchymal disease that is not within the planned resection and that would not allow for an adequate future liver remnant (FLR) is identified, changing the planned operation into a two-stage approach should be considered. For patients with bilateral disease, this would mean immediately addressing tumors within the left liver (the planned FLR), followed by right portal vein embolization and subsequent second-stage right or extended right hepatectomy. However, if resection to negative margins is no longer considered feasible even with portal vein embolization and/or two-stage hepatectomy, resection should not be pursued. Similarly, if tumor involvement of a major vascular structure that would not allow for adequate inflow and outflow of the planned FLR is identified, resection should be aborted.

Technical Aspects

Abdominal inspection

On entry into the peritoneum, a systematic visual and manual/instrumental inspection to exclude unplanned and unresectable extrahepatic disease should be performed, focusing particular attention on the common sites of radiographically occult disease

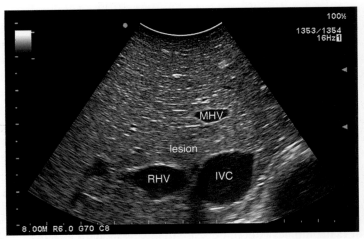

FIGURE 6-1   This intraoperative ultrasound shows a colorectal liver metastasis lesion between the middle and right hepatic veins. This is nonpalpable, so the only way to delineate the margins of its planned resection is via ultrasound. IVC: inferior vena cava; MHV: middle hepatic vein; RHV: right hepatic vein.

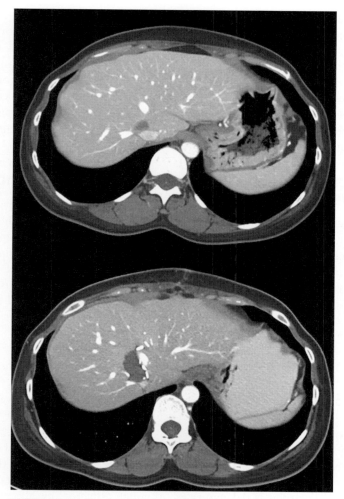

FIGURE 6-2 The preoperative (*top*) and postoperative (*bottom*) CT scans for a planned nonanatomic resection of a colorectal liver metastasis lesion between the middle and right hepatic veins. The preoperative image matches the intraoperative ultrasound image from Figure 6-1.

including omentum, peritoneal surfaces including the bilateral diaphragms and the (intact or resected) primary tumor quadrant, bowel serosa, mesentery, and portal (stations 12 and 8) nodes. If macroscopic disease is detected, a tissue biopsy should be collected and sent for immediate histopathologic analysis. Although there is no required "order" to this systematic approach, intraoperative systematic evaluation for radiographically occult disease is critical.

Intraoperative ultrasound

A variety of liver ultrasound technologies can be used intraoperatively by either the surgeon or radiologist, including either a minimally invasive or open ultrasound probe. The liver should be evaluated in a systematic fashion, including the hepatic vein confluence, portal vein divisions, and associated bile ducts. The relationship of all metastatic lesions to the FLR, portal pedicles, and/or hepatic veins is critical to assess in order to determine resectability. Ultrasound can also be used to define and measure both parenchymal and vascular margins and can be used throughout the operation to guide the parenchymal transection.

2. RESECTION OF PLANNED LESIONS TO MACROSCOPICALLY NEGATIVE MARGINS

Recommendation: All metastatic lesions planned for resection should be resected either individually or en bloc with the goal of obtaining negative macroscopic (R0/R1) parenchymal and vascular margins while simultaneously preserving maximal functional volume in the FLR. Portal lymphadenectomy should not be performed routinely. Lymphadenectomy can be considered in highly selected patients for whom there is either suspicion of or known metastatic lymphadenopathy and the goal of clearing all macroscopic disease has been established within the context of a multimodality plan.

Type of Data: Retrospective reports, case series, or case-control studies

Strength of Recommendation: Strong recommendation, medium-level evidence

Rationale

Resection of CLM with a positive margin is associated with a high risk of local recurrence (defined as recurrence within the same segment or within the bed of the previous resection site) and short overall survival.[13,66–68] Thus, resection with a putative goal of "negative" (R0) margins is recommended, although a microscopically positive (R1) margin is acceptable if this is identified incidentally on final pathology or if the tumor has been cleanly detached from major vascular structures (contemporarily defined as an "R1-vascular" margin).[69–71] Thoughtful planning of the extent of liver resection for CLM should carefully consider the balance between margin clearance and extent/volume of parenchymal resection and its associated morbidity. Any planned "debulking," or macroscopically incomplete (R2) resection, is ineffective and should not be performed unless part of a planned two-stage resection.

Specimen orientation and margin assessment

Following resection of each specimen, if a concern for an R1 parenchymal margin exists and it is technically possible to resect additional hepatic parenchyma, the surgical specimen should be oriented and sent for immediate gross assessment. If the immediate intraoperative margin is grossly positive, additional tissue clearance may be attempted, taking into consideration the anticipated FLR after additional resection and the location of the tumor. Retrospectively, there is no definite evidence that re-resection of a positive microscopic margin is associated with a reduction in local recurrence, any-site recurrence, or overall survival. Rather, microscopically positive margins are thought to be more representative of underlying tumor biology (e.g., RAS mutation status) rather than surgical technique.[72,73] In recent studies, RAS mutation tumors were more likely to have positive microscopic margins owing to satellite cancer cells found further away from the tumor despite macroscopically negative margins. However, re-resection in these studies did not reduce recurrence in that liver segment, in another segment, or outside the liver, thus representing the poor biology of RAS mutation tumors. Therefore, routine frozen section margin assessment is not recommended if the margin is grossly negative. If there is no intention or possibility of additional resection for further margin clearance (e.g., already detached from a hepatic vein), there is no need for any immediate (gross or frozen microscopic) intraoperative pathologic evaluation.

Nodal resection

The rate of portal lymph node involvement in patients with CLM has been reported to range between 4% and 20%. Although patients with metastatic portal lymphadenopathy are known to have a poor prognosis relative to patients without metastatic nodes, the presence of cancer in portal lymph nodes is not an absolute contraindication to surgery. Several series have reported long-term survival following resection in well-selected patients.[61,74,75]

Limited data exist regarding the benefit of routine versus selective portal lymphadenectomy.[61,76,77] Therefore, routine portal (hepatoduodenal ligament) lymphadenectomy is not recommended or required. But in well-selected patients, portal lymphadenectomy may be performed if clinical suspicion of nodal involvement exists, on the basis of either preoperative imaging or intraoperative findings. This decision should be made in the context of a multidisciplinary plan (with systemic therapy) and in a setting of macroscopic clearance of all radiographically evident disease.

Importantly, celiac, retropancreatic, and para-aortic nodes have a poor prognosis in general with overall survival rates below 5% at 5 years. In most cases, liver resection is contraindicated in this setting.

Technical Aspects

Access approach

Within high-volume centers, minimally invasive and traditional open resection for CLM can be performed with similar oncologic outcomes and equivalent margin status.[78,79] A recently reported randomized controlled trial comparing candidates for laparoscopic and open parenchyma-sparing liver resection for CLM (OSLO-COMET) found a decrease in postoperative morbidity in the laparoscopic group (19% vs. 31%), with equivalent margin negativity rates and similar overall survival to open surgery.[78] Therefore, either approach is considered acceptable if it can be performed safely and a macroscopically margin-negative resection can be achieved.

Parenchymal transection

A complete discussion regarding the specific method of parenchymal transection (e.g., crush and clamp, ultrasonic tissue dissectors, energy devices, surgical staplers) with or without intermittent inflow occlusion is not the objective of this chapter. A number of studies have attempted to determine which technique is superior. Although the data generally support choice of transection technique based on surgeon experience, a meticulous dissection of parenchymal structures with ultrasonic dissection or crush-clamp is recommended to minimize blood loss. Ultrasound should be used to measure and delineate the intended surgical margin. When necessary, tumor(s) may be dissected directly off major vascular structures (such as the middle and right hepatic veins seen in Fig. 6-2) to preserve parenchyma, reduce postoperative morbidity, and increase the opportunity for future therapies, including repeat hepatectomy.

Portal lymphadenectomy

If portal nodes are known to be clinically positive before surgery or are concerning on palpation during the liver resection, they can be resected with a standardized technique—with the aforementioned caveat that surgery should be within the context of a multidisciplinary plan that includes systemic therapy and clearance of all radiographic disease. Portal lymph nodes include the stations for the common hepatic artery (station 8 with 8a [anterior] and 8p [posterior]) and the hepatoduodenal ligament (station 12 with 12a [artery], 12b [bile duct], and 12p [portal vein]). Unless there is direct concern about posterior pancreatic head nodes (station 13), there is typically no need for a full Kocher maneuver to clear the hepatoduodenal ligament. However, a partial Kocher maneuver can give some laxity to the hepatoduodenal ligament and open up the shorter-than-expected space between the central liver and duodenum. Station 8 nodes can be cleared by identifying and skeletonizing the common hepatic artery from the hepatic artery bifurcation back toward the celiac axis. Station 12 can be approached from either left (12a) to right or from right (12p) to left by skeletonizing the lymphatic tissue off the artery, duct, and portal vein.

CHAPTER 15

Liver Resection for Hepatocellular Carcinoma

CRITICAL ELEMENTS

- Laparoscopic or Open Inspection of the Abdomen and Liver
- All Lesions Should Be Resected to Macroscopically Negative Margins

1. LAPAROSCOPIC OR OPEN INSPECTION OF THE ABDOMEN AND LIVER

Recommendation: The liver parenchyma should be evaluated thoroughly for the presence of fibrosis and/or cirrhosis. Portal hypertension should be excluded. Inspection and/or palpation of the liver (to rule out intrahepatic metastases or multifocal disease) and peritoneal cavity is critical. Intraoperative ultrasound is recommended to evaluate and confirm the relationship of any identified lesion(s) to the vascular and biliary pedicles and to guide parenchymal transection.

Type of Data: Retrospective reports, case series, or case-control studies

Strength of Recommendation: Strong recommendation, low-quality evidence

Rationale

Although liver protocol (thin cuts with arterial and venous phases) computed tomography (CT) and hepatobiliary contrasted magnetic resonance imaging (MRI) have been significantly refined in the past two decades, some limitations to their use in staging of hepatocellular carcinoma (HCC) still exist. The most accurate and current standard for intraoperative staging of HCC is laparoscopy or laparotomy with intraoperative ultrasound.[80–82] Rates of identification of clinically occult lesions or relevant anomalies in tumor anatomy are far lower than they were prior to the widespread use of liver protocol CT and MRI, but ultrasonographic evaluation of the liver is still mandatory prior to planned resection.[83,84]

In addition to a thorough inspection of all metastatic lesions and critical inflow and outflow structures, the underlying health and size of the future liver remnant (FLR) should also be evaluated. Approximately 80% of HCC arise in the setting of cirrhosis, so delineation of the underlying liver function is critical prior to resection. Many preoperative methods exist to evaluate the health and function of the liver prior to surgery. These methods include measurement of indocyanine green excretion, MRI elastography, and evaluation of random liver biopsies. Less objective, but more common, indicators of liver dysfunction include high Childs-Pugh score, abnormalities in liver function tests, and thrombocytopenia. Furthermore, evidence of cirrhosis with radiographic evidence of portal hypertension such as splenomegaly, esophageal varices, a recanalized umbilical vein, rounding of the segment 2/3 liver edge, an enlarged caudate lobe, a generally shrunken and/or scalloped liver, and ascites are stigmata of advanced liver disease that may preclude safe liver resection. Almost all of these factors can and should be assessed prior to entry into the operating room. If concern for portal hypertension persists following other attempts at measuring liver dysfunction, transhepatic portal pressure gradients can be measured preoperatively. Despite the plethora of methods available to assess liver function preoperatively, the extent of liver cirrhosis may be more advanced than anticipated on thorough abdominal exploration.

Despite a thorough preoperative staging workup, unexpected disease can be found intraoperatively in the form of peritoneal metastases, an inadequate FLR, cirrhosis worse than preoperatively thought, bilateral intrahepatic metastases, main portal vein or inferior vena cava invasion, and/or adjacent organ invasion.[84] Previous concern for peritoneal tumoral hemorrhage should be addressed at this time by inspecting for tumoral spread. Except in well-selected cases of limited macrovascular invasion, such findings preclude resection of HCC.

Technical Aspects

Laparoscopic versus open inspection

As in many other disease processes, initiating an operative intervention with laparoscopy (as opposed to full laparotomy) carries many potential benefits. For HCC, beginning a procedure with laparoscopy allows the operating surgeon to evaluate the liver and peritoneal cavity to an extent similar to that accomplished by open laparotomy but with a reduction in the morbidity and operative time if the inspection leads to an aborted resection. Laparoscopic evaluation should include visual inspection of the peritoneal cavity for extrahepatic disease, especially along the diaphragm, and the appearance of the liver, particularly if the degree of cirrhosis is unclear from preoperative evaluation (Fig. 6-3). If the surgeon feels that histopathologic sampling of the nontumoral FLR needs to be performed to assess the degree of fibrosis or cirrhosis and if this information would affect deciding whether to proceed, this biopsy should be sent for permanent section and the operation canceled until that result is finalized.

Intraoperative ultrasound

The liver should be evaluated via ultrasonography using a systematic approach. The hepatic vein confluence, portal vein divisions, and associated bile ducts should each

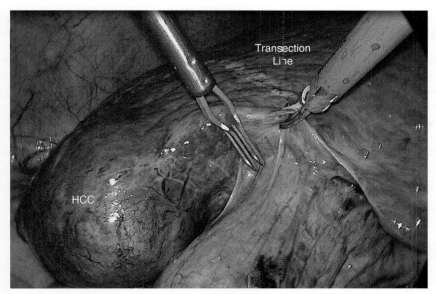

FIGURE 6-3 This laparoscopic image shows the planned transection line (created using cautery but directed by intraoperative ultrasound to ensure adequate margins. The purpose of this initial pretransection inspection includes examining the diaphragm, peritoneum, and the liver itself. HCC: hepatocellular cancer.

be identified. The relationship of all lesions to the FLR, Glissonian pedicles, and/or hepatic veins is critical to assess in order to confirm resectability. Ultrasound should be used to define and mark (using surface cautery) both parenchymal and vascular margins and should be used liberally throughout the resection to guide the parenchymal transection (Fig. 6-4).

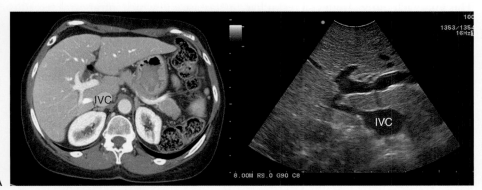

FIGURE 6-4 This intraoperative ultrasound shows the Glissonian pedicle to the right anterior sector, showing the pedicles for subsegments 8 ventral and 8 dorsal. The preoperative CT (**A**) should be viewed as an overlay while in the operating room alongside the intraoperative ultrasound CT (**B**) to identify the targeted pedicle for the hepatocellular cancer in segment 8. IVC: inferior vena cava.

2. ALL LESIONS SHOULD BE RESECTED TO MACROSCOPICALLY NEGATIVE MARGINS

Recommendation: All lesions should be resected either individually or en bloc in order to obtain negative margins on the parenchyma, hepatic vein (or tributaries), and Glissonian pedicle or branches while ensuring adequate FLR. Glissonian pedicle–based "anatomic" resection is preferred. When a "nonanatomic" resection technique is performed, gross margins of 1 to 2 cm should be sought. The specimen should be oriented and sent for immediate gross evaluation if concern exists for a positive margin. If the tumor is visible at the resection margin (grossly positive), re-resection of the margin should be considered if technically feasible and the volume of the FLR is sufficient. Portal lymphadenectomy is not recommended routinely, but selective lymphadenectomy should be considered in patients for whom suspicion of metastatic lymphadenopathy exists.

Type of Data: Retrospective reports, case series, or case-control studies

Strength of Recommendation: Strong recommendation, low-quality evidence

Rationale

Definition of margins

The oncologic goal of negative margins must be balanced with the simultaneous need to preserve an FLR with adequate regenerative capacity and function to survive the postoperative recovery period.

HCCs are known for intraportal metastases (Fig. 6-5) that follow the portal drainage flow from the tumor.[85] This drainage pattern can lie entirely within a single segment or can bridge two or three segments' territories. Thus, anatomic-based resection, which removes all segmental portal pedicles, is preferred. When an anatomic resection is used, margin is based on the segments resected rather than parenchymal distance. This approach differs from colorectal liver metastases, in which intraportal spread is uncommon and margin planning is based only on distance from each tumor. That is why colorectal liver metastases are routinely resected using a parenchymal-sparing nonanatomic approach.

When a nonanatomic approach for HCC is chosen (instead of anatomic pedicle-based resection), wide margins should be planned because microvascular invasion cannot be determined by gross liver surface examination or radiographic staging and can only be assessed on final pathology. Prospective and multi-institutional data suggest that when the technique of nonanatomic resection is used, a wider margin is better than a narrower margin, especially in patients with microvascular invasion (intraportal tumor microscopic thrombi) in order to encompass small, regional intraportal structures that may harbor metastases.[86] A gross margin of at least 1 to 2 cm should be taken when technically feasible.[87,88] Supporting this concept, closer margin width was not associated with any adverse oncologic outcomes in patients undergoing anatomic resection (because the appropriate anatomic portal drainage was followed

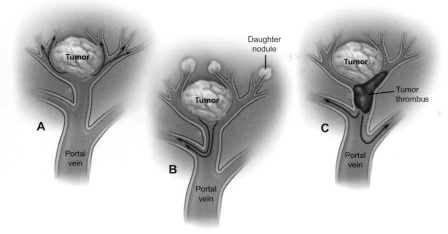

FIGURE 6-5 This illustration shows the putative reason for either a segment-based anatomic resection or a wide nonanatomic resection. Hepatocellular carcinoma is known for intraportal metastases beyond its immediate margins (**A**). Tumor cells can travel within the portal distribution for that tumor (**B**). Tumor thrombus can even develop from this intraportal tumor cell invasion (**C**). Thus, resection of the tumor-bearing portal drainage territory is the goal rather than just enucleating the gross tumor.

rather than an arbitrary margin distance), but empirically planned wider margins were important when choosing the technique of nonanatomic resections, in terms of both recurrence-free and overall survival.[88]

The anatomic rationale described above explains the existing controversy regarding routine anatomic versus nonanatomic resection for HCC. A recent meta-analysis and several large retrospective series argue for routine anatomic resection, but there are many studies that argue against routine anatomic resection as simply diagrammed in Figure 6-5. Detractors of anatomic resection correctly point out that not all tumors are conveniently located in the center of a Couinaud segment.[89,90] Additionally, measuring parenchymal margin oversimplifies liver anatomy to assume that each tumor is surrounded only by parenchyma. In some instances, vascular structures need to be considered preserved for functional reasons.[91] In summary, current data support that both portal pedicle anatomic-based resections and nonanatomic resections with wide margins of at least 1 to 2 cm are associated with improved oncologic outcome.

Nodal sampling
Patients with histologically positive (or radiographically enlarged) portal lymph nodes should undergo lymphadenectomy, as various studies report improved long-term survival with lymph node dissection in certain patients with clinically involved nodal disease, especially fibrolamellar HCC.[61,74,75,92] In those patients, the radiographically positive lymph node basins should be cleared. Otherwise, in patients without preoperative suspicion of nodal disease, routine lymph node sampling is not recommended.[51]

Technical Aspects

First introduced by Makuuchi et al.,[85] the concept of Glissonian pedicle–based anatomic resection (defined as resecting all associated tumor-draining portal territory for
potential microthrombi [Fig. 6-6]) has been favored over nonanatomic resection (defined as widely aiming for a negative parenchymal resection without following portal
territories).[89,93] As noted above, the concept of portal pedicle–based anatomic resection is misunderstood and often confused with performing unnecessary formal hemihepatectomies or formal segmentectomies, sacrificing hepatic parenchyma and raising
risks for postoperative liver failure–related death. Even subsegmental anatomic resections can be performed with appropriate planning. For example, a central tumor in
segment 8 ventral may drain into both segment 8 ventral and 4A Glissonian pedicles
and can be anatomically resected with a combined segment 8 ventral plus 4A subsegmental resection. This approach would be more appropriate (and safer in preserving
liver function) than a larger formal total segment 8 plus 4 bisegment resection, central
hepatectomy, or extended right/left hepatectomy.

Anatomic resection is accomplished via selective ligation of the inflow portal vessels (hepatic artery and portal vein) with the associated draining bile duct (all three
making up the Glissonian pedicle), followed by ligation of outflow hepatic vein(s) associated with the territory to be resected. The resection can be performed as an open
procedure or via minimally invasive surgery (MIS). Various mapping techniques in-
jecting indocyanine green or methylene blue can assist with coloring the parenchyma
supplied and drained by the associated Glissonian pedicle.

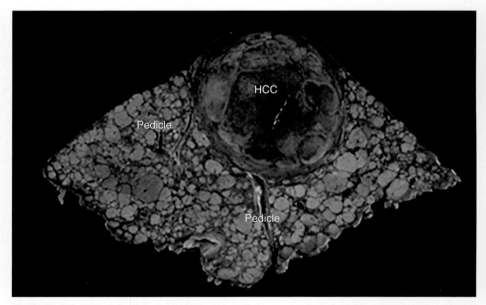

FIGURE 6-6   This is a cut image of a hepatocellular cancer (HCC) with green coloration, which
is pathognomonic for HCC. This cross-section shows the resection of the tumor-draining portal
pedicle cut in cross-section directly under the tumor at the 6 o'clock position and smaller pedicle
at the 9 o'clock position.

Nonanatomic resection can adequately resect the draining territory of an HCC if the gross parenchymal margin is mapped out to encompass the appropriate Couinaud segment or confluence of subsegments. In plain terms, the non-Glissonian nonanatomic approach is simply cutting down to the eventual Glissonian pedicle, rather than ligating it early as in the Glissonian method. It can be seen that this nonanatomic approach can be less exact and be at risk of leaving tumor-draining territory and thus the recommendation for grossly wide 1 to 2 cm margins when a nonanatomic approach is the surgeon's technical preference. Multifocal disease should be resected en bloc if the multiple tumors are simply satellites of a main tumor or separately resected if truly multicentric.

Parenchymal transection can be performed using myriad techniques. These include the following: crush and clamp technique, ultrasonic tissue dissector, various energy devices, and/or vascular staplers. There are no convincing data to suggest that any one technique is superior to another, and tumor location, underlying health of the liver, potential operative blood loss, and operating room time must be considered when deciding which modality to use. Perhaps most importantly, the preference and comfort level of the surgeon with the technique of choice should usually guide the operative plan.[54,95]

The role of subsequent laparoscopic or robotic-assisted (MIS) resection for HCC is emerging. Data suggest that MIS resection is both feasible and safe. Furthermore, postoperative morbidity and blood loss appear to be significantly reduced with an MIS approach compared with traditional "open" resections in a pooled systematic review of multiple retrospective studies.[96] Nonetheless, whether resection should be conducted via an MIS or open approach is surgeon dependent and ultimately depends on patient safety and ability to obtain an adequate oncologic resection. MIS resection should only be performed in experienced hands owing to the technical demand of the procedures.[97–101]

Following resection, the surgical specimen should be oriented. If there is concern for adequacy of the margin, especially with nonanatomic approaches when the initial parenchymal transection lines are planned by estimating a 1- to 2-cm distance, the specimen should be sent for immediate intraoperative histopathologic evaluation if there is potential for additional parenchymal resection. If an insufficient liver remnant or the location of the tumor precludes further re-resection, there is no need for immediate pathology review. If the margin is microscopically positive (tumors within 1 mm of the inked margin), an additional margin should be resected if the FLR volume is sufficient and if there is high degree of confidence regarding the focality or sidedness of the positive microscopic margin. The second point about focality relates to orientation of the specimen. If there is no certainty on the exact close margin, there is no point in blindly resecting more liver. In any decisions on margin re-resection, it must be kept in mind that each additional volume of liver resection is directly reducing the liver remnant on which the patient must survive the operation, with adequate liver function for quality of life and/or future therapies. Finally, if the permanent pathology margin comes back narrow or positive, no indication exists for return to the operating room to clear further tissue.

Final pathologic evaluation of the tumor can be in the form of one specimen or multiple specimens and should include margin distance, tumor differentiation and histology, size, and micro- or macrovascular invasion. Based on prognostic information from the final pathology report, further treatment recommendations and surveillance decisions can be made with a multidisciplinary team.[102]

CHAPTER 16

Cholangiocarcinoma

CRITICAL ELEMENTS

- Resection of Primary Tumor to Microscopically Negative Margins
- Routine Portal Lymphadenectomy with Selective Sampling of Aortocaval and Retroperitoneal Nodes

1. RESECTION OF PRIMARY TUMOR TO MICROSCOPICALLY NEGATIVE MARGINS

Recommendation: Local excision of the bile duct alone represents inadequate oncologic surgery for patients with hilar cholangiocarcinoma. En bloc hemihepatectomy is, therefore, recommended in all operations conducted with curative intent. Resection and reconstruction of the portal vein is justified when the vein is directly involved by cancer and an R0 resection is otherwise anticipated. Resection of intrahepatic cholangiocarcinoma (ICC) consists of removal of the involved liver to microscopically negative (R0) parenchymal, biliary, and vascular margins.

Type of Data: Retrospective reports, case series, or case-control studies

Strength of Recommendation: Strong recommendation, low-quality evidence

Rationale

Hilar cholangiocarcinoma
Surgery remains the only potentially curative treatment option for hilar cholangiocarcinoma. The principal objective of surgery is a microscopically margin-negative (R0) resection,[103] as margin status is the most important prognostic factor for patients with this disease, independent of stage.[104] If surgery is planned, the surgeon should feel reasonably certain that an R0 resection is possible, as a planned R1/R2 resection is not indicated.

440

R0 resection can be difficult to achieve in patients with hilar cholangiocarcinoma, owing to the proximity of the tumor and associated biliary radicals to nearby portal vein and hepatic artery branches. Published series have documented that R0 resection rates can be achieved in 63% to 78% of patients.[105-113] A microscopically positive (R1) resection has been found to be associated with shorter overall survival than that associated with an R0 resection.[105,106,113,114] Nagino et al.[113] reviewed 574 patients who underwent surgical resection for hilar cholangiocarcinoma and noted that macroscopically or microscopically positive margins were associated with shorter overall survival (risk ratio, 1.59; 95% confidence interval [CI], 1.18 to 2.15; $P = .002$). Similar findings were reported in a multicenter Italian study involving 440 patients, which reported that R0 resection was associated with improved overall survival (hazard ratio, 0.65; 95% CI, 0.45 to 0.94; $P = .02$) and disease-free survival (hazard ratio, 0.59; 95% CI, 0.40 to 0.85; $P = .005$).[112] More recently, Tran et al.[106] reported that R1 resection was adversely associated with actual 5-year survival in a multi-institutional data set from the United States. It is generally thought that patients who undergo R1 resection have survival outcomes that are indistinguishable from those with locally advanced cancer who do not undergo resection.[115]

Hilar cholangiocarcinoma is known to spread via perineural and lymphovascular invasion, frequently extending up to 2 cm beyond the palpable tumor into the liver parenchyma and porta hepatis.[116-118] For this reason, hemihepatectomy is recommended en bloc with bile duct excision. This approach has been associated with a higher rate of R0 resection over bile duct excision alone. In fact, extrahepatic bile duct excision alone has been noted to yield a margin-positive resection in over two-thirds of patients.[116] Consequently, hemihepatectomy en bloc with bile duct excision has been demonstrated to yield superior survival outcomes than bile duct excision alone, owing to a lower risk of local recurrence at the surgical margin. This is particularly relevant given that hilar cholangiocarcinoma has been previously shown to recur locoregionally in most resected patients who experience recurrence.[119] Van Gulik et al.[120] reported that the use of extended resections for perihilar tumors was associated with higher rates of R0 resection (13% vs. 59%; $P < .05$) and greater 5-year overall survival (20% ± 3% vs. 33% ± 9%; $P < .05$). Similarly, Ito et al.[121] examined a series of patients who were operated in the era of major liver resection and compared their outcomes to those of patients who were operated in the earlier era of bile duct excision alone. They noted a higher rate of R0 resection (85% vs. 39%; $P = .006$), longer durations of disease-specific survival (65 vs. 31 months; $P = .005$) and disease-free survival (55 vs. 23 months; $P = .005$), as well as a decreased incidence of initial recurrence in the liver (5% vs. 33%; $P = .031$). Finally, a systematic review of 15 relevant studies[122] demonstrated that a greater rate of R0 resection was achievable with combined liver and bile duct resection compared with bile duct excision alone. For these reasons, local excision of the bile duct alone represents inadequate oncologic therapy for patients with hilar cholangiocarcinoma, and hemihepatectomy is recommended en bloc at all operations with curative intent. A very select subset of patients with true mid-duct cholangiocarcinoma below the hilum at the level of the cystic duct may be offered a bile duct excision alone, but these patients typically have misdiagnosed gallbladder cancer, not hilar cholangiocarcinoma.

For advanced hilar cholangiocarcinoma with vascular involvement, resection and reconstruction of the portal vein is justified if it facilitates R0 resection. A systematic review of portal vein resection in this setting examined 11 relevant studies.[123] A higher perioperative mortality rate was associated with portal vein resection, although this association was not found among subgroups of patients treated more recently and in high-volume centers. Nonetheless, R0 rates and overall survival following resection of the portal vein were similar to those of patients with less invasive disease and vascular invasion, for whom portal vein resection was not performed.[123] Additional data from a large multi-institutional series of 305 patients who underwent resection suggest that the addition of portal vein resection to radical surgery for hilar cholangiocarcinoma was associated with a higher 90-day mortality rate (17.6% vs. 10.6%; $P < .001$) but a comparable rate of R0 resection and no difference in overall survival.[124] More recently, other retrospective data from a US consortium of academic centers found no increase in perioperative complications and 30-day mortality following vascular resection in a subset of 201 patients who underwent resection for hilar cholangiocarcinoma.[125] In addition, no significant association was noted between vascular resection and survival on multivariate analysis. The absence of association between portal vein resection and survival was corroborated in another series of 674 patients with perihilar cholangiocarcinoma who were treated with either surgery or palliative approaches.[126]

Thus, there remains little debate regarding the role of portal vein resection for hilar cholangiocarcinoma with vascular invasion when vascular involvement by tumor is all that prohibits the performance of an R0 resection. However, controversy continues to exist in the literature regarding the role of routine "unconditional," no-touch, en bloc excision of the portal vein bifurcation with the tumor[127] as well as the practice of hepatic artery resection and reconstruction.[125,128] Both of these techniques have vocal proponents who have published technical descriptions and encouraging perioperative and survival outcomes data. At present, these techniques have not been uniformly adopted among North American liver surgeons, their relative merits continue to be evaluated in the literature,[126,129–131] and their use is not recommended.

Intrahepatic cholangiocarcinoma

Multiple retrospective studies have shown that resection to microscopically negative margins is also an important predictor of survival and recurrence among patients with ICC.[132–136] A large multi-institutional study evaluating the impact of margin status on oncologic outcome demonstrated that the presence of a grossly or microscopically positive surgical margin was an independent predictor of poor overall survival.[136] Although some small studies have not corroborated this association,[137] the overwhelming consensus is that margin status is associated with outcome.[138–140] Therefore, surgeons should strive for negative parenchymal, biliary, and vascular margins in all operations for ICC conducted with curative intent.

Although there is general consensus on the impact of margin status on outcomes, the "margin width" that is optimal for survival is less well defined. In a study by

Murakami et al.,[141] among patients who had undergone R0 resection, a width of 5 mm or less of normal hepatic parenchyma between cancer and the true margin was no worse than a width greater than 5 mm in terms of outcome. In contrast, in a multi-institutional study by Spolverato et al.,[136] patients who had a 1 cm or greater tumor-free margin had longer recurrence-free and overall survival durations than patients with a thinner tumor-free margin. The margin width and margin status (R0 vs. R1) may be influenced by multiple factors, including infiltrative growth, the tumor's proximity to vital vascular structures, and future liver remnant size. Therefore, given that R0 resection status has been associated with an improvement in 5-year overall survival relative to a positive margin ranging from 28% through 63%,[134,142,143] resection to microscopically negative margins, irrespective of "margin width," should be the primary goal of curative surgery. Extended resection with vascular and/or biliary reconstruction at experienced centers is reasonable if it facilitates R0 resection of advanced tumors.

Technical Aspects

In order to maximize the likelihood of R0 resection of hilar cholangiocarcinoma, the involved hemiliver, biliary confluence, and extrahepatic bile ducts should be resected. For most hilar lesions, an extended right hepatectomy en bloc with the caudate lobe, extrahepatic bile ducts, and porta hepatis lymph nodes as well as connective tissue clearance is the preferable operation. This choice of procedure is advantageous because the left hepatic duct (2 to 3 cm) is typically longer than the right hepatic duct (<1 cm), thus allowing for a more radical resection onto the future liver remnant.[127] In contrast, for tumors extending into the left hepatic duct, a left hepatectomy (or extended left hepatectomy) is typically preferred.

Following exploration of the abdomen to rule out metastatic disease, the procedure typically should be started with the dissection and preparation of the hepatoduodenal ligament. In the case of a planned (extended) right hepatectomy, the base of the umbilical fissure should be fully dissected, exposing and encircling the left portal vein. The left hepatic duct can also be assessed. Resectability can thus be assessed before division of the distal bile duct or liver parenchymal transection. Regional lymphadenectomy should be performed. The common and proper hepatic arteries should be skeletonized. The left hepatic artery and the segment 4 middle hepatic artery should also be fully dissected up to the base of the liver. The origin of the right hepatic artery should be dissected. The main portal vein should be dissected and skeletonized. The common bile duct should be divided at the level of the pancreas and reflected cranially. The right hepatic artery and segment 4 middle hepatic artery can then be ligated and divided. The right portal vein should be similarly ligated. The left hepatic duct should then be divided sharply, and a frozen section of the margin should be sent to rule out neoplastic cells. The remainder of the operation should follow the standard steps of an (extended) right hepatectomy, including dissection and division of the right hepatic vein, mobilization of the right liver, and parenchymal transection (Fig. 6-7). At the conclusion of the resection, biliary reconstruction via a

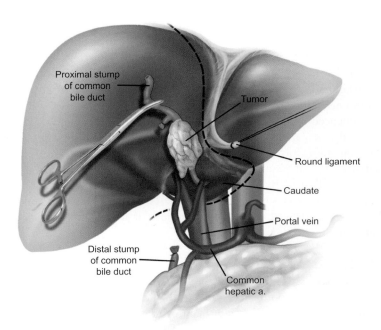

FIGURE 6-7   At this step, the distal common bile duct has been divided and lifted upward to expose the portal vein and hepatic artery bifurcation to determine resectability. The proposed line of transection for an extended right hepatectomy plus caudate resection is marked with the *dashed black line*.

Roux-en-Y hepaticojejunostomy should be performed, and a surgical drain typically should be left near the anastomosis.

If a portal vein resection is required, it can typically be performed prior to liver parenchymal transection, although occasionally, resection and reconstruction after transection may be preferred if exposure is difficult. To do so, the main portal vein should be encircled and isolated. The distal portal vein should be fully dissected up to the segmental divisions. In isolating the left portal vein, caudate branches from the left portal vein must be secured and divided, to allow maximal mobility of the vein. The main and lobar portal veins can then be clamped and divided, leaving the portal vein bifurcation with the tumor. An end-to-end primary anastomosis can then be fashioned, and consideration can be given to tying the suture of the anastomosis with a growth factor to allow full expansion of the vein and anastamosis.[144] An interposition graft is rarely needed (Fig. 6-8).

Hepatectomy for ICC follows the same technique as any parenchymal lesion (primary or metastatic). Vasculobiliary invasion mandates en bloc resection; however, bile duct resection is only needed in case of involvement of the biliary confluence.

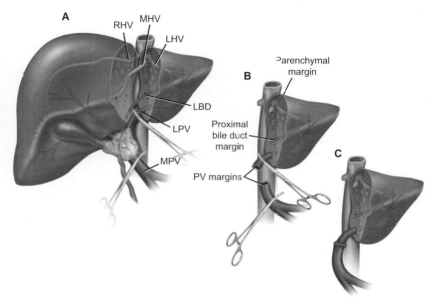

FIGURE 6-8   Depiction of resection and reconstruction of the portal vein (PV) during extended right hepatectomy. Transection depicted (**A**). Once the liver has been fully mobilized and divided, vascular clamps should be placed on the main portal vein (MPV) and left portal vein (LPV) (**B**). The left hepatic duct should be divided, and the margin should be sent for frozen section. The PV to the remnant liver should then be anastomosed in an end-to-end fashion with a "growth stitch" (**C**). LBD: left biliary duct: LHV: left hepatic vein; MHV: main hepatic vein; RHV: right hepatic vein.

2. ROUTINE PORTAL LYMPHADENECTOMY WITH SELECTIVE SAMPLING OF AORTOCAVAL AND RETROPERITONEAL NODES

Recommendation

- For hilar cholangiocarcinoma, a complete lymphadenectomy of the basins within the hepatoduodenal ligament to resect the hilar, cystic duct, choledochal, hepatic artery, portal vein, and posterior pancreaticoduodenal lymph nodes should be routinely performed.
- For ICC, lymphadenectomy should routinely include the lymph nodes in the hepatoduodenal ligament; for tumors in the left liver, lymphadenectomy should also include the nodes at the right cardia and lesser curvature; and for tumors in the right liver, lymphadenectomy should also include the retropancreatic nodes.
- In all cases, suspicious periaortic, pericaval, superior mesenteric artery, and celiac artery lymph nodes should be sampled; if positive for metastatic cancer, resection should be aborted.

Type of Data: Retrospective reports, case series, or case-control studies

Strength of Recommendation: Strong recommendation, low-quality evidence

Rationale

Hilar cholangiocarcinoma

Lymph node metastasis is one of the principal prognostic factors for patients with hilar cholangiocarcinoma. Routine lymphadenectomy (along with margin-negative hepatic resection and resection of the extrahepatic bile duct) is accepted to be a key technical aspect of surgery for hilar cholangiocarcinoma; however, the optimal anatomic extent of nodal dissection and the value of extended lymphadenectomy remain unsettled. Likewise, the number of lymph nodes that are required to adequately stage patients with hilar cholangiocarcinoma, as well the prognostic significance of the location of positive lymph nodes, remains unclear.

Hilar cholangiocarcinoma frequently metastasizes to regional lymph nodes. In a recent systematic review, the rate of nodal involvement in patients with resected perihilar tumors ranged from 31% to 58%.[145] Despite advances in surgical technique and adjuvant therapy, overall survival following curative-intent surgery remains guarded, and the reported 5-year overall survival rate is 20% to 42%.[146] Lymph node status has consistently been shown to predict the survival of patients with resected hilar cholangiocarcinoma.[111,114,147–156] Although lymph node involvement does not preclude the possibility of long-term survival, the reported 5-year overall survival in node-positive patients is only 0% through 25%.[111,151–153,157–159]

The *AJCC Cancer Staging Manual*, Eighth Edition, defines the hilar, cystic duct, common bile duct, portal, hepatic artery, portal vein, and posterior pancreaticoduodenal nodes as regional nodes for hilar cholangiocarcinoma.[3] Involvement of lymph nodes outside the hepatoduodenal ligament, including the celiac artery, superior mesenteric artery, periaortic, and pericaval nodes, is considered metastatic (M1) disease.[3] In the *AJCC Cancer Staging Manual*, Eighth Edition, N status is assigned according to the number of positive nodes: cancer metastatic to one to three nodes is designated N1 disease and to at least four nodes is designated N2 disease.[3] In the previous edition (seventh edition) of the *AJCC Cancer Staging Manual*, N stage was assigned based on nodal location, with involvement of the aforementioned distant nodes being defined as N2 disease.[160] Both the National Comprehensive Cancer Network guidelines and the Japan Society of Hepato-Biliary-Pancreatic Surgery consensus guidelines consider periaortic node metastasis a contraindication to radical resection.[161]

Within the literature, debate continues on the value of extended lymphadenectomy of stations outside the porta hepatis for hilar tumors.[30,105,147,151,162,163] The lymphatic network surrounding the perihilar region is complex. Lymphatic flow has been shown to go from the choledochal nodes to the posterior pancreatic, retroportal, posterior common hepatic artery, and periaortic nodes.[164,165]

Several retrospective single-center series have been published with respect to extended lymphadenectomy. In one report, the choledochal nodes were the most commonly involved (42.7%), and positive nodes were more commonly located in the periaortic rather than posterior pancreaticoduodenal stations (17.3% vs. 14.5%).[151] Long-term survival was possible in patients who had involvement of distant nodes; however, the prognosis was improved for patients with only microscopically positive rather than macroscopically positive periaortic lymph nodes at the time of surgery (5-year overall survival, 28.6% vs. 0%; median survival, 22.1 vs. 7.6 months; $P < .001$).[151] In a more recent retrospective study, extended lymphadenectomy was not associated with improved overall survival; its authors advocated for aborting surgery when positive celiac, superior mesenteric artery, or periaortic nodes were encountered.[30]

Only one prospective randomized trial of extended lymphadenectomy exists; that study included a cohort of patients with distal cholangiocarcinoma treated with pancreatoduodenectomy.[166] This study failed to reveal a survival benefit of extended lymphadenectomy in the entire cohort and in patients with cholangiocarcinoma specifically.[166] Further studies may be warranted to clarify the role of extended lymphadenectomy in hilar cholangiocarcinoma for patients with macroscopically negative, distant nodes. However, at present, routine extended lymphadenectomy outside the porta hepatis is not indicated. Distant nodal sampling yielding a diagnosis of metastatic cancer should preclude curative resection.

The number of resected nodes that constitutes an adequate lymphadenectomy remains controversial. Various single-center, multi-institutional, and large database studies have attempted to define a desired total lymph node count. Numerous, divergent recommendations have been made, ranging from ≥4 to ≥13 nodes.[56,114,147,150,152–154,156] In general, the aforementioned studies demonstrate that the total lymph node count has little impact on the outcome of patients with lymph node–positive cancer. Conversely, for patients with N0 cancer, a low total lymph node count is associated with poor survival, presumably owing to understaging of patients with occult, node-positive disease.[156]

The only guideline that attempts to define the number of resected lymph nodes necessary for adequate staging of hilar cholangiocarcinoma is that published by the International Union Against Cancer.[158] The *AJCC Cancer Staging Manual*, Eighth Edition, defines six nodes as an adequate lymphadenectomy for gallbladder malignancies but does not specifically define criteria for total lymph node count.[3] The International Union Against Cancer, in contrast, defines an adequate lymphadenectomy as a total lymph node count of 15 or more. This number is criticized as being unobtainable in the setting of a standard lymphadenectomy. DeOliveira et al.[114] published a systematic review detailing that the median total lymph node count, as reported in 20 studies, ranged between 2 and 24.[114] However, a median total lymph node count of 15 or more was only achieved in 9% of patients undergoing resection of hilar cholangiocarcinoma and exclusively in those patients who underwent an extended lymphadenectomy.

Intrahepatic cholangiocarcinoma

Among patients with ICC, lymph node status remains one of the most important determinants of long-term cancer-recurrence and overall survival following resection.[167] Multiple retrospective studies have highlighted that lymph node status is the most important prognostic characteristic among patients undergoing resection.[168] In addition, information on lymph node involvement may influence decision-making regarding adjuvant therapies,[169] and lymphadenectomy may improve locoregional disease control.[170] Although there is little data to suggest that lymphadenectomy directly leads to a survival benefit, given its prognostic importance and influence on treatment decision-making, a concurrent, formal lymphadenectomy is recommended at the time of surgical resection.[92]

The seventh edition of the *AJCC Cancer Staging Manual* was the first to include a traditional tumor-node-metastasis staging-based system specifically for ICC, acknowledging the prognostic importance of lymph node sampling.[160] The *AJCC Cancer Staging Manual*, Eighth Edition, has recently been updated to recommend a minimum of six lymph nodes harvested for adequate staging.[3,104] The European Society for Medical Oncology, Liver Cancer Study Group of Japan, and Americas Hepato-Pancreato-Biliary Association similarly recommend performing lymphadenectomy at the time of resection.[139,140,171] Conversely, the National Comprehensive Cancer Network states that a portal lymphadenectomy is only "reasonable," whereas the European Association for the Study of the Liver guidelines suggest that lymphadenectomy should be "strongly considered."[138,172]

The lymphatic drainage of the liver has been extensively described and follows two pathways—a superficial lymphatic system, found beneath the Glisson capsule, and a deep lymphatic system.[173] The deep lymphatic drainage flows to the hilar lymph nodes and then to the lymph nodes of the hepatoduodenal ligament. Two main lymph node chains are present within the hepatoduodenal ligament: those along the hepatic artery and the posterior periportal chain. The former drains from the common hepatic artery nodes to the celiac artery nodes and then to the cisterna chyli, whereas the latter drains from the portocaval nodes to the retropancreatic nodes and then to aortocaval nodes before the cisterna chyli.

These anatomic considerations are important to the definition of a proper lymphadenectomy. Some have postulated divergent draining patterns of the left and right hemilivers such that left-sided tumors are more likely to drain into the gastrohepatic ligament, whereas right-sided tumors are more likely to drain through the hepatoduodenal ligament into the retropancreatic lymph nodes.[174,175] However, the evidence to support this assertion is overall limited, and "crossover" can occur.[176] Therefore, it remains controversial whether the extent of lymphadenectomy should be modified based on the location of the tumor. At present, formal portal hepatis lymphadenectomy should routinely include the lymph nodes in the hepatoduodenal ligament, including the hilar, hepatic artery, and portocaval lymph nodes, and be extended to include the right cardia and lesser curvature nodes for tumors in the left liver or retropancreatic nodes for tumors in the right liver. In general, positive lymph nodes beyond the regional nodal basins (e.g., aortocaval or celiac axis) are considered metastatic disease and represent a contraindication to surgical resection.[177]

Limited evidence suggests that lymphadenectomy should be performed routinely for patients with any morphologic subtype of ICC regardless of the presence of cirrhosis and even when surgery is performed in a minimally invasive fashion.[178] Nevertheless, despite improving trends in recent years, most resections performed in the United States do not sample any lymph nodes, and few harvest at least six lymph nodes.[179]

Technical Aspects

Prior to any attempt at hepatic resection, a thorough assessment for systemic metastases and involvement of the distant nodal stations is mandatory. To evaluate the periaortic and pericaval lymph nodes and enable adequate exposure of the posterior pancreaticoduodenal space, a generous Kocher maneuver is required. The duodenum should be mobilized as far as to enable visualization of the left renal vein as it crosses the aorta. Careful palpation of the aortocaval space for abnormal lymph nodes, followed by sampling and frozen section analysis of macroscopically abnormal tissue, should ensue. This process should be repeated for lymph nodes along the celiac and superior mesenteric arteries. If involvement of distant lymph nodes is confirmed on frozen section analysis, resection of the primary should be abandoned.[129,139,151]

In the absence of distant lymph node involvement, regional lymphadenectomy should be performed in a methodical fashion. Technically, this consists of resecting all lymphatic tissue from the hepatoduodenal ligament (station 12). The portal vein and hepatic artery should be skeletonized and stripped of all lymphatic tissue medial to the common bile duct (station 8). This should be achieved in an en bloc fashion with resection of the extra-hepatic bile duct and involved hemiliver when indicated for hilar cholangiocarcinoma. For ICCs in the left liver, the lymphadenectomy should also include the nodes at the right cardia and lesser curvature (stations 1 and 3). For tumors in the right liver, it should include the retropancreatic nodes (station 13), which is facilitated by fully mobilizing the duodenum to enable exposure of these lymph node stations. In all cases, suspicious periaortic, pericaval, superior mesenteric artery, and celiac artery lymph nodes should be sampled. If positive for metastatic cancer, resection should be aborted (Fig. 6-9).

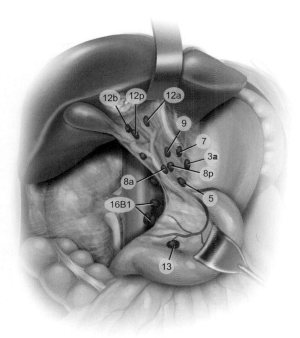

FIGURE 6-9 This illustration depicts the lymph node stations exposed via a Kocher maneuver. Portal lymph nodes consist of those in the hepatoduodenal ligament (station 12) and common hepatic artery (station 8). Lesser curve (station 3) and left gastric nodes (station 7) should be collected for left-sided tumors. Nodes behind the pancreatic head (station 13) can be involved for right-sided tumors. Celiac (station 9) and aortocaval (station 16) are markers of more advanced disease, typically precluding curative resection when positive.

In patients undergoing curative resection for perihilar cholangiocarcinoma (PHC), is caudate resection superior to caudate preservation with regard to improved margin clearance and overall survival (OS)?

INTRODUCTION

Surgical resection of PHC is challenging, in part owing to the tight anatomic boundaries and infiltrative growth pattern resulting in tumor growth to include intrahepatic biliary ducts and adjacent vascular structures. For the subgroup of patients who are eligible for curative surgical resection, surgery consists of en bloc hepatectomy with resection of the extrahepatic biliary tree and locoregional lymphadenectomy. Excision of the bile duct alone has been largely abandoned.

Margin-negative resection (R0) is the strongest prognostic factor following surgical resection, independent of stage.[103,129] Evidence suggests that patients who undergo a microscopically margin-positive resection (R1) have comparable survival to those who do not undergo surgery at all.[112] However, achieving an R0 resection in patients with PHC proves challenging given the frequent involvement of vascular structures in the porta hepatis as well as the extension along the biliary tree both proximally and distally. Additionally, some surgeons propose that routine resection of the caudate lobe (irrespective of obvious tumor involvement of the caudate duct) is a critical element in surgical resection of PHC.[180,181]

The biliary drainage of the caudate is highly variable but typically involves at least four bile ducts with a dominant left draining branch.[182,183] Owing to its anatomic location, the caudate is frequently involved in PHC, especially in Bismuth-Corlette IIIb and IV lesions. Retrospective series have demonstrated microscopic invasion of the caudate bile duct in 24% to 98% of patients with PHC.[180,184,185] Caudate lobe resection (CLR) is clearly justified when tumor involvement is suspected; however, in situations in which no obvious caudate lobe invasion exists, its role remains unclear. Several studies have suggested that routine CLR improves the likelihood of R0 resection.[129,186] Although technically feasible, resection of the caudate comes at added risk because of its close approximation to the inferior vena cava, the portal inflow, and middle and left hepatic veins. Currently, a robust synthesis of the data supporting routine resection of the caudate in patients with PHC does not exist. The purpose of this work was to evaluate whether routine CLR improves margin status and OS while considering postoperative morbidity in patients undergoing curative resection for PHC compared with caudate preservation.

METHODOLOGY

A systematic search of MEDLINE, EMBASE, and Cochrane databases was performed from inception to September 2019 using a predetermined search strategy. The protocol for this review was registered with the International Prospective Register of Systematic

Reviews (PROSPERO registration: 156145). The search strategy comprised Medical Subject Headings (MeSH) terms and keywords relevant to PHC, surgical resection for cholangiocarcinoma, and CLR, including "Klatskin tumor," "Cholangiocarcinoma," "Bile duct neoplasm," and "Hepatectomy."

No language restrictions were used. The reference list of each included publication was subsequently reviewed for omitted citations.

Eligible studies included adult patients with PHC undergoing curative intent surgery consisting of hepatectomy and resection of the extrahepatic bile duct. Studies that included patients undergoing isolated bile duct excision, exclusive of hepatectomy in the control group, were excluded from analysis. The intervention of interest was CLR in addition to en bloc hepatectomy and extrahepatic bile duct resection. The outcomes of interest were the proportion of patients achieving R0 resection and 5-year OS. Secondary outcomes included postoperative morbidity and mortality. Findings are reported in accordance with the Preferred Reporting Items for Systematic Reviews and Meta-Analyses (PRISMA).[187]

Both interventional (randomized control trials) and observational studies (prospective or retrospective cohort studies and cross-sectional studies) met inclusion criteria for abstract review. Case reports, case series with fewer than 20 patients, editorial letters, and review articles were excluded from analysis.

The initial search yielded 1,054 publications (Fig. 6-10). After 283 duplicates were removed, 771 abstracts were reviewed independently by two authors, of which 714 were excluded. Studies that passed the abstract review were retrieved for full-text review. Of these 57 studies, 51 were excluded because they were the wrong study design, wrong patient population, wrong comparator, or duplicate study population.

Two studies were performed on a similar patient cohort. Kow et al.[188] was a study of a subset of the patient cohort included in Song et al.[189] Kow et al.[188] was included in this review and Song et al.[189] was excluded, as the former had both a more comprehensive reporting of outcomes and a higher score when evaluated with the MINORS criteria (18 vs. 7).

Six studies were included in the qualitative systematic review (Table 6-6). Data extraction of the six articles was completed in duplicate by two authors using a preestablished data extraction form. Each article was reviewed and assigned a quality of evidence based on the Grading of Recommendations, Assessment, Development, and Evaluation (GRADE) system.[193,194]

Three of the studies (Cheng et al.,[190] Kow et al.,[188] Wahab et al.[192]) were considered of moderate grade of evidence, whereas three studies (Rea et al.,[191] Dinant et al.,[186] Nuzzo et al.[112]) were considered of low grade of evidence. Only Cheng et al.[190] reported prospectively collected data.

There were no randomized control trials included in the six studies. A total of 917 patients were included for analysis. The cohort size was variable, with two studies (Rea et al.,[191] Dinant et al.[186]) having under 100 patients, three studies having between 100 and 200 patients (Cheng et al.,[190] Kow et al.,[188] Wahab et al.[192]), and only one having greater than 300 patients (Nuzzo et al.[112]). The proportion of patients undergoing the intervention of interest was also variable across studies. In four studies, the majority of participants underwent CLR (Cheng et al.,[190] Kow et al.,[188] Nuzzo et al.,[112] Wahab et al.[192]).

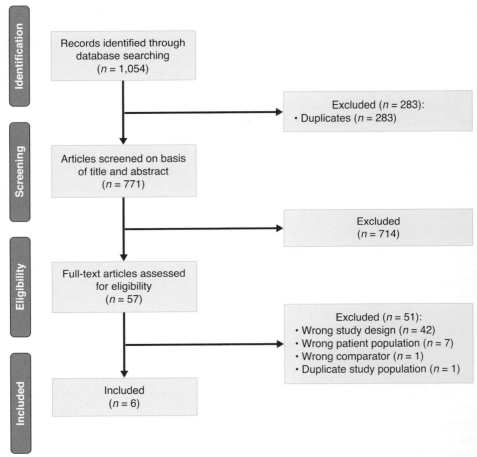

FIGURE 6-10   Preferred Reporting Items for Systematic Reviews and Meta-Analyses diagram for caudate resection in patients undergoing curative resection for perihilar cholangiocarcinoma.

FINDINGS

The characteristics of the included studies are presented in Table 6-6. Only three studies characterized the extent of tumor involvement, all using the Bismuth-Corlette classification (Rea et al.,[191] Cheng et al.,[190] Kow et al.[188]). Two studies limited the study population by Bismuth-Corlette class. Cheng et al.[190] included only patients with class III and class IV tumors, whereas Kow et al.[188] included only patients with class III tumors.

All studies reported the type of liver resection performed, with right and left hepatectomies comprising most cases in all studies. Preoperative biliary decompression was reported in four studies (Rea et al.,[191] Cheng et al.,[190] Kow et al.,[188] Wahab et al.[192]), with 42% to 76% of patients undergoing preoperative drainage. Other relevant perioperative variables were poorly reported across the included studies, with only two

TABLE 6-6   Studies Assessing R0 Resection and Overall Survival of Perihilar Cholangiocarcinoma in Patients Undergoing Liver Resection with or without Caudate Lobe Resection

Authors, Year	Country of Origin	Number of Patients	CLR, No. (%)	Type of Surgery, No. (%)	R0 Resection, No. (%)	Overall Survival, mo	5-Year Overall Survival, %	Grade of Evidence*
Cheng et al.,[190] 2012	China	171	137 (80.1)	Left hepatectomy 107 (62.6) Right hepatectomy 24 (14) Left trisegmentectomy 15 (8.8) Right trisegmentectomy 17 (9.9) Other 8 (4.7)	CLR 122 (89) No CLR 12 (35) $P < .01$	CLR median, 30 No CLR median, 17 $P < .01$	CLR 16 No CLR 6	+++
Dinant et al.,[186] 2006	Netherlands	38	15 (39.5)	Left hepatectomy 19 (50) Right hepatectomy 5 (13.2) Left trisegmentectomy — Right trisegmentectomy 14 (36.8) Uther —	CLR 10 (66.7) No CLR 5 (21.7) $P < .01$	CLR 44.3 No CLR 50 $P = NS$	NR	++
Kow et al.,[188] 2012	South Korea	127	70 (55.1)	Left hepatectomy 24 (18.9) Right hepatectomy 48 (37.8) Left trisegmentectomy 10 (7.9) Right trisegmentectomy 35 (27.6) Other 10 (7.9)	CLR 64 (91) No CLR 48 (84) $P = NS$	CLR median, 64 No CLR median, 34.6 $P < .01$	CLR 66 No CLR 30	+++

(continued)

TABLE 6-6   Studies Assessing R0 Resection and Overall Survival of Perihilar Cholangiocarcinoma in Patients Undergoing Liver Resection with or without Caudate Lobe Resection (continued)

Authors, Year	Country of Origin	Number of Patients	CLR, No. (%)	Type of Surgery, No. (%)	R0 Resection, No. (%)	Overall Survival, mo	5-Year Overall Survival, %	Grade of Evidence*
Nuzzo et al.,[112] 2012	Italy	376	293 (77.9)	Left hepatectomy 179 (47.6) Right hepatectomy 69 (18.4) Left trisegmentectomy 3 (0.8) Right trisegmentectomy 103 (27.4) Other 22 (5.9)	NR	CLR median, 24 No CLR median, 27 P = NR	CLR 26.3 No CLR 27.4	++
Rea et al.,[191] 2004	United States	46	18 (39.1)	Left hepatectomy 25 (54) Right hepatectomy 17 (37) Left trisegmentectomy — Right trisegmentectomy 4 (9) Other —	CLR 18 (100) No CLR 19 (67.9) P = NR	CLR 39 No CLR 21 P = NR	CLR 28 No CLR 25	++
Wahab et al.,[192] 2012	Egypt	159	80 (50.3)	Left hepatectomy 104 (65.4) Right hepatectomy 55 (34.6) Left trisegmentectomy — Right trisegmentectomy — Other —	CLR 57 (71) No CLR 30 (38) P = .001	CLR median, 39.8 No CLR median, 23.1 P < .001	CLR 28 No CLR 5	+++

CLR: caudate lobe resection; NR: not reported; NS: nonsignificant.
*Grade: ++ low; +++ moderate.

studies reporting preoperative portal vein embolization (Cheng et al.,[190] Kow et al.[188]), operative time (Kow et al.,[188] Wahab et al.[192]), and blood transfusion (Cheng et al.,[190] Wahab et al.[192]).

R0 Resection

All included studies, with the exception of Nuzzo et al.,[112] reported data on the proportion of patients achieving R0 resection in both the CLR and no CLR groups. The proportion of patients who had an R0 resection ranged from 66.7% through 100% in the CLR group as compared with 21.7% through 84% in the no CLR group (Table 6-6). Three studies reported a statistically significant increased likelihood of achieving an R0 resection in the patients who underwent CLR,[186,190,192] whereas in two studies, the difference failed to reach statistical significance.[188,191]

Survival

OS was reported by all included studies, with most studies conveying median OS (Table 6-6). The median OS ranged from 24 through 64 months to 17 through 50 months in the CLR and no CLR groups, respectively. Wahab et al.,[192] Cheng et al.,[190] and Kow et al.[188] all reported a statistically significantly improved survival in the cohort who underwent CLR. For example, Wahab et al.[192] reported on a cohort of 159 patients, with 50.3% having undergone CLR. The 5-year OS was 28% in those who had resection of the caudate as compared with 5% in those who did not. Both Cheng et al.[190] and Kow et al.[188] also reported statistically improved 5-year OS with CLR: 16% versus 6% and 66% versus 30%, respectively.[188,190] However, the largest study in this review, by Nuzzo et al.,[112] which included 376 patients, did not demonstrate any improvement in OS (24 vs. 27 months) or 5-year OS (26.3% vs. 27.4%).[112]

Perioperative Morbidity

Perioperative morbidity was inconsistently reported and was defined using discordant definitions. As a result, the proportion of patients who were reported as having had a complication ranged from 4.3% to 60% in the CLR group and 8.8% to 72.7% in the no CLR group. Of the four studies that described surgical complications, no study reported a statistically significant difference between patients undergoing CLR and those who did not.[186,188,190,192]

Perioperative complications felt to be potentially specific to CLR, including blood loss, bile leak, and liver failure, were examined, but data pertaining to any of these outcomes were reported in only two studies. Wahab et al.[192] demonstrated no significant difference between the CLR and no CLR groups in terms of rates of blood transfusions of more than 3 units (30.4% vs. 33.8%, respectively; P = NS). Wahab et al.[192] reported the proportion of patients developing a biliary leak was 6.3% of patients in both CLR and no CLR groups, whereas Kow et al.[188] reported bile leaks in 2.8% of patients who underwent CLR and no leaks in the group without CLR (P = NS). Incidence of liver failure was reported in only one study.[192] This study demonstrated that 15% of patients undergoing CLR developed postoperative liver failure, compared with 11.4% of patients who did not have CLR (P = NS).

Perioperative mortality was variably described in four studies, with both 30-day and 90-day mortality being reported.[186,188,190,192] The incidence of perioperative mortality in the CLR cohort was between 1% and 13.3%, whereas the incidence of mortality in the non-CLR cohort was between 4% and 27.3%. No studies reported a statistically significant difference between groups.

CONCLUSION

The results of this systematic review support routine caudate lobectomy in addition to hepatic resection and extrahepatic bile duct resection in the surgical management of PHC. Routine CLR appears to be associated with an increased likelihood of achieving an R0 resection and improved OS. Further studies are needed to specifically address the paucity of robust data pertaining to additive surgical morbidity associated with caudate resection in PHC.

A limitation of this systematic review is the lack of available high-quality, prospectively collected, randomized data comparing hepatic resection including the caudate with hepatic resection alone. This limitation is commonplace across the surgical literature owing to the scarcity of randomized controlled trials comparing different surgical techniques. Specifically, given the retrospective nature of the data, it is not possible to evaluate why an individual patient underwent caudate resection. It is plausible that many of the patients who underwent CLR may have had preoperative imaging findings that suggested involvement of the caudate biliary drainage, thereby necessitating a caudate resection. The high proportion of patients who underwent a left or extended left hepatectomy in the included studies suggests that the patient populations may have been already subselected to require a caudate resection.

In patients undergoing resection of perihilar cholangiocarcinoma (PHC), does intraoperative re-resection of positive margins based on frozen section analysis improve overall survival (OS) compared with clinical assessment of margins?

INTRODUCTION

PHC is an aggressive malignancy in which complete surgical resection with microscopic negative margins (R0) remains the best option for long-term OS and potential for cure. Although improvements in systemic therapy may have reduced the impact of surgical margins in some cancers, margin positivity remains a significant negative prognostic factor following resection for PHC.[195] Along with tumor grade, stage, vascular invasion, and lymph node involvement, positive margins remain a significant predictor of local recurrence and disease-free survival and OS.[196,197] Cholangiocarcinoma, especially the mass-forming and sclerosing/periductal infiltrating subtypes, is prone to extension along the bile duct and surrounding neural and lymphatic structures. This extension is difficult to assess on preoperative radiographic imaging. The periductal growth pattern poses significant challenges in both the pre- and intraoperative assessment of where to transect the duct and parenchyma and leads to significant rates of resections with positive microscopic (R1) margins. As a result, routine assessment of the proximal and distal duct margins intraoperatively by frozen section with the intent of further resection in the event of a positive margin to obtain complete tumor clearance has been proposed. However, interpretation of margins on frozen section is not always reliable, especially in the setting of biliary stents or previous cholangitis. Published series demonstrate low sensitivity (68% to 75%) and specificity (46% to 97%), with a false-negative rate of up to 16%, limiting its clinical effectiveness.[198,199] To add to this uncertainty, the outcome of patients with carcinoma in situ at the margin appears similar to patients with negative margins (R0) when compared with those with invasive cancer at the proximal margin.[200] Owing to the anatomic complexity of PHC, there are operative safety factors that limit wide tumor clearance and further bile duct resection, which could further reduce the size and function of the future liver remnant. Theoretically, the transection of the bile duct through areas with microscopic cancer invasion can disrupt the tumor plane, leading to potential dissemination as well. Thus, it is unclear if further resection in the event of an intraoperative positive margin has any oncologic benefit.

Owing to the relative rarity of PHC, large clinical experiences are limited to a relatively few centers internationally. Recent multicenter randomized trials of adjuvant therapy for biliary tract cancers have had either negative results (ACCORD-PRODIGE)[201] or very limited benefit (BILCAP),[30] placing a continued emphasis on the role of margins in PHC. However, no randomized trials exist specific to operative techniques and/or margin management in PHC. As such, the literature that guides the surgical management of PHC comprises retrospective single- and multicenter studies.

Despite this, a number of publications have addressed the issue of positive margins in PHC and specifically the outcomes of patients who had an upfront R0 resection compared with patients who had an R1 resection and with those who underwent further resection for an intraoperative positive margin. It bears mentioning that surgical risk implications are different for a positive proximal margin (requiring additional duct resection and sometimes parenchymal resection) as compared with a positive distal margin (requiring a pancreatoduodenectomy).

The purpose of this work was to evaluate whether intraoperative re-resection of positive margins based on frozen section analysis leads to superior OS in patients undergoing resection of PHC compared with clinical assessment of margins.

METHODOLOGY

A systematic search of the PubMed database was performed from inception to December 1, 2019, using a predetermined search strategy. This search strategy was composed of Medical Subject Headings (MeSH) terms and keywords relevant to PHC, surgical resection for cholangiocarcinoma, and margins. MeSH terms included "Klatskin tumor," "Cholangiocarcinoma," "Bile duct neoplasm," "Hepatectomy," "Margin," There were no language or date restrictions. The reference list of each included publication was subsequently reviewed for omitted citations. Findings are reported in accordance with the Preferred Reporting Items for Systematic Reviews and Meta-Analyses (PRISMA).[187]

The initial search generated 852 unique articles (Fig. 6-11). From this, 687 articles were excluded after preliminary review because they did not address the study question or because an abstract in English was not available. Full abstracts of 165 manuscripts were reviewed, after which 137 manuscripts were excluded as they did not address the question of interest. Twenty-eight full-text articles were reviewed, of which 21 were excluded for inadequate study design and for failing to report sufficient data on margin status and outcomes. Seven studies described the outcome of patients following R0 or R1 resection, as well as cases in which intraoperative revision of margins resulted in a secondary R0 margin, and therefore met all the criteria for inclusion in this systematic review (Table 6-7). The primary outcome assessed was OS. Each article was reviewed by and assigned a quality of evidence based on the Grading of Recommendations, Assessment, Development, and Evaluation (GRADE) system.[193,194] Overall, the quality of evidence ranged from very low to moderate.

FINDINGS

Distal Bile Duct Margin

In a Japanese cohort, Otsuka et al.[204] reported their experience focusing on the distal bile duct margin and the role of concomitant hepatic and pancreaticoduodenal resection. Over a 14-year experience (2001 to 2015), 74 out of 558 patients who had combined liver and bile duct resection had an initial positive margin in the operating room. Patients who underwent re-resection ($n = 53$) had superior outcomes compared with those who did not. However, the subset of patients who were not re-resected had a variety of adverse factors including positive proximal or radial margins, positive lymph

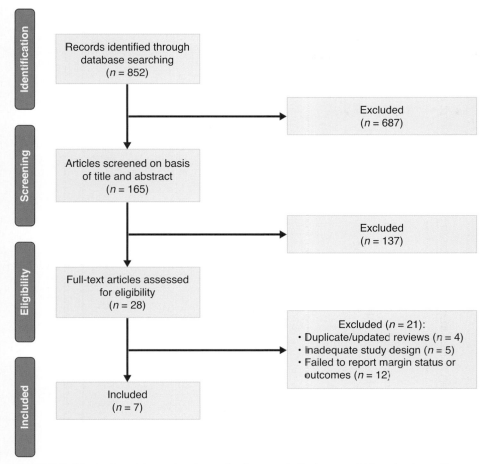

FIGURE 6-11 Preferred Reporting Items for Systematic Reviews and Meta-Analyses diagram for intraoperative re-resection of positive margins based on frozen section analysis in patients undergoing resection of perihilar cholangiocarcinoma.

nodes, or patient factors that discouraged further aggressive resection. Among patients with initial positive margins, negative lymph node status and additional resection (bile duct resection or pancreaticoduodenectomy) were associated with improved OS.

In a multicenter North American series by Zhang et al.,[207] patients who underwent re-resection and secondary R0 status had a median survival and 5-year OS of 30.6 months and 44%, respectively, which was comparable to patients with a primary R0 margin and superior to those with a final R1 margin. This series reported on patients with positive proximal margin ($n = 57$), distal margin ($n = 11$), and both ($n = 12$). Twenty-nine patients were rendered margin-negative following re-resection. However, in keeping with practice patterns in Western centers, combined hepatectomy and pancreaticoduodenectomy was rarely performed (3/29), and none (0/3) of these cases achieved a secondary R0 margin.

TABLE 6-7   Studies Assessing Proximal or Distal Margin Assessment with Frozen Section to Convert an R1 to R0 Resection

Authors, Year	Total Patients, No.	Margins Assessed	Initial Positive Margin n, No. (%)	Re-resection, No.	Secondary R0, no.	Final R1, No.	Overall Survival				Grade of Evidence*
							Outcome	Primary R0	Secondary R0	R1	
Endo et al.,[115] 2008	101	PD	20 (20)	15	9	19	Median 5-y	56 mo 43%	38 mo 18%†	32 mo	+
Lee et al.,[202] 2012	162	PD	37 (22.8)	15	6	31	3-y 5-y	55.5% 44.5%	—	39.5‡ 34.9	++
Ma et al.,[203] 2018	228	PD	44 (19.3)	37	21	23	Median	23 mo	21 mo	10.5 mo	++
Otsuka et al.,[204] 2019	558	DD	74 (13.3)	53	30	44	5-y	NR	38%	22%	+++
Ribero et al.,[205] 2011	67	PD	19 (28)	18	13	8	Median 5-y	29.3 mo 31%	30.6 mo 50%	14.9 mo 0%	+
Shingu et al.,[206] 2010	138	PD	17 (12)	12	8	20	3-y 5-y	56% 40%	0% 0%	39% 21%	+
Zhang et al.,[207] 2018	215	PD, DD	80 (37.2)	58	29	51	Median 5-y	22.3 mo 23.3%	30.6 mo 44.3%	18.5 mo 7.9%	+++

DD: distal bile duct; NR, not reported; PD: proximal bile duct.
*Grade: + very low; ++ low; +++ moderate.
†Included 19 patients with a negative intraoperative margin who had a positive margin on the specimen, referred to as "narrow" margin.
‡Patients with secondary R0 were included in R1 group for the survival analysis.

Proximal Bile Duct Margin

The role of re-resection of a proximal bile duct margin in patients with PHC has been specifically examined in retrospective series, with contrasting conclusions. Shingu et al.[206] reported the experience from Nagoya, Japan, examining outcomes in 303 patients, of whom 138 had undergone frozen section analysis with 28 patients having a positive margin (11 carcinoma in situ and 17 with invasive cancer). Twelve of the patients who were margin positive for invasive cancer underwent re-resection, and eight of these ultimately had R0 margins on final pathology. Of note, the additional margin that could be resected was less than 5 mm in all cases. In patients with a secondary R0 margin, the survival was similar to patients with a positive margin on final pathology who had not undergone re-resection and significantly worse than patients with a primary R0 margin or R1 with carcinoma in situ. These findings, in a very limited number of patients, led the investigators to conclude that additional resection of a positive proximal margin on frozen section was not associated with a survival benefit.

Endo et al.[115] described a single-center series of 101 patients who underwent resections for PHC, of whom 20 had a proximal bile duct margin that was positive or suspicious for invasive cancer on frozen section. Of this group, re-resection of the proximal margins was attempted in 15, and a secondary negative margin was achieved in 9 patients. Furthermore, of the 81 patients with negative intraoperative margins, 8 were found to be positive (false negative) on permanent section analysis. The authors then reported outcomes of patients according to the status of the intraoperative frozen section and the specimen margins. Fifty-four patients with negative intraoperative and specimen margins (wide R0) had a median survival of 56 months and 5-year OS of 43%. Twenty-eight patients with "narrow" margins included patients with a negative intraoperative margin but a positive specimen margin ($n = 19$) and patients who had a positive intraoperative margin that was revised to a secondary R0 margin ($n = 9$). The "narrow" margin group had a median and 5-year survival of 38 months and 18%, respectively, which was not statistically different from patients with a final R1 margin.

Contrary to the previous two studies, Ribero et al.[205] found that re-resection of positive proximal margins was associated with improved survival in their cohort of 75 patients who underwent resection for PHC. Of these, 67 patients eventually were classified as R0, with 54 patients having an initial R0 resection and 13 patients with a secondary R0 resection following margin re-resection in 18 patients. Patients with primary and secondary R0 resections had similar median survival (primary 29.3 months and secondary 30.6 months), which was significantly better than patients with R1 margins (14.9 months). Importantly, these investigators also evaluated the pattern of recurrence, given the theoretical potential of dissemination of cancer cells when cutting across a positive margin, and found patients with primary and secondary R0 resections had similar patterns of recurrence. An additional finding of this series, however, was that re-resection was associated with an increased biliary fistula rate (44.4% vs. 17.5%), highlighting the potential morbidity of chasing the frozen section margin.

Lee et al.[202] reported a series of 162 patients who underwent resection for PHC. Frozen section of the proximal bile duct margin showed 119 patients with negative margins (R0), 6 (4%) patients with carcinoma in situ, and 37 (22.8%) patients with invasive cancer at the margin, Re-excision was performed in 16 patients (15 with invasive cancer and 1 with carcinoma in situ), and a secondary negative margin was achieved in 7 (44%). In the survival analysis, patients with secondary R0 margins were analyzed with the R1 subgroup, and there were no significant differences in survival between patients with R0 and R1 resection status.

As noted above, a recent evaluation of a multicenter retrospective database by Zhang et al.[207] demonstrated an improved survival in those patients who had either primary or secondary R0 margins, which both were superior to patients with R1 margins. Importantly in this series, in which 58 patients underwent re-resection (including both proximal and distal margins), the incidence of biliary fistula (and other complications) was not increased as compared with patients who had not undergone margin re-resection.

Ma et al.[203] also recently reported outcomes for patients who had undergone re-resection of a positive proximal margin. Patients with a secondary R0 margin were found to be comparable to initial R0 patients (21 vs. 23 months), and both had superior outcomes compared with patients with an R1 margin (10.5 months).

Proximal and Distal Margins

Mantel et al.[198] reported their experience with analysis of surgical margins using intraoperative frozen section in 67 patients, of whom 17 (25%) had positive margins. Of patients with positive margins, 10 of 17 underwent margin revision, 3 of 10 achieved secondary R0, 1 patient had negative biliary margins on re-resection but had persistent radial margins, and 4 patients had persistent positive margins. Unfortunately, outcomes of patients with re-resection and secondary R0 were not reported.

CONCLUSION

Overall, series examining the outcome for patients following resection of a positive distal or proximal margin in the setting of resection for PHC are limited to small retrospective cohorts. The persistent negative effect of positive margin status in these series, and previous surgical series, coupled with the lack of highly active adjuvant therapies would suggest that frozen section evaluation of margins during resection of PHC, and re-resection if technically and safely feasible, is reasonable.

CHAPTER 17

Gallbladder Cancer

CRITICAL ELEMENTS

- Selective Staging Laparoscopy Prior to Resection of Gallbladder Cancer
- Microscopically Complete (R0) Resection of Local Tumor
- Routine Portal Lymphadenectomy, with Selective Sampling of Aortocaval and Retroperitoneal Nodes
- Port Site Excision Need Not Be Performed Routinely for Incidentally Discovered Gallbladder Cancer

1. SELECTIVE STAGING LAPAROSCOPY PRIOR TO RESECTION OF GALLBLADDER CANCER

Recommendation: Staging laparoscopy should be considered prior to definitive resection in selected patients in whom gallbladder cancer was identified incidentally at prior cholecystectomy. Staging laparoscopy should be performed routinely in patients with per primum gallbladder cancer to assess for radiographically occult metastatic disease prior to committing to oncologic resection. In either case, if metastatic disease is identified on exploration, resection should not be pursued.

Type of Data: Retrospective reports, case series, or case-control studies; prospective clinical trials

Strength of Recommendation: Strong recommendation, low-level evidence

Rationale

Because of its insidious onset, gallbladder cancer often presents with advanced disease that is not amenable to surgical resection. Additionally, lesions on the surface of the liver and smaller deposits of carcinomatosis are difficult to identify on preoperative

463

imaging computed tomography (CT), magnetic resonance imaging (MRI), and positron emission tomography (PET) scans. In general, detection of lesions smaller than 0.8 to 1 cm is challenging. Some studies report that, despite appropriate preoperative imaging, only 46% to 75% of patients undergoing surgery for hepatobiliary cancers have the potential for a curative resection, as many have occult disease identified at exploration that precludes rational resection.[208-214]

Staging laparoscopy is a useful modality to identify radiographically occult metastatic disease in various gastrointestinal malignancies. The identification of peritoneal or surface liver lesions using a minimally invasive approach can spare patients a nontherapeutic laparotomy. However, staging laparoscopy can often fail to identify small liver parenchymal tumors or nodal metastases, and it is not suitable to characterize local resectability. For these reasons, it is possible for a patient to undergo a "negative" staging laparoscopy despite lymph node metastasis or local disease extent that precludes safe resection at subsequent laparotomy.

Although there are benefits to the smaller incisions and fast recovery of staging laparoscopy, the addition of a second procedure does increase the time and cost of surgery, and it requires the use of additional operating room resources.[215] Furthermore, controversies exist as to whether staging laparoscopy should be performed on all patients, when it should ideally be performed (i.e., as a separate procedure or under the same anesthetic as the intended resection), and whether it should be used for patients in whom cancer was discovered incidentally in a prior cholecystectomy specimen. To optimize its value, staging laparoscopy would ideally be limited to patients most likely to harbor occult residual disease that would alter management if found prior to intended resection.

Incidental gallbladder cancer

In patients in whom gallbladder cancer was identified incidentally in a cholecystectomy specimen, the benefit of diagnostic laparoscopy has not been established. By definition, these patients have already undergone some degree of abdominal exploration, so the chances of identifying disease on subsequent staging laparoscopy may be low. Furthermore, adhesions from the prior cholecystectomy may hinder the ability to conduct a thorough staging procedure laparoscopically, especially if the index operation was performed via a subcostal incision owing to excessive inflammation.

Weber et al.[216] reported in 2002 that, although the yield and accuracy of staging laparoscopy prior to primary resection of gallbladder cancer was 56%, in patients having previously undergone cholecystectomy, the yield of staging laparoscopy was only 20%. This low yield of staging laparoscopy prior to definitive surgery for incidentally discovered lesions was confirmed in a study by Butte et al.[217] in which the yield of staging laparoscopy was only 4.3% (Table 6-8).

Given these data, use of staging laparoscopy in this setting should be selective based on the likelihood of occult metastatic or unresectable cancer. In 2007, a study by Pawlik et al.[220] found that nearly 60% of patients with incidentally discovered gallbladder cancer were found to have residual disease on subsequent exploration.

TABLE 6-8   Yield and Accuracy of Staging Laparoscopy for Hepatobiliary and Gallbladder Malignancy

Authors, Year	Years	Type of Gallbladder Cancer	Diagnostic Laparoscopy, No.	Yield* of SL	Accuracy† of SL for Unresectable Disease	Accuracy of SL for Detectable Lesions	Findings
Agarwal et al.,[218] 2013	2006–2011	Primary	409	95/409 (23%)	95/170 overall (56%)	95/101 94%	More patients with T1/T2 gallbladder cancer had higher rate of resectability, but there was no difference in the yield or accuracy of SL.
Butte et al.,[217] 2011	1998–2009	Incidental	46/136	2/46 (4.3%)	2/19%	—	SL at time of definitive resection in 45/46 patients Only T3 tumors were associate with + diagnostic laparoscopy. Multivariate analysis associated predictors of unresectable disease • Positive margins cholecystectomy • Poorly differentiated tumor
D'Angelica et al.,[219] 2003	1997–2001	Primary	50	50%	50/79 (63%)	—	Hepatobiliary series of 401 patients
Goere et al.,[210] 2006	2002–2004	Primary	8	5/8 (62%)	5/6 (83%)	—	Part of 39-patient study with biliary cancers
Vollmer et al.,[214] 2002	1996–1999	Primary	11	6/11 (55%)	6/12 (50%)	100%	Part of a series on hepatobiliary malignancies
Weber et al.,[216] 2002	1997–2001	Both	100	21/44 (48%)	21/36 (58%)	87.5%	Hepatobiliary series with 44 gallbladder malignancy

*Yield: number of patients detected to have unresectable disease via staging laparoscopy (SL) divided by number of patients undergoing SL.
†Accuracy: number of patients detected to have unresectable disease via SL divided by number of patients with unresectable disease.

Increasing T stage and the presence of a positive cystic duct margin were significantly associated with the identification of residual disease. Butte et al.[217] further evaluated patients found to have disseminated disease at the time of definitive surgery for gallbladder cancer and found that the likelihood of disseminated disease correlated with a positive cystic duct margin at cholecystectomy, T3 stage, and a poorly differentiated tumor. Of the 10 patients found to have disseminated disease, only 2 were diagnosed on laparoscopy.

In 2017, Ethun et al.[221] described a pathology-based preoperative risk score to define patients at increased risk of both locoregional and distant disease after discovery of incidental gallbladder cancer. Advanced T stage, grade, and presence of both lymphovascular and perineural invasion on the original gallbladder specimen were all associated with increased rates of persistent disease following cholecystectomy. Increased risk score was associated not only with increased likelihood of finding locoregional and distant disease but also with a short duration of overall survival.[221] Although not yet validated, a risk score may be a useful tool to improve selection of patients with incidental gallbladder cancer for staging laparoscopy prior to definitive surgery.

Per primum gallbladder cancer

Gallbladder cancer is known to spread frequently to peritoneal surfaces, the liver, and locoregional and distant lymph nodes with nontherapeutic surgical exploration in 38% to 62% of patients.[210] Although there are limits to the detection of distant lymph nodes and local unresectability, staging laparoscopy can detect between 17% and 55% of distant lesions, thereby preventing nontherapeutic laparotomy in many patients (Table 6-8).[214,216,218,222] Some attempts have been made to define patients most likely to have detectable lesions at the time of diagnostic laparoscopy, such as those with locally advanced tumors, a high level of bilirubin or carbohydrate antigen 19-9, or a low level of albumin. However, staging laparoscopy is currently recommended prior to definitive oncologic resection for all patients with per primum gallbladder cancer. This recommendation is consistent with both the 2014 American Hepato-Pancreato-Biliary Association Consensus Statement for Gallbladder Cancer and the National Comprehensive Cancer Network Guidelines for Gallbladder Cancer.[12,223]

Technical Aspects

Access to the abdomen should be obtained via either an optical trocar peritoneal entry into the left upper quadrant or a periumbilical Hasson or Veress technique. The abdomen should be insufflated with carbon dioxide, and a 30° scope should be introduced into the abdomen. In order to get a thorough exploration and to facilitate biopsies, a second 5-mm port may be placed. The four quadrants of the abdomen and pelvis should be thoroughly explored. Both diaphragms, the undersurface of the liver, the omentum, and serosal surfaces of the abdominal organs should be diligently inspected (Fig. 6-12). Any suspicious nodules should be biopsied and sent for immediate histopathologic analysis. Definitive surgical resection should be aborted if a positive frozen section reveals metastatic disease.

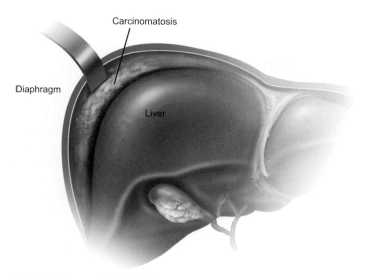

FIGURE 6-12 The field of inspection during laparoscopy for gallbladder cancer includes the diaphragm and liver surface where peritoneal spread for carcinomatosis can be found.

2. MICROSCOPICALLY COMPLETE (R0) RESECTION OF LOCAL TUMOR

Recommendation: Resection of per primum gallbladder cancer should be performed by resection of the gallbladder en bloc with either formal IVb and V segmentectomy or wedge resection of the tumor-bearing liver. For gallbladder cancer incidentally identified in a cholecystectomy specimen, re-resection is not justified for patients with Tis and T1a disease in whom cystic duct margin is negative. For patients with T1b or greater disease, either wedge resection of the gallbladder bed or formal IVb and V segmentectomy is indicated. In all cases, a microscopically complete (R0) resection should be sought. The cystic duct margin should be sent for intraoperative assessment of involvement by carcinoma. Routine common bile duct excision should not be performed unless necessary to achieve an R0 resection.

Type of Data: Retrospective reports, case series, or case-control studies; prospective clinical trials

Strength of Recommendation: Moderate recommendation, low-quality evidence

Rationale

Patients in whom Tis or T1a gallbladder cancer was discovered incidentally in a cholecystectomy specimen and in whom the cystic duct margin is negative have been definitively treated with simple cholecystectomy alone, and radical re-resection is not justified.[224,225]

However, multiple retrospective analyses have demonstrated an improvement in 5-year overall survival following re-resection of T2 gallbladder cancer relative to cholecystectomy alone.[224] For patients with T1b tumors or greater, radical re-resection should be routinely performed, as the evidence suggests patients with T1b tumors may have an incidence of residual disease similar to that of patients with T2 tumors.[12,225,226] The frequency of residual disease identified at radical re-resection increases with advanced T stages (T1: 30%, T2: 61%, T3: 85%, T4: 100%).[11] For patients with gallbladder cancers found incidentally following cholecystectomy for benign diagnoses, a scenario representative of roughly 60% of all gallbladder cancer cases, there does not appear to be any survival difference between patients who are discovered to have cancer intraoperatively and are immediately converted to an open radical resection and patients who are discovered to have cancer following histopathologic analysis of the surgical specimen and are taken for a re-resection at a later date.[226]

Anatomic IVb and V segmentectomy versus wedge resection of the gallbladder bed

In a retrospective analysis of extent of resection for adenocarcinoma of the gallbladder, D'Angelica et al.[227] demonstrated no significant difference in survival outcomes between patients who underwent a "major hepatectomy" versus those who did not. However, a microscopically complete (R0) resection has been demonstrated in multiple studies to be significantly associated with improved survival.[12,220,228,229] Therefore, for both re-resection after incidentally discovered gallbladder cancer and for per primum gallbladder cancer, a wedge resection of the gallbladder bed or a formal anatomic segmentectomy of IVb and V are both acceptable surgical strategies, as long as an R0 resection is obtained. If a wedge resection is performed, it has been recommended that the hepatic resection margin width should measure approximately 2 to 3 cm intraoperatively, but there is no universal consensus or specific data to support this recommendation.[230]

Bile duct resection

In a retrospective analysis of the extent of resection that should be performed for adenocarcinoma of the gallbladder, D'Angelica et al.[227] demonstrated no significant difference in survival outcomes between those patients who underwent common bile duct excision versus those who did not. A similar analysis was performed by Shih et al.,[226] who compared those patients who underwent hepatic resection and lymphadenectomy with or without "biliary tree resection." No significant difference in survival was found between the two cohorts.[226] Gani et al.[231] performed a retrospective analysis of 449 gallbladder cancer patients and found that those who underwent excision of the common bile duct had shorter survival than those who did not. However, after controlling for confounding variables such as margin status, presence of lymph node metastasis, and T stage, the authors concluded that bile duct excision did not affect overall survival. Rather, the presence of disease at the surgical margin (R1/2 resection) was independently associated with shorter overall survival (hazard ratio [HR], 3.11; 95% confidence interval [CI], 1.22 to 7.96; $P = .010$). Pawlik et al.[220] arrived at similar conclusions and suggested that bile duct excision should be performed only when it is necessary to achieve an R0 resection.[12,220,231]

It has previously been argued that excision of the common bile duct may be beneficial, regardless of cystic duct margin status, because it may allow more complete lymph node collection. However, multiple studies have now been published that suggest that bile duct excision has no impact on the number of lymph nodes harvested.[12,227,231] Importantly, studies have demonstrated that common bile duct excision is associated with increase in postoperative complications (60% vs. 23%, $P = .0001$, in one study). D'Angelica et al.[227] even estimated a 33% incidence of grade 3 or 4 morbidity in patients who underwent bile duct excision and reconstruction.

In contrast, cystic duct margin status does appear to be a reliable predictor of residual disease in the common bile duct (negative cystic duct 4.3% vs. positive cystic duct 42.1%; $P = .01$).[220] Therefore, to the extent that an R0 resection should be sought in all cases conducted with curative intent, a positive intraoperative cystic duct margin, either on the initial cholecystectomy specimen or on intraoperative biopsy of the cystic duct stump during an operation for per primum gallbladder cancer, indicates a common bile duct excision is warranted.[220,227,232] In cases of both re-resection for incidentally discovered gallbladder cancer or elective extended cholecystectomies for per primum gallbladder cancer, the cystic duct margin should be sent for intraoperative assessment of involvement by carcinoma. If the cystic duct margin is negative for cancer, no common bile duct excision is required.

Technical Aspects

The extent of hepatectomy should be marked on the liver surface using cautery and intraoperative ultrasound. Regardless of the extent, the entire cystic plate to the level of the hilar plate should be included. If a formal IVb/V hepatectomy is planned, the boundaries should span from the umbilical fissure to the most distal aspect of the right hepatic vein. The cranial border of the resection should be determined by ultrasound to encompass the vasculobiliary pedicles to segments IVb/V. The liver parenchyma should then be divided by the surgeon's method of choice, again with the goal of an adequate margin of tissue around the tumor.

3. ROUTINE PORTAL LYMPHADENECTOMY, WITH SELECTIVE SAMPLING OF AORTOCAVAL AND RETROPERITONEAL NODES

Recommendation: Lymphadenectomy comprising the nodes in the hepatoduodenal ligament (12) along the common hepatic artery (8) and behind the pancreas (13) should be routinely performed. Selective sampling of lymph nodes in the aortocaval space (16) should be performed if there is clinical suspicion. An attempt should be made to ensure three to six nodes in the specimen for staging purposes.

Type of Data: Retrospective reports, case series, or case-control studies; prospective clinical trials

Strength of Recommendation: Moderate recommendation, low-quality evidence

Rationale

Among all patients with gallbladder cancer, those with lymph node metastasis have an increased risk of disease recurrence (HR, 2.28; 95% CI, 1.37 to 3.80; $P = .002$) and death (HR, 1.87; 95% CI, 1.24 to 2.82; $P = .003$). The rate of lymph node metastases increases with increasing T stage (T1a, <2.5%; T1b, 12.5%; T2, 31.3%; T3, 45.5%).[220,224,230]

In a 2009 study of T1b and T2 gallbladder cancers conducted using the Surveillance, Epidemiology, and End Results database, patients who underwent radical resection plus lymphadenectomy lived longer than those who underwent radical resection alone.[233] Therefore, performance of a lymph node dissection during radical cholecystectomy has become standard of care. In a large study of patients who underwent operative treatment of T1b and beyond gallbladder cancer who underwent radical resections, pathologic evaluation of at least one lymph node was associated with a significant improvement in median overall survival compared with evaluation of zero lymph nodes (T1b and T2: 123 vs. 22 months, $P < .0001$; T3: 12 vs. 7 months, $P = .014$). Additionally, radical resection without lymph node evaluation was associated with similar overall survival as cholecystectomy alone (T1b and T2: 22 vs. 23 months, $P = $ NS; T3: 7 vs. 6 months, $P = $ NS).[234] Downing et al.[235] demonstrated that resection of five or more lymph nodes was associated with a survival benefit over resection of one to four lymph nodes, and that resection of one to four lymph nodes was associated with a survival benefit over having no lymphadenectomy. Mayo et al.[236] found that lymphadenectomy with resection of three or more nodes was independently associated with increased survival.

However, consensus around the extent of adequate lymphadenectomy for gallbladder cancer does not exist. Although the American Joint Committee on Cancer (*AJCC*) *Cancer Staging Manual*, Sixth Edition, stated that more than three lymph nodes are required to adequately determine the N stage, this point was deleted in the seventh edition.[230,237,238] Despite lack of consensus guidelines, many surgeons advocate that adequate lymphadenectomy includes assessment of any suspicious regional nodes, evaluation of the aortocaval nodal basin, and a goal recovery of at least three to six nodes for pathologic examination.[12,230]

A point of clarification is that the *AJCC Cancer Staging Manual*, Sixth Edition, defines regional group 1 (N1) as comprising the cystic duct lymph node, common bile duct lymph node, and lymph nodes around the hepatoduodenal ligament (hepatic artery lymph node and portal vein lymph node).[237] In contrast, the posterior pancreaticoduodenal lymph node, celiac artery lymph node, superior mesenteric artery lymph node, para-aortic lymph node, and pericaval lymph node are classified as belonging to regional lymph node group 2 (N2).[230] Involvement of the N2 nodal basins with disease should be interpreted as indicating distant metastasis: patients with confirmed metastases to the N2 nodal stations do not benefit from radical resection and should receive systemic and/or palliative treatments, not surgery.[12,230] This recommendation is clarified in the *AJCC Cancer Staging Manual*, Eighth Edition, wherein N1 disease denotes one to three positive lymph nodes, N2 denotes four or more positive nodes, and positive lymph nodes in the celiac and para-aortic regions confer a diagnosis of distant metastatic disease.[3]

Technical Aspects

Portal lymphadenectomy should begin with mobilization of the duodenum via a generous Kocher maneuver. This allows for exposure of the entire bile duct in the porta hepatis. This should be followed by palpation of the aortocaval space for distant nodal metastases (station 16). If metastasis to this station is confirmed, the remainder of the procedure should be aborted. Retroportal and retropancreatic lymphadenectomy should be performed (station 13). Next, all lymphatic tissue from the hepatoduodenal ligament (station 12) should be harvested. The portal vein and hepatic artery should be skeletonized and stripped of all lymphatic tissue medial to the common bile duct (station 8).

4. PORT SITE EXCISION NEED NOT BE PERFORMED ROUTINELY FOR INCIDENTALLY DISCOVERED GALLBLADDER CANCER

Recommendation: Routine excision of port sites during curative reoperation for incidentally discovered gallbladder cancer does not add a survival benefit and should be avoided.

Type of Data: Retrospective reports, case series, or case-control studies

Strength of Recommendation: Strong recommendation, low-quality evidence

Rationale

Most gallbladder cancers are discovered incidentally after cholecystectomy performed for presumed benign disease. As minimally invasive cholecystectomy techniques began to supplant the traditional open approach, seeding of trocar sites during the index operation was a concern. The first review of data during this early period of minimally invasive cholecystectomy suggested a port site metastasis rate of up to 30%.[239] Recent review suggests this rate has decreased to 10%, with the extraction site being the most commonly implanted.[240] However, it was unknown if routine port site excision (PSE), given these high metastatic rates, would affect survival, or if the presence of port site metastasis was simply a poor prognostic indicator. The Memorial Sloan Kettering group attempted to answer this question in a retrospective review of 113 patients treated at their institution between 1992 and 2009, 69 (61%) of whom underwent PSE. After adjusting for R0 resection, T stage, and N stage of tumor, a PSE was not associated with a difference in overall survival.[241] They concluded that port site metastasis was likely a marker of disseminated peritoneal disease and routine PSE should not be performed. Two multi-institutional retrospective reviews followed this report and had similar findings. In 2013, a French consortium reported their results of 148 patients with incidentally discovered gallbladder cancer who underwent re-resection, 54 with concomitant PSE, from 1998 through 2008. They found no difference in 1-, 3-, or 5-year overall survival but did report a 15% incisional hernia rate associated with PSE.[242] This study was followed by a similar 2017 US consortium report of 193 patients undergoing re-resection, 47 with concomitant PSE, from 2000 through 2015. These authors found only tumor grade and T stage were associated with decreased overall survival on multivariate analysis, again suggesting routine PSE has no impact on overall survival.[243] Although port site metastasis may occur in up to 10% of patients with incidentally discovered gallbladder cancer, routine resection of these port sites is not likely to affect overall survival and should not be performed.

REFERENCES

1. Vatandoust S, Price TJ, Karapetis CS. Colorectal cancer: metastases to a single organ. *World J Gastroenterol.* 2015;21(41):11767-11776. doi:10.3748/wjg.v21.i41.11767
2. Tzeng CD, Aloia TA. Colorectal liver metastases. *J Gastrointest Surg.* 2013;17(1):195-202. doi:10.1007/s11605-012-2022-3
3. Amin MB, Edge SB, Green FL, et al. *AJCC Cancer Staging Manual.* 8th ed. Springer; 2017.
4. Melstrom LG, Tzeng CD. Metastatic colorectal cancer: the reality of the present and the optimism of the future. *J Surg Oncol.* 2019;119(5):547-548. doi:10.1002/jso.25427
5. Forner A, Llovet JM, Bruix J. Hepatocellular carcinoma. *Lancet.* 2012;379(9822):1245-1255. doi:10.1016/S0140-6736(11)61347-0
6. Llovet JM, Schwartz M, Mazzaferro V. Resection and liver transplantation for hepatocellular carcinoma. *Semin Liver Dis.* 2005;25(2):181-200. doi:10.1055/s-2005-871198
7. Vogl TJ, Schwarz WO, Heller M, et al. Staging of Klatskin tumours (hilar cholangiocarcinomas): comparison of MR cholangiography, MR imaging, and endoscopic retrograde cholangiography. *Eur Radiol.* 2006;16(10):2317-2325. doi:10.1007/s00330-005-0139-4
8. Saha SK, Zhu AX, Fuchs CS, Brooks GA. Forty-year trends in cholangiocarcinoma incidence in the U.S.: intrahepatic disease on the rise. *Oncologist.* 2016;21(5):594-599. doi:10.1634/theoncologist.2015-0446
9. Tyson GL, El-Serag HB. Risk factors for cholangiocarcinoma. *Hepatology.* 2011;54(1):173-184. doi:10.1002/hep.24351
10. Hsing AW, Gao YT, Han TQ, et al. Gallstones and the risk of biliary tract cancer: a population-based study in China. *Br J Cancer.* 2007;97(11):1577-1582. doi:10.1038/sj.bjc.6604047
11. Duffy A, Capanu M, Abou-Alfa GK, et al. Gallbladder cancer (GBC): 10-year experience at Memorial Sloan-Kettering Cancer Centre (MSKCC). *J Surg Oncol.* 2008;98(7):485-489. doi:10.1002/jso.21141
12. Aloia TA, Járufe N, Javle M, et al. Gallbladder cancer: expert consensus statement. *HPB (Oxford).* 2015;17(8):681-690. doi:10.1111/hpb.12444
13. Fong Y, Fortner J, Sun RL, Brennan MF, Blumgart LH. Clinical score for predicting recurrence after hepatic resection for metastatic colorectal cancer: analysis of 1001 consecutive cases. *Ann Surg.* 1999;230(3):309-321. doi:10.1097/00000658-199909000-00004
14. Brudvik KW, Jones RP, Giuliante F, et al. RAS mutation clinical risk score to predict survival after resection of colorectal liver metastases. *Ann Surg.* 2019;269(1):120-126. doi:10.1097/SLA.0000000000002319
15. Kopetz S, Chang GJ, Overman MJ, et al. Improved survival in metastatic colorectal cancer is associated with adoption of hepatic resection and improved chemotherapy. *J Clin Oncol.* 2009;27(22):3677-3683. doi:10.1200/JCO.2008.20.5278
16. Nordlinger B, Sorbye H, Glimelius B, et al. Perioperative chemotherapy with FOLFOX4 and surgery versus surgery alone for resectable liver metastases from colorectal cancer (EORTC Intergroup Trial 40983): a randomised controlled trial. *Lancet.* 2008;371(9617):1007-1016. doi:10.1016/S0140-6736(08)60455-9
17. Sorbye H, Mauer M, Gruenberger T, et al. Predictive factors for the benefit of perioperative FOLFOX for resectable liver metastasis in colorectal cancer patients (EORTC Intergroup Trial 40983). *Ann Surg.* 2012;255(3):534-539. doi:10.1097/SLA.0b013e3182456aa2
18. Shindoh J, Tzeng CD, Aloia TA, et al. Portal vein embolization improves rate of resection of extensive colorectal liver metastases without worsening survival. *Br J Surg.* 2013;100(13):1777-1783. doi:10.1002/bjs.9317
19. Shindoh J, Truty MJ, Aloia TA, et al. Kinetic growth rate after portal vein embolization predicts posthepatectomy outcomes: toward zero liver-related mortality in patients with colorectal liver metastases and small future liver remnant. *J Am Coll Surg.* 2013;216(2):201-209. doi:10.1016/j.jamcollsurg.2012.10.018
20. Torzilli G, Nagino M, Tzeng CD, et al. SSAT State-of-the-Art Conference: new frontiers in liver surgery. *J Gastrointest Surg.* 2017;21(1):175-185. doi:10.1007/s11605-016-3193-0

21. Fessas P, Kaseb A, Wang Y, et al. Post-registration experience of nivolumab in advanced hepatocellular carcinoma: an international study. *J Immunother Cancer*. 2020;8(2):e001033. doi:10.1136/jitc-2020-001033

22. Demir T, Lee SS, Kaseb AO. Systemic therapy of liver cancer. *Adv Cancer Res*. 2021;149:257-294. doi:10.1016/bs.acr.2020.12.001

23. Finn RS, Qin S, Ikeda M, et al. Atezolizumab plus bevacizumab in unresectable hepatocellular carcinoma. *N Engl J Med*. 2020;382(20):1894-1905. doi:10.1056/NEJMoa1915745

24. Rea DJ, Heimbach JK, Rosen CB, et al. Liver transplantation with neoadjuvant chemoradiation is more effective than resection for hilar cholangiocarcinoma. *Ann Surg*. 2005;242(3):451-461. doi:10.1097/01.sla.0000179678.13285.fa

25. Kipp BR, Stadheim LM, Halling SA, et al. A comparison of routine cytology and fluorescence in situ hybridization for the detection of malignant bile duct strictures. *Am J Gastroenterol*. 2004;99(9):1675-1681. doi:10.1111/j.1572-0241.2004.30281.x

26. Rosen CB, Darwish Murad S, Heimbach JK, Nyberg SL, Nagorney DM, Gores GJ. Neoadjuvant therapy and liver transplantation for hilar cholangiocarcinoma: is pretreatment pathological confirmation of diagnosis necessary? *J Am Coll Surg*. 2012;215(1):31-40. doi:10.1016/j.jamcollsurg.2012.03.014

27. Rahnemai-Azar AA, Pawlik TM. Cholangiocarcinoma: shedding light on the most promising drugs in clinical development. *Expert Opin Investig Drugs*. 2021;30(4):419-427. doi:10.1080/13543784.2021.1897103

28. DiPeri TP, Javle MM, Meric-Bernstam F. Next generation sequencing for biliary tract cancers. *Expert Rev Gastroenterol Hepatol*. 2021;15(5):471-474. doi:10.1080/17474124.2021.1896967

29. Akateh C, Ejaz AM, Pawlik TM, Cloyd JM. Neoadjuvant treatment strategies for intrahepatic cholangiocarcinoma. *World J Hepatol*. 2020;12(10):693-708 doi:10.4254/wjh.v12.i10.693

30. Primrose JN, Fox RP, Palmer DH, et al. Capecitabine compared with observation in resected biliary tract cancer (BILCAP): a randomised, controlled, multicentre, phase 3 study. *Lancet Oncol*. 2019;20(5):663-673. doi:10.1016/S1470-2045(18)30915-X

31. Ben-Josef E, Guthrie KA, El-Khoueiry AB, et al. SWOG S0809: a phase II intergroup trial of adjuvant capecitabine and gemcitabine followed by radiotherapy and concurrent capecitabine in extrahepatic cholangiocarcinoma and gallbladder carcinoma. *J Clin Oncol*. 2015;33(24):2617-2622. doi:10.1200/JCO.2014.60.2219

32. Tzeng CD, Fleming JB, Lee JE, et al. Defined clinical classifications are associated with outcome of patients with anatomically resectable pancreatic adenocarcinoma treated with neoadjuvant therapy. *Ann Surg Oncol*. 2012;19(6):2045-2053. doi:10.1245/s10434-011-2211-4

33. Isaji S, Mizuno S, Windsor JA, et al. International consensus on definition and criteria of borderline resectable pancreatic ductal adenocarcinoma 2017. *Pancreatology*. 2018;18(1):2-11. doi:10.1016/j.pan.2017.11.011

34. Ribero D, Abdalla EK, Madoff DC, Donadon M, Loyer EM, Vauthey JN. Portal vein embolization before major hepatectomy and its effects on regeneration, resectability and outcome. *Br J Surg*. 2007;94(11):1386-1394. doi:10.1002/bjs.5836

35. Abdalla EK, Denys A, Chevalier P, Nemr RA, Vauthey JN. Total and segmental liver volume variations: implications for liver surgery. *Surgery*. 2004;135(4):404-410. doi:10.1016/j.surg.2003.08.024

36. Vauthey JN, Pawlik TM, Ribero D, et al. Chemotherapy regimen predicts steatohepatitis and an increase in 90-day mortality after surgery for hepatic colorectal metastases. *J Clin Oncol*. 2006;24(13):2065-2072. doi:10.1200/JCO.2005.05.3074

37. Creasy JM, Sadot E, Koerkamp BG, et al. Actual 10-year survival after hepatic resection of colorectal liver metastases: what factors preclude cure? *Surgery*. 2018;163(6):1238-1244. doi:10.1016/j.surg.2018.01.004

38. Berzigotti A, Reig M, Abraldes JG, Bosch J, Bruix J. Portal hypertension and the outcome of surgery for hepatocellular carcinoma in compensated cirrhosis: a systematic review and meta-analysis. *Hepatology*. 2015;61(2):526-536. doi:10.1002/hep.27431

39. Abdalla EK, Barnett CC, Doherty D, Curley SA, Vauthey JN. Extended hepatectomy in patients with hepatobiliary malignancies with and without preoperative portal vein embolization. *Arch Surg*. 2002;137(6):675-681. doi:10.1001/archsurg.137.6.675

40. Mullen JT, Ribero D, Reddy SK, et al. Hepatic insufficiency and mortality in 1,059 noncirrhotic patients undergoing major hepatectomy. *J Am Coll Surg*. 2007;204(5):854-864.

41. Farges O, Regimbeau JM, Fuks D, et al. Multicentre European study of preoperative biliary drainage for hilar cholangiocarcinoma. *Br J Surg*. 2013;100(2):274-283. doi:10.1002/bjs.8950

42. Hochwald SN, Burke EC, Jarnagin WR, Fong Y, Blumgart LH. Association of preoperative biliary stenting with increased postoperative infectious complications in proximal cholangiocarcinoma. *Arch Surg.* 1999;134(3):261-266. doi:10.1001/archsurg.134.3.261

43. Kawakami H, Kondo S, Kuwatani M, et al. Preoperative biliary drainage for hilar cholangiocarcinoma: which stent should be selected? *J Hepatobiliary Pancreat Sci.* 2011;18(5):630-635. doi:10.1007/s00534-011-0404-7

44. Ethun CG, Postlewait LM, Le N, et al. Association of optimal time interval to re-resection for incidental gallbladder cancer with overall survival: a multi-institution analysis from the US extrahepatic biliary malignancy consortium. *JAMA Surg.* 2017;152(2):143-149. doi:10.1001/jamasurg.2016.3642

45. Day RW, Brudvik KW, Vauthey JN, et al. Advances in hepatectomy technique: toward zero transfusions in the modern era of liver surgery. *Surgery.* 2016;159(3):793-801. doi:10.1016/j.surg.2015.10.006

46. Aloia TA, Zorzi D, Abdalla EK, Vauthey JN. Two-surgeon technique for hepatic parenchymal transection of the noncirrhotic liver using saline-linked cautery and ultrasonic dissection. *Ann Surg.* 2005;242(2):172-177. doi:10.1097/01.sla.0000171300.62318.f4

47. Moggia E, Rouse B, Simillis C, et al. Methods to decrease blood loss during liver resection: a network meta-analysis. *Cochrane Database Syst Rev.* 2016;10(10):CD010683. doi:10.1002/14651858.CD010683.pub3

48. Correa-Gallego C, Berman A, Denis SC, et al. Renal function after low central venous pressure-assisted liver resection: assessment of 2116 cases. *HPB (Oxford).* 2015;17(3):258-264. doi:10.1111/hpb.12347

49. Correa-Gallego C, Tan KS, Arslan-Carlon V, et al. Goal-directed fluid therapy using stroke volume variation for resuscitation after low central venous pressure-assisted liver resection: a randomized clinical trial. *J Am Coll Surg.* 2015;221(2):591-601. doi:10.1016/j.jamcollsurg.2015.03.050

50. Zimmitti G, Vauthey JN, Shindoh J, et al. Systematic use of an intraoperative air leak test at the time of major liver resection reduces the rate of postoperative biliary complications. *J Am Coll Surg.* 2013;217(6):1028-1037. doi:10.1016/j.jamcollsurg.2013.07.392

51. Kemp Bohan PM, O'Shea AE, Lee AJ, et al. Lymph node sampling in resectable hepatocellular carcinoma: national practice patterns and predictors of positive lymph nodes. *Surg Oncol.* 2021;36:138-146. doi:10.1016/j.suronc.2020.12.011

52. Kemp Bohan PM, O'Shea AE, Ellis OV, et al. Rates, predictors, and outcomes of portal lymphadenectomy for resectable gallbladder cancer. *Ann Surg Oncol.* 2021;28(6):2960-2972. doi:10.1245/s10434-021-09667-8

53. Lee AJ, Chiang YJ, Lee JE, et al. Validation of American Joint Committee on Cancer eighth staging system for gallbladder cancer and its lymphadenectomy guidelines. *J Surg Res.* 2018;230:148-154. doi:10.1016/j.jss.2018.04.067

54. Bagante F, Spolverato G, Weiss M, et al. Assessment of the lymph node status in patients undergoing liver resection for intrahepatic cholangiocarcinoma: the New Eighth Edition AJCC Staging System. *J Gastrointest Surg.* 2018;22(1):52-59. doi:10.1007/s11605-017-3426-x

55. Zhang XF, Xue F, Dong DH, et al. Number and station of lymph node metastasis after curative—intent resection of intrahepatic cholangiocarcinoma impact prognosis. *Ann Surg.* Published online January 14, 2020. doi:10.1097/SLA.0000000000003788

56. Bagante F, Tran T, Spolverato G, et al. Perihilar cholangiocarcinoma: number of nodes examined and optimal lymph node prognostic scheme. *J Am Coll Surg.* 2016;222(5):750-759.e2. doi:10.1016/j.jamcollsurg.2016.02.012

57. Bickenbach KA, Dematteo RP, Fong Y, et al. Risk of occult irresectable disease at liver resection for hepatic colorectal cancer metastases: a contemporary analysis. *Ann Surg Oncol.* 2013;20(6):2029-2034. doi:10.1245/s10434-012-2813-5

58. Hariharan D, Constantinides V, Kocher HM, Tekkis PP. The role of laparoscopy and laparoscopic ultrasound in the preoperative staging of patients with resectable colorectal liver metastases: a meta-analysis. *Am J Surg.* 2012;204(1):84-92. doi:10.1016/j.amjsurg.2011.07.018

59. Quenet F, Elias D, Roca L, et al. A UNICANCER phase III trial of hyperthermic intra-peritoneal chemotherapy (HIPEC) for colorectal peritoneal carcinomatosis (PC): PRODIGE 7. *J Clin Oncol.* 2018;36(18 suppl):LBA3503-LBA3503.

60. Verwaal VJ, Bruin S, Boot H, van Slooten G, van Tinteren H. 8-Year follow-up of randomized trial: cytoreduction and hyperthermic intraperitoneal chemotherapy versus systemic chemotherapy in patients with peritoneal carcinomatosis of colorectal cancer. *Ann Surg Oncol.* 2008;15(9):2426-2432. doi:10.1245/s10434-008-9966-2

61. Adam R, de Haas RJ, Wicherts DA, et al. Is hepatic resection justified after chemotherapy in patients with colorectal liver metastases and lymph node involvement? *J Clin Oncol.* 2008;26(22):3672-3680. doi:10.1200/JCO.2007.15.7297

62. Adam R, de Haas RJ, Wicherts DA, et al. Concomitant extrahepatic disease in patients with colorectal liver metastases: when is there a place for surgery? *Ann Surg.* 2011;253(2):349-359. doi:10.1097/SLA.0b013e318207bf2c

63. Chua TC, Saxena A, Liauw W, Chu F, Morris DL. Hepatectomy and resection of concomitant extrahepatic disease for colorectal liver metastases—a systematic review. *Eur J Cancer.* 2012;48(12):1757-1765. doi:10.1016/j.ejca.2011.10.034

64. Bonanni L, de'Liguori Carino N, Deshpande R, et al. A comparison of diagnostic imaging modalities for colorectal liver metastases. *Eur J Surg Oncol.* 2014;40(5):545-550. doi:10.1016/j.ejso.2013.12.023

65. Hoch G, Croise-Laurent V, Germain A, Brunaud L, Bresler L, Ayav A. Is intraoperative ultrasound still useful for the detection of colorectal cancer liver metastases? *HPB (Oxford).* 2015;17(6):514-519. doi:10.1111/hpb.12393

66. Pawlik TM, Scoggins CR, Zorzi D, et al. Effect of surgical margin status on survival and site of recurrence after hepatic resection for colorectal metastases. *Ann Surg.* 2005;241(5):715-724. doi:10.1097/01.sla.0000160703.75808.7d

67. Zorzi D, Mullen JT, Abdalla EK, et al. Comparison between hepatic wedge resection and anatomic resection for colorectal liver metastases. *J Gastrointest Surg.* 2006;10(1):86-94. doi:10.1016/j.gassur.2005.07.022

68. Choti MA, Sitzmann JV, Tiburi MF, et al. Trends in long-term survival following liver resection for hepatic colorectal metastases. *Ann Surg.* 2002;235(6):759-766. doi:10.1097/00000658-200206000-00002

69. Charnsangavej C, Clary B, Fong Y, Grothey A, Pawlik TM, Choti MA. Selection of patients for resection of hepatic colorectal metastases: expert consensus statement. *Ann Surg Oncol.* 2006;13(10):1261-1268. doi:10.1245/s10434-006-9023-y

70. Benson AB III, Venook AP, Cederquist L, et al. Colon Cancer, Version 1.2017, NCCN Clinical Practice Guidelines in Oncology. *J Natl Compr Canc Netw.* 2017;15(3):370-398. doi:10.6004/jnccn.2017.0036

71. Adam R, de Gramont A, Figueras J, et al. Managing synchronous liver metastases from colorectal cancer: a multidisciplinary international consensus. *Cancer Treat Rev.* 2015;41(9):729-741. doi:10.1016/j.ctrv.2015.06.006

72. Brudvik KW, Mise Y, Chung MH, et al. RAS mutation predicts positive resection margins and narrower resection margins in patients undergoing resection of colorectal liver metastases. *Ann Surg Oncol.* 2016;23(8):2635-2643. doi:10.1245/s10434-015-5187-2

73. Yamashita S, Chun YS, Kopetz SE, Vauthey JN. Biomarkers in colorectal liver metastases. *Br J Surg.* 2018;105(6):618-627. doi:10.1002/bjs.10834

74. Leung U, Gönen M, Allen PJ, et al. Colorectal cancer liver metastases and concurrent extrahepatic disease treated with resection. *Ann Surg.* 2017;265(1):158-165. doi:10.1097/SLA.0000000000001624

75. Pulitanò C, Bodingbauer M, Aldrighetti L, et al. Colorectal liver metastasis in the setting of lymph node metastasis: defining the benefit of surgical resection. *Ann Surg Oncol.* 2012;19(2):435-442. doi:10.1245/s10434-011-1902-1

76. Pindak D, Pavlendova J, Tomas M, Dolnik J, Duchon R, Pechan J. Selective versus routine lymphadenectomy in the treatment of liver metastasis from colorectal cancer: a retrospective cohort study. *BMC Surg.* 2017;17(1):34. doi:10.1186/s12893-017-0233-y

77. Gurusamy KS, Imber C, Davidson BR. Management of the hepatic lymph nodes during resection of liver metastases from colorectal cancer: a systematic review. *HPB Surg.* 2008;2008:684150. doi:10.1155/2008/684150

78. Fretland ÅA, Dagenborg VJ, Bjørnelv GMW, et al. Laparoscopic versus open resection for colorectal liver metastases: the OSLO-COMET randomized controlled trial. *Ann Surg.* 2018;267(2):199-207. doi:10.1097/SLA.0000000000002353

79. Martínez-Cecilia D, Cipriani F, Shelat V, et al. Laparoscopic versus open liver resection for colorectal metastases in elderly and octogenarian patients: a multicenter propensity score based analysis of short- and long-term outcomes. *Ann Surg.* 2017;265(6):1192-1200. doi:10.1097/SLA.0000000000002147

80. Donadon M, Torzilli G. Intraoperative ultrasound in patients with hepatocellular carcinoma: from daily practice to future trends. *Liver Cancer.* 2013;2(1):16-24. doi:10.1159/000346421

81. Torzilli G. Intraoperative ultrasound in surgery for hepatocellular carcinoma. *Ann Ital Chir.* 2008;79(2):99-106.
82. Takayama T, Kosuge T, Yamamoto J, et al. Intraoperative ultrasound for the diagnosis of hepatocellular carcinoma. Article in Japanese. *Nihon Rinsho.* 1991;49(8):1764-1767.
83. Lo CM, Lai EC, Liu CL, Fan ST, Wong J. Laparoscopy and laparoscopic ultrasonography avoid exploratory laparotomy in patients with hepatocellular carcinoma. *Ann Surg.* 1998;227(4):527-532. doi:10.1097/00000658-199804000-00013
84. Montorsi M, Santambrogio R, Bianchi P, et al. Laparoscopy with laparoscopic ultrasound for pretreatment staging of hepatocellular carcinoma: a prospective study. *J Gastrointest Surg.* 2001;5(3):312-315. doi:10.1016/s1091-255x(01)80053-6
85. Makuuchi M, Hasegawa H, Yamazaki S. Ultrasonically guided subsegmentectomy. *Surg Gynecol Obstet.* 1985;161(4):346-350.
86. Han J, Li ZL, Xing H, et al. The impact of resection margin and microvascular invasion on long-term prognosis after curative resection of hepatocellular carcinoma: a multi-institutional study. *HPB (Oxford).* 2019;21(8):962-971. doi:10.1016/j.hpb.2018.11.005
87. Shi M, Guo RP, Lin XJ, et al. Partial hepatectomy with wide versus narrow resection margin for solitary hepatocellular carcinoma: a prospective randomized trial. *Ann Surg.* 2007;245(1):36-43. doi:10.1097/01.sla.0000231758.07868.71
88. Tsilimigras DI, Sahara K, Moris D, et al. Effect of surgical margin width on patterns of recurrence among patients undergoing R0 hepatectomy for T1 hepatocellular carcinoma: an international multi-institutional analysis. *J Gastrointest Surg.* 2020;24(7):1552-1560. doi:10.1007/s11605-019-04275-0
89. Moris D, Tsilimigras DI, Kostakis ID, et al. Anatomic versus non-anatomic resection for hepatocellular carcinoma: a systematic review and meta-analysis. *Eur J Surg Oncol.* 2018;44(7):927-938. doi:10.1016/j.ejso.2018.04.018
90. Kaibori M, Kon M, Kitawaki T, et al. Comparison of anatomic and non-anatomic hepatic resection for hepatocellular carcinoma. *J Hepatobiliary Pancreat Sci.* 2017;24(11):616-626. doi:10.1002/jhbp.502
91. Donadon M, Terrone A, Procopio F, et al. Is R1 vascular hepatectomy for hepatocellular carcinoma oncologically adequate? Analysis of 327 consecutive patients. *Surgery.* 2019;165(5):897-904. doi:10.1016/j.surg.2018.12.002
92. Amini N, Ejaz A, Spolverato G, Maithel SK, Kim Y, Pawlik TM. Management of lymph nodes during resection of hepatocellular carcinoma and intrahepatic cholangiocarcinoma: a systematic review. *J Gastrointest Surg.* 2014;18(12):2136-2148. doi:10.1007/s11605-014-2667-1
93. Tan Y, Zhang W, Jiang L, Yang J, Yan L. Efficacy and safety of anatomic resection versus nonanatomic resection in patients with hepatocellular carcinoma: a systemic review and meta-analysis. *PloS One.* 2017;12(10):e0186930. doi:10.1371/journal.pone.0186930
94. Simillis C, Li T, Vaughan J, Becker LA, Davidson BR, Gurusamy KS. A Cochrane systematic review and network meta-analysis comparing treatment strategies aiming to decrease blood loss during liver resection. *Int J Surg.* 2015;23(pt A):128-136. doi:10.1016/j.ijsu.2015.09.064
95. Alexiou VG, Tsitsias T, Mavros MN, Robertson GS, Pawlik TM. Technology-assisted versus clamp-crush liver resection: a systematic review and meta-analysis. *Surg Innov.* 2013;20(4):414-428. doi:10.1177/1553350612468510
96. Yin Z, Fan X, Ye H, Yin D, Wang J. Short- and long-term outcomes after laparoscopic and open hepatectomy for hepatocellular carcinoma: a global systematic review and meta-analysis. *Ann Surg Oncol.* 2013;20(4):1203-1215. doi:10.1245/s10434-012-2705-8
97. Yoon YI, Kim KH, Cho HD, et al. Long-term perioperative outcomes of pure laparoscopic liver resection versus open liver resection for hepatocellular carcinoma: a retrospective study. *Surg Endosc.* 2020;34(2):796-805. doi:10.1007/s00464-019-06831-w
98. Wu X, Huang Z, Lau WY, et al. Perioperative and long-term outcomes of laparoscopic versus open liver resection for hepatocellular carcinoma with well-preserved liver function and cirrhotic background: a propensity score matching study. *Surg Endosc.* 2019;33(1):206-215. doi:10.1007/s00464-018-6296-8
99. Cho CW, Choi GS, Kim JM, Kwon CHD, Joh JW. Long-term oncological outcomes of laparoscopic liver resection for solitary hepatocellular carcinoma: comparison of anatomical and nonanatomical resection using propensity score matching analysis. *J Laparoendosc Adv Surg Tech A.* 2019;29(6):752-758. doi:10.1089/lap.2018.0600
100. Molina V, Sampson-Dávila J, Ferrer J, et al. Benefits of laparoscopic liver resection in patients with hepatocellular carcinoma and portal hypertension: a case-matched study. *Surg Endosc.* 2018;32(5):2345-2354. doi:10.1007/s00464-017-5930-1

101. Guro H, Cho JY, Han HS, et al. Outcomes of major laparoscopic liver resection for hepatocellular carcinoma. *Surg Oncol*. 2018;27(1):31-35. doi:10.1016/j.suronc.2017.11.006

102. Kamarajah SK, Frankel TL, Sonnenday C, Cho CS, Nathan H. Critical evaluation of the American Joint Commission on Cancer (AJCC) 8th edition staging system for patients with hepatocellular carcinoma (HCC): a Surveillance, Epidemiology, End Results (SEER) analysis. *J Surg Oncol*. 2018;117(4):644-650. doi:10.1002/jso.24908

103. Rocha FG, Matsuo K, Blumgart LH, Jarnagin WR. Hilar cholangiocarcinoma: the Memorial Sloan-Kettering Cancer Center experience. *J Hepatobiliary Pancreat Sci*. 2010;17(4):490-496. doi:10.1007/s00534-009-0205-4

104. Amin MB, Greene FL, Edge SB, et al. The Eighth Edition AJCC Cancer Staging Manual: continuing to build a bridge from a population-based to a more "personalized" approach to cancer staging. *CA Cancer J Clin*. 2017;67(2):93-99. doi:10 3322/caac.21388

105. Groot Koerkamp B, Wiggers JK, Gonen M, et al. Survival after resection of perihilar cholangiocarcinoma—development and external validation of a prognostic nomogram. *Ann Oncol*. 2015;26(9):1930-1935. doi:10.1093/annonc/mdv279

106. Tran TB, Ethun CG, Pawlik TM, et al. Actual 5-year survivors after surgical resection of hilar cholangiocarcinoma. *Ann Surg Oncol*. 2019;26(2):611-618 doi:10.1245/s10434-018-7075-4

107. Buettner S, Margonis GA, Kim Y, et al. Conditional probability of long-term survival after resection of hilar cholangiocarcinoma. *HPB (Oxford)*. 2016;18(6):510-517. doi:10.1016/j.hpb.2016.04.001

108. Matsuo K, Rocha FG, Ito K, et al. The Blumgart preoperative staging system for hilar cholangiocarcinoma: analysis of resectability and outcomes in 380 patients. *J Am Coll Surg*. 2012;215(3):343-355. doi:10.1016/j.jamcollsurg.2012.05.025

109. Murakami Y, Uemura K, Sudo T, et al. Prognostic factors after surgical resection for intrahepatic, hilar, and distal cholangiocarcinoma. *Ann Surg Oncol*. 2011;18(3):651-658. doi:10.1245/s10434-010-1325-4

110. Jarnagin WR, Fong Y, DeMatteo RP, et al. Staging, resectability, and outcome in 225 patients with hilar cholangiocarcinoma. *Ann Surg*. 2001;234(4):507-519. doi:10.1097/00000658-200110000-00010

111. Nishio H, Nagino M, Nimura Y. Surgical management of hilar cholangiocarcinoma: the Nagoya experience. *HPB (Oxford)*. 2005;7(4):259-262. doi:10.1080/13651820500373010

112. Nuzzo G, Giuliante F, Ardito F, et al. Improvement in perioperative and long-term outcome after surgical treatment of hilar cholangiocarcinoma: results of an Italian multicenter analysis of 440 patients. *Arch Surg*. 2012;147(1):26-34. doi:10.1001/archsurg.2011.771

113. Nagino M, Ebata T, Yokoyama Y, et al. Evolution of surgical treatment for perihilar cholangiocarcinoma: a single-center 34-year review of 574 consecutive resections. *Ann Surg*. 2013;258(1):129-140. doi:10.1097/SLA.0b013e3182708b57

114. DeOliveira ML, Cunningham SC, Cameron JL, et al. Cholangiocarcinoma: thirty-one-year experience with 564 patients at a single institution. *Ann Surg*. 2007;245(5):755-762. doi:10.1097/01.sla.0000251366.62632.d3

115. Endo I, House MG, Klimstra DS, et al. Clinical significance of intraoperative bile duct margin assessment for hilar cholangiocarcinoma. *Ann Surg Oncol*. 2008;15(8):2104-2112. doi:10.1245/s10434-008-0003-2

116. Pichlmayr R, Ringe B, Lauchart W, Bechstein WO, Gubernatis G, Wagner E. Radical resection and liver grafting as the two main components of surgical strategy in the treatment of proximal bile duct cancer. *World J Surg*. 1988;12(1):68-77. doi:10.1007/BF01658489

117. Bhuiya MR, Nimura Y, Kamiya J, et al. Clinicopathologic studies on perineural invasion of bile duct carcinoma. *Ann Surg*. 1992;215(4):344-349. doi:10.1097/00000658-199204000-00007

118. Ouchi K, Suzuki M, Hashimoto L, Sato T. Histologic findings and prognostic factors in carcinoma of the upper bile duct. *Am J Surg*. 1989;157(6):552-556.

119. Jarnagin WR, Ruo L, Little SA, et al. Patterns of initial disease recurrence after resection of gallbladder carcinoma and hilar cholangiocarcinoma: implications for adjuvant therapeutic strategies. *Cancer*. 2003;98(8):1689-1700. doi:10.1002/cncr.11699

120. van Gulik TM, Kloek JJ, Ruys AT, et al. Multidisciplinary management of hilar cholangiocarcinoma (Klatskin tumor): extended resection is associated with improved survival. *Eur J Surg Oncol*. 2011;37(1):65-71. doi:10.1016/j.ejso.2010.11.008

121. Ito F, Agni R, Rettammel RJ, et al. Resection of hilar cholangiocarcinoma: concomitant liver resection decreases hepatic recurrence. *Ann Surg*. 2008;248(2):273-279. doi:10.1097/SLA.0b013e31817f2bfd

122. Capussotti L, Vigano L, Ferrero A, Muratore A. Local surgical resection of hilar cholangiocarcinoma: is there still a place? *HPB (Oxford)*. 2008;10(3):174-178. doi:10.1080/13651820801992534

123. Wu XS, Dong P, Gu J, et al. Combined portal vein resection for hilar cholangiocarcinoma: a meta-analysis of comparative studies. *J Gastrointest Surg*. 2013;17(6):1107-1115. doi:10.1007/s11605-013-2202-9

124. de Jong MC, Marques H, Clary BM, et al. The impact of portal vein resection on outcomes for hilar cholangiocarcinoma: a multi-institutional analysis of 305 cases. *Cancer*. 2012;118(19):4737-4747. doi:10.1002/cncr.27492

125. Schimizzi GV, Jin LX, Davidson JT IV, et al. Outcomes after vascular resection during curative-intent resection for hilar cholangiocarcinoma: a multi-institution study from the US extrahepatic biliary malignancy consortium. *HPB (Oxford)*. 2018;20(4):332-339. doi:10.1016/j.hpb.2017.10.003

126. van Vugt JLA, Gaspersz MP, Coelen RJS, et al. The prognostic value of portal vein and hepatic artery involvement in patients with perihilar cholangiocarcinoma. *HPB (Oxford)*. 2018;20(1):83-92. doi:10.1016/j.hpb.2017.08.025

127. Neuhaus P, Thelen A, Jonas S, et al. Oncological superiority of hilar en bloc resection for the treatment of hilar cholangiocarcinoma. *Ann Surg Oncol*. 2012;19(5):1602-1608. doi:10.1245/s10434-011-2077-5

128. Nagino M, Nimura Y, Nishio H, et al. Hepatectomy with simultaneous resection of the portal vein and hepatic artery for advanced perihilar cholangiocarcinoma: an audit of 50 consecutive cases. *Ann Surg*. 2010;252(1):115-123. doi:10.1097/SLA.0b013e3181e463a7

129. Rassam F, Roos E, van Lienden KP, et al. Modern work-up and extended resection in perihilar cholangiocarcinoma: the AMC experience. *Langenbecks Arch Surg*. 2018;403(3):289-307. doi:10.1007/s00423-018-1649-2

130. Abbas S, Sandroussi C. Systematic review and meta-analysis of the role of vascular resection in the treatment of hilar cholangiocarcinoma. *HPB (Oxford)*. 2013;15(7):492-503. doi:10.1111/j.1477-2574.2012.00616.x

131. Groeschl RT, Nagorney DM. Portal vein reconstruction during surgery for cholangiocarcinoma. *Curr Opin Gastroenterol*. 2016;32(3):216-224. doi:10.1097/MOG.0000000000000259

132. Farges O, Fuks D, Boleslawski E, et al. Influence of surgical margins on outcome in patients with intrahepatic cholangiocarcinoma: a multicenter study by the AFC-IHCC-2009 study group. *Ann Surg*. 2011;254(5):824-830. doi:10.1097/SLA.0b013e318236c21d

133. Jonas S, Thelen A, Benckert C, et al. Extended liver resection for intrahepatic cholangiocarcinoma: a comparison of the prognostic accuracy of the fifth and sixth editions of the TNM classification. *Ann Surg*. 2009;249(2):303-309. doi:10.1097/SLA.0b013e318195e164

134. Luo X, Yuan L, Wang Y, Ge R, Sun Y, Wei G. Survival outcomes and prognostic factors of surgical therapy for all potentially resectable intrahepatic cholangiocarcinoma: a large single-center cohort study. *J Gastrointest Surg*. 2014;18(3):562-572. doi:10.1007/s11605-013-2447-3

135. Sonbare DJ. Influence of surgical margins on outcome in patients with intrahepatic cholangiocarcinoma: a multicenter study by the AFC-IHCC-2009 Study Group. *Ann Surg*. 2014;259(2):e36. doi:10.1097/SLA.0b013e3182a5c985

136. Spolverato G, Yakoob MY, Kim Y, et al. The impact of surgical margin status on long-term outcome after resection for intrahepatic cholangiocarcinoma. *Ann Surg Oncol*. 2015;22(12):4020-4028. doi:10.1245/s10434-015-4472-9

137. Tamandl D, Herberger B, Gruenberger B, Puhalla H, Klinger M, Gruenberger T. Influence of hepatic resection margin on recurrence and survival in intrahepatic cholangiocarcinoma. *Ann Surg Oncol*. 2008;15(10):2787-2794. doi:10.1245/s10434-008-0081-1

138. Benson AB, D'Angelica MI, Abbott DE, et al. Guidelines Insights: Hepatobiliary Cancers, Version 2.2019. *J Natl Compr Canc Netw*. 2019;17(4):302-310. doi:10.6004/jnccn.2019.0019

139. Valle JW, Borbath I, Khan SA, et al. Biliary cancer: ESMO Clinical Practice Guidelines for diagnosis, treatment and follow-up. *Ann Oncol*. 2016;27(suppl 5):v28-v37. doi:10.1093/annonc/mdw324

140. Weber SM, Ribero D, O'Reilly EM, Kokudo N, Miyazaki M, Pawlik TM. Intrahepatic cholangiocarcinoma: expert consensus statement. *HPB (Oxford)*. 2015;17(8):669-680. doi:10.1111/hpb.12441

141. Murakami S, Ajiki T, Okazaki T, et al. Factors affecting survival after resection of intrahepatic cholangiocarcinoma. *Surg Today*. 2014;44(10):1847-1854. doi:10.1007/s00595-013-0825-9

142. Ali SM, Clark CJ, Zaydfudim VM, Que FG, Nagorney DM. Role of major vascular resection in patients with intrahepatic cholangiocarcinoma. *Ann Surg Oncol*. 2013;20(6):2023-2028. doi:10.1245/s10434-012-2808-2

143. Lang H, Sotiropoulos GC, Sgourakis G, et al. Operations for intrahepatic cholangiocarcinoma: single-institution experience of 158 patients. *J Am Coll Surg.* 2009;208(2):218-228. doi:10.1016 /j.jamcollsurg.2008.10.017

144. Starzl TE, Iwatsuki S, Shaw BW Jr. A growth factor in fine vascular anastomoses. *Surg Gynecol Obstet.* 1984;159(2):164-165.

145. Kambakamba P, Linecker M, Slankamenac K, DeOliveira ML. Lymph node dissection in resectable perihilar cholangiocarcinoma: a systematic review. *Am J Surg.* 2015;210(4):694-701. doi:10.1016/j.amjsurg.2015.05.015

146. Akamatsu N, Sugawara Y, Hashimoto D. Surgical strategy for bile duct cancer: advances and current limitations. *World J Clin Oncol.* 2011;2(2):94-107. doi:10.5306/wjco.v2.i2.94

147. Mao K, Liu J, Sun J, et al. Patterns and prognostic value of lymph node dissection for resected perihilar cholangiocarcinoma. *J Gastroenterol Hepatol.* 2016;31(2):417-426. doi:10.1111 /jgh.13072

148. Kawasaki S, Imamura H, Kobayashi A, Noike T, Miwa S, Miyagawa S. Results of surgical resection for patients with hilar bile duct cancer: application of extended hepatectomy after biliary drainage and hemihepatic portal vein embolization. *Ann Surg.* 2003;238(1):84-92. doi:10.1097/01.SLA.0000074984.83031.02

149. Seyama Y, Kubota K, Sano K, et al. Long-term outcome of extended hemihepatectomy for hilar bile duct cancer with no mortality and high survival rate. *Ann Surg.* 2003;238(1):73-83. doi:10.1097/01.SLA.0000074960.55004.72

150. Schwarz RE, Smith DD. Lymph node dissection impact on staging and survival of extrahepatic cholangiocarcinomas, based on U.S. population data. *J Gastrointest Surg.* 2007;11(2):158-165. doi:10.1007/s11605-006-0018-6

151. Kitagawa Y, Nagino M, Kamiya J, et al. Lymph node metastasis from hilar cholangiocarcinoma: audit of 110 patients who underwent regional and paraaortic node dissection. *Ann Surg.* 2001;233(3):385-392. doi:10.1097/00000658-200103000-00013

152. Conci S, Ruzzenente A, Sandri M, et al. What is the most accurate lymph node staging method for perihilar cholangiocarcinoma? Comparison of UICC/AJCC pN stage, number of metastatic lymph nodes, lymph node ratio, and log odds of metastatic lymph nodes. *Eur J Surg Oncol.* 2017;43(4):743-750. doi:10.1016/j.ejso.2016.12.007

153. Guglielmi A, Ruzzenente A, Campagnaro T, et al. Prognostic significance of lymph node ratio after resection of peri-hilar cholangiocarcinoma. *HPB (Oxford).* 2011;13(4):240-245. doi:10.1111/j.1477-2574.2010.00277.x

154. Ito K, Ito H, Allen PJ, et al. Adequate lymph node assessment for extrahepatic bile duct adenocarcinoma. *Ann Surg.* 2010;251(4):675-681. doi:10.1097/SLA.0b013e3181d3d2b2

155. Hakeem AR, Marangoni G, Chapman SJ, et al. Does the extent of lymphadenectomy, number of lymph nodes, positive lymph node ratio and neutrophil-lymphocyte ratio impact surgical outcome of perihilar cholangiocarcinoma? *Eur J Gastroenterol Hepatol.* 2014;26(9):1047-1054. doi:10.1097/MEG.0000000000000162

156. Giuliante F, Ardito F, Guglielmi A, et al. Association of lymph node status with survival in patients after liver resection for hilar cholangiocarcinoma in an Italian multicenter analysis. *JAMA Surg.* 2016;151(10):916-922. doi:10.1001/jamasurg.2016.1769

157. Buettner S, van Vugt JLA, Gaspersz MP, et al. Survival after resection of perihilar cholangiocarcinoma in patients with lymph node metastases. *HPB (Oxford).* 2017;19(8):735-740. doi:10.1016/j.hpb.2017.04.014

158. Lai EC, Lau WY. Aggressive surgical resection for hilar cholangiocarcinoma. *ANZ J Surg.* 2005;75(11):981-985. doi:10.1111/j.1445-2197.2005.03595.x

159. Nagakawa T, Kayahara M, Ikeda S, et al. Biliary tract cancer treatment: results from the Biliary Tract Cancer Statistics Registry in Japan. *J Hepatobiliary Pancreat Surg.* 2002;9(5):569-575. doi:10.1007/s005340200076

160. Edge SB, Compton CC. The American Joint Committee on Cancer: the 7th edition of the AJCC Cancer Staging Manual and the future of TNM. *Ann Surg Oncol.* 2010;17(6):1471-1474. doi:10.1245/s10434-010-0985-4

161. Miyazaki M, Yoshitomi H, Miyakawa S, et al. Clinical practice guidelines for the management of biliary tract cancers 2015: the 2nd English edition. *J Hepatobiliary Pancreat Sci.* 2015;22(4):249-273. doi:10.1002/jhbp.233

162. Murakami Y, Uemura K, Sudo T, et al. Is para-aortic lymph node metastasis a contraindication for radical resection in biliary carcinoma? *World J Surg.* 2011;35(5):1085-1093. doi:10.1007 /s00268-011-1036-4

163. Aoba T, Ebata T, Yokoyama Y, et al. Assessment of nodal status for perihilar cholangiocarcinoma: location, number, or ratio of involved nodes. *Ann Surg.* 2013;257(4):718-725. doi:10.1097/SLA.0b013e3182822277

164. Ito M, Mishima Y, Sato T. An anatomical study of the lymphatic drainage of the gallbladder. *Surg Radiol Anat.* 1991;13(2):89-104. doi:10.1007/BF01623880

165. Shirai Y, Yoshida K, Tsukada K, Ohtani T, Muto T. Identification of the regional lymphatic system of the gallbladder by vital staining. *Br J Surg.* 1992;79(7):659-662. doi:10.1002/bjs.1800790721

166. Yeo CJ, Cameron JL, Lillemoe KD, et al. Pancreaticoduodenectomy with or without distal gastrectomy and extended retroperitoneal lymphadenectomy for periampullary adenocarcinoma, part 2: randomized controlled trial evaluating survival, morbidity, and mortality. *Ann Surg.* 2002;236(3):355-368.

167. de Jong MC, Nathan H, Sotiropoulos GC, et al. Intrahepatic cholangiocarcinoma: an international multi-institutional analysis of prognostic factors and lymph node assessment. *J Clin Oncol.* 2011;29(23):3140-3145. doi:10.1200/JCO.2011.35.6519

168. Bagante F, Spolverato G, Merath K, et al. Intrahepatic cholangiocarcinoma tumor burden: a classification and regression tree model to define prognostic groups after resection. *Surgery.* 2019;166(6):983-990. doi:10.1016/j.surg.2019.06.005

169. Horgan AM, Amir E, Walter T, Knox JJ. Adjuvant therapy in the treatment of biliary tract cancer: a systematic review and meta-analysis. *J Clin Oncol.* 2012;30(16):1934-1940. doi:10.1200/JCO.2011.40.5381

170. Shimada K, Sano T, Nara S, et al. Therapeutic value of lymph node dissection during hepatectomy in patients with intrahepatic cholangiocellular carcinoma with negative lymph node involvement. *Surgery.* 2009;145(4):411-416.

171. Kokudo N, Makuuchi M. Extent of resection and outcome after curative resection for intrahepatic cholangiocarcinoma. *Surg Oncol Clin N Am.* 2002;11(4):969-983. doi:10.1016/s1055-3207(02)00040-6

172. Bridgewater J, Galle PR, Khan SA, et al. Guidelines for the diagnosis and management of intrahepatic cholangiocarcinoma. *J Hepatol.* 2014;60(6):1268-1289. doi:10.1016/j.jhep.2014.01.021

173. Harisinghani MG. *Atlas of Lymph Node Anatomy.* Springer; 2013.

174. Shirabe K, Shimada M, Harimoto N, et al. Intrahepatic cholangiocarcinoma: its mode of spreading and therapeutic modalities. *Surgery.* 2002;131(1 suppl):S159-S164.

175. Tsuji T, Hiraoka T, Kanemitsu K, Takamori H, Tanabe D, Tashiro S. Lymphatic spreading pattern of intrahepatic cholangiocarcinoma. *Surgery.* 2001;129(4):401-407. doi:10.1067/msy.2001.111873

176. Okami J, Dono K, Sakon M, et al. Patterns of regional lymph node involvement in intrahepatic cholangiocarcinoma of the left lobe. *J Gastrointest Surg.* 2003;7(7):850-856. doi:10.1007/s11605-003-0029-5

177. Gu J, Xia L, Xu B, et al. Clinical prognostic significance of regional and extended lymphadenectomy for biliary cancer with para-aortic lymph node metastasis: a systematic review and meta-analysis. *Dig Liver Dis.* 2016;48(7):717-725. doi:10.1016/j.dld.2016.03.019

178. Ratti F, Fiorentini G, Cipriani F, Paganelli M, Catena M, Aldrighetti L. Perioperative and long-term outcomes of laparoscopic versus open lymphadenectomy for biliary tumors: a propensity-score-based, case-matched analysis. *Ann Surg Oncol.* 2019;26(2):564-575. doi:10.1245/s10434-018-6811-0

179. Zhang XF, Chen Q, Kimbrough CW, et al. Lymphadenectomy for intrahepatic cholangiocarcinoma: has nodal evaluation been increasingly adopted by surgeons over time? A National Database Analysis. *J Gastrointest Surg.* 2018;22(4):668-675. doi:10.1007/s11605-017-3652-2

180. Nimura Y, Hayakawa N, Kamiya J, Kondo S, Shionoya S. Hepatic segmentectomy with caudate lobe resection for bile duct carcinoma of the hepatic hilus. *World J Surg.* 1990;14(4):535-544. doi:10.1007/BF01658686

181. Popescu I, Dumitrascu T. Curative-intent surgery for hilar cholangiocarcinoma: prognostic factors for clinical decision making. *Langenbecks Arch Surg.* 2014;399(6):693-705. doi:10.1007/s00423-014-1210-x

182. Abdalla EK, Vauthey JN, Couinaud C. The caudate lobe of the liver: implications of embryology and anatomy for surgery. *Surg Oncol Clin N Am.* 2002;11(4):835-848. doi:10.1016/s1055-3207(02)00035-2

183. Mizumoto R, Suzuki H. Surgical anatomy of the hepatic hilum with special reference to the caudate lobe. *World J Surg.* 1988;12(1):2-10. doi:10.1007/BF01658479

184. Ogura Y, Mizumoto R, Tabata M, Matsuda S, Kusuda T. Surgical treatment of carcinoma of the hepatic duct confluence: analysis of 55 resected carcinomas. *World J Surg.* 1993;17(1):85-93. doi:10.1007/BF01655714

185. Tsao JI, Nimura Y, Kamiya J, et al. Management of hilar cholangiocarcinoma: comparison of an American and a Japanese experience. *Ann Surg.* 2000;232(2):166-174. doi:10.1097/00000658-200008000-00003

186. Dinant S, Gerhards MF, Rauws EA, Busch OR, Gouma DJ, van Gulik TM. Improved outcome of resection of hilar cholangiocarcinoma (Klatskin tumor). *Ann Surg Oncol.* 2006;13(6):872-880. doi:10.1245/ASO.2006.05.053

187. Moher D, Liberati A, Tetzlaff J, Altman DG; PRISMA Group. Preferred reporting items for systematic reviews and meta-analyses: the PRISMA statement. *BMJ.* 2009;339:b2535. doi:10.1136/bmj.b2535

188. Kow AW, Wook CD, Song SC, et al. Role of caudate lobectomy in type III A and III B hilar cholangiocarcinoma: a 15-year experience in a tertiary institution. *World J Surg.* 2012;36(5):1112-1121. doi:10.1007/s00268-012-1497-0

189. Song SC, Choi DW, Kow AW, et al. Surgical outcomes of 230 resected hilar cholangiocarcinoma in a single centre. *ANZ J Surg.* 2013;83(4):268-274. doi:10.1111/j.1445-2197.2012.06195.x

190. Cheng QB, Yi B, Wang JH, et al. Resection with total caudate lobectomy confers survival benefit in hilar cholangiocarcinoma of Bismuth type III and IV. *Eur J Surg Oncol.* 2012;38(12):1197-1203. doi:10.1016/j.ejso.2012.08.009

191. Rea DJ, Munoz-Juarez M, Farnell MB, et al. Major hepatic resection for hilar cholangiocarcinoma: analysis of 46 patients. *Arch Surg.* 2004;139(5):514-525. doi:10.1001/archsurg.139.5.514

192. Wahab MA, Sultan AM, Salah T, et al. Caudate lobe resection with major hepatectomy for central cholangiocarcinoma: is it of value? *Hepatogastroenterology.* 2012;59(114):321-324. doi:10.5754/hge11999

193. Atkins D, Best D, Briss PA, et al. Grading quality of evidence and strength of recommendations. *BMJ.* 2004;328(7454):1490. doi:10.1136/bmj.328.7454.1490

194. Atkins D, Eccles M, Flottorp S, et al. Systems for grading the quality of evidence and the strength of recommendations I: critical appraisal of existing approaches The GRADE Working Group. *BMC Health Serv Res.* 2004;4(1):38. doi:10.1186/1472-6963-4-38

195. Hemming AW, Reed AI, Fujita S, Foley DP, Howard RJ. Surgical management of hilar cholangiocarcinoma. *Ann Surg.* 2005;241(5):693-702. doi:10.1097/01.sla.0000160701.38945.82

196. Komaya K, Ebata T, Yokoyama Y, et al. Recurrence after curative-intent resection of perihilar cholangiocarcinoma: analysis of a large cohort with a close postoperative follow-up approach. *Surgery.* 2018;163(4):732-738. doi:10.1016/j.surg.2017.08.011

197. Tang Z, Yang Y, Zhao Z, Wei K, Meng W, Li X. The clinicopathological factors associated with prognosis of patients with resectable perihilar cholangiocarcinoma: a systematic review and meta-analysis. *Medicine (Baltimore).* 2018;97(34):e11999. doi:10.1097/MD.0000000000011999

198. Mantel HT, Westerkamp AC, Sieders E, et al. Intraoperative frozen section analysis of the proximal bile ducts in hilar cholangiocarcinoma is of limited value. *Cancer Med.* 2016;5(7):1373-1380. doi:10.1002/cam4.693

199. Okazaki Y, Horimi T, Kotaka M, Morita S, Takasaki M. Study of the intrahepatic surgical margin of hilar bile duct carcinoma. *Hepatogastroenterology.* 2002;49(45):625-627.

200. Sasaki R, Takeda Y, Funato O, et al. Significance of ductal margin status in patients undergoing surgical resection for extrahepatic cholangiocarcinoma. *World J Surg.* 2007;31(9):1788-1796. doi:10.1007/s00268-007-9102-7

201. Edeline J, Benabdelghani M, Bertaut A, et al. Gemcitabine and oxaliplatin chemotherapy or surveillance in resected biliary tract cancer (PRODIGE 12-ACCORD 18-UNICANCER GI): a randomized phase III study. *J Clin Oncol.* 2019;37(8):658-667. doi:10.1200/JCO.18.00050

202. Lee JH, Hwang DW, Lee SY, Park KM, Lee YJ. The proximal margin of resected hilar cholangiocarcinoma: the effect of microscopic positive margin on long-term survival. *Am Surg.* 2012;78(4):471-477.

203. Ma WJ, Wu ZR, Shrestha A, et al. Effectiveness of additional resection of the invasive cancer-positive proximal bile duct margin in cases of hilar cholangiocarcinoma. *Hepatobiliary Surg Nutr.* 2018;7(4):251-269. doi:10.21037/hbsn.2018.03.14

204. Otsuka S, Ebata T, Yokoyama Y, et al. Clinical value of additional resection of a margin-positive distal bile duct in perihilar cholangiocarcinoma. *Br J Surg.* 2019;106(6):774-782. doi:10.1002/bjs.11125

205. Ribero D, Amisano M, Lo Tesoriere R, Rosso S, Ferrero A, Capussotti L. Additional resection of an intraoperative margin-positive proximal bile duct improves survival in patients with hilar cholangiocarcinoma. *Ann Surg.* 2011;254(5):776-783. doi:10.1097/SLA.0b013e3182368f85

206. Shingu Y, Ebata T, Nishio H, Igami T, Shimoyama Y, Nagino M. Clinical value of additional resection of a margin-positive proximal bile duct in hilar cholangiocarcinoma. *Surgery*. 2010;147(1):49-56. doi:10.1016/j.surg.2009.06.030

207. Zhang XF, Squires MH III, Bagante F, et al. The impact of intraoperative re-resection of a positive bile duct margin on clinical outcomes for hilar cholangiocarcinoma. *Ann Surg Oncol*. 2018;25(5):1140-1149. doi:10.1245/s10434-018-6382-0

208. Bartlett DL, Fong Y, Fortner JG, Brennan MF, Blumgart LH. Long-term results after resection for gallbladder cancer. Implications for staging and management. *Ann Surg*. 1996;224(5):639-646. doi:10.1097/00000658-199611000-00008

209. Burke EC, Jarnagin WR, Hochwald SN, Pisters PW, Fong Y, Blumgart LH. Hilar cholangiocarcinoma: patterns of spread, the importance of hepatic resection for curative operation, and a presurgical clinical staging system. *Ann Surg*. 1998;228(3):385-394. doi:10.1097/00000658-199809000-00011

210. Goere D, Wagholikar GD, Pessaux P, et al. Utility of staging laparoscopy in subsets of biliary cancers: laparoscopy is a powerful diagnostic tool in patients with intrahepatic and gallbladder carcinoma. *Surg Endosc*. 2006;20(5):721-725. doi:10.1007/s00464-005-0583-x

211. Jarnagin WR, Fong Y, Blumgart LH. The current management of hilar cholangiocarcinoma. *Adv Surg*. 1999;33:345-373.

212. Klempnauer J, Ridder GJ, von Wasielewski R, Werner M, Weimann A, Pichlmayr R. Resectional surgery of hilar cholangiocarcinoma: a multivariate analysis of prognostic factors. *J Clin Oncol*. 1997;15(3):947-954. doi:10.1200/JCO.1997.15.3.947

213. Kosuge T, Sano K, Shimada K, Yamamoto J, Yamasaki S, Makuuchi M. Should the bile duct be preserved or removed in radical surgery for gallbladder cancer? *Hepatogastroenterology*. 1999;46(28):2133-2137.

214. Vollmer CM, Drebin JA, Middleton WD, et al. Utility of staging laparoscopy in subsets of peripancreatic and biliary malignancies. *Ann Surg*. 2002;235(1):1-7. doi:10.1097/00000658-200201000-00001

215. Tapper E, Kalb B, Martin DR, Kooby D, Adsay NV, Sarmiento JM. Staging laparoscopy for proximal pancreatic cancer in a magnetic resonance imaging-driven practice: what's it worth? *HPB (Oxford)*. 2011;13(10):732-737. doi:10.1111/j.1477-2574.2011.00366.x

216. Weber SM, DeMatteo RP, Fong Y, Blumgart LH, Jarnagin WR. Staging laparoscopy in patients with extrahepatic biliary carcinoma. Analysis of 100 patients. *Ann Surg*. 2002;235(3):392-399. doi:10.1097/00000658-200203000-00011

217. Butte JM, Gönen M, Allen PJ, et al. The role of laparoscopic staging in patients with incidental gallbladder cancer. *HPB (Oxford)*. 2011;13(7):463-472. doi:10.1111/j.1477-2574.2011.00325.x

218. Agarwal AK, Kalayarasan R, Javed A, Gupta N, Nag HH. The role of staging laparoscopy in primary gall bladder cancer—an analysis of 409 patients: a prospective study to evaluate the role of staging laparoscopy in the management of gallbladder cancer. *Ann Surg*. 2013;258(2):318-323. doi:10.1097/SLA.0b013e318271497e

219. D'Angelica M, Fong Y, Weber S, et al. The role of staging laparoscopy in hepatobiliary malignancy: prospective analysis of 401 cases. *Ann Surg Oncol*. 2003;10(2):183-189. doi:10.1245/aso.2003.03.091

220. Pawlik TM, Gleisner AL, Vigano L, et al. Incidence of finding residual disease for incidental gallbladder carcinoma: implications for re-resection. *J Gastrointest Surg*. 2007;11(11):1478-1487. doi:10.1007/s11605-007-0309-6

221. Ethun CG, Postlewait LM, Le N, et al. A novel pathology-based preoperative risk score to predict locoregional residual and distant disease and survival for incidental gallbladder cancer: a 10-institution study from the U.S. extrahepatic biliary malignancy consortium. *Ann Surg Oncol*. 2017;24(5):1343-1350. doi:10.1245/s10434-016-5637-x

222. Davidson JT IV, Jin LX, Krasnick B, et al. Staging laparoscopy among three subtypes of extra-hepatic biliary malignancy: a 15-year experience from 10 institutions. *J Surg Oncol*. 2019;119(3):288-294. doi:10.1002/jso.25323

223. Benson AB III, D'Angelica MI, Abbott DE, et al. NCCN Guidelines Insights: Hepatobiliary Cancers, Version 1.2017. *J Natl Compr Canc Netw*. 2017;15(5):563-573. doi:10.6004/jnccn.2017.0059

224. Pilgrim C, Usatoff V, Evans PM. A review of the surgical strategies for the management of gallbladder carcinoma based on T stage and growth type of the tumour. *Eur J Surg Oncol*. 2009;35(9):903-907. doi:10.1016/j.ejso.2009.02.005

225. Rathanaswamy S, Misra S, Kumar V, et al. Incidentally detected gallbladder cancer—the controversies and algorithmic approach to management. *Indian J Surg*. 2012;74(3):248-254. doi:10.1007/s12262-012-0592-7

226. Shih SP, Schulick RD, Cameron JL, et al. Gallbladder cancer: the role of laparoscopy and radical resection. *Ann Surg.* 2007;245(6):893-901. doi:10.1097/SLA.0b013e31806beec2

227. D'Angelica M, Dalal KM, DeMatteo RP, Fong Y, Blumgart LH, Jarnagin WR. Analysis of the extent of resection for adenocarcinoma of the gallbladder. *Ann Surg Oncol.* 2008;16(4):806-816. doi:10.1245/s10434-008-0189-3

228. Butte JM, Matsuo K, Gönen M, et al. Gallbladder cancer: differences in presentation, surgical treatment, and survival in patients treated at centers in three countries. *J Am Coll Surg.* 2011;212(1):50-61.

229. Dixon E, Vollmer CM Jr, Sahajpal A, et al. An aggressive surgical approach leads to improved survival in patients with gallbladder cancer. *Ann Surg.* 2005;241(3):385-394. doi:10.1097/01 .sla.0000154118.07704.ef

230. Lee SE, Kim KS, Kim WB, et al. Practical guidelines for the surgical treatment of gallbladder cancer. *J Korean Med Sci.* 2014;29(10):1333-1340.

231. Gani F, Buettner S, Margonis GA, et al. Assessing the impact of common bile duct resection in the surgical management of gallbladder cancer. *J Surg Oncol.* 2016;114(2):176-180. doi:10.1002 /jso.24283

232. Pawlik TM, Choti MA. Biology dictates prognosis following resection of gallbladder carcinoma: sometimes less is more. *Ann Surg Oncol.* 2009;16(4):787-788. doi:10.1245/s10434-009-0319-6

233. Ørntoft TF, Vestergaard EM, Holmes E, et al. Influence of Lewis α 1-3/4-L-fucosyltransferase (FUT3) gene mutations on enzyme activity, erythrocyte phenotyping, and circulating tumor marker sialyl-Lewis a levels. *J Biol Chem.* 1996;271(50):32260-32268. doi:10.1074 /jbc.271.50.32260

234. Jensen EH, Abraham A, Jarosek S, et al. Lymph node evaluation is associated with improved survival after surgery for early stage gallbladder cancer. *Surgery.* 2009;146(4):706-713. doi:10.1016/j.surg.2009.06.056

235. Downing SR, Cadogan KA, Ortega G, et al. Early-stage gallbladder cancer in the surveillance, epidemiology, and end results database. *Arch Surg.* 2011;146(6):734-738. doi:10.1001 /archsurg.2011.128

236. Mayo SC, Shore AD, Nathan H, et al. National trends in the management and survival of surgically managed gallbladder adenocarcinoma over 15 years: a population-based analysis. *J Gastrointest Surg.* 2010;14(10):1578-1591. doi:10.1007/s11605-010-1335-3

237. Edge SB, Byrd DR, Compton CC, Fritz AG, Greene FL, Trotti A, eds. *AJCC Cancer Staging Manual.* 7th ed. Springer; 2010.

238. Greene FL, Page DL, Fleming ID, et al, eds. *AJCC Cancer Staging Manual.* 6th ed. Springer; 2002.

239. Paolucci V. Port site recurrences after laparoscopic cholecystectomy. *J Hepatobiliary Pancreat Surg.* 2001;8(6):535-543. doi:10.1007/s005340100022

240. Berger-Richardson D, Chesney TR, Englesakis M, Govindarajan A, Cleary SP, Swallow CJ. Trends in port-site metastasis after laparoscopic resection of incidental gallbladder cancer: a systematic review. *Surgery.* 2017;161(3):618-627. doi:10.1016/j.surg.2016.08.007

241. Maker AV, Butte JM, Oxenberg J, et al. Is port site resection necessary in the surgical management of gallbladder cancer? *Ann Surg Oncol.* 2012;19(2):409-417. doi:10.1245/s10434 -011-1850-9

242. Fuks D, Regimbeau JM, Pessaux P, et al. Is port-site resection necessary in the surgical management of gallbladder cancer? *J Visc Surg.* 2013;150(4):277-284. doi:10.1016/j.jviscsurg.2013.03.006

243. Ethun CG, Postlewait LM, Le N, et al. Routine port-site excision in incidentally discovered gallbladder cancer is not associated with improved survival: a multi-institution analysis from the US Extrahepatic Biliary Malignancy Consortium. *J Surg Oncol.* 2017;115(7):805-811. doi:10.1002/jso.24591

Synoptic Operative Report: Gallbladder Cancer

Date of procedure _____ Surgeon(s) _____

_____

Preoperative

Type
- ☐ Incidental
- ☐ In situ

Preoperative T stage
- ☐ X
- ☐ 0
- ☐ Is
- ☐ 1a
- ☐ 1b
- ☐ 2a
- ☐ 2b
- ☐ 3
- ☐ 4

Preoperative N stage
- ☐ X
- ☐ 0
- ☐ 1
- ☐ 2

Preoperative therapy
- ☐ Yes
- ☐ No

Cystic duct margin
- ☐ Positive
- ☐ Negative
- ☐ Unknown

Synoptic Operative Report: Gallbladder Cancer

Date of procedure _____   Surgeon(s) _____

_____

Intraoperative

Hepatectomy type

☐ Cystic plate
☐ Wedge
☐ IVb/V

Approach

☐ Open
☐ Laparoscopic
☐ Robotic

Lymphadenectomy

☐ Yes
   ☐ Portal
   ☐ Aortocaval
   ☐ Other _____
☐ No

Bile duct resection

☐ Yes
☐ No

Synoptic Operative Report: Hepatocellular Carcinoma

Date of procedure _____　Surgeon(s) _____

_____

Preoperative

Cirrhosis
- ☐ Yes
- ☐ No

Portal hypertension
- ☐ Yes
- ☐ No

Preoperative therapy
- ☐ TACE
- ☐ Y90
- ☐ Ablation
- ☐ Chemotherapy
- ☐ Immunotherapy

Embolization procedure for hypertrophy
- ☐ Yes
- ☐ No

Intraoperative

Hepatectomy type
- ☐ Left
- ☐ Extended left
- ☐ Right
- ☐ Extended right
- ☐ Posterior section
- ☐ Anterior section
- ☐ Left lateral section
- ☐ Wedge

Technique
- ☐ Open
- ☐ Laparoscopic
- ☐ Robotic

Lymphadenectomy
- ☐ Yes
  - ☐ Portal
  - ☐ Other _____
- ☐ No

Synoptic Operative Report: Hilar Cholangiocarcinoma

Date of procedure _____   Surgeon(s) _____

_____

Preoperative

Stenting
- ☐ Yes
  - ☐ Percutaneous
  - ☐ Endoscopic
  - ☐ Both
- ☐ No

Embolization procedure for hypertrophy
- ☐ Yes
- ☐ No

Intraoperative

Hepatectomy extent
- ☐ Left
- ☐ Extended left
- ☐ Right
- ☐ Extended right

Caudate resection
- ☐ Yes
- ☐ No

Lymphadenectomy
- ☐ Yes
  - ☐ Portal
  - ☐ Aortocaval
  - ☐ Other _____
- ☐ No

Frozen section
- ☐ Yes
  - ☐ Distal bile duct
  - ☐ Proximal hepatic duct
  - ☐ Other _____
- ☐ No

Portal vein resection
- ☐ Yes
- ☐ No

Synoptic Operative Report: Intrahepatic Cholangiocarcinoma

Date of procedure _____ Surgeon(s) _____

_____

Preoperative

Preoperative therapy
- ☐ Yes
- ☐ No

Stenting
- ☐ Yes
  - ☐ Percutaneous
  - ☐ Endoscopic
  - ☐ Both
- ☐ No

Embolization procedure for hypertrophy
- ☐ Yes
- ☐ No

Intraoperative

Hepatectomy type
- ☐ Major
- ☐ Minor
- ☐ Left
- ☐ Extended left
- ☐ Right
- ☐ Extended right
- ☐ Posterior section
- ☐ Anterior section
- ☐ Left lateral section
- ☐ Nonanatomic

Approach
- ☐ Open
- ☐ Laparoscopic
- ☐ Robotic

Synoptic Operative Report:
Intrahepatic Cholangiocarcinoma

Date of procedure _____   Surgeon(s) _____

_____

Lymphadenectomy
☐ Yes
☐ Portal
☐ Other _____
☐ No

Bile duct resection
☐ Yes
☐ No

Synoptic Operative Report: Metastatic Colon Cancer

Date of procedure _____ Surgeon(s) _____

_____

Preoperative

Preoperative therapy
☐ Yes
☐ No

Agent(s) _____

Number of doses _____

Presentation
☐ Synchronous ($\geq$1 y)
☐ Metachronous

Embolization procedure for
hypertrophy
☐ Yes
☐ No

Intraoperative

Hepatectomy extent
☐ Left
☐ Extended left
☐ Right
☐ Extended right
☐ Posterior section
☐ Anterior section
☐ Left lateral section
☐ Nonanatomic resections

Technique
☐ Open
☐ Laparoscopic
☐ Robotic

Lymphadenectomy
☐ Yes
  ☐ Portal
  ☐ Other _____
☐ No

Ablation
☐ Yes
☐ No

COMMENTARY: HEPATOBILIARY SECTION

Reid B. Adams, MD
S. Hurt Watts Professor and Chair
Chief, Hepatobiliary and Pancreatic Surgery
Department of Surgery
Chief Medical Officer
University of Virginia Health System

The hepatobiliary section in *Operative Standards for Cancer Surgery*, Volume 3, covers staging, preoperative care, and intraoperative management of patients with liver metastasis from colorectal cancer (CRM), hepatocellular carcinoma (HCC), cholangiocarcinoma (CCA), and gallbladder adenocarcinoma (GC). The introduction reviews recent changes in staging, the importance of multidisciplinary care, the central issues in perioperative care, and the critical nature of preoperative imaging to assess resectability. Subsequent chapters focus on the technical details to consider when treating each disease process.

The authors have done yeoman's work in preparing this section, working to provide insight and advice for each disease while recognizing there often is little in the way of high-quality data to clearly guide us. We continue to suffer in the Hepatopancreatobiliary realm from a dearth of prospective randomized controlled trials to direct our care with respect to a number of thorny issues; as a result, they remain unresolved. Hence, much of what we use in daily practice and is outlined in this section is guided by expert opinion and case series. Therefore, the authors' emphasis on the role of multidisciplinary teams and conferences in guiding the care for these complex patients is a crucial takeaway message from this section. Knowing and understanding the information in these chapters is critical, as surgeons should continue to lead the integration of multimodal therapy approaches for the treatment of each of these malignancies. I will highlight some common themes for all these diagnoses, followed by a few specifics for the various diseases.

Comments on several of the technical aspects addressed by the authors including some common themes as well as specific differences between the various diagnoses follow.

Multidisciplinary Care

Colorectal Cancer Metastasis: Treatment of CRM to the liver has evolved significantly over the past two decades with the advent of more effective systemic therapy and an improved understanding of the technical issues allowing a more broad application of hepatic resection.[1-3] These have led to considerably more patients being eligible for hepatic resection for their CRM. Stage IV disease treatment sequencing (systemic prior to resection, after, or at all) remains debated and a clear standard unresolved. This is even more complex when the primary tumor is intact at the time metastatic disease is discovered. These complex decisions on treatment options and sequence illustrate the absolute necessity of a multidisciplinary team approach to managing these patients.

Hepatocellular Carcinoma: Advances in treatment of HCC revolve less around systemic therapies and more on locoregional or resectional options. Critical to the treatment decisions are hepatologist, oncology-focused interventional radiologist, and liver transplant teams. Multidisciplinary team discussions are ideal for the complex decision-making required to determine the best treatment option for these patients. Although resection may be appropriate for some, the significant degree of parenchymal injury and subsequent hepatocellular dysfunction frequently necessitates chemo- or radioembolization, thermal ablation, or transplantation approaches as better alternatives.

Cholangiocarcinoma: Histologic diagnosis of perihilar CCA can be elusive and treatment decisions often are made based on presentation and imaging as a clear tissue diagnosis often is absent. The role for high-quality imaging and multidisciplinary input, therefore, is critical to optimize treatment decisions and outcomes in these patients. Those deemed unresectable due to locally advanced disease may be candidates for liver transplantation, necessitating this team's involvement. Advances in understanding the biology of intrahepatic CCA have elucidated several targetable mutations and systemic therapy options. These recent findings, again, illustrate the crucial role of multidisciplinary input in determining treatment plans for those with intrahepatic CCA.

Gallbladder Carcinoma: Despite considerable investigative efforts, GC continues to have few good nonsurgical therapies for treatment. Nonetheless, multidisciplinary discussions are important in deciding the treatment course for those with node-positive disease, bile spillage from an incidental cholecystotomy during the initial cholecystectomy, or positive margins post resection.

Perioperative Care

The authors emphasize the critical nature of high-quality imaging to determine disease extent and develop a sound operative plan. Although debate persists regarding the optimal modality, both computed tomography (CT) and magnetic resonance imaging (MRI) offer high-resolution images. We strongly favor MRI in our own practice as it is excellent in determining the extent of the lesion(s) in the liver/biliary tract and it gives superb anatomic detail of both the vascular and biliary structures. Finally, MRI characteristics often are crucial for distinguishing the nature of an intraparenchymal lesion. With today's outstanding imaging, a clear operative plan can be developed preoperatively, and one should expect relatively few significant changes once in the operating room. The role of intraoperative ultrasound (IOUS) is discussed later.

The second commonality addressed by the authors is determining hepatic parenchymal function and ensuring an adequately sized future liver remnant based on its size and relationship to any parenchymal dysfunction. This is a critical determinate of a patient's candidacy for resection and, if they are, the extent of hepatectomy they will tolerate. If resection will result in a future liver remnant that is too small, consideration of preoperative portal vein embolization, a two-staged hepatectomy, or another complex approach is important.

For CRM, RAS mutation status is an important determinate in resection decisions. Mutated RAS is an independent predictor of poor outcome, consequently influencing resection planning.[4]

Imaging of CRM or HCC that shows tumor abutment of intrahepatic vascular structures typically led to hepatectomy planning that included vascular resection, and therefore, larger parenchymal resections in an effort to achieve a negative margin. Recent studies report that vascular resection is not critical in some of these situations and does not decrease recurrence or improve survival.[5,6] This allows adequate resection while preserving hepatic parenchyma.

Regarding perihilar CCA, I view some of the issues differently than the authors. Although debate persists on the role of preoperative biliary drainage in these patients, practically speaking, nearly all patients come to surgical assessment already having biliary intervention. In those without biliary intervention, the bilirubin typically is elevated and preoperative biliary drainage is desirable to allow for safe preoperative portal vein embolization and/or optimal hepatic function post resection. We prefer endobiliary drainage when possible. Similarly, an extended hepatectomy *is not* almost always required to achieve tumor clearance. This issue is discussed below.

Our pathologists review every incidentally discovered GC referred for evaluation. This is critical to understand the depth of invasion and cystic duct margin involvement, as both guide treatment. A careful review of the operative note or a conversation with the surgeon is critical to determine any intraoperative findings that will influence treatment decisions. For instance, bile spillage or cholecystotomy should merit consideration of preoperative systemic therapy prior to laparoscopy and resection due to the risk of intraperitoneal disease.

Finally, the authors emphasize careful perioperative planning, including involvement of the anesthesia team, ensuring their understanding of the plan, and the need for low central venous pressure fluid management and goal-directed fluid administration to minimize bleeding during parenchymal transection. This facet of preparation and intraoperative care is as equally important as all the other issues discussed.

Operative Care

Frequently debated issues in hepatic surgery involve the role of laparoscopy, IOUS, and parenchymal transection techniques. These issues are common to all the entities discussed herein. I use staging laparoscopy routinely, performed at the time of definitive resection, and not at a separate procedure. It allows excellent abdominal exploration and uniform staging. It is easy and quick and provides additional information not available by preoperative imaging. It can be combined with laparoscopic ultrasonography, if necessary, to answer uncertainties remaining from the preoperative evaluation. There is little downside to laparoscopy prior to laparotomy. In CRM, CCA or GC, interfaces such as the liver surface may have metastatic foci not seen on preoperative imaging. Likewise, small peritoneal metastasis in all three of these diseases may be present and identified only on laparoscopy. Finally, liver parenchymal quality can be assessed, allowing liver biopsy if necessary.

IOUS is an essential part of all hepatic surgery. Although the likelihood of identifying unknown lesions with today's high resolution imaging is much smaller than in the past, IOUS continues to play a critical role in assessing, and reassessing, the resection as it proceeds. The fine detail seen on IOUS can modify the resection plan, particularly if lesions abut vascular or biliary structures. Real-time imaging can optimize parenchymal preservation and assure adequate margins are maintained as the transection proceeds.

All approaches, open, laparoscopically, and robotically, have been described for each of these malignancies. Assuming standard resection principles are followed and an oncologically appropriate resection can be achieved, any of these approaches are reasonable.

A variety of parenchymal transection techniques exist, and they have increased over time as new technology becomes available. Several studies have compared the various techniques/tools without any shown to be superior. A common theme in these studies is that the crush-clamp technique is quick and easy, requires no advanced/sophisticated equipment, and is associated with similar or lower blood loss than other techniques. As a result, it is less costly. As a general rule, it is best to use what you are familiar, and proficient, with for transection. The one caveat we impart to all our trainees is to be sure you know how to do a transection using the "low tech" method as one's more advanced/thermal equipment inevitability will fail as some point.

Hepatocellular Carcinoma: IOUS is particularly critical during resection, particularly to identify any satellite lesions and ensure resection of the entire portal distribution of the tumor bearing area. As the authors emphasize, this minimizes the parenchymal resection compared to the need for larger margins in nonanatomic resections.

In patients with parenchymal injury, particularly cirrhosis, strong consideration for transplantation should be given, if the patient is a candidate. In patients with multifocal HCC, unless these are satellite lesions within the primary tumor's portal distribution, resection should not be done as the outcomes are very poor; instead, transplantation should be considered.

Cholangiocarcinoma: Perihilar CCA has been described as a disease of millimeters. As such, the goal is to extend the bile duct transection site as far up on the liver side as feasible while allowing a successful reconstruction. Using this as a principle, many of the debatable issues surrounding CCA subside. First, an R0 resection is critical to affect a cure. However, obtaining an R0 resection does not routinely require an extended hepatectomy. For Bismuth type I, II, and IIIa tumors, an equivalent resection can be achieved with a right hepatectomy that includes the portion of segment IV anterior to the hilum without the need for a formal segment IV resection. Resection of this portion of segment IV extended over to the base of the umbilical fissure allows clearance of the hepatic parenchyma adjacent to the hilum. Typically, this type of resection also includes the caudate process and paracaval portion of the caudate, leaving the Spiegel lobe to the left of the vena cava intact and resulting in a caudate resection that allows clearance around the hilum.[7] If necessary, the Spiegel lobe can be resected as part of the specimen. Finally, this type of resection helps one resect the fullest extent of the left hepatic duct as it begins to traverse ventrally into the umbilical fissure. Done in this fashion, one typically transects the duct just as the segment II/III/IV ducts come together. Depending on the individual's anatomy, this may result in multiple orifices requiring reconstruction to a single orifice for anastomosis. This concept is nicely illustrated by the work of Hirose et al.[8] We typically transect the left hepatic duct following completion of the parenchymal transection, as this allows duct transection as far to the left as possible, typically just to the right of the umbilical portion of the left portal vein or just anterior (behind) it. If one resects the duct to its fullest extent, it obviates the need for frozen sections of the margin, as no additional duct can be safely resected. Some authors describe transecting the duct to the left of the umbilical portion of the left portal vein, necessitating formal resection of segment IV. This is not our usual practice. Finally, if one uses the approach of a partial segment I resection, it is critical that you carefully inspect the transected caudate surface and ligate any disconnected bile ducts emerging from the transected edge to prevent a bile leak.

As described by the authors, we also begin with dissection of the hepatoduodenal ligament to ensure resectability. In our experience, this can be done without transecting the bile duct before resectability is determined, avoiding a nontherapeutic anastomosis in unresectable patients.

Intrahepatic CCA has regional lymph node metastases in a significant minority of patients. As a result, we routinely do a portal lymphadenectomy in conjunction with the hepatic resection. This allows accurate staging, better prognostication, and facilitates the decision for systemic therapy. Whether lymphadenectomy outside the hepatoduodenal ligament is appropriate and useful remains unknown.

Gallbladder Carcinoma: The issue of staging laparoscopy for GC is affected by the context. I agree with the authors that it should be done at the time of the definitive resection for an intact GC. Patients with incidentally discovered GC and a low risk of occult or metastatic disease can forgo laparoscopy if the definitive resection is done within a few weeks of the initial cholecystectomy. If done later than 4 to 6 weeks, we typically do laparoscopy at the same time as the definitive re-resection. If the patient had an incidental cholecystotomy and/or bile spillage during the index cholecystectomy, we consider preoperative systemic therapy for 6 to 8 weeks followed by staging laparoscopy done at the time of the planned re-resection.

An R0 resection is paramount to improve survival. Although data suggests no difference in outcomes of a formal IVb/V resection versus a "wedge" resection of the hepatic parenchyma around the cystic plate, one should be conscious of the location of the primary. Those along the cystic plate wall low in the fossa (adjacent to the hilum) should be excised with caution. Doing a "wedge" resection in this circumstance can lead to "cheating" during the parenchyma transection adjacent to the hilum due to concern for injury to the perihilar structures. Hence, one should ensure an adequate resection of this area or risk a positive margin.

Data supports no role for routine bile duct resection. Although data shows worse outcomes in patients with a positive cystic duct margin, when present, an R0 resection often is achievable by resecting the remaining cystic duct without necessitating resection of the common bile/hepatic ducts. This is particularly so, as many surgeons leave very long cystic duct stumps following laparoscopic cholecystectomy.

To conclude, the authors have provided an excellent summary of the pre- and intraoperative issues for evaluating and treating a number of hepatic and biliary malignancies. They discuss the data supporting their recommendations and acknowledge its limitations. They illustrate there are a numerous areas that require additional investigation if we are going to truly practice evidence-based care for these diseases. It is a pleasure to have the opportunity to provide commentary on this superb piece of work.

REFERENCES

1. de Haas RJ, Wicherts DA, Flores E, Azoulay D, Castaing D, Adam R. R1 resection by necessity for colorectal liver metastases: is it still a contraindication to surgery? *Ann Surg.* 2008;248(4):626-637. doi:10.1097/SLA.0b013e31818a07f1
2. Andreou A, Aloia TA, Brouquet A, et al. Margin status remains an important determinant of survival after surgical resection of colorectal liver metastases in the era of modern chemotherapy. *Ann Surg.* 2013;257(7):1079-1088. doi:10.1097/SLA.0b013e318283a4d1
3. Passot G, Chun YS, Kopetz SE, et al. Predictors of safety and efficacy of 2-stage hepatectomy for bilateral colorectal liver metastases. *J Am Coll Surg.* 2016;223(1):99-108. doi:10.1016/j.jamcollsurg.2015.12.057
4. Brudvik KW, Mise Y, Chung MH, et al. RAS mutation predicts positive resection margins and narrower resection margins in patients undergoing resection of colorectal liver metastases. *Ann Surg Oncol.* 2016;23(8):2635-2643. doi:10.1245/s10434-016-5187-2
5. Viganò L, Procopio F, Cimino MM, et al. Is tumor detachment from vascular structures equivalent to R0 resection in surgery for colorectal liver metastases? An observational cohort. *Ann Surg Oncol.* 2016;23(4):1352-1360. doi:10.1245/s10434-015-5009-y
6. Matsui Y, Terakawa N, Satoi S, et al. Postoperative outcomes in patients with hepatocellular carcinomas resected with exposure of the tumor surface: clinical role of the no-margin resection. *Arch Surg.* 2007;142(7):596-602, discussion 603. doi:10.1001/archsurg.142.7.596
7. Kumon M. Anatomical study of the caudate lobe with special reference to portal venous and biliary branches using corrosion liver casts and clinical application. *Liver Cancer.* 2017;6(2):161-170. doi:10.1159/000454682
8. Hirose T, Igami T, Ebata T, et al. Surgical and radiological studies on the length of the hepatic ducts. *World J Surg.* 2015;39(12):2983-2989. doi:10.1007/s00268-015-3201-7

A page number followed by *f* indicates figures; *t* indicates tables.

A

Abdominal inspection
  for colorectal liver metastases, 426–429
  for hepatocellular carcinoma, 433–435
Abdominal recurrence-free survival (ARFS), 10
Abdominal visceral resections, for peritoneal
    malignancies, 239–248
  cholecystectomy in, 245, 247
  enteric, 239–240, 242–244, 242*f*–243*f*
  hepatic, 240–241, 241*f*, 245–247, 245*f*, 246*f*
  pancreatectomy in, 241, 248
  pelvic peritonectomy in, 233–239, 237*f*, 238*f*
  within pelvis, 233–239
  rationale for, 239–241
  recommendation for, 239
  right upper quadrant in, 247
  splenectomy in, 241, 248
  technical aspects of, 242–248
ACC. *See* Adrenocortical carcinoma
Adams, Reid B., 491–496
Adrenalectomy, 78–79, 83–102
  en bloc resection of adjacent organs invaded
    by cancer in, 88–89
  exposure and line of dissection in, 86, 86*f*–87*f*
  incisions for, 84, 85*f*
  incomplete resection in, problems with, 83–84
  laparoscopic, 91–102
    advantages and disadvantages of, 102*t*
    findings, 98–101
    methodology, 91–98
    systematic reviews and meta-analyses of,
      91–92, 92*f*, 93*t*–97*t*
  left, 87–88, 87*f*
  multivisceral resection with, 83–102
  open *versus* minimally invasive, 91–102, 92*f*,
    93*t*–97*t*, 102*t*
  prophylactic lymphadenectomy with,
    120–128
  rationale for, 83–84, 88–89
  recommendations for, 83, 88
  renal involvement in, 87–89, 90*f*
  resection of primary tumor to microscopically
    negative margins in, 83–88
  right, 85–87, 86*f*
  technical aspects of, 84–88, 89
Adrenal hormone excess
  medications for, 79, 80*t*
  signs and symptoms of, 76–77
  testing for, 76–78, 77*t*

Adrenal malignancies, 74–142. *See
    also* Adrenocortical carcinoma;
    Pheochromocytoma
Adrenal neuroendocrine tumors, 145
Adrenocortical carcinoma (ACC), 74–142
  adrenalectomy for, 78–79, 83–102
    en bloc resection of adjacent organs
      invaded by cancer in, 88–89
    exposure and line of dissection in, 86,
      86*f*–87*f*
    incisions for, 84, 85*f*
    incomplete resection in, problems with,
      83–84
    left, 87–88, 87*f*
    multivisceral resection with, 83–102
    open *versus* minimally invasive, 91–102,
      92*f*, 93*t*–97*t*, 102*t*
    prophylactic lymphadenectomy with,
      120–128
    rationale for, 83–84, 88–89
    recommendations, 83, 88
    renal involvement in, 87–89, 90*f*
    resection of primary tumor to microscopically
      negative margins in, 83–88
    right, 85–87, 86*f*
    technical aspects of, 84–88, 89
  adrenalectomy for, laparoscopic, 91–102
    advantages and disadvantages of, 102*t*
    findings, 98–101
    methodology, 91–98
    systematic reviews and meta-analyses of,
      91–92, 92*f*, 93*t*–97*t*
  biopsy of, 77*t*
  clinical staging of, 74, 75*t*, 113, 141–142
  commentary on, 141–142
  diagnostic evaluation for, 76–78, 77*t*
  epidemiology of, 74
  genetic conditions associated with, 74, 76
  imaging of, 77–78, 77*t*, 142
  lymph nodes involved in, 117–118, 117*f*–118*f*
  metastases from, 78, 142
  metastatic, lymphadenectomy for, 116–128
    prophylactic, 120–128, 121*f*, 122*t*–126*t*
    rationale for, 116–118
    recommendation, 116
    technical aspects of, 119
  metastatic (stage IV), surgery for, 110–115
    findings, 113–115
    methodology, 110–111

Adrenocortical carcinoma (ACC) (*continued*)
  systematic reviews and meta-analyses,
    110–111, 111*f*, 112*t*
  multidisciplinary care for, 75–76
  perioperative care for, 76–82
  postoperative adjuvant therapy for, 82
  quality measures for, 82
  surgical decision on, 78–79
  surgical expertise required for, 79
  synoptic operative report on, 79, 135–140
  synoptic pathologic report on, 79
  vascular invasion by, 103–109
    en bloc resection of adjacent blood vessels,
      103–109
    extent of tumor thrombus in, 106*f*
    extraction of tumor thrombus in, 108–109
    hypothermic perfusion of liver in, 107, 108*f*
    IVC exposure in, 105
    IVC reconstruction in, 109
    IVC resection in, 103–108
    recommendation for, 103
    resection rationale for, 103–105
    technical aspects of resection, 105–109
    vascular control in, 106–108, 107*f*
    venovenous bypass in, 107, 107*f*
AJCC. *See* American Joint Committee on
    Cancer staging system
Aldosterone excess, medications for, 80*t*
Aldosterone-secreting ACC, 77
Alexander, H. Richard, Jr., 286–289
Alpha-blockade, of pheochromocytoma,
    79–82, 81*t*
ALTs. *See* Atypical lipomatous tumors/well-
    differentiated liposarcomas
American Association of Clinical
    Endocrinologists, 98
American Association of Endocrine Surgeons, 98
American Joint Committee on Cancer (AJCC)
    staging system
  for ACC, 74, 75*t*, 113, 141–142
  for appendiceal neoplasms, 217, 217*t*–218*t*
  for bladder cancer, 295*t*–296*t*
  for cholangiocarcinoma, intrahepatic, 417,
    419*t*, 447–448
  for cholangiocarcinoma, perihilar, 415–417,
    418*t*, 448
  for colorectal cancer, 219
  for colorectal liver metastases, 414, 415*t*
  for gallbladder cancer, 421*t*, 470
  for gastric carcinoma, 219
  for hepatocellular cancer, 414, 416*t*
  for neuroendocrine neoplasms, 147, 148*t*–152*t*
  for soft tissue sarcoma, 2–9, 2*t*–9*t*, 28
  for upper urinary tract cancer, 297*t*–298*t*
  for urethral cancer, 298*t*–300*t*
American Urological Association (AUA),
    300–302, 335
Amiloride, 80*t*
Ampulla of Vater, neuroendocrine tumors of,
    147, 148*t*–149*t*
Amputation, for soft tissue sarcoma, 10, 18, 22

Anastrozole, 80*t*
Androgen blockade, for adrenal malignancies, 80*t*
Angiosarcoma, breast, 18, 25, 26*f*
Aortocaval node sampling
  for cholangiocarcinoma, 445–449
  for gallbladder cancer, 469–471
Appendiceal neoplasms
  clinical staging of, 216–218, 217*t*–218*t*
  diagnosis of, 221
  patient history and physical findings of, 220
  peritoneal metastases from, 216–219, 220
    (*See also* Peritoneal malignancies)
  PCI limit in, 262*t*–263*t*, 267
ARFS. *See* Abdominal recurrence-free survival
Assessment of Multiple Systematic Reviews 2
    (AMSTAR 2), 356, 358, 361*t*, 362–363
Association for Urologic Oncology of the
    German Cancer Society, 331
Atezolizumab, 420
Atypical lipomatous tumors/well-differentiated
    liposarcomas (ALTs), 18, 24

B

Beta-blockade, of pheochromocytoma, 79–82,
    81*t*
Bile duct cancer. *See* Cholangiocarcinoma
Biopsy. *See also* Sentinel lymph node biopsy
  adrenal, 77*t*
  perihilar cholangiocarcinoma, 420–422
  soft tissue sarcoma, 12–13
    of extremity and trunk, 12–17
    orientation of tract and incision in, 15,
      16*f*–17*f*
    rationale for, 14–15
    technical aspects of, 15–17, 16*f*–17*f*
  urothelial, 308, 309, 310
Bladder. *See* Gallbladder; Urinary bladder
Blue light cystoscopy, 304, 304*f*
Bone, in resection of soft tissue sarcoma, 20*f*,
    21–22, 45
Breast angiosarcomas, 18, 25, 26*f*
Budd-Chiari syndrome, 103

C

Calcium channel blockers, for
    pheochromocytoma, 79–82, 81*t*
Capecitabine, for gallbladder cancer, 422
Carcinoid syndrome, 145, 152–153, 154
Carcinoma in situ (CIS), urinary bladder,
    316–317
Caudate lobe resection (CLR), for perihilar
    cholangiocarcinoma, 450–456
  findings, 452–456
  methodology, 450–451
  overall survival rates in, 453*t*–454*t*, 455
  perioperative morbidity in, 455–456
  R0 resection in, 455
  systematic reviews and meta-analyses, 451,
    452*f*, 453*t*–454*t*
Central pancreatectomy, 182–183

Chemoradiation
  for colorectal liver metastases, 420
  for perihilar cholangiocarcinoma, 420
  for urothelial carcinoma, 301
Chemotherapy
  for adrenocortical carcinoma, 79, 82, 89
  for gallbladder cancer, 422
  hyperthermic intraperitoneal, 216, 216t,
    219–222, 249–253
  for intrahepatic cholangiocarcinoma, 422
  intravesical
    perioperative instillation of, 375–376
    postoperative instillation of, 311–312, 409
  for neuroendocrine neoplasms, 153–154
  for pheochromocytoma, 82
  for soft tissue sarcoma, 11
  for urothelial carcinoma, 300–301
Chest radiography, for soft tissue sarcoma, 12, 13
Cholangiocarcinoma, 440–462
  commentary on, 491–496
  portal lymphadenectomy/nodal sampling for,
    430, 431, 432, 445–449, 449f, 495
  resection of primary tumor to
    microscopically negative margins,
    440–444, 444f, 445f, 494–495
Cholangiocarcinoma, intrahepatic
  clinical staging of, 417, 419t, 447–448
  commentary on, 491–496
  epidemiology of, 417
  future liver remnant in, 422, 423
  lymphadenectomy for, 425
  multidisciplinary care for, 422, 492
  perioperative care/preoperative decision-
    making for, 423, 492–493
  portal lymphadenectomy/nodal sampling
    for, 495
    rationale for, 447–448
    recommendation for, 445
    technical aspects of, 448–449, 449f
  quality measures in, 424–425
  resection of primary tumor to
    microscopically negative margins
    rationale for, 442–443
    recommendation for, 440
    technical aspects of, 444
  synoptic operative report on, 488–489
Cholangiocarcinoma, perihilar
  bile duct margins in
    distal, 458–459, 461
      positive, intraoperative re-resection based
        on frozen section analysis in, 457–462,
        459f, 460t
      proximal, 461–462
  caudate lobe resection for, 450–456
    findings, 452–456
    methodology, 450–451
    overall survival rates in, 453t–454t, 455
    perioperative morbidity in, 455–456
    R0 resection in, 455
    systematic reviews and meta-analyses, 451,
      452f, 453t–454t

clinical staging of, 415–417, 418t, 448
commentary on, 491–496
endoscopic biopsy of, 420–422
future liver remnant in, 423–424
lymphadenectomy for, 425
multidisciplinary care for, 420–422, 492
perioperative care/preoperative decision-
  making for, 423–424, 492–493
portal lymphadenectomy/nodal sampling for
  rationale for, 446–447
  recommendation for, 445
  technical aspects of, 448–449, 449f
portal vein resection and reconstruction in,
  442, 444, 445f
quality measures in, 424–425
resection of primary tumor to microscopically
  negative margins, 494–495
  rationale for, 440–442
  recommendation for, 440
  technical aspects of, 443–444, 444f, 445f
Cholecystectomy
  for gallbladder cancer, 424, 467–468
  incidental cancer findings in, 417–418, 424,
    463–468
  for peritoneal malignancies, 245, 247
  prophylactic, for NETs, 165, 166–173, 212
    findings, 167–173
    methodology, 166
    systematic reviews and meta-analyses, 166,
      167f 168t–170t
Cirrhosis, and HCC surgery, 433–435, 494
Cisplatin, for urothelial carcinoma, 300–301,
  409
CLM. See Colorectal liver metastases
Colon. See Large bowel, peritoneal
  malignancies involving
Colorectal cancer
  metastases from (See Colorectal liver
    metastases; Colorectal peritoneal
    metastases)
  patient history and physical findings of, 220
  quality measures in, 424–425
Colorectal liver metastases
  clinical staging of, 414, 415t
  commentary on, 491–496
  extraregional nodal disease with, 426–427
  liver resection for, 426–432
    access approach in, 431
    critical elements of, 426
    evaluation of liver quality for, 427
    future liver remnant in, 423, 428, 430–431
    intraoperative ultrasound in, 426, 428,
      428f, 429f, 430
    open parenchyma-sparing, 431
    parenchymal transection in, 432
    quality measures in, 424–425
    rationale for, 426–428, 430–431
    recommendations for, 426, 430
    resection of planned lesions to
      macroscopically negative margins in,
      430–432

Colorectal liver metastases (*continued*)
  specimen orientation and margin
     assessment in, 430–431
  systematic abdominal inspection in, 426–429
  technical aspects of, 428–430, 431–432
  multidisciplinary care for, 420, 491–492
  perioperative care/preoperative decision-
     making for, 423, 492–493
  perioperative chemotherapy for, 420
  peritoneal metastases with, 426–427
  staging laparoscopy for, 427
  synoptic operative report on, 490
Colorectal peritoneal metastases, 216,
     216*t*, 219, 220. *See also* Peritoneal
     malignancies
  cytoreduction plus HIPEC for, survival
     versus complications in, 269–273, 270*f*,
     271*t*
  with metastatic hepatic disease, 426–427
  PCI limit in, 256–267, 258*t*–261*t*
Commentary
  adrenal, 141–142
  hepatobiliary, 491–496
  neuroendocrine tumors, 211–213
  peritoneal, 286–289
  sarcoma, 71–72
  urothelial, 409–411
Completeness of cytoreduction (CC) score, 254
Computed tomography (CT)
  for adrenal malignancies, 77–78, 77*t*
  for colorectal liver metastases, 426
  for gallbladder cancer, 420, 463–464
  for hepatobiliary malignancies, 492
  for hepatocellular cancer, 433
  for intrahepatic cholangiocarcinoma, 417
  for neuroendocrine neoplasms, 147
  for perihilar cholangiocarcinoma, 417
  for peritoneal malignancies, 220–221
  for soft tissue sarcoma, 12, 13
Continent cutaneous diversion, 332–334
Core needle biopsy, percutaneous, of soft tissue
     sarcoma, 12
  extremity and trunk, 12–13, 15, 16*f*–17*f*
Cortisol excess, medications for, 80*t*
Cortisol-secreting ACCs, 77
CRS. *See* Cytoreductive surgery
CT. *See* Computed tomography
Cushing syndrome, 76, 79
Cyproheptadine, 152
Cystectomy, organ-sparing, 323–329
  in females, 294–300, 323–325, 326*f*, 327*f*
     patient selection for, 325
     rationale for, 324–325
     recommendation for, 323
     technical aspects of, 326*f*, 328
  in males, 326–328
     patient selection for, 326–327
     rationale for, 326–327
     recommendation for, 323
     technical aspects of, 328, 329*f*

Cystectomy, partial, 300, 313–318
  commentary on, 410
  contraindications to, 316–317, 317*f*
  critical elements of, 313
  intraoperative localization of tumor in,
     313–314, 315*f*
  margin status in, 316
  as organ-sparing alternative, 318
  rationale for, 313–316
  recommendations for, 313, 314–315
  recurrence rates after, 316
  resection to adequate margins in, 314–317
  synoptic operative report on, 405–408
  technical aspects of, 314, 315*f*, 317–318,
     318*f*
  ureteral implantation in, 316
Cystectomy, radical, 292, 294–301, 319–353
  bladder removal to negative resection
     margins in, 319–323
     rationale for, 319–320
     recommendation for, 319
     technical aspects of, 320–323, 321*f*, 322*f*,
        323*f*, 324*f*
  bladder-sparing chemoradiation *versus*, 301
  chemotherapy with, 300–301
  commentary on, 409–410
  concomitant pelvic organ management in,
     323–329
  critical elements of, 319
  in females
     organ-sparing, 294–300, 323–325, 326*f*,
        327*f*
     rationale for, 324, 325*f*
     recommendation for, 323
     urethral management in, 321, 326*f*
     urinary diversion in, 321, 324 328, 333–334
  in males
     organ-sparing, 326–328, 329*f*
     recommendation for, 323
     urethral management in, 322–323
     urinary diversion in, 333
  minimally invasive *versus* open, 322–323,
     324*f*, 354–363
  partial cystectomy *versus*, 318
  pelvic lymph node dissection with, 319–320,
     330–332
     anatomic extent of, 330–331, 331*f*
     count (yield) in, 330, 336–337, 339*t*–349*t*,
        350–352
     discussion, 351–353
     extended, 330–331, 331*f*, 335
     findings, 336–351
     limited, 330–331, 331*f*, 335
     methodology, 336
     rationale for, 330–331
     recommendation for, 330
     standard, 330–332, 331*f*, 335
     standard *versus* extended, 335–353, 337*f*,
        338*t*, 346*t*–349*t*
     superextended, 330, 331*f*, 335

systematic reviews and meta-analyses, 336,
337f, 338t–349t
technical aspects of, 331–332
timing of, 331
perioperative care in, 301–302
rectum management in, 321, 323f
robot-assisted, 322–323, 354–363
AMSTAR 2 criteria for studies, 356, 358,
361t, 362–363
diffusion of technology, 354
discussion, 360–363
findings, 357–360
methodology, 355–356
studies excluded from review of, 356, 358t
systematic reviews and meta-analyses,
355–356, 357f, 359t
synoptic operative report on, 396–399
urachal resection in, 320, 321f
ureteral resection in, 321, 322f
urethrectomy with, 321–322
urinary diversion following, 300, 332–334,
410
rationale for, 332–333
recommendation for, 332
Cystoprostatectomy, radical, 294
Cystoscopy
blue light, 304, 304f
diagnostic, 303–306, 304f, 305f, 314
intraoperative, 314, 315f, 317, 318f
in nephroureterectomy, 368–370
photodynamic, 303, 304–305, 304f, 305f, 306
white light, 303, 304–305, 304f, 305f, 306
Cystostomy, 317
Cytoreductive surgery (CRS)
for hepatic metastases from NETs, 173–178,
176f, 177t
for peritoneal malignancies, 216, 216t,
219–248
abdominal visceral resections in, 239–248
cholecystectomy in, 245, 247
commentary on, 286–289
completeness score in, 254
critical elements of, 223
diaphragmatic, 228–233, 229f, 230f, 232f
enteric resection in, 239–240, 242–244,
242f–243f
full-thickness resection of diaphragm in,
232–233
hepatic resection in, 240–241, 241f,
245–247, 245f, 246f
HIPEC following, 249–253
HIPEC with, survival *versus* complications
in, 269–273, 270f, 271t
hysterectomy in, 234–237, 238f
lesser omentectomy in, 224–227, 226f
pancreatectomy for, 241, 248
PCI score and outcome of, 254–268
pelvic peritonectomy in, 233–239, 237f, 238f
within pelvis, 233–239
quality measures for, 221–222

rectosigmoid resection in, 237–238, 238f
resection of mesenteric disease in,
227–228, 228f
small bowel mesenteric peritonectomy in,
228, 228f
splenectomy for, 241, 248
subdiaphragmatic peritonectomy in,
231–232, 232f
supracolic greater omentectomy in,
225–227, 226f
visceral peritonectomy of right upper
quadrant in, 247

D

Deep venous thromboembolism (DVT), radical
cystectomy and, 301
Dermatofibrosarcoma protuberans (DFSP), 18,
24–25
Desmoid tumors
extra-abdominal, 18, 24
retroperitoneal and intra-abdominal, 47
DFSP. *See* Dermatofibrosarcoma protuberans
Diaphragm
cytoreduction of, 228–233
complete, 229, 230f
rationale for, 229–231
recommendation for, 228
subdiaphragmatic peritonectomy in,
231–232, 232f
technical aspects of, 231–233
full-thickness resection of, 232–233
redistribution phenomenon in, 229, 230f
Dinney, Colin P. N., 409–411
Distal ureterectomy, 294, 366, 368–371
Doxazosin, 81t
Drains, for sarcoma resection, 26, 27f
Duodenotomy, 158
Duodenum, neuroendocrine tumors of
clinical staging of, 147, 148t–149t
intraoperative exploration for, 157–160
location of nodal metastases, 161, 162f
regional lymphadenectomy for, 160–164
resection of primary tumor, 164–165

E

Eilber, Fritz C., 71–72
Enhanced Recovery After Surgery (ERAS)
protocols, 301
ENSAT. *See* European Network for the Study
of Adrenal Tumors
Enteric resection, for peritoneal malignancies
rationale for, 239–240
technical aspects of, 242–244, 242f–243f
Enucleation, of pancreatic NETs, 180–183
indications/criteria for, 180–181, 181f
intraoperative ultrasound prior to, 179–180
rationale for, 180–182
recommendation for, 180
technical aspects of, 182

Eplerenone, 80*t*
Estrogen blockade, for adrenal malignancies, 80*t*
Etomidate, 80*t*
European Association of Urology (EAU), 335
European Network for the Study of Adrenal
  Tumors (ENSAT), 74, 75*t*, 98, 113
European Neuroendocrine Tumor Society, 155
European Society of Endocrinology, 98
Everolimus, 152, 153
Extended lymph node dissection (eLND),
  pelvic, 330–331, 331*f*
  findings, 336–351
  methodology, 336
  standard *versus*, 335–353
  systematic reviews and meta-analyses, 336,
    337*f*, 338*t*, 346*t*–349*t*
Extended resection, of retroperitoneal sarcoma,
  48–61
Extra-abdominal desmoid tumors, 18, 24
Extraperitoneal parietal peritonectomy, 231
Extremity sarcoma (soft tissue)
  amputation indications for, 9, 18, 22
  biopsy of, 12–17
    orientation of tract and incision in, 15,
      16*f*–17*f*
    rationale for, 14–15
    technical aspects of, 15–17, 16*f*–17*f*
  clinical staging of, 2*t*–4*t*
  limb-salvage surgery for, 10, 18, 22, 24
  postoperative care and follow-up for, 13
  preoperative clinical and imaging evaluation
    of, 11
  resection of, 14–39
    clip placement for postoperative radiation
      planning in, 22, 23*f*
    considerations for specific histologic
      subtypes, 18, 24–25
    en bloc, of biopsy tract, 18–19
    intraoperative frozen section in, 17, 19
    macroscopically complete, of primary
      tumor, 17–25
    management of bone and tendons in, 20*f*,
      21–22
    management of neurovascular bundles in,
      20–21, 20*f*
    rationale for, 18–19
    recommendation for, 17
    reconstruction in, 23–24
    surgical drain placement in, 26, 27*f*
    surgical margins in, 19, 20*f*
    technical aspects of, 20–25
  sentinel lymph node biopsy for, 28–39
    findings, 30–38, 33*t*–37*t*
    impact on patient outcomes, 33*t*–37*t*, 38–39
    methodology, 28–30, 29*f*
    positive, complete lymph node dissection
      after, 39
    qualitative systematic review, 30, 31*t*–32*t*
  synoptic operative report, 68–70
  treatment guidelines for, 9

F

Falciform ligament
  in hepatic resection, 241, 241*f*, 245, 246*f*
  in visceral peritonectomy of right upper
    quadrant, 247
FDG-PET. *See* ^{18}F-fluoro-deoxy-D-glucose
  positron emission tomography, for
  adrenal malignancies
Fédération Nationale des Centres de Lutte
  Contre le Cancer, 2
[18]F-fluoro-deoxy-D-glucose positron emission
  tomography (FDG-PET), for adrenal
  malignancies, 77*t*, 78, 142
Fibrosarcomatous-DFSP, 25
Field-cancerization hypothesis, 409
FLR. *See* Future liver remnant
FOLFOX, for colorectal liver metastases, 420
Frozen section, intraoperative, soft tissue
  sarcoma, 17, 19
Future liver remnant (FLR), 422–424, 492–493
  in colorectal liver metastases, 423, 428,
    430–431
  in gallbladder cancer, 424
  in hepatocellular cancer, 423, 434–436, 439
  in intrahepatic cholangiocarcinoma, 422, 423
  in perihilar cholangiocarcinoma, 423–424

G

^{68}Ga-DOTATE-PET/CT
  for adrenal malignancies, 78
  for neuroendocrine neoplasms, 147, 153–154
Gallbladder
  peritoneal malignancies involving, 245, 247
  surgical removal of
    for gallbladder cancer, 424, 467–468
    incidental cancer findings in, 417–418,
      424, 463–468
    for peritoneal malignancies, 245, 247
    prophylactic, for NETs, 165, 166–173,
      167*f*, 168*t*–170*t*
Gallbladder cancer, 463–472
  anatomic IVb and V segmentectomy *versus*
    wedge resection of gallbladder bed for,
    468, 496
  bile duct resection for, 468–469, 496
  chemotherapy for, 422
  cholecystectomy alone *versus* re-resection for,
    467–468
  clinical staging of, 417–420, 421*t*, 470
  commentary on, 491–496
  critical elements of approach for, 463
  future liver remnant in, 424
  incidental, 417–420, 463–468, 471–472
  lymphadenectomy for, 425
  microscopically complete resection of local
    tumor in, 467–469, 496
    rationale for, 467–469
    recommendation for, 467
    technical aspects of, 469

multidisciplinary care for, 422, 492
perioperative care/preoperative decision-
    making for, 424, 492–493
per primum, 463, 466, 467
portal lymphadenectomy/nodal sampling for,
    469–471
port site excision for, routine, 471–472
    rationale for, 471–472
    recommendation for, 471
quality measures in, 424–425
risk factors for, 417
selective staging laparoscopy prior to
    resection of, 463–466, 495
    rationale for, 463–466
    recommendation for, 463
    technical aspects of, 466, 467f
synoptic operative report on, 484–485
Gallstones, NETs and, 166–173
Gastric cancer. See also specific types and tumors
    clinical staging of, 219
    patient history and physical findings of, 220
    peritoneal metastases from, 216, 216t, 219,
        220 (See also Peritoneal malignancies)
        cytoreduction plus HIPEC for, survival
            versus complications in, 269–273, 270f,
            271t
        PCI limit in, 264t–265t, 267–268
Gastric GISTs, clinical staging of, 4t–5t
Gastrinoma
    intraoperative exploration for, 157–160, 157f
    location of nodal metastases, 161, 162f
    regional lymphadenectomy for, 160–164
Gastrinoma triangle, 157, 157f, 159
Gastrointestinal stromal tumors (GISTs)
    biopsy of, 13
    chemotherapy for, 10
    clinical staging of, 4t–7t
    postoperative care and follow-up for, 13
    preoperative clinical and imaging evaluation
        of, 11
    resection of, 46–47
        laparoscopic, 47, 47f
        macroscopically complete, of primary
            tumor without disruption of tumor
            capsule, 40–41
        rationale for, 40–41
        recommendation for, 40
    rupture of, 41
Gemcitabine, intravesical, postoperative,
    311–312, 409
Gerota fascia, in adrenalectomy, 86, 87f, 88
Gibson incision, 41, 42f
Gleevec, for soft tissue sarcoma, 11
Glissonian pedicle–based liver resection, 436,
    437f, 438–439, 438f
Glucocorticoids, for adrenal hormone excess,
    79, 80t
Greater omentectomy, supracolic, 223–227
    indications for, 224
    rationale for, 223–225

recommendation for, 223
technical aspects of, 225–227, 226f
Greater omentum
    anatomy and physiology of, 223
    peritoneal malignancies involving, 223–227,
        224f
    as "policeman of the abdomen," 223

H

HCC. See Hepatocellular cancer
Hepatectomy. See Liver resection
Hepatic metastases, colorectal. See Colorectal
    liver metastases
Hepatobiliary malignancies, 414–496. See
    also Cholangiocarcinoma; Colorectal
    liver metastases; Gallbladder cancer;
    Hepatocellular cancer
    clinical staging of, 414–420
    commentary on, 491–496
    lymphadenectomy for, 425
    multidisciplinary care for, 420–422, 491–492
    perioperative care for, 422–424, 492–494
    preoperative decision-making for
        resectability of, 422
    quality measures in, 424–425
    synoptic operative reports on, 484–490
Hepatocellular cancer (HCC)
    clinical staging of, 414, 416t
    commentary on, 491–496
    immunotherapy for, 420
    intraportal metastases from, 436–437, 437f
    liver resection for, 414, 433–439, 494
        critical elements of, 433
        future liver remnant in, 423, 434–436, 439
        Glissonian pedicle–based (anatomic), 436,
            437f, 438–439, 438f
        inspection of abdomen and liver in,
            433–435
        intraoperative ultrasound in, 433–435,
            435f
        laparoscopic versus open inspection in,
            434, 435f
        to macroscopically negative margins,
            436–439
        margin definition in, 436–437, 437f
        minimally invasive, 438, 439
        nodal sampling in, 437
        nonanatomic, 436–437, 437f, 439
        parenchymal transection in, 439
        rationale for, 433–434, 436–437
        recommendations for, 433, 436
        robot-assisted, 439
        specimen orientation in, 439
        technical aspects of, 434–435, 438–439,
            438f
    liver transplant for, 414, 494
    multidisciplinary care for, 420, 492
    perioperative care/preoperative decision-
        making for, 423, 492–493

Hilar cholangiocarcinoma. *See* Perihilar
  cholangiocarcinoma
HIPEC. *See* Hyperthermic intraperitoneal
  chemotherapy
Howe, James R., 211–213
Hydrocortisone, for adrenal hormone excess,
  79, 80*t*
Hyperthermic intraperitoneal chemotherapy
  (HIPEC), 216, 216*t*, 219–222, 249–253
  administration standards for, 251–252
  commentary on, 286–289
  with (following) cytoreduction, 249–253
  with cytoreduction, survival *versus*
    complications in, 269–273, 270*f*, 271*t*
  exposure precautions for, 252
  open *versus* closed technique, 250, 251, 252*f*
  patient management and monitoring in, 253
  PCI score and outcome of, 254–268
  perfusion system for, 251, 251*f*
  quality measures for, 221–222
  rationale for, 249–250
  recommendation for, 249
  systematic reviews and meta-analyses of,
    269, 270*f*, 271*t*
  technical aspects of, 250–253
  temperature requirements for, 253
Hysterectomy
  minimally invasive *versus* open, 354
  peritoneal malignancies involving uterus,
    234–237, 238*f*

I

ICC. *See* Intrahepatic cholangiocarcinoma
Ileal conduit, 332–333
Ileum, neuroendocrine tumors of
  clinical staging of, 147, 149*t*–150*t*
  intraoperative exploration for, 158, 160
  regional lymphadenectomy for, 160–164
  resection of primary tumor, 164–165
Imatinib mesylate (Gleevec), for soft tissue
  sarcoma, 11
Immunotherapy
  for hepatocellular cancer, 420
  for urothelial carcinoma, 301
Incidental gallbladder cancer, 417–420,
  463–468, 471–472
Inferior vena cava (IVC)
  adrenalectomy and, 86–87, 88, 89
  adrenal malignancies and resection of,
    103–109
    exposure in, 105
    extent of tumor thrombus in, 106*f*
    extraction of tumor thrombus in, 108–109
    hypothermic perfusion of liver in, 107, 108*f*
    infracardiac and intra-atrial, 107–108
    infrahepatic, 106
    reconstruction of IVC in, 109
    retro- and suprahepatic but below
      diaphragm, 107

technical aspects of, 105–109
vascular control in, 106–108
venovenous bypass in, 107, 107*f*
lymphadenectomy and, 119
in visceral peritonectomy of right upper
  quadrant, 247
Intra-abdominal sarcoma. *See also*
  Gastrointestinal stromal tumors
  resection of, 40–67
    considerations for specific histologic
      subtypes, 45–46
    en bloc, of invaded organs, 43–47, 44*f*,
      46*f*
    extended, 48–61
    macroscopically complete, of primary
      tumor without disruption of tumor
      capsule, 40–41
    management of bony structures in, 45
    management of neurovascular bundles
      in, 45
    psoas resection in, 45
    rationale for, 40–41, 43–44
    recommendation for, 40
    technical aspects of, 41, 45–47
Intrahepatic cholangiocarcinoma (ICC)
  clinical staging of, 417, 419*t*, 447–448
  commentary on, 491–496
  epidemiology of, 417
  future liver remnant in, 422, 423
  lymphadenectomy for, 425
  multidisciplinary care for, 422, 492
  perioperative care/preoperative decision-
    making for, 423, 492–493
  portal lymphadenectomy/nodal sampling
    for, 495
  rationale for, 447–448
  recommendation for, 445
  technical aspects of, 448–449, 449*f*
  quality measures in, 424–425
  resection of primary tumor to
    microscopically negative margins
    rationale for, 442–443
    recommendation for, 440
    technical aspects of, 444
  synoptic operative report on, 488–489
Intramuscular sarcoma, oncologic barrier in, 19
Intraoperative ultrasound (IOUS)
  for colorectal liver metastases, 426, 428,
    428*f*, 429*f*, 430
  for hepatobiliary malignancies, 493–494
  for hepatocellular carcinoma, 433–435,
    435*f*, 494
  for neuroendocrine neoplasms, 158, 159,
    179–180
Intravesical chemotherapy
  perioperative instillation of, 375–376
  postoperative instillation of, 311–312, 409
IOUS. *See* Intraoperative ultrasound
Ipilimumab, 420
IVC. *See* Inferior vena cava

J

Jejunum, neuroendocrine tumors of
 clinical staging of, 147, 149*t*–150*t*
 intraoperative exploration for, 158, 160
 regional lymphadenectomy for, 160–164
 resection of primary tumor, 164–165

K

Ketoconazole, 80*t*, 141
Kidney(s)
 adrenal malignancies invading, 88–89
 removal, in urothelial carcinoma, 364–376
  (*See also* Nephroureterectomy)
Klatskin tumor. *See* Perihilar cholangiocarcinoma
Kocher maneuver, 85, 432, 448, 449*f*

L

Lanreotide, for NETs, 152–154
 frequency of gallstones in patients treated
  with, 172–173
 pathogenesis of gallstones secondary to, 171
 prophylactic cholecystectomy with, 166–173
Laparoscopic adrenalectomy, 91–102
 advantages and disadvantages of, 102*t*
 findings, 98–101
 methodology, 91–98
 systematic reviews and meta-analyses of,
  91–92, 92*f*, 93*t*–97*t*
Laparoscopic inspection, in HCC, 434, 435*f*
Laparoscopic nephroureterectomy, 365–366, 367
Laparoscopic resection, of GISTs, 47, 47*f*
Laparoscopic staging
 for colorectal liver metastases, 427
 for gallbladder cancer, 463–466
Laparoscopy, peritoneal, 221
Large bowel, peritoneal malignancies involving,
 239–240, 242–244
Large bowel resection, for peritoneal
 malignancies
 rationale for, 234–235
 technical aspects of, 242–244
Leiomyosarcoma, retroperitoneal, 45
Lenvatinib, 420
Lesser omentectomy, 224–227, 226*f*
Ligamentum teres hepatis
 in hepatic resection, 241, 241*f*, 245, 246*f*
 in visceral peritonectomy of right upper
  quadrant, 247
Limb-salvage surgery, for soft tissue sarcoma,
 10, 18, 22, 24
Limited lymph node dissection, pelvic,
 330–331, 331*f*, 335
Liposarcoma
 retroperitoneal, 44*f*, 45
 well-differentiated, 18
Liver
 adrenal malignancies invading, 88–89
 colorectal metastases to (*See* Colorectal liver
  metastases)

hypothermic perfusion of, 107, 108*f*
NETs metastatic to
 hepatic debulking for, 174–178, 176*f*, 177*t*
 treatment options for, 174–175
 peritoneal malignancies involving, 240–241,
  245–247
Liver remnant, future. *See* Future liver remnant
Liver resection
 for cholangiocarcinoma, 440–462
  caudate lobe, 450–456
  critical elements of, 440
  future liver remnant in, 422, 423–424
  portal lymphadenectomy/nodal sampling
   with, 430, 431, 432, 445–449, 495
  rationale for, 440–442, 440–443
  recommendations for, 440
  resection of primary tumor to microscopically
   negative margins in, 440–444
  technical aspects of, 443–444, 444*f*, 445*f*
 for colorectal liver metastases, 426–432
  access approach in, 431
  critical elements of, 426
  evaluation of liver quality for, 427
  future liver remnant in, 423, 428, 430–431
  intraoperative ultrasound in, 426, 428,
   428*f*, 429*f*, 430
  open parenchyma-sparing, 431
  parenchymal transection in, 432
  quality measures in, 424–425
  rationale for, 426–428, 430–431
  recommendations for, 426, 430
  resection of planned lesions to
   macroscopically negative margins in,
   430–432
  specimen orientation and margin
   assessment in, 430–431
  systematic abdominal inspection in,
   426–429
  technical aspects of, 428–430, 431–432
 for hepatocellular cancer, 414, 433–439, 494
  critical elements of, 433
  future liver remnant in, 423, 434–436, 439
  Glissonian pedicle–based (anatomic), 436,
   437*f*, 438–439, 438*f*
  inspection of abdomen and liver in, 433–435
  intraoperative ultrasound in, 433–435, 435*f*
  laparoscopic *versus* open inspection in,
   434, 435*f*
  to macroscopically negative margins,
   436–439
  margin definition in, 436–437, 437*f*
  minimally invasive, 438, 439
  nodal sampling in, 437
  nonanatomic, 436–437, 437*f*, 439
  parenchymal transection in, 439
  rationale for, 433–434, 436–437
  recommendations for, 433, 436
  robot-assisted, 439
  specimen orientation in, 439
  technical aspects of, 434–435, 438–439, 438*f*

Liver resection (*continued*)
    indications for, 414
    for peritoneal malignancies
        falciform ligament and ligamentum teres
            hepatis in, 241, 241*f*, 245, 246*f*
        rationale for, 240–241
        technical aspects of, 245–247, 245*f*, 246*f*
Liver transplant, for hepatocellular cancer, 414,
    494
LNC. *See* Lymph node count
Lungs, neuroendocrine tumors of, 145, 147
Lymphadenectomy, for ACC, 116–128
    prophylactic, 120–128
        findings, 127–128
        methodology, 120–127
        systematic reviews and meta-analyses,
            120–127, 121*f*, 122*t*–126*t*
    rationale for, 116–118
    recommendation, 116
    technical aspects of, 119
Lymphadenectomy, for colorectal liver
        metastases, 430, 431, 432
Lymphadenectomy, for gallbladder cancer, 425
Lymphadenectomy, for hepatocellular cancer,
    437
Lymphadenectomy, for pancreatic NETs, 183–198
    findings, 187–198
        impact on overall survival, 197–198
        impact on recurrence-free survival, 187–197
    methodology, 186–187
    systematic reviews and meta-analyses,
        186–187, 186*f*, 188*t*–196*t*
Lymphadenectomy, for small bowel NETs
    rationale for, 160–162
    recommendation, 160
    regional, along segmental vessels, 160–164, 163*f*
Lymphadenectomy, for upper tract urothelial
        cancer, 372–375
    rationale for, 372–375
    recommendation for, 372
    technical aspects of, 375
    templates for, 372–374, 373*f*, 374*f*
Lymphadenectomy, pelvic, with radical
        cystectomy, 319–320, 330–332
    anatomic extent of, 330–331, 331*f*
    count (yield) in, 330, 336–337, 339*t*–349*t*,
        350–352
    discussion, 351–353
    extended, 330–331, 331*f*, 335
    findings, 336–351
    limited, 330–331, 331*f*, 335
    methodology, 336
    rationale for, 330–331
    recommendation for, 330
    standard, 330–332, 331*f*, 335
    standard *versus* extended, 335–353, 337*f*,
        338*t*, 346*t*–349*t*
    superextended, 330, 331*f*, 335
    systematic reviews and meta-analyses, 336,
        337*f*, 338*t*–349*t*

technical aspects of, 331–332
    timing of, 331
Lymphadenectomy, portal
    for cholangiocarcinoma, 430, 431, 432,
        445–449, 495
        lymph node count in, 447
        rationale for, 446–448
        recommendation for, 445
        technical aspects of, 448–449, 449*f*
    for gallbladder cancer, 469–471
        rationale for, 470
        recommendation for, 469
        technical aspects of, 470
Lymph node biopsy. *See* Sentinel lymph node
        biopsy
Lymph node count (LNC)
    in hepatobiliary malignancies, 425, 447, 470
    in pelvic dissection, 330, 336–337, 339*t*–349*t*,
        350–352

M

Macroscopically negative margins. *See also*
        specific procedures
    for colorectal liver metastases, 430–432
    for hepatocellular cancer, 436–439
    for soft tissue sarcoma, 17–25, 40–41
Magnetic resonance cholangiopancreatography
        (MRCP), 417
Magnetic resonance imaging (MRI)
    for adrenal malignancies, 77*t*, 78
    for colorectal liver metastases, 426
    for gallbladder cancer, 420
    for hepatobiliary malignancies, 492
    for hepatocellular cancer, 433
    for intrahepatic cholangiocarcinoma, 417
    for neuroendocrine neoplasms, 147
    for perihilar cholangiocarcinoma, 417
    for soft tissue sarcoma, 12, 13
    for urothelial carcinoma, 293
Makuuchi incision, 84, 85*f*
Makuuchi incision, modified, 41
Margins. *See* Negative margins; *specific
        procedures*
Mastectomy, for sarcoma (angiosarcoma), 25,
        26*f*
Mayo, William, 142
Mayo protocol, 420
Mesenteric resection, for peritoneal
        malignancies, 227–228
    rationale for, 227–228
    recommendation for, 227
    technical aspects of, 228, 228*f*
Mesothelioma, peritoneal, 216
    clinical staging of, 219
    metastases from, 216, 216*t*
    patient history and physical findings of,
        220
Metyrapone, 80*t*, 141
Metyrosine, 81*t*

Microscopically negative margins. *See also specific procedures*
for adrenal malignancies, 83–88
for cholangiocarcinoma, intrahepatic, 440, 442–443, 444
for cholangiocarcinoma, perihilar, 440–444, 444f, 445f, 494–495
for gallbladder cancer, 467–469, 496
Midline incision, for adrenalectomy, 84, 85f
Midline laparotomy, 41
Miest, Tanner S., 409–411
Mifepristone, 80t
Mitomycin, intravesical
perioperative, 375–376
postoperative, 311–312, 409
Mitotane, 80t, 82
Mitotic rate
of GISTs, 5t–7t, 13
of neuroendocrine neoplasms, 144t
Mitra, Anirban P., 409–411
Mixed adeno-neuroendocrine carcinoma, 147
Mohs micrographic surgery, 24
MRCP (magnetic resonance cholangiopancreatography), 417
MRI. *See* Magnetic resonance imaging
Muscle-invasive bladder cancer (MIBC), 292, 294. *See also* Urinary bladder cancer
pelvic lymph node dissection, standard *versus* extended, 335–353
robot-assisted radical cystectomy for, 354–363
Myxofibrosarcoma, 18, 25

N
Narrow band imaging (NBI), 303, 304–305, 305f
National Comprehensive Cancer Network (NCCN) guidelines
for cholangiocarcinoma, 446, 448
for colorectal liver metastases, 269
for gallbladder cancer, 466
for neuroendocrine neoplasms, 155, 185
for soft tissue sarcoma, 9
for urothelial carcinoma, 301
NECs. *See* Neuroendocrine carcinomas
Negative margins. *See also specific procedures*
macroscopically
for colorectal liver metastases, 430–432
for hepatocellular cancer, 436–439
for soft tissue sarcoma, 17–25, 40–41
microscopically
for adrenal malignancies, 83–88
for cholangiocarcinoma, intrahepatic, 440, 442–443, 444
for cholangiocarcinoma, perihilar, 440–444, 444f, 445f, 494–495
for gallbladder cancer, 467–469, 496
Neobladder (orthotopic diversion), 332–334
Nephrectomy, for invasive adrenal malignancy, 89

Nephroureterectomy, 294, 364–376
commentary on, 410–411
critical elements of, 364
distal ureteral resection in, 366, 368–371
distal ureter/cuff management in, 368–371
endoscopic, 368–370
extravesical approach for, 368, 370, 371f
intravesical approach for, 371
pluck technique for, 368, 369
rationale for, 368–369
recommendation for, 368
studies/reviews of, 369–370
technical aspects of, 370–371, 371f
transvesical approach for, 368, 369
kidney-sparing approach *versus*, 311
laparoscopic, 365–366, 367
lymphadenectomy with, 372–375
rationale for, 372–375
recommendation for, 372
technical aspects of, 375
templates for, 372–374, 373f, 374f
minimally invasive, 365–366, 367
open, 365–367
optimal surgical approach to, 365–366
perioperative intravesical chemotherapy with, 375–376
removal of kidney and ureter in, 364–368
rationale for, 364–365
recommendation for, 364
technical aspects of, 366–368
robot-assisted, 365–366, 367
segmental ureteral resection in, 366, 367–368
sex-related outcomes of, 370
single-incision approach in, 366
surgical extirpation in, 364, 365f
synoptic operative report on, 400–404
two-incision approach in, 366
NETs. *See* Neuroendocrine tumors
Neuroendocrine carcinomas (NECs), 144, 146–147
classification of, 144, 144t
clinical staging of, 147
extrapulmonary, 146
genetics of, 146
large cell, 144t
mixed, 144t, 147
small cell, 144t
Neuroendocrine neoplasms (NENs), 144, 144t. *See also* Neuroendocrine tumors
carcinoid syndrome with, 145, 152–153, 154
clinical staging of, 147, 148t–152t
hereditary syndrome associated with, 145, 146t
locally advanced and metastatic, 153–154
multidisciplinary care for, 147–154
perioperative care for, 154
quality measures, 155
Neuroendocrine tumors (NETs), 144–145
classification of, 144, 144t
clinical staging of, 147, 148t–152t
commentary on, 211–213

Neuroendocrine tumors (NETs) (*continued*)
  grades/grading of, 144, 144*t*
  hereditary syndromes associated with, 145,
      146*t*
  location and behavior of, 145
  metastatic to liver
      hepatic debulking for, 174–178, 176*f*, 177*t*
      treatment options for, 174–175
  perioperative care for, 154
  quality measures, 155
  underlying setting and development of, 145
Neuroendocrine tumors (NETs), pancreatic
    behavior of, 145
  central and spleen-preserving distal
      pancreatectomy for, 182–183
  clinical staging for, 147, 151*t*–152*t*
  commentary on, 211–213
  hereditary syndromes associated with, 146,
      146*t*
  intraoperative ultrasound prior to
      enucleation of, 179–180
      rationale for, 179–180
      recommendation for, 179
      technical aspects for, 180
  locally advanced and metastatic, 153–154
  lymphadenectomy for, 183–198
      findings, 187–198
      impact on overall survival, 197–198
      impact on recurrence-free survival,
          187–197
      methodology, 186–187
      systematic reviews and meta-analyses,
          186–187, 186*f*, 188*t*–196*t*
  NCCN guidelines for, 185
  parenchyma-preserving pancreatectomy for,
      179–198
  regional lymph node sampling for, 183–184,
      184*f*
  resection of primary tumor, 180–183
      indications/criteria for enucleation,
          180–181, 181*f*
      rationale for, 180–182
      recommendation for, 180
      technical aspects of, 182–183
  synoptic operative report on, 209
Neuroendocrine tumors (NETs), small bowel,
    156–173
  clinical staging of, 147, 148*t*–150*t*
  commentary on, 211–213
  intraoperative evaluation and identification
      of primary tumors, 156–160, 159*f*
  location of nodal metastases, 161, 162*f*
  lymphatic mapping of, 160, 161*f*
  prophylactic cholecystectomy for, 165,
      166–173, 167*f*, 168*t*–170*t*, 212
  recommendations for, 156, 160, 164
  regional lymphadenectomy along segmental
      vessels for, 160–164, 163*f*
  resection of primary tumor, 164–165
  synoptic operative report on, 210

Neurovascular bundles, in resection of soft
    tissue sarcoma, 20–21, 20*f*, 45
Nicardipine, 79–82, 81*t*
Nivolumab, 420
Non-muscle-invasive bladder cancer (NMIBC),
    292, 294, 305, 311–312. *See also*
    Urinary bladder cancer
  pelvic lymph node dissection, standard
      versus extended, 335–353
  robot-assisted radical cystectomy for, 354–363
North American Neuroendocrine Tumor
    Society, 142, 155

O

Octreotide, for NETs, 152–154
  frequency of gallstones in patients treated
      with, 172–173
  pathogenesis of gallstones secondary to, 171
  prophylactic cholecystectomy with, 166–173
Omental caking, 221
Omental GISTs, clinical staging of, 4*t*–5*t*
Omentectomy. *See* Greater omentectomy,
    supracolic; Lesser omentectomy
Ondansetron, 152
Oophorectomy, for peritoneal malignancies
    involving ovaries, 233, 235
Open parenchyma-sparing liver resection for
    CLM (OSLO-COMET), 431
Organ-sparing cystectomy (OSC), 323–329
  in females, 294–300, 323–325, 326*f*, 327*f*
      patient selection for, 325
      rationale for, 324–325
      recommendation for, 323
      technical aspects of, 326*f*, 328
  in males, 326–328
      patient selection for, 326–327
      rationale for, 326–327
      recommendation for, 323
      technical aspects of, 328, 329*f*
Orthotopic diversion, 319, 320, 321, 324, 328,
    332–334
OSC. *See* Organ-sparing cystectomy
Osilodrostat, 80*t*
Ovarian cancer, peritoneal metastases from,
    216, 216*t*
Ovaries, peritoneal malignancies involving,
    234–235
Ovary-sparing cystectomy, 324–325, 326*f*, 328

P

Pancreas
  adrenal malignancies invading, 88–89
  peritoneal malignancies involving, 241, 248
Pancreatectomy
  for NETs
      central and spleen-preserving, 182–183
      parenchyma-sparing, 179–198
  for peritoneal malignancies, 241, 248

Pancreatic neuroendocrine tumors (pNETs)
  behavior of, 145
  central and spleen-preserving distal
    pancreatectomy for, 182–183
  clinical staging for, 147, 151t–152t
  commentary on, 211–213
  hereditary syndromes associated with, 146, 146t
  intraoperative ultrasound prior to
    enucleation of, 179–180
    rationale for, 179–180
    recommendation for, 179
    technical aspects for, 180
  locally advanced and metastatic, 153–154
  lymphadenectomy for, 183–198
    findings, 187–198
    impact on overall survival, 197–198
    impact on recurrence-free survival, 187–197
    methodology, 186–187
    systematic reviews and meta-analyses,
      186–187, 186f, 188t–196t
  NCCN guidelines for, 185
  parenchyma-preserving pancreatectomy for,
    179–198
  regional lymph node sampling for, 183–184,
    184f
  resection of primary tumor, 180–183
    indications/criteria for enucleation,
      180–181, 181f
    rationale for, 180–182
    recommendation for, 180
    technical aspects of, 182–183
  synoptic operative report on, 209
Paragangliomas, 74
Partial cystectomy, 300, 313–318
  commentary on, 410
  contraindications to, 316–317, 317f
  critical elements of, 313
  intraoperative localization of tumor in,
    313–314, 315f
  margin status in, 316
  as organ-sparing alternative, 318
  rationale for, 313–316
  recommendations for, 313, 314–315
  recurrence rates after, 316
  resection to adequate margins in, 314–317
  synoptic operative report on, 405–408
  technical aspects of, 314, 315f, 317–318, 318f
  ureteral implantation in, 316
PCI. See Peritoneal cancer index
Pelvic lymph node dissection (PLND), with
    radical cystectomy, 319–320, 330–332
  anatomic extent of, 330–331, 331f
  count (yield) in, 330, 336–337, 339t–349t,
    350–352
  discussion, 351–353
  extended, 330–331, 331f, 335
  findings, 336–351
  limited, 330–331, 331f, 335
  methodology, 336
  rationale for, 330–331

  recommendation for, 330
  standard, 330–332, 331f, 335
  standard *versus* extended, 335–353, 337f,
    338t, 346t–349t
  superextended, 330, 331f, 335
  systematic reviews and meta-analyses, 336,
    337f, 338t–349t
  technical aspects of, 331–332
  timing of, 331
Pelvic peritonectomy, 233–239
  rationale for, 233–236
  recommendation for, 233
  technical aspects of, 236, 237f, 238f
Pelvis
  anatomy of, 233, 234f
  cytoreduction within, 233–239
    rationale for, 233–236
    recommendation for, 233
Peptide receptor radionuclide therapy (PRRT),
    152, 153–154
Perihilar cholangiocarcinoma (PHC)
  bile duct margins in
    distal, 458–459, 461
    positive, intraoperative re-resection based
      on frozen section analysis in, 457–462,
      459f, 460t
    proximal, 461–462
  caudate lobe resection for, 450–456
    findings, 452–456
    methodology, 450–451
    overall survival rates in, 453t–454t, 455
    perioperative morbidity in, 455–456
    R0 resection in, 455
    systematic reviews and meta-analyses, 451,
      452f, 453t–454t
  clinical staging of, 415–417, 418t, 448
  commentary on, 491–496
  endoscopic biopsy of, 420–422
  future liver remnant in, 423–424
  lymphadenectomy for, 425
  multidisciplinary care for, 420–422, 492
  perioperative care/preoperative decision-
    making for, 423–424, 492–493
  portal lymphadenectomy/nodal sampling for
    rationale for, 446–447
    recommendation for, 445
    technical aspects of, 448–449, 449f
  portal vein resection and reconstruction in,
    442, 444, 445f
  quality measures in, 424–425
  resection of primary tumor to microscopically
    negative margins, 494–495
    rationale for, 440–442
    recommendation for, 440
    technical aspects of, 443–444, 444f, 445f
Peritoneal cancer index (PCI), 216, 219, 254, 255t
  optimal limit of, 254–268
    methodology on, 255
    in PSD associated with appendiceal cancer/
      pseudomyxoma peritonei, 262t–263t, 267

Peritoneal cancer index (PCI) (*continued*)
  in PSD associated with colorectal cancer, 256–267, 258*t*–261*t*
  in PSD associated with gastric cancer, 264*t*–265*t*, 267–268
  systematic reviews and meta-analyses of, 255*t*, 258*t*–265*t*
Peritoneal malignancies, 216–289
  clinical staging of, 216–219
  commentary on, 286–289
  cytoreductive surgery for, 216, 216*t*, 219–248
    abdominal visceral resections in, 239–248
    cholecystectomy in, 245, 247
    critical elements of, 223
    diaphragmatic, 228–233, 229*f*, 230*f*, 232*f*
    enteric resection in, 239–240, 242–244, 242*f*–243*f*
    full-thickness resection of diaphragm in, 232–233
    hepatic resection in, 240–241, 241*f*, 245–247, 245*f*, 246*f*
    HIPEC following, 249–253
    HIPEC with, survival *versus* complications in, 269–273, 270*f*, 271*t*
    hysterectomy in, 234–237, 238*f*
    lesser omentectomy in, 224–227, 226*f*
    pancreatectomy for, 241, 248
    PCI score and outcome of, 254–268
    pelvic peritonectomy in, 233–239, 237*f*, 238*f*
    within pelvis, 233–239
    quality measures for, 221–222
    rectosigmoid resection in, 237–238, 238*f*
    resection of mesenteric disease in, 227–228, 228*f*
    small bowel mesenteric peritonectomy in, 228, 228*f*
    splenectomy for, 241, 248
    subdiaphragmatic peritonectomy in, 231–232, 232*f*
    supracolic greater omentectomy in, 223–227, 226*f*
    visceral peritonectomy of right upper quadrant in, 247
  diagnosis of, 221
  hyperthermic intraperitoneal chemotherapy for, 216, 216*t*, 219–222, 249–253
    administration standards for, 251–252
    commentary on, 286–289
    with (following) cytoreduction, 249–253
    with cytoreduction, survival *versus* complications in, 269–273, 270*f*, 271*t*
    exposure precautions for, 252
    open *versus* closed technique, 250, 251, 252*f*
    patient management and monitoring in, 253
    PCI score and outcome of, 254–268
    perfusion system for, 251, 251*f*
    quality measures for, 221–222
    rationale for, 249–250
    recommendation for, 249
    systematic reviews and meta-analyses of, 269, 270*f*, 271*t*
    technical aspects of, 250–253
    temperature requirements for, 253
  imaging of, 220–221
  lesion size score of, 216
  metastatic, 216–219
  multidisciplinary care for, 216, 219
  omental caking with, 221
  patient history and physical findings in, 220
  perioperative care for, 220–221
  postoperative care for, 221
  quality measures for, 221–222
  survival rate, 219
  synoptic operative report on, 284–285
  tumor markers of, 220
Peritoneal reflections, 233, 234*f*
Peritoneal Surface Oncology Group International, 216–217
Peritonectomy
  extraperitoneal parietal, 231
  pelvic, 233–239, 237*f*, 238*f*
  small bowel mesenteric, 227–228, 228*f*
  subdiaphragmatic, 228, 231–232, 232*f*
  subphrenic, 231
  visceral, of right upper quadrant, 247
Per primum gallbladder cancer, 463, 466, 467
Perrier, Nancy D., 141–142
PET. *See* Positron emission tomography
PHC. *See* Perihilar cholangiocarcinoma
Phenoxybenzamine, 79, 81*t*
Pheochromocytoma, 74–102
  adrenalectomy for, 78–79, 83–102
    disruption of surgical capsule in, 84
    en bloc resection of adjacent organs invaded by cancer in, 88–89
    radicality of, 84
    resection of primary tumor to microscopically negative margins in, 83–88
  biopsy of, 77*t*
  diagnostic evaluation for, 76–78, 77*t*
  epidemiology of, 74
  genetic conditions associated with, 74
  imaging of, 77–78, 77*t*
  metastases from, 78, 82
  multidisciplinary care for, 75–76
  perioperative care for, 76–82
  preoperative blockade of, 79–82, 81*t*
  quality measures for, 82
  surgical expertise required for, 79
  synoptic operative report on, 79, 135–140
  synoptic pathologic report on, 79
  vascular invasion by, en bloc resection of adjacent blood vessels, 103–109
Pheochromocytomatosis, 84
Photodynamic cystoscopy, 303, 304–305, 306
PLND. *See* Pelvic lymph node dissection

pNETs. *See* Pancreatic neuroendocrine tumors
Portal lymphadenectomy
  for cholangiocarcinoma, 430, 431, 432,
    445–449, 495
    lymph node count in, 447
    rationale for, 446–448
    recommendation for, 445
    technical aspects of, 448–449, 449*f*
  for gallbladder cancer, 469–471
    rationale for, 470
    recommendation for, 469
    technical aspects of, 471
Portal vein, in perihilar cholangiocarcinoma,
  442, 444, 445*f*
Positron emission tomography (PET)
  for adrenal malignancies, 78, 142
  for neuroendocrine neoplasms, 147
  for urothelial carcinoma, 292
Prazosin, 81*t*
Pringle maneuver, 107
Prostate cancer, urothelial
  clinical staging of, 293
  epidemiology of, 292
Prostatectomy, radical, robot-assisted, 354
Prostate-sparing cystectomy, 326–327, 328,
  329*f*
PRRT. *See* Peptide receptor radionuclide
  therapy
Pseudomyxoma peritonei, PCI limit in
  peritoneal surface disease associated
  with, 262*t*–263*t*, 267
Psoas resection, 45
Pulmonary embolism
  radical cystectomy and, 301
  tumor thrombus and, 103

R
Radical cystectomy (RC), 292, 294–301,
  319–353
  bladder removal to negative resection
    margins in, 319–323
    rationale for, 319–320
    recommendation for, 319
    technical aspects of, 320–323, 321*f*, 322*f*,
    323*f*, 324*f*
  bladder-sparing chemoradiation *versus*, 301
  chemotherapy with, 300–301
  commentary on, 409–410
  concomitant pelvic organ management in,
    323–329
  critical elements of, 319
  in females
    organ-sparing, 294–300, 323–325, 326*f*,
    327*f*
    rationale for, 324, 325*f*
    recommendation for, 323
    urethral management in, 321, 326*f*
    urinary diversion in, 321, 324–325, 328,
    333–334

  in males
    organ-sparing, 326–328, 329*f*
    recommendation for, 323
    urethral management in, 322–323
    urinary diversion in, 333
  minimally invasive *versus* open, 322–323,
    324*f*, 354–363
  partial cystectomy *versus*, 318
  pelvic lymph node dissection with, 319–320,
    330–332
    anatomic extent of, 330–331, 331*f*
    count (yield) in, 330, 336–337, 339*t*–349*t*,
    350–352
    discussion, 351–353
    extended, 330–331, 331*f*, 335
    findings, 336–351
    limited, 330–331, 331*f*, 335
    methodology, 336
    rationale for, 330–331
    recommendation for, 330
    standard, 330–332, 331*f*, 335
    standard *versus* extended, 335–353, 337*f*,
    338*t*, 346*t*–349*t*
    superextended, 330, 331*f*, 335
    systematic reviews and meta-analyses, 336,
    337*f*, 338*t*–349*t*
    technical aspects of, 331–332
    timing of, 331
  perioperative care in, 301–302
  rectum management in, 321, 323*f*
  robot-assisted, 322–323, 354–363
    AMSTAR 2 criteria for studies, 356, 358,
    361*t*, 362–363
    diffusion of technology, 354
    discussion, 360–363
    findings, 357–360
    methodology, 355–356
    studies excluded from review of, 356, 358*t*
    systematic reviews and meta-analyses,
    355–356, 357*f*, 359*t*
  synoptic operative report on, 396–399
  urachal resection in, 320, 321*f*
  ureteral resection in, 321, 322*f*
  urethrectomy with, 321–322
  urinary diversion following, 300, 332–334,
    410
    rationale for, 332–333
    recommendation for, 332
Radical cystoprostatectomy, 294
Radical nephroureterectomy. *See*
  Nephroureterectomy
Radical prostatectomy, robot-assisted, 354
"Radical TURBT," 300
Radiotherapy
  postoperative, clip placement for planning,
    22, 23*f*
  for soft tissue sarcoma, 10
  for urothelial carcinoma, 301
RARC. *See* Robot-assisted radical cystectomy
RC. *See* Radical cystectomy

Rectosigmoid resection, 237–238, 238f
Rectum
    cancer of (*See* Colorectal cancer)
    management in radical cystectomy, 321, 323f
Renal artery, adrenal malignancies involving,
        103–105
Renal vein, adrenal malignancies involving,
        103–105
Resection. *See also specific organs,*
        malignancies, and procedures
    abdominal visceral, for peritoneal
            malignancies, 239–248
        cholecystectomy in, 245, 247
        enteric, 239–240, 242–244, 242f–243f
        hepatic, 240–241, 241f, 245–247, 245f,
            246f
        pancreatectomy in, 241, 248
        pelvic peritonectomy in, 233–239, 237f,
            238f
        within pelvis, 233–239
        rationale for, 239–241
        recommendation for, 239
        right upper quadrant in, 247
        splenectomy in, 241, 248
        technical aspects of, 242–248
    of adrenal malignancies
        en bloc, of adjacent blood vessels, 103–109
        en bloc, of adjacent organs invaded by
            cancer, 88–89
        laparoscopic, 91–102, 92f, 93t–97t
        metastatic (stage IV) ACC, 110–115, 111f,
            112t
        primary tumor, to microscopically negative
            margins, 83–88
    liver
        for cholangiocarcinoma, 440–462
        for colorectal liver metastases, 426–432
        for hepatocellular cancer, 414, 433–439,
            494
        indications for, 414
        for peritoneal malignancies, 240–241,
            241f, 245–247, 245f, 246f
    small bowel, for NETs, 156–178
    of soft tissue sarcoma
        extremity and trunk, 14–39
        rationale for, 18–19, 40–41
        recommendations for, 17, 40, 43
        retroperitoneal and intra-abdominal,
            40–67
        surgical margins in, 9, 19, 20f
        technical aspects of, 20–25, 45–47
Retroperitoneal node sampling
    for cholangiocarcinoma, 445–449
    for gallbladder cancer, 469–471
Retroperitoneal sarcoma
    abdominal recurrence-free survival in, 10
    clinical staging of, 7t–9t
    postoperative care and follow-up for, 13
    preoperative clinical and imaging evaluation
        of, 12

resection of, 40–67
    considerations for specific histologic
        subtypes, 45–46
    en bloc, of invaded organs to obtain
        complete gross resection, 43–47, 44f,
        46f
    Gibson incision for, 41, 42f
    macroscopically complete, of primary
        tumor without disruption of tumor
        capsule, 40–41
    management of bony structures in, 45
    management of neurovascular bundles
        in, 45
    psoas resection in, 45
    rationale for, 40–41, 43–44
    recommendation for, 40
    technical aspects of, 41, 45–47
resection of, extended, 48–61
    definition of extent, 50
    findings, 50–61
    impact of extent on local recurrence, 61
    impact of extent on multivisceral resection,
        50–61
    methodology, 48–50, 49f
    outcomes of, 57t–60t, 61
    qualitative systematic review, 50, 51t–60t
    treatment guidelines for, 10
    tumor rupture, 41
Robot-assisted hysterectomy, 354
Robot-assisted liver resection, 439
Robot-assisted nephroureterectomy, 365–366,
        367
Robot-assisted radical cystectomy (RARC),
        322–323, 354–363
    AMSTAR 2 criteria for studies, 356, 358,
        361t, 362–363
    diffusion of technology, 354
    discussion, 360–363
    findings, 357–360
    methodology, 355–356
    studies excluded from review of, 356, 358t
    systematic reviews and meta-analyses,
        355–356, 357f, 359t
Robot-assisted radical prostatectomy, 354
Roux-en-Y hepaticojejunostomy, 443–444

S

Salpingo-oophorectomy, for ovarian metastases
        from peritoneal surface, 235
Sarcoma Meta-Analysis Collaboration, 11
SBNETs. *See* Small bowel NETs
Scandinavian Sarcoma Group, 11
Segmental ureterectomy, 366, 367–368
Sentinel lymph node biopsy (SLNB), for soft
        tissue sarcoma
    extremity and trunk, 28–39
    findings, 30–38, 33t–37t
    impact on patient outcomes, 33t–37t, 38–39
    methodology, 28–30, 29f

positive, complete lymph node dissection
    after, 39
qualitative systematic review, 30, 31t–32t
Sexual function, organ-sparing cystectomy and
    in females, 324–325, 326f, 327f, 328
    in males, 326–328, 329f
SLNB. *See* Sentinel lymph node biopsy
Small bowel, peritoneal malignancies involving,
    227–228, 239–240, 242–244
Small bowel mesenteric peritonectomy,
    227–228, 228f
Small bowel NETs, 156–173
    clinical staging of, 147, 148t–150t
    commentary on, 211–213
    intraoperative evaluation and identification
        of primary tumors, 156–160, 159f
    location of nodal metastases, 161, 162f
    lymphatic mapping of, 160, 161f
    prophylactic cholecystectomy for, 165,
        166–173, 167f, 168t–170t, 212
    recommendations for, 156, 160, 164
    regional lymphadenectomy along segmental
        vessels for, 160–164, 163f
    resection of primary tumor, 164–165
    synoptic operative report on, 210
Small bowel resection, for peritoneal
        malignancies
    rationale for, 239–240
    technical aspects of, 242–244, 242f–243f
Soft tissue sarcomas
    aggressiveness of, understanding, 71
    amputation indications for, 9, 18, 22
    biopsy of, 12–13
        extremity and trunk, 12–17
        orientation of tract and incision in, 15,
            16f–17f
        rationale for, 14–15
        technical aspects of, 15–17, 16f–17f
    clinical staging of, 2–9, 2t–9t, 28
        for GISTs, 4t–7t
        for retroperitoneal sarcomas, 7t–9t
        for sarcoma of trunk and extremities, 2t–4t
    commentary on, 71–72
    heterogeneous family of, 2
    histological grading of, 2, 9
    limb-salvage surgery for, 10, 18, 22, 24
    metastases from, 10–11, 28, 30–38
    multidisciplinary care for, 9–11
    perioperative care for, 11–13
    postoperative care and follow-up for, 13
    preoperative clinical and imaging evaluation
        of, 11
    resection of
        clip placement for postoperative radiation
            planning in, 22, 23f
        considerations for specific histologic
            subtypes, 18, 24–25, 45–46
        en bloc, of biopsy tract, 18–19
        en bloc, of invaded organs, 43–47, 44f,
            46f

extended, 48–61
extremity and trunk, 14–39
intraoperative frozen section in, 17, 19
macroscopically complete, of primary
    tumor, 17–25, 40–41
management of bone and tendons in, 20f,
    21–22, 45
management of neurovascular bundles in,
    20–21, 20f, 45
rationale for, 18–19, 40–41, 43–44
recommendations for, 17, 40, 43
reconstruction in, 23–24
retroperitoneal and intra-abdominal,
    40–57
surgical drain placement in, 26, 27f
surgical margins in, 9, 19, 20f
technical aspects of, 20–25, 45–47
sentinel lymph node biopsy for, 28–39
    findings, 30–38, 33t–37t
    impact on patient outcomes, 33t–37t,
        38–39
    methodology, 28–30, 29f
    positive, complete lymph node dissection
        after, 39
    qualitative systematic review, 30, 31t–32t
synoptic operative report, 68–70
unnecessary radical or morbid operation for,
    71–72
Somatostatin analogues, for NETs, 152–154
    frequency of gallstones in patients treated
        with, 172–173
    pathogenesis of gallstones secondary to, 171
    prophylactic cholecystectomy with, 166–173
Sorafenib, 420
Spironolactone, 80t
Spleen
    adrenal malignancies invading, 88–89
    peritoneal malignancies involving, 241, 248
Spleen-preserving distal pancreatectomy,
    182–183
Splenectomy, for peritoneal malignancies
    involving spleen, 241
SpyGlass biopsies, 420–422
Staging, clinical
    of adrenocortical carcinoma, 74, 75t, 113,
        141–142
    of appendiceal neoplasms, 216–218,
        217t–218t
    of cholangiocarcinoma, intrahepatic, 417,
        419t, 447–448
    of cholangiocarcinoma, perihilar, 415–417,
        418t, 448
    of colorectal liver metastases, 414, 415t
    of gallbladder cancer, 417–420, 421t, 470
    of gastric cancer, 219
    of hepatobiliary malignancies, 414–420
    of hepatocellular cancer, 414, 416t
    of neuroendocrine carcinomas, 147
    of neuroendocrine neoplasms, 147,
        148t–152t

Staging, clinical (*continued*)
  of neuroendocrine tumors, 147, 148*t*–152*t*
  of peritoneal malignancies, 216–219
  of upper tract urothelial carcinoma,
      292–293, 294*f*, 297*t*–298*t*, 409
  of urinary bladder cancer, 292–293, 293*f*,
      295*t*–296*t*, 303–304
  of urothelial carcinoma, 292–293, 293*f*,
      294*f*, 295*t*–300*t*, 303–304, 409
Staging laparoscopy
  for colorectal liver metastases, 427
  for gallbladder cancer, 463–466, 495
  for hepatobiliary malignancies, 493–494
Staging systems
  AJCC
    for ACC, 74, 75*t*, 113, 141–142
    for appendiceal neoplasms, 217,
      217*t*–218*t*
    for cholangiocarcinoma, intrahepatic, 417,
      419*t*, 447–448
    for cholangiocarcinoma, perihilar,
      415–417, 418*t*, 448
    for colorectal cancer, 219
    for colorectal liver metastases, 414, 415*t*
    for gallbladder cancer, 421*t*, 470
    for gastric carcinoma, 219
    for hepatocellular cancer, 414, 416*t*
    for neuroendocrine neoplasms, 147,
      148*t*–152*t*
    for soft tissue sarcomas, 2–9, 2*t*–9*t*, 28
    for upper urinary tract cancer, 297*t*–298*t*
    for urethral cancer, 298*t*–300*t*
  ENSAT, 74, 75*t*, 113
  TNM
    for adrenal malignancies, 75*t*
    for appendiceal neoplasms, 217–218,
      218*t*
    for cholangiocarcinoma, intrahepatic,
      419*t*, 447–448
    for cholangiocarcinoma, perihilar, 418*t*,
      447
    for colorectal liver metastases, 415*t*
    for gallbladder cancer, 420, 421*t*, 470
    for hepatocellular cancer, 416*t*
    for neuroendocrine tumors, 147,
      148*t*–151*t*
    for peritoneal mesothelioma, 219
    for soft tissue sarcoma, 2–9, 2*t*–9*t*
    for urothelial carcinoma, 293, 295*t*–300*t*,
      409
Standard lymph node dissection (sLND),
    pelvic, 330–332, 331*f*
  definition of, 335
  extended *versus*, 335–353, 337*f*, 338*t*–349*t*
  findings, 336–351
  methodology, 336
  systematic reviews and meta-analyses, 336,
    337*f*, 338*t*, 346*t*–349*t*
Stomach, neuroendocrine tumors of, 147
STRASS trial, 10

Subcostal incision, for adrenalectomy, 84, 85*f*
Subdiaphragmatic peritonectomy, 228,
    231–232, 232*f*
Subphrenic peritonectomy, 231
Sunitinib, 153
Superextended lymph node dissection (seLND),
    pelvic, 330, 331*f*, 335
Supracolic greater omentectomy, 223–227
  indications for, 224
  rationale for, 223–225
  recommendation for, 223
  technical aspects of, 225–227, 226*f*
Surgical drains, for sarcoma resection, 26, 27*f*
Synoptic operative report
  adrenal, 79, 135–140
  colorectal liver metastases, 490
  extremity sarcoma, 68–70
  gallbladder cancer, 484–485
  hepatobiliary, 484–490
  hepatocellular cancer, 486–487
  pancreatic NET, 209
  peritoneal, 284–285
  small bowel NET, 210
  urothelial (nephroureterectomy), 400–404
  urothelial (partial cystectomy), 405–408
  urothelial (radical cystectomy), 396–399
  urothelial (TURBT), 392–395
Synoptic pathologic report, adrenal
    malignancies, 79

T

Telotristat ethyl, 152–153
Tendon(s), in resection of soft tissue sarcoma,
    21–22
Terazosin, 81*t*
Thoracoabdominal incision, for adrenalectomy,
    84, 85*f*
Thrombus, tumor, adrenal malignancy and,
    103–109, 106*f*
Transurethral resection of bladder tumor
    (TURBT), 306–308
  complete and thorough, as criterion
    standard, 308
  conventional staged approach in, 308
  en bloc, 308
  imaging/diagnostic techniques in, 304–306
  intravesical chemotherapy after, 311–312
  monopolar *versus* bipolar energy in, 308
  quality measures for, 302
  "radical," 300
  rationale for, 307
  recommendation for, 306
  staging in, 292, 307
  synoptic operative report on, 392–395
  technical aspects of, 307–308
  therapeutic goals of, 307
  in trimodal therapy, 301
Transurethral resection (TUR) syndrome, 308
Trimodal therapy, for urothelial carcinoma, 301

Truncal sarcoma
  biopsy of, 12–17
    orientation of tract and incision in, 15
    rationale for, 14–15
    technical aspects of, 15–17
  clinical staging of, 2t–4t, 28
  postoperative care and follow-up for, 13
  preoperative clinical and imaging evaluation
    of, 12
  resection of, 14–39
    clip placement for postoperative radiation
      planning in, 22
    considerations for specific histologic
      subtypes, 18, 24–25
    en bloc, of biopsy tract, 18–19
    intraoperative frozen section in, 17, 19
    macroscopically complete, of primary
      tumor, 17–25
    management of bone and tendons in, 21–22
    management of neurovascular bundles in,
      20–21
    rationale for, 18–19
    recommendation for, 17
    reconstruction in, 23–24
    surgical drain placement in, 26
    surgical margins in, 19
    technical aspects of, 20–25
  sentinel lymph node biopsy for, 28–39
    findings, 30–38, 33t–37t
    impact on patient outcomes, 33t–37t, 38–39
    methodology, 28–30, 29f
    positive, complete lymph node dissection
      after, 39
    qualitative systematic review, 30, 31t–32t
  treatment guidelines for, 10
Tumor-node-metastasis (TNM) staging
  for adrenal malignancies, 75t
  for appendiceal neoplasms, 217–218, 218t
  for cholangiocarcinoma, intrahepatic, 419t,
    447–448
  for cholangiocarcinoma, perihilar, 418t, 447
  for colorectal liver metastases, 415t
  for gallbladder cancer, 420, 421t, 470
  for hepatocellular cancer, 416t
  for neuroendocrine tumors, 147, 148t–151t
  for peritoneal mesothelioma, 219
  for soft tissue sarcoma, 2–9, 2t–9t
  for urothelial carcinoma, 293, 295t–300t, 409
Tumor thrombus, adrenal malignancy and,
  103–109, 106f
TURBT. See Transurethral resection of bladder
  tumor

U

Ultrasound
  intraoperative
    for colorectal liver metastases, 426, 428,
      428f, 429f, 430
    for hepatobiliary malignancies, 493–494

  for hepatocellular carcinoma, 433–435,
    435f, 494
  for neuroendocrine neoplasms, 158, 159,
    179–180
  for neuroendocrine neoplasms, 147
Upper tract urothelial carcinoma (UTUC)
  biopsy of, 310
  bladder cancer versus, 294
  chemotherapy for, 301
  clinical staging of, 292–293, 294f, 297t–298t,
    409
  commentary on, 409–411
  endoscopic management of, 292, 309–311
    ablative, 309, 311
    diagnostic versus therapeutic, 309
    kidney-sparing, 311
    rationale for, 309
    recommendation for, 309
    technical aspects of, 309–311, 310f
  epidemiology of, 292
  multidisciplinary care for, 294–301
  nephroureterectomy for, 294, 364–376
    commentary on, 410–411
    critical elements of, 364
    distal ureteral resection in, 366, 368–371
    distal ureter/cuff management in,
      368–371, 371f
    kidney-sparing approach versus, 311
    laparoscopic, 365–366, 367
    lymphadenectomy with, 372–375, 373f,
      374f
    minimally invasive, 365–366, 367
    open, 365–367
    optimal surgical approach to, 365–366
    perioperative intravesical chemotherapy
      with, 375–376
    removal of kidney and ureter in, 364–368
    robot-assisted, 365–366, 367
    segmental ureteral resection in, 366,
      367–368
    sex-related outcomes of, 370
    single-incision approach in, 366
    surgical extirpation in, 364, 365f
    synoptic operative report on, 400–404
    two-incision approach in, 366
Upper Tract Urothelial Carcinoma
  Collaboration, 372
Ureteral cancer. See also Upper tract urothelial
    carcinoma
  biopsy of, 310
  clinical staging of, 293
  distal ureterectomy for, 294
  endoscopic management of, 309–311
    ablative, 309, 311
    diagnostic versus therapeutic, 309
    rationale for, 309
    recommendation for, 309
    technical aspects of, 309–311, 310f
  epidemiology of, 292
  nephroureterectomy for, 294, 364–376

Ureteral metastases, from peritoneal surface, 235–236
Ureteral reimplantation, 294, 316
Ureteral resection
in nephroureterectomy, 366
in radical cystectomy, 321, 322*f*
Ureteral stripping, 369
Ureterectomy
distal, 294, 366, 368–371
segmental, 366, 367–368
Ureteroscopy, 309–311
percutaneous renal access in, 309
rationale for, 309
recommendation for, 309
technical aspects of, 309–311, 310*f*
Ureter removal, in urothelial carcinoma, 364–376. *See also* Nephroureterectomy
Urethral cancer
chemotherapy for, 301
clinical staging of, 293, 298*t*–300*t*
endoscopic evaluation of, 303–306
endoscopic management of, 303–308
epidemiology of, 292
radical prostatectomy for, 294
Urethral-sparing cystectomy, 319
Urethrectomy, with radical cystectomy, 321–322
Urinary bladder
chemotherapy for, 300–301
metastases from peritoneal surface to, 234–236
surgical removal of (*See* Cystectomy)
Urinary bladder cancer, 292–411
biopsy of, 308
carcinoma in situ, 316–317
clinical staging of, 292–293, 293*f*, 295*t*–296*t*, 303–304
commentary on, 409–411
endoscopic evaluation of, 303–306, 304*f*, 305*f*, 314
endoscopic management of, 292, 303–308
postoperative intravesical chemotherapy with, 311–312
immunotherapy for, 301
multidisciplinary care for, 294–301
muscle-invasive of, 292, 294
narrow band imaging of, 303, 304–305, 305*f*
non-muscle-invasive, 292, 294, 305, 311–312
organ-sparing cystectomy for, 323–329
in females, 294–300, 323–325, 326*f*, 327*f*, 328
in males, 326–328, 329*f*
patient selection for, 325, 326–327
rationale for, 324–325, 326–327
recommendations for, 323
technical aspects of, 326*f*, 328, 329*f*
partial cystectomy for, 300, 313–318
commentary on, 410
contraindications to, 316–317, 317*f*
critical elements of, 313

intraoperative localization of tumor in, 313–314, 315*f*
margin status in, 316
as organ-sparing alternative, 318
rationale for, 313–316
recommendations for, 313, 314–315
recurrence rates after, 316
resection to adequate margins in, 314–317
synoptic operative report on, 405–408
technical aspects of, 314, 315*f*, 317–318, 318*f*
ureteral implantation in, 316
pelvic lymph node dissection for, 319–320, 330–332
anatomic extent of, 330–331, 331*f*
count (yield) in, 330, 336–337, 339*t*–349*t*, 350–352
discussion, 351–353
extended, 330–331, 331*f*, 335
findings, 336–351
limited, 330–331, 331*f*, 335
methodology, 336
rationale for, 330–331
recommendation for, 330
standard, 330–332, 331*f*, 335
standard *versus* extended, 335–353, 337*f*, 338*t*, 346*t*–349*t*
superextended, 330, 331*f*, 335
systematic reviews and meta-analyses, 336, 337*f*, 338*t*–349*t*
technical aspects of, 331–332
timing of, 331
photodynamic cystoscopy of, 303, 304–305, 304*f*, 305*f*
quality measures for, 302
radical cystectomy for, 292, 294–301, 319–363, 409–410
bladder removal to negative resection margins in, 319–323, 321*f*, 322*f*, 323*f*, 324*f*
bladder-sparing chemoradiation *versus*, 301
chemotherapy with, 300–301
concomitant pelvic organ management in, 323–329
critical elements of, 319
minimally invasive *versus* open, 322–323, 324*f*, 354–363
partial cystectomy *versus*, 318
perioperative care in, 301–302
rationale for, 319–320
recommendation for, 319
rectum management in, 321, 323*f*
synoptic operative report on, 396–399
technical aspects of, 320–323, 321*f*, 322*f*, 323*f*, 324*f*
urachal resection in, 320, 321*f*
ureteral resection in, 321, 322*f*
urethrectomy with, 321–322
urinary diversion following, 300, 332–334, 410

radical cystectomy for, robot-assisted, 322–323, 354–363
  AMSTAR 2 criteria for studies, 356, 358, 361t, 362–363
  diffusion of technology, 354
  discussion, 360–363
  findings, 357–360
  methodology, 355–356
  studies excluded from review of, 356, 358t
  systematic reviews and meta-analyses, 355–356, 357f, 359t
recurrent, 292
surveillance measures for, 302, 302t
transurethral resection of tumor in, 306–308
  complete and thorough, as criterion standard, 308
  conventional staged approach in, 308
  en bloc, 308
  imaging/diagnostic techniques in, 304–306
  intravesical chemotherapy after, 311–312
  monopolar versus bipolar energy in, 308
  quality measures for, 302
  "radical," 300
  rationale for, 307
  recommendation for, 306
  staging in, 292, 307
  synoptic operative report on, 392–395
  technical aspects of, 307–308
  therapeutic goals of, 307
  in trimodal therapy, 301
trimodal therapy for, 301
UTUC versus, 294
Urinary diversion procedures, 300, 332–334, 410
  continent cutaneous, 332–334
  in females, 321, 324, 328, 333–334
  ileal conduit, 332–333
  in males, 319, 320, 333
  options and contraindications, 332–333
  orthotopic, 319, 320, 321, 328, 332–334
  rationale for, 332–333
  recommendation for, 332
  technical aspects of, 333–334
Urothelial carcinoma, 292–411
  biopsy of, 308, 309, 310
  chemotherapy for, 300–301
  clinical staging of, 292–293, 293f, 294f, 295t–300t, 303–304, 409
  commentary on, 409–411
  endoscopic evaluation of, 303–306, 304f, 305f, 314
    rationale for, 303–305
    recommendation for, 303
    technical aspects of, 306
  endoscopic management of, 292, 303–312
    critical elements of, 303
    postoperative intravesical chemotherapy with, 311–312
    upper tract, 292, 309–311
  epidemiology of, 292
  immunotherapy for, 301
  multidisciplinary care for, 294–301
  narrow band imaging of, 303, 304–305, 305f
  nephroureterectomy for, 294, 364–376, 410–411
    critical elements of, 364
    distal ureteral resection in, 366, 368–371
    distal ureter/cuff management in, 368–371, 371f
    kidney-sparing approach versus, 311
    laparoscopic, 365–366, 367
    lymphadenectomy with, 372–375, 373f, 374f
    minimally invasive, 365–366, 367
    open, 365–367
    optimal surgical approach to, 365–366
    perioperative intravesical chemotherapy with, 375–376
    removal of kidney and ureter in, 364–368
    robot-assisted, 365–366, 367
    segmental ureteral resection in, 366, 367–368
    sex-related outcomes of, 370
    single-incision approach in, 366
    surgical extirpation in, 364, 365f
    synoptic operative report on, 400–404
    two-incision approach in, 366
  organ-sparing cystectomy for, 323–329
    in females, 294–300, 323–325, 326f, 327f, 328
    in males, 326–328, 329f
    patient selection for, 325, 326–327
    rationale for, 324–325, 326–327
    recommendations for, 323
    technical aspects of, 326f, 328, 329f
  partial cystectomy for, 300, 313–318
    commentary on, 410
    contraindications to, 316–317, 317f
    critical elements of, 313
    intraoperative localization of tumor in, 313–314, 315f
    margin status in, 316
    as organ-sparing alternative, 318
    rationale for, 313–316
    recommendations for, 313, 314–315
    recurrence rates after, 316
    resection to adequate margins in, 314–317
    synoptic operative report on, 405–408
    technical aspects of, 314, 315f, 317–318, 318f
    ureteral implantation in, 316
  pelvic lymph node dissection for, 319–320, 330–332
    anatomic extent of, 330–331, 331f
    count (yield) in, 330, 336–337, 339t–349t, 350–352
    discussion, 351–353
    extended, 330–331, 331f, 335
    findings, 336–351
    limited, 330–331, 331f, 335
    methodology, 336

Urothelial carcinoma (*continued*)
    rationale for, 330–331
    recommendation for, 330
    standard, 330–332, 331*f*, 335
    standard *versus* extended, 335–353, 337*f*, 338*t*, 346*t*–349*t*
    superextended, 330, 331*f*, 335
    systematic reviews and meta-analyses, 336, 337*f*, 338*t*–349*t*
    technical aspects of, 331–332
    timing of, 331
  photodynamic cystoscopy of, 303, 304–305, 304*f*, 305*f*
  quality measures for, 302
  radical cystectomy for, 292, 294–301, 319–363, 409–410
    bladder removal to negative resection margins in, 319–323, 321*f*, 322*f*, 323*f*, 324*f*
    bladder-sparing chemoradiation *versus*, 301
    chemotherapy with, 300–301
    concomitant pelvic organ management in, 323–329
    critical elements of, 319
    minimally invasive *versus* open, 322–323, 324*f*, 354–363
    partial cystectomy *versus*, 318
    perioperative care in, 301–302
    rationale for, 319–320
    recommendations for, 319
    rectum management in, 321, 323*f*
    synoptic operative report on, 396–399
    technical aspects of, 320–323, 321*f*, 322*f*, 323*f*, 324*f*
    urachal resection in, 320, 321*f*
    ureteral resection in, 321, 322*f*
    urethrectomy with, 321–322
    urinary diversion following, 300, 332–334, 410
  radical cystectomy for, robot-assisted, 322–323, 354–363
    AMSTAR 2 criteria for studies, 356, 358, 361*t*, 362–363
    diffusion of technology, 354
    discussion, 360–363
    findings, 357–360
    methodology, 355–356
    studies excluded from review of, 356, 358*t*
    systematic reviews and meta-analyses, 355–356, 357*f*, 359*t*
  radical cystoprostatectomy for, 294
  surveillance measures for, 302, 302*t*
  transurethral resection of bladder tumor for, 306–308
    complete and thorough, as criterion standard, 308
    conventional staged approach in, 308
    en bloc, 308
    imaging/diagnostic techniques in, 304–306
    intravesical chemotherapy after, 311–312
    monopolar *versus* bipolar energy in, 308
    quality measures for, 302
    "radical," 300
    rationale for, 307
    recommendation for, 306
    staging in, 292, 307
    synoptic operative report on, 392–395
    technical aspects of, 307–308
    therapeutic goals of, 307
    in trimodal therapy, 301
  trimodal therapy for, 301
  upper tract, 292
Uterine metastases, from peritoneal surface, 234–237, 238*f*
Uterus-sparing cystectomy, 324–325, 327*f*, 328
UTUC. *See* Upper tract urothelial carcinoma

V

Vacuum-assisted closure therapy, 24
Vaginal-sparing cystectomy, 294–300, 324–325, 326*f*, 328
Vascular invasion, by ACC, 103–109
    en bloc resection of adjacent blood vessels, 103–109
    extent of tumor thrombus in, 106*f*
    extraction of tumor thrombus in, 108–109
    hypothermic perfusion of liver in, 107
    IVC exposure in, 105
    IVC reconstruction in, 109
    IVC resection in, 103–108
    recommendation for, 103
    resection rationale for, 103–105
    technical aspects of resection, 105–109
    vascular control in, 106–108, 107*f*
    venovenous bypass in, 107, 107*f*
Vena cava. *See* Inferior vena cava
Venovenous bypass circuit, 107, 107*f*
Visceral peritonectomy, of right upper quadrant, 247

W

Wedge resection, for gallbladder cancer, 468, 496
White light cystoscopy, 303, 304–305, 304*f*, 305*f*, 306
World Health Organization (WHO), classification of neuroendocrine neoplasms, 144, 144*t*

Z

Zollinger-Ellison syndrome, 157